Volume 1

Overview and Basic Concepts 1

Back 2

Upper Limb 3

Thorax 4

Volume 2

Abdomen 5

Pelvis and Perineum 6

Lower Limb 7

Volume 3

Head 8

Neck 9

Summary of Cranial Nerves 10

Moore's CLINICALLY ORIENTED ANATOMY

Volume 3

Second South Asian Edition

As per the Indian Competency-Based Medical Curriculum

SAE Editors

S. Aruna, MS (Anatomy)
Professor and Head
Department of Anatomy
Indira Gandhi Medical College and Research Institute
Puducherry, India

N. Isai Vani, MS, DNB (Anatomy)
Associate Professor
Department of Anatomy
Indira Gandhi Medical College and Research Institute
Puducherry, India

International Editors

Arthur F. Dalley II, PhD, FAAA
Professor, Department of Cell and Developmental Biology
Adjunct Professor, Department of Orthopaedic Surgery
Co-Director, Brain, Behavior, and Movement
Vanderbilt University School of Medicine
Adjunct Professor of Anatomy
Belmont University School of Physical Therapy
Nashville, Tennessee

Anne M. R. Agur, BSc (OT), MSc, PhD
Professor, Division of Anatomy, Department of Surgery, Faculty of Medicine
Division of Physical Medicine and Rehabilitation, Department of Medicine
Department of Physical Therapy, Department of Occupational Science & Occupational Therapy
Division of Biomedical Communications, Institute of Medical Science
Rehabilitation Sciences Institute, Graduate Department of Dentistry
University of Toronto
Toronto, Ontario, Canada

Wolters Kluwer

Senior Publishing Manager: Sangeetha P
Development Editor: Nayan Gogoi
Senior Content Management Analyst: Amit Rai
Asstt. Manager Manufacturing: Sumit Johry

3rd Floor, Tower B, Building No. 10, Phase – II, DLF Cyber City
Gurgaon, Haryana - 122002

First South Asian Edition, 2018
Second South Asian Edition, 2022

ISBN: 978-93-93553-43-0

Authorised for sale only in South Asia

Published by Wolters Kluwer (India) Pvt. Ltd., New Delhi
Compositor: Design Modus, New Delhi (www.designmodus.in)
Printed and bound at Gopsons Papers Pvt. Ltd.

For product enquiry, please contact– Marketing Department (marketing@wolterskluwerindia.co.in) or log on to our website www.wolterskluwerindia.co.in.

Dr. Keith Leon Moore (1925–2019)

by Dr. Arthur F. Dalley II and Dr. Anne M. R. Agur

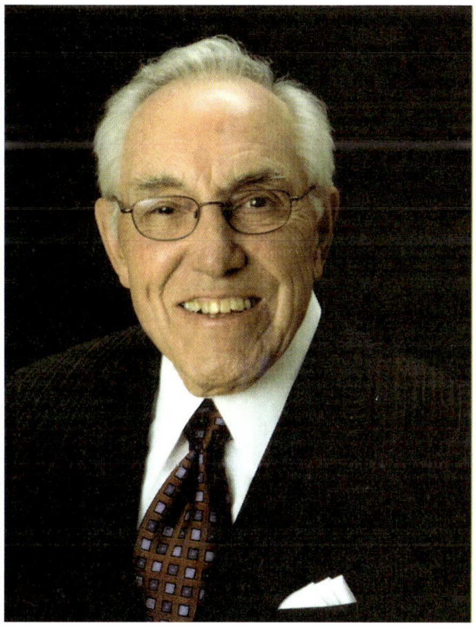

Dr. Keith Leon Moore
BA, MSc, PhD, Hon. DSc (OSU), Hon. DSc (WU)
FIAC, FRSM, FAAA

One of the most world-renowned anatomists of our time, Dr. Keith Leon Moore, passed away at age 94 on November 25, 2019. Keith was the founding author of *Clinically Oriented Anatomy* (COA) in 1980 and founding co-author, with Anne Agur, of *Essential Clinical Anatomy* (ECA) in 1996, both in the vanguard of *Clinically Oriented Anatomy* textbooks. Keith was the sole author for the fi rst three editions of COA, bringing on Arthur Dalley as co-author starting with the fourth edition and Anne starting with the sixth edi-tion. Keith and Anne brought me on as co-author for ECA starting with the fourth edition. Keith mentored Anne and me well, with COA now in its ninth edition, and ECA in its sixth. The retitling of COA and ECA as "Moore's" pays trib-ute to Keith's foundational work on the books and the legacy they represent. Keith was also the author/co-author of four clinically oriented embryology texts.

Dr. Moore was born in Brantford, Canada, on October 5, 1925. Keith joined the Canadian Navy during World War II. He was a Sick Birth Attendant on Vancouver Island and was trained as a radiology technician. When the war was over, he went to the Western University, where he received his BA, MSc, and PhD degrees. Keith married Marion McDermid in 1949, and together they had five children and nine grandchildren. Marion was the typist, offering the "initial critique" for the first three editions of COA.

In 1956, Keith accepted the position of assistant professor at the University of Manitoba in Winnipeg. In 1965, he was pro-moted to the Head of Anatomy. In 1976, he became the chair of anatomy and then the associate dean of the Basic Medical Sciences at the University of Toronto. After retirement in 1991, Keith continued to work on his textbooks, give guest lectures, and attend anatomy meetings for more than two decades.

Keith was the recipient of many prestigious awards and recognitions. He received the highest awards for excel-lence in human anatomy education at the medical, dental, graduate, and undergraduate levels—and for his remark-able record of textbook publications in Clinically Oriented Anatomy and Embryology—from both the American Association of Anatomists (Henry Gray Distinguished Educator Award, 2007) and the American Association of Clinical Anatomists (AACA Honored Member Award, 1994). In 2012, Dr. Moore received honorary Doctor of Science degrees from The Ohio State University and the University of Western Ontario, the Queen Elizabeth II Diamond Jubilee Medal honoring significant contribu-tions and achievements by Canadians, and the R. Benton Adkins, Jr., Distinguished Service Award for his outstand-ing record of service to the AACA.

Preface

Clinically Oriented Anatomy by late Keith L Moore continues to fascinate students and faculty of medicine and allied subjects for the last four decades. This is because of its marked evolution since its inception, a reflection of changes in the clinical application of anatomy, new imaging technologies that reveal living anatomy in new ways, and improvements in graphic and publication technology that enable superior demonstration of this information.

The second South Asian Edition of *Moore's Clinically Oriented Anatomy* provides necessary updates that incorporate the rapid advances in the clinical application of anatomy. The first edition was reviewed by students, anatomists, and clinicians for accuracy and relevance, and based on the feedback, the second edition is revised with significant new changes and updates.

Key Features

Moore's Clinically Oriented Anatomy has been widely acclaimed for the relevance of its clinical correlations. As in previous editions, this edition places clinical emphasis on anatomy that is important in physical diagnosis for primary care, interpretation of diagnostic imaging, and understanding the anatomical basis of clinical conditions and surgical procedures. Special attention has been directed toward assisting students in learning the anatomy they will need to know in the 21st century and to meet the changes in medical curriculum, and to this end, new features have been added and existing features updated.

COMPETENCY-BASED LEARNING

The National Medical Commission (NMC) of India has laid out Competency-Based Medical Education (CBME) with outcome-based learning and assessment methods. To cater to this, competencies to be achieved have been integrated with the text where it is addressed. The competencies to be achieved as prescribed by the NMC along with the competency number and reference page number have been listed at the beginning of each chapter. The appropriate competency numbers have also been aligned with the description of the text within the chapters.

Clinical anatomy videos have been provided online to explore the selected clinical applications.

RELEVANT REFERENCES WITHIN THE TEXT

To accomplish certain competencies and to make it all inclusive, appropriate references have also been given from South Asian Editions of *Langman's Medical Embryology*, *diFiore's Atlas of Histology with Functional Correlations*, *Snell's Clinical Neuroanatomy*, and *Snell's Clinical Anatomy*.

STUDENT-CENTERED LEARNING

Three new topics along with illustrations have been added:

- Summary of nerves of upper limb
- Summary of arteries of lower limb
- Summary of peripheral nerves of lower limb

This will help the students to have a comprehensive idea about the vascularity and innervation of the limbs so that they can recollect and remember better.

EXTENSIVE ART PROGRAM

New simplified line diagrams are introduced for branches and distribution of nerves of upper limb. This will aid in easy understanding and reproducibility of the pictures in examinations.

CLINICAL BLUE BOXES

Widely known as "blue boxes," the highlighted clinical correlations are titled "Clinical Boxes." They have evolved with changes in practice and many of them are supported by photographs and/or dynamic color illustrations to help with understanding the practical value of anatomy. In this edition, the clinical boxes have undergone extensive review and revision and reflect many recent medical advances.

Topics in the Clinical Boxes are classified by the following icons to indicate the type of clinical information covered:

Anatomical variations feature anatomical variations that may be encountered in the dissection lab or in practice, emphasizing the clinical importance of awareness of such variations.

Life cycle boxes emphasize prenatal developmental factors that affect postnatal anatomy and anatomical phenomena specifically associated with stages of life—childhood, adolescence, adult, and advanced age.

Trauma boxes feature the effects of traumatic events—such as fractures of bones or dislocations of joints—on normal anatomy and the clinical manifestations and dysfunction resulting from such injuries.

Diagnostic procedures discuss the anatomical features and observations that play a role in physical diagnosis.

Surgical procedures address such topics as the anatomical basis of surgical procedures, such as the planning of incisions, and the anatomical basis of regional anesthesia.

Pathology boxes cover the effects of disease on normal anatomy, such as cancer of the breast, and anatomical structures or principles involved in the confinement or dissemination of disease within the body.

BOTTOM LINE SUMMARIES

Frequent "The Bottom Line" boxes summarize the preceding information, ensuring that primary concepts do not become lost in the many details necessary for thorough understanding. These summaries provide a convenient means of ongoing review and underscore the "big picture" point of view.

SURFACE ANATOMY AND MEDICAL IMAGING

Surface anatomy and medical imaging, formerly presented separately, are integrated into the chapter, presented at the time each region is being discussed, clearly demonstrating anatomy's relationship to physical examination and diagnosis. Both natural views of unobstructed surface anatomy and illustrations superimposing anatomical structures on surface anatomy photographs are components of each regional chapter. Medical images, focusing on normal anatomy, include plain and contrast radiographic, MRI, CT, and ultrasonography studies, often with correlative line art as well as explanatory text, to help prepare future professionals who need to be familiar with diagnostic images.

MULTIPLE CHOICE QUESTIONS

The NMC has also introduced the Early Clinical Exposure program that discusses some aspects of clinical context of patient care in the first year of UG Teaching Program. In tune with this objective, *Moore's Clinically Oriented Anatomy* makes learning anatomy more relevant to clinical practice, with reasoning questions added along with multiple-choice questions at the end of each chapter.

For undergraduates, this will facilitate early clinical exposure, problem-solving skills, application of anatomy knowledge in clinical scenarios and self-assessment. This will also prepare them for the competency-based assessment methods introduced in the new curriculum. For postgraduates, this will serve as a tool in preparation for competitive examinations.

Student Case Study, wherein case-based scenarios with questions and detailed explanations relevant for each chapter, has been given at the end of book as *Appendix*.

TERMINOLOGY

The terminology fully adheres to *Terminologia Anatomica: International Anatomical Nomenclature* (1998), generated by the Federative International Program on Anatomical Terminology (FIPAT) and approved by the International Federation of Associations of Anatomists (IFAA). Although the official English-equivalent terms are used throughout the book, when new terms are introduced, the Latin form, used in Europe, Asia, and other parts of the world, is often provided. The roots and derivations of terms are provided to help students understand meaning and increase retention. Eponyms, although not endorsed by the IFAA, appear in parentheses in this edition—for example, sternal angle (angle of Louis)—to assist students who will hear eponymous terms during their clinical studies. The terminology is available online at http://www.unifr.ch/ifaa.

IMPROVED FEATURES

- Routine facts (such as muscle attachments, innervations, and actions) presented in tables organized to demonstrate shared qualities and illustrated to demonstrate the provided information. *Moore's Clinically Oriented Anatomy* provides more tables than any other anatomy textbook
- Illustrated clinical correlations that not only describe but also show anatomy as it is applied clinically
- Illustrations that reflect the diversity of both those using the textbook and the patients they will be treating
- Illustrations that facilitate orientation. Many orientation figures have been added, along with arrows to indicate the locations of the inset figures (areas shown in close-up

views) and viewing sequences. Labels have been placed to minimize the distance between label and object, with leader lines running the most direct course possible.

- Equitable focus on female as well as male anatomy. Traditionally, texts have been thorough regarding the presentation of the male phallus and insufficient on treatment of the female external genitalia, implying that the clitoris is merely a much smaller version of the penis. This edition provides a thorough presentation of the anatomy of the clitoris, showing that its anatomy is distinct and clearly not a miniature version of the penis.
- **Bold face type** indicates the main entries of anatomical terms when they are introduced and defined. In the index, the page numbers of these main entries also appear in boldface type, so that the main entries can be easily located. Boldface type is also used to introduce clinical terms in the clinical blue boxes.
- *Italic type* indicates anatomical terms important to the topic and region of study or labeled in an illustration that is being referenced.
- Useful content outlines appear at the beginning of every chapter.

This edition has a lot of distinctive changes to make this book more student friendly and pertinent to the changing times and to the changing trends in medical education.

S. Aruna
N. Isai Vani

Acknowledgments

"Above all, we bow down to GOD, for everything we do flows from HIM"

We are eternally grateful to our teachers, who were monumental in kindling interest in Anatomy and inspiring us to teach.

We appreciate all the faculty and students for their honest and valid feedback on the first South Asian Edition, which served as a platform to plan for the improvement of the second South Asian Edition.

Our sincere thanks to the Director and Dean of Indira Gandhi Medical College and Research Institute, Puducherry, faculty and staff of the Department of Anatomy for their kind co-operation.

Our sincere thanks and acknowledgment to Dr M Sivakumar for his contribution to the first South Asian Edition.

Moreover, we would like to thank the publisher, Wolters Kluwer India Private Limited, for giving us this wonderful opportunity to edit *Moore's Clinically Oriented Anatomy*, first South Asian Edition, the most renowned textbook of Anatomy widely preferred by medical fraternity; and in particular Sangeetha Parthasarathy (Senior Publishing Manager), Nayan Gogoi (Development Editor), and Amit Rai (Senior Content Management Analyst) for their relentless support in this project. Their guidance and suggestions helped us in successfully completing this project.

Last but not the least, we express our heartfelt gratitude to our family members for their encouragement and constant support.

S. Aruna
N. Isai Vani

List of Reviewers*

Adari Raja
Senior Resident
Department of Anatomy
NRI Institute of Medical Sciences
Visakhapatnam, Andhra Pradesh

Alok Tripathi
Associate Professor
Department of Anatomy
Subharti Medical College
Meerut, Uttar Pradesh

T S R Anjana
Associate Professor
Department of Anatomy
Omadurar Government Medical College
Chennai, Tamil Nadu

Anjana Mittal
Professor and Head
Department of Anatomy
MMU Medical College
Mullana, Haryana

Anju Yadav
Professor
Department of Anatomy
Lady Hardinge Medical College
New Delhi

Asha K R
Professor and Head
Department of Anatomy
Siddaganga Medical College and Research Institute
Tumakuru, Karnataka

Asha Latha
Professor
Department of Anatomy
Siddhartha Medical College
Vijayawada, Andhra Pradesh

S Babu Rao
Professor and Head
Department of Anatomy
Malla Reddy Medical College for Women
Hyderabad, Telangana

Balachandra N
Professor and Head
Department of Anatomy
East Point College of Medical Sciences
Bengaluru, Karnataka

Ch N V Bharath
Associate Professor
Department of Anatomy
Alluri Sitarama Raju Academy of Medical Sciences
Eluru, Andhra Pradesh

Chada Jayashree
Assistant Professor
Department of Anatomy
Surabhi Institute of medical Sciences
Siddipet, Telangana

Chandra Philip
Professor and Head
Department of Anatomy
Mahatma Gandhi Medical College and Research Institute
Puducherry

M S Farooqi
Dean and Professor
Department of Anatomy
NIMRA Institute of Medical Sciences
Vijayawada, Andhra Pradesh

TLS Gowri
Associate Professor
Department of Anatomy
Government Medical College
Sangareddy, Telangana

*The names are arranged alphabetically as per the first name.

Hannah Sugirthabai Rajila R
Professor and Head
Department of Anatomy
Chettinad Hospital and Research Institute
Chennai, Tamil Nadu

Jami Sagar Prusty
Professor and Head
Department of Anatomy
Saheed Laxman Nayak Medical College and Hospital
Koraput, Odisha

V Janaki
Professor and Head
Department of Anatomy
Osmania Medical College
Hyderabad, Telangana

Joy A Ghoshal
Dean and Head
Department of Anatomy
All India Institute of Medical Sciences
Mangalagiri, Andhra Pradesh

Jyoti Arora
Director Professor and Head
Department of Anatomy
Atal Bihari Vajpayee Institute of Medical Sciences and Dr. Ram Manohar Lohia Hospital
New Delhi

Julie Christy A
Assistant Professor
Department of Anatomy
Shri Sathya Sai Medical College and Research Centre
Chennai, Tamil Nadu

Kanagavalli P
Associate Professor
Department of Anatomy
Madras Medical College
Chennai, Tamil Nadu

S Karthick
Professor and Head
Department of Anatomy
Melmaruvathur Adhiparasakthi Institute of Medical Sciences and Research
Melmaruvathur, Tamil Nadu

Komala Nagaraja
Professor and Head
Department of Anatomy
BGS Global Institute of Medical Sciences
Bengaluru, Karnataka

Kumar Satish Ravi
Additional Professor
Department of Anatomy
All India Institute of Medical Sciences
Rishikesh, Uttarakhand

Lalitha Chandra
Professor and Head
Department of Anatomy
Kempegowda Institute of Medical Sciences
Bengaluru, Karnataka

Martin Lucas
Professor and Head
Department of Anatomy
Dr Chandramma Dayananda Sagar Institute of Medical Education and Research (CDSIMER)
Devarakaggalahalli, Karnataka

Minkashi Malhotra
Associate Professor
Department of Anatomy
Lady Hardinge Medical College
New Delhi

T Nava Kalyani
Professor and Head
Department of Anatomy
Government Medical College
Mahabubnagar, Telangana

Nirmala
Professor and Head
Department of Anatomy
Karpagam Medical College and Hospital
Coimbatore, Tamil Nadu

V Padmaja
Associate Professor
Department of Anatomy
Kakatiya Medical College
Warangal, Telangana

G Prabavathy
Professor
Department of Anatomy
Mahatma Gandhi Medical College and Research Institute
Puducherry

Praveen Kumar
Assistant Professor
Department of Anatomy
Trichy SRM Medical College Hospital and Research Centre
Trichy, Tamil Nadu

Priya Ranganath
Professor and Head
Department of Anatomy
Bangalore Medical College and Research Institute
Bengaluru, Karnataka

Pushpalatha K
Professor and Head
Department of Anatomy
JSS Medical College
Mysuru, Karnataka

T Rajan
Professor and Head cum Vice Principal
Department of Anatomy
Aarupadai Veedu Medical College
Puducherry

Rajanigandha Vadgaonkar
Professor and Head
Department of Anatomy
Kasturba Medical College
Mangalore, Karnataka

V Raja Priya
Professor and Head
Department of Anatomy
Government Medical College
Tiruvallur, Tamil Nadu

Rajeshwari C. Eligar
Professor and Head
Department of Anatomy
Karnataka Institute of Medical Sciences
Hubballi, Karnataka

Ravichandran Doraiswamy
Professor and Head
Department of Anatomy
Dhanalakshmi Srinivasan Medical College and Hospital
Trichy, Tamil Nadu

Rudragouda S Bulagouda
Professor and Head
Department of Anatomy
BLDE (DU) Shri B M Patil Medical College
Vijayapura, Karnataka

Sadhu Lokanadham
Associate Professor
Department of Anatomy
Santhiram Medical College
Nandyal, Andhra Pradesh

Samata Roshini
Professor and Head
Department of Anatomy
Surabhi Institute of medical Sciences
Siddipet, Telangana

Sangeeta M
Professor and Head
Department of Anatomy
MVJ Medical College and Research Hospital
Bengaluru, Karnataka

Sanjeev Kolagi
Professor and Head,
Department of Anatomy
Coordinator, Medical Education
S. Nijalingappa Medical College and Research Centre
Navanagar, Bagalkot

Santhini Arulselvi
Professor and Head
Department of Anatomy
Vinayaka Missions Medical College
Karaikal, Puducherry

Satyam Khare
Professor and Head
Department of Anatomy
Subharti Medical College
Meerut, Uttar Pradesh

Shailaja Shetty
Professor and Head
Department of Anatomy
M. S. Ramaiah Medical College
Bengaluru, Karnataka

Shanthi K C
Professor and Head
Department of Anatomy
Vinayaka Mission's Kirupananda Variyar Medical College & Hospital
Salem, Tamil Nadu

Sheetal Joshi
Associate Professor
Department of Anatomy
Lady Hardinge Medical College
New Delhi

Shilpi Jain
Professor
Department of Anatomy
Subharti Medical College
Meerut, Uttar Pradesh

Shruthi B N
Professor and Head
Raja Rajeswari Medical College and Hospital
Bengaluru, Karnataka

Shruthy K M
Associate Professor
Department of Anatomy
A.C.S Medical College and Hospital
Chennai, Tamil Nadu

S Sreelatha
Professor
Department of Anatomy
Malla Reddy Medical College for Women
Hyderabad, Telangana

Sreevidya J
Associate Professor
Department of Anatomy
Madras Medical College
Chennai, Tamil Nadu

Sridevi N S
Professor and Head
Department of Anatomy
Sri Devaraj Urs Academy of Higher Education and Research
Kolar, Karnataka

Suma H Y
Professor and Head
Department of Anatomy
Jawaharlal Institute of Postgraduate Medical Education & Research (JIPMER)
Puducherry

Swathi Poornima
Professor and Head
Department of Anatomy
Pinnamaneni Siddhartha Institute of Medical Sciences
Vijayawada, Andhra Pradesh

Tejaswi Hiremarali Lokanathan
Professor
Department of Anatomy
Adichunchanagiri Institute of Medical Sciences
BG Nagara, Karnataka

Thotakura Balaji
Professor
Department of Anatomy
Chettinad Hospital and Research Institute
Chennai, Tamil Nadu

Varsha Mokashi
Professor and Head
Department of Anatomy
Vydehi Institute of Medical Sciences and Research Centre
Bengaluru, Karnataka

Vasudha Kulkarni
Professor and Head
Department of Anatomy
Akash Institute of Medical Sciences and Research Center
Bengaluru, Karnataka

Vijaya R
Associate Professor
Department of Anatomy
All India Institute of Medical Sciences
Madurai, Tamil Nadu

Vijisha Phalgunan
Professor and Head
Department of Anatomy
Sri Lakshmi Narayana Institute of Medical Sciences
Puducherry

Contents

Preface / vii
Acknowledgments / x
List of Reviewers / xi
Clinical Anatomy Videos / xx
Abbreviations / xx
CBME Topics / xxi

Volume 1

1 OVERVIEW AND BASIC CONCEPTS 1

Approaches to Studying Anatomy / 2
Regional Anatomy / 2
Systemic Anatomy / 4
Clinical Anatomy / 5
ANATOMICOMEDICAL TERMINOLOGY / 5
Anatomical Position / 6
Anatomical Planes / 6
Terms of Relationship and Comparison / 7
Terms of Laterality / 9
Terms of Movement / 9
ANATOMICAL VARIATIONS / 12
INTEGUMENTARY SYSTEM / 12
FASCIAS, FASCIAL COMPARTMENTS, BURSAE, AND POTENTIAL SPACES / 17
SKELETAL SYSTEM / 19
Cartilage and Bones / 20
Classification of Bones / 21
Bone Markings and Formations / 21
Bone Development / 22
Vasculature and Innervation of Bones / 23
Joints / 25
MUSCLE TISSUE AND MUSCULAR SYSTEM / 29
Types of Muscle (Muscle Tissue) / 29
Skeletal Muscles / 31
Cardiac Striated Muscle / 37
Smooth Muscle / 37
CARDIOVASCULAR SYSTEM / 38
Vascular Circuits / 38
Blood Vessels / 39
LYMPHOID SYSTEM / 43
NERVOUS SYSTEM / 46
Central Nervous System / 47
Peripheral Nervous System / 47
Somatic Nervous System / 58
Autonomic Nervous System / 58
MEDICAL IMAGING TECHNIQUES / 67
Conventional Radiography / 67
Computed Tomography / 68
Ultrasonography / **69**
Magnetic Resonance Imaging / **69**
Nuclear Medicine Imaging / **71**
Multiple-Choice Questions / 72

2 BACK 73

OVERVIEW OF BACK AND VERTEBRAL COLUMN / 74
VERTEBRAE / 74
Structure and Function of Vertebrae / 75
Regional Characteristics of Vertebrae / 77
Ossification of Vertebrae / 87
Variations in Vertebrae / 89
VERTEBRAL COLUMN / 97
Joints of Vertebral Column / 97
Movements of Vertebral Column / 103
Curvatures of Vertebral Column / 104
Vasculature of Vertebral Column / 106
Nerves of Vertebral Column / 107
MUSCLES OF BACK / 118
Extrinsic Back Muscles / 118
Intrinsic Back Muscles / 119

Surface Anatomy of Back Muscles / **126**
Suboccipital and Deep Neck Muscles / **126**

CONTENTS OF VERTEBRAL CANAL / 130
Spinal Cord / **130**
Spinal Nerves and Nerve Roots / **130**
Spinal Meninges and Cerebrospinal Fluid (CSF) / **132**
Vasculature of Spinal Cord and Spinal Nerve Roots / **137**
Multiple-Choice Questions / 142

3 UPPER LIMB 144

OVERVIEW OF UPPER LIMB / 147
COMPARISON OF UPPER AND LOWER LIMBS / 147
BONES OF UPPER LIMB / 148
Clavicle / 148
Scapula / 150
Humerus / 151
Bones of Forearm / 152
Bones of Hand / 153
Surface Anatomy of Upper Limb Bones / 156

FASCIA, EFFERENT VESSELS, CUTANEOUS INNERVATION, AND MYOTOMES OF UPPER LIMB / 164
Fascia of Upper Limb / 164
Venous Drainage of Upper Limb / 165
Lymphatic Drainage of Upper Limb / 167
Summary of Peripheral Nerves of Upper Limb / 167
Cutaneous Innervation of Upper Limb / 169
Motor Innervation (Myotomes) of Upper Limb / 171

PECTORAL AND SCAPULAR REGIONS / 176
Anterior Axio-Appendicular Muscles / 176
Posterior Axio-Appendicular and Scapulohumeral Muscles **/ 179**
Surface Anatomy of Pectoral, Scapular, and Deltoid Regions / 186

AXILLA / 193
Axillary Artery / 195
Axillary Vein / 198
Axillary Lymph Nodes / 198
Brachial Plexus / 199

ARM / 212
Muscles of Arm / 212
Brachial Artery / 217
Veins of Arm / 217
Nerves of Arm / 218
Cubital Fossa / 220
Surface Anatomy of Arm and Cubital Fossa / 221

FOREARM / 228
Compartments of Forearm / 228
Muscles of Forearm / 228
Arteries of Forearm / 241
Veins of Forearm / 243
Nerves of Forearm / 244
Surface Anatomy of Forearm / 247

HAND / 254
Fascia and Compartments of Palm / 254
Muscles of Hand / 256
Long Flexor Tendons and Tendon Sheaths in Hand **/ 262**
Arteries of Hand / 262
Veins of Hand / 265
Nerves of Hand / 265
Surface Anatomy of Hand / 269

JOINTS OF UPPER LIMB / 276
Sternoclavicular Joint / 277
Acromioclavicular Joint / 279
Glenohumeral Joint / 279
Elbow Joint **/ 284**
Proximal Radio-Ulnar Joint / 287
Distal Radio-Ulnar Joint / 289
Wrist Joint / 291
Intercarpal Joints / 291
Carpometacarpal and Intermetacarpal Joints / 294
Metacarpophalangeal and Interphalangeal Joints / 295
Multiple-Choice Questions / 303

4 THORAX 306

OVERVIEW OF THORAX / 308
THORACIC WALL / 308
Skeleton of Thoracic Wall / 310
Thoracic Apertures / 314
Joints of Thoracic Wall / 315
Movements of Thoracic Wall / 317
Muscles of Thoracic Wall / 322
Fascia of Thoracic Wall / 324
Nerves of Thoracic Wall / 327
Vasculature of Thoracic Wall / 330
Breasts / 332
Surface Anatomy of Thoracic Wall / 335

VISCERA OF THORACIC CAVITY / 343
Pleurae, Lungs, and Tracheobronchial Tree / 344
Overview of Mediastinum / 367
Pericardium / 367
Heart / 375
Superior Mediastinum and Great Vessels **/ 402**
Posterior Mediastinum / 408
Anterior Mediastinum / 414
Surface Anatomy of Heart and Mediastinal Viscera / 414
Auscultatory Areas / 415
Multiple-Choice Questions / 425

APPENDIX A: Student Case Study / A-1
APPENDIX B: References and Suggested Reading / B-1
INDEX / I-1

ONLINE RESOURCES
- **eBook**
- **Clinical Anatomy Videos**
- **Multiple-Choice Questions**

Volume 2

5 ABDOMEN 428

OVERVIEW: WALLS, CAVITIES, REGIONS, AND PLANES / 432

ANTEROLATERAL ABDOMINAL WALL / 434
- Fascia of Anterolateral Abdominal Wall / 434
- Muscles of Anterolateral Abdominal Wall / 435
- Neurovasculature of Anterolateral Abdominal Wall / 441
- Internal Surface of Anterolateral Abdominal Wall / 449
- Inguinal Region / 450
- Spermatic Cord, Scrotum, and Testes / 454
- Surface Anatomy of Anterolateral Abdominal Wall / 458

PERITONEUM AND PERITONEAL CAVITY / 465
- Embryology of Peritoneal Cavity / 466
- Peritoneal Formations / 467
- Subdivisions of Peritoneal Cavity / 469

ABDOMINAL VISCERA / 474
- Overview of Abdominal Viscera and Digestive Tract / 474
- Esophagus / 477
- Stomach / 478
- Small Intestine / 487
- Large Intestine / 494
- Spleen / 513
- Pancreas / 514
- Liver / 517
- Biliary Ducts and Gallbladder / 527
- Kidneys, Ureters, and Suprarenal Glands / 541
- Summary of Innervation of Abdominal Viscera / 553

DIAPHRAGM / 559
- Vessels and Nerves of Diaphragm / 560
- Diaphragmatic Apertures / 561
- Actions of Diaphragm / 562

POSTERIOR ABDOMINAL WALL / 563
- Fascia of Posterior Abdominal Wall / 563
- Muscles of Posterior Abdominal Wall / 565
- Nerves of Posterior Abdominal Wall / 566
- Vessels of Posterior Abdominal Wall / 567

SECTIONAL MEDICAL IMAGING OF ABDOMEN / 575
- ***Multiple-Choice Questions*** / 579

6 PELVIS AND PERINEUM 583

INTRODUCTION TO PELVIS AND PERINEUM / 585

PELVIC GIRDLE / 585
- Bones and Features of Pelvic Girdle / 585
- Orientation of Pelvic Girdle / 589
- Pelvic Girdle Sexual Differences / 589
- Joints and Ligaments of Pelvic Girdle / 589

PELVIC CAVITY / 596
- Walls and Floor of Pelvic Cavity / 596
- Peritoneum and Peritoneal Cavity of Pelvis / 601
- Pelvic Fascia / 603

NEUROVASCULAR STRUCTURES OF PELVIS / 607
- Pelvic Arteries / 607
- Pelvic Veins / 613
- Lymph Nodes of Pelvis / 613
- Pelvic Nerves / 614

PELVIC VISCERA / 620
- Urinary Organs / 620
- Rectum / 626
- Male Internal Genital Organs / 634
- Female Internal Genital Organs / 640
- Lymphatic Drainage of Pelvic Viscera / 658

PERINEUM / 661
- Fasciae and Pouches of Urogenital Triangle / 664
- Features of Anal Triangle / 668
- Male Urogenital Triangle / 677
- Female Urogenital Triangle / 687

SECTIONAL IMAGING OF PELVIS AND PERINEUM / 693
- Magnetic Resonance Imaging **/ 693**
- ***Multiple-Choice Questions* / 698**

7 LOWER LIMB 701

OVERVIEW OF LOWER LIMB / 704

DEVELOPMENT OF LOWER LIMB / 705

BONES OF LOWER LIMB / 705
- Arrangement of Lower Limb Bones / 707
- Hip Bone / 708
- Ilium / 709
- Femur / 711
- Patella / 715
- Tibia and Fibula / 715
- Bones of Foot / 718
- Surface Anatomy of Bones of Foot / 720

FASCIA, VEINS, LYMPHATICS, EFFERENT VESSELS, AND CUTANEOUS NERVES OF LOWER LIMB / 728
- Subcutaneous Tissue and Fascia / 728

OVERVIEW OF VESSELS AND NERVES OF LOWER LIMB / 728
- Arterial Supply of Lower Limb / 728
- Venous Drainage of Lower Limb / 731
- Lymphatic Drainage of Lower Limb / 733
- Cutaneous Innervation of Lower Limb / 734
- Motor Innervation of Lower Limb / 734
- Peripheral Nerves of Lower Limb / 734

POSTURE AND GAIT / 743
- Standing at Ease / 743
- Walking: The Gait Cycle / 743

ANTERIOR AND MEDIAL REGIONS OF THIGH / 745
- Organization of Proximal Lower Limb / 745
- Anterior Thigh Muscles / 746
- Medial Thigh Muscles / 749

Neurovascular Structures and Relationships in Anteromedial Thigh / **752**
Surface Anatomy of Anterior and Medial Regions of Thigh / 757
GLUTEAL AND POSTERIOR THIGH REGIONS / 763
Gluteal Region: Buttocks and Hip Region / 763
Muscles of Gluteal Region / 764
Posterior Thigh Region / 770
Neurovascular Structures of Gluteal and Posterior Thigh Regions / 773
Surface Anatomy of Gluteal and Posterior Thigh Regions / 779
POPLITEAL FOSSA AND LEG / 785
Popliteal Region / 785
Anterior Compartment of Leg / 789
Lateral Compartment of Leg / 794
Posterior Compartment of Leg / 798
Surface Anatomy of Leg / 805
FOOT / 811
Skin and Fascia of Foot / 812
Muscles of Foot / 812
Neurovascular Structures and Relationships in Foot / 816
Surface Anatomy of Ankle and Foot Regions / **824**
JOINTS OF LOWER LIMB / 828
Hip Joint / 828
Knee Joint / 836
Tibiofibular Joints / 845
Ankle Joint / 849
Foot Joints / 851
Surface Anatomy of Joints of Knee, Ankle, and Foot / 859
Multiple-Choice Questions / 872

APPENDIX A: Student Case Study / A-1
APPENDIX B: References and Suggested Reading / B-1
INDEX / I-1

ONLINE RESOURCES
- **eBook**
- **Clinical Anatomy Videos**
- **Multiple-Choice Questions**

Volume 3

8 HEAD 876

OVERVIEW OF HEAD / 879
CRANIUM / 879
Facial Aspect of Cranium / 882
Lateral Aspect of Cranium / 886
Occipital Aspect of Cranium / 886
Superior Aspect of Cranium / 887
External Surface of Cranial Base / 887
Internal Surface of Cranial Base / 890
Walls of Cranial Cavity / 893
Regions of Head / 894
FACE AND SCALP / 900
Face / 900
Scalp / 900
Muscles of Face and Scalp / 901
Nerves of Face and Scalp / 906
Superficial Vasculature of Face and Scalp / 912
Surface Anatomy of Face / 915
CRANIAL MENINGES / 922
Dura Mater / 922
Arachnoid Mater and Pia Mater / 929
Meningeal Spaces / 929
BRAIN / 935
Parts of Brain / 935
Ventricular System of Brain / 935
Arterial Blood Supply to Brain / 939
Venous Drainage of Brain / 940
EYE, ORBIT, ORBITAL REGION, AND EYEBALL / 946
Orbits / 946
Eyelids and Lacrimal Apparatus / 948
Eyeball / 951
Extra-Ocular Muscles of Orbit / 955
Nerves of Orbit / 962
Vasculature of Orbit / 963
Surface Anatomy of Eye and Lacrimal Apparatus / 965
PAROTID AND TEMPORAL REGIONS, INFRATEMPORAL FOSSA, AND TEMPOROMANDIBULAR JOINT / 973
Parotid Region / 973
Temporal Region / 975
Infratemporal Fossa / 975
ORAL REGION / 987
Oral Cavity / 987
Lips, Cheeks, and Gingivae / 987
Teeth / 989
Palate / 993
Tongue / 997
Salivary Glands / 1002
PTERYGOPALATINE FOSSA / 1011
Pterygopalatine Part of Maxillary Artery / 1011
Maxillary Nerve / 1011
NOSE / 1015
External Nose / 1015
Nasal Cavities / 1016
Vasculature and Innervation of Nose / 1019
Paranasal Sinuses / 1020
EAR / 1026
External Ear / 1026
Middle Ear / 1027
Internal Ear / 1033
Multiple-Choice Questions / 1042

9 NECK 1045

OVERVIEW / 1047

BONES OF NECK / 1047
- Cervical Vertebrae / 1047
- Hyoid Bone / 1049

FASCIA OF NECK / 1050
- Cervical Subcutaneous Tissue and Platysma / 1050
- Deep Cervical Fascia / 1052

SUPERFICIAL STRUCTURES OF NECK: CERVICAL REGIONS / 1054
- Sternocleidomastoid Region / 1054
- Posterior Cervical Region / 1057
- Lateral Cervical Region / 1057
- Anterior Cervical Region / 1064
- Surface Anatomy of Cervical Regions and Triangles of Neck / 1070

DEEP STRUCTURES OF NECK / 1077
- Prevertebral Muscles / 1077
- Root of Neck / 1077

VISCERA OF NECK / 1083
- Endocrine Layer of Cervical Viscera / 1083
- Respiratory Layer of Cervical Viscera / 1087
- Alimentary Layer of Cervical Viscera / 1097
- Surface Anatomy of Endocrine and Respiratory Layers of Cervical Viscera **/ 1104**

LYMPHATICS OF NECK / 1105
- ***Multiple-Choice Questions*** / 1117

10 SUMMARY OF CRANIAL NERVES 1119

OVERVIEW / 1120

OLFACTORY NERVE (CN I) / 1127

OPTIC NERVE (CN II) / 1128

OCULOMOTOR NERVE (CN III) / 1129

TROCHLEAR NERVE (CN IV) / 1132

TRIGEMINAL NERVE (CN V) / 1133
- Ophthalmic Nerve (CN V1) / 1135
- Maxillary Nerve (CN V2) / 1135
- Mandibular Nerve (CN V3) / 1135

ABDUCENT NERVE (CN VI) / 1135

FACIAL NERVE (CN VII) / 1138
- Somatic (Branchial) Motor / 1140
- Visceral (Parasympathetic) Motor / 1140
- Somatic (General) Sensory / 1140
- Special Sensory (Taste) / 1140

VESTIBULOCOCHLEAR NERVE (CN VIII) / 1140

GLOSSOPHARYNGEAL NERVE (CN IX) / 1142
- Somatic (Branchial) Motor / 1142
- Visceral (Parasympathetic) Motor / 1142
- Somatic (General) Sensory / 1142
- Special Sensory (Taste) / 1142
- Visceral Sensory / 1142

VAGUS NERVE (CN X) / 1143

SPINAL ACCESSORY NERVE (CN XI) / 1146

HYPOGLOSSAL NERVE (CN XII) / 1148
- ***Multiple-Choice Questions*** / 1157

APPENDIX A: Student Case Study / A-1

APPENDIX B: References and Suggested Reading / B-1

INDEX / I-1

ONLINE RESOURCES
- eBook
- Clinical Anatomy Videos
- Multiple-Choice Questions

Clinical Anatomy Videos*

S.No	Video title	Competency number and description	Chapter number/ Page number
1	Facial nerve palsy	**AN28.7** Explain the anatomical basis of facial nerve palsy	Chapter 8/918, 920
2	Laryngeal nerve injury	**AN38.3** Describe anatomical basis of recurrent laryngeal nerve injury	Chapter 9/1109
3	Carpel tunnel syndrome	**AN12.4** Explain the anatomical basis of carpal tunnel syndrome	Chapter 3/251, 273
4	Carcinoma of breast	**AN9.2** Describe the applied anatomy of breast	Chapter 4/340
5	Lumbar puncture	**AN50.3** Describe lumbar puncture (site, direction of the needle, structures pierced during the lumbar puncture)	Chapter 2/140
6	Benign prostatic hyperplasia	**AN48.7** Mention the lobes involved in benign prostatic hypertrophy and prostatic cancer	Chapter 6/639
7	Ankle injuries	**AN20.1** Describe and demonstrate the type, articular surfaces, capsule, synovial membrane, ligaments, relations, movements and muscles involved, blood and nerve supply of ankle joint	Chapter 7/868
8	Inguinal hernia	**AN44.5** Explain the anatomical basis of inguinal hernia	Chapter 5/453, 460

Abbreviations

a., aa.	artery, arteries
abd.	abdomen, abductor
acc.	accessory
ACL	anterior cruciate ligament
add.	adductor
ANS	autonomic nervous system
ant.	anterior
ASIS	anterior superior iliac spine
AV	atrioventricular
C	cervical
CCA	common carotid artery
CN	cranial nerve
CNS	central nervous system
Co	coccygeal
CSF	cerebrospinal fluid
ECA	external carotid artery
e.g.	for example
EJV	external jugular vein
ENS	enteric nervous system
et al.	and others
ext.	extensor, external
flex.	flexor
Fr.	French
G.	Greek
GI	gastrointestinal
ICA	internal carotid artery
i.e.	that is
IJV	internal jugular vein
inf.	inferior
int.	internal
IVC	internal vena cava
l.	left
L	liter, lumbar
L.	Latin
LA	left atrium
lat.	lateral
LCA	left coronary artery
lev.	levator
LLQ	left lower quadrant
LRV	left renal vein
LUQ	left upper quadrant
LV	left ventricle
m., mm.	muscle, muscles
med.	medial
PCL	posterior cruciate ligament
PNS	peripheral nervous system
post.	posterior
PSIS	posterior superior iliac spine
PSNS	parasympathetic nervous system
PV	hepatic portal vein
r.	right
RA	right atrium
RCA	right coronary artery
RLQ	right lower quadrant
RUQ	right upper quadrant
RV	right ventricle
S	sacral
SA	sinu-atrial
SCM	sternocleidomastoid
SNS	sensory nervous system
sp.	spinal
SPNS	sympathetic nervous system
sup.	superior
supf.	superficial
SV	sinoventricular
SVC	superior vena cava
T	thoracic
TA	Terminologia Anatomica
TMJ	temporomandibular joint
v., vv.	vein, veins
vs.	versus
yo	years old

*Online Resource

CBME Topics

Competency Based Undergraduate Curriculum Topics: Page-Wise Coverage

Number	Competencies	Page/s
AN1.1	Demonstrate normal anatomical position, various planes, relation, comparison, laterality and movement in our body	6
AN1.2	Describe composition of bone and bone marrow	20
AN2.1	Describe parts, blood and nerve supply of a long bone	23
AN2.2	Enumerate laws of ossification	23
AN2.3	Enumerate special features of a sesamoid bone	21
AN2.4	Describe various types of cartilage with its structure and distribution in body	20
AN2.5	Describe various joints with subtypes and examples	25
AN2.6	Explain the concept of nerve supply of joints and Hilton's law	28
AN3.1	Classify muscle tissue according to structure and action	29
AN3.2	Enumerate parts of skeletal muscle and differentiate between tendons and aponeuroses with examples	31
AN3.3	Explain shunt and spurt muscles	35
AN4.1	Describe different types of skin and dermatomes in body	13, 52
AN4.2	Describe structure and function of skin with its appendages	12, 13
AN4.3	Describe superficial fascia along with fat distribution in body	17
AN4.4	Describe modifications of deep fascia with its functions	17
AN4.5	Explain principles of skin incisions	15
AN5.1	Differentiate between blood vascular and lymphatic system	38
AN5.2	Differentiate between pulmonary and systemic circulation	38
AN5.3	List general differences between arteries and veins	30
AN5.4	Explain functional difference between elastic, muscular arteries and arterioles	39
AN5.5	Describe portal system giving examples	38, 42
AN5.6	Describe the concept of anastomoses and collateral circulation with significance of end-arteries	41
AN5.7	Explain function of meta-arterioles, precapillary sphincters, arterio-venous anastomoses	41
AN5.8	Define thrombosis, infarction and aneurysm	42
AN6.1	List the components and functions of the lymphatic system	43
AN6.2	Describe structure of lymph capillaries and mechanism of lymph circulation	43
AN6.3	Explain the concept of lymphoedema and spread of tumors via lymphatics and venous system	45
AN7.1	Describe general plan of nervous system with components of central, peripheral and autonomic nervous systems	46
AN7.2	List components of nervous tissue and their functions	46
AN7.3	Describe parts of a neuron and classify them based on number of neurites, size and function	46
AN7.4	Describe structure of a typical spinal nerve	50
AN7.5	Describe principles of sensory and motor innervation of muscles	52
AN7.6	Describe concept of loss of innervation of a muscle with its applied anatomy	58
AN7.7	Describe various type of synapse	52
AN7.8	Describe differences between sympathetic and spinal ganglia	58
AN8.1	Identify the given bone, its side, important features and keep it in anatomical position	148
AN8.2	Identify and describe joints formed by the given bone	148
AN8.3	Enumerate peculiarities of clavicle	148, 159
AN8.4	Demonstrate important muscle attachment on the given bone	148, 179, 183, 215, 231, 234, 259
AN8.5	Identify and name various bones in articulated hand, specify the parts of metacarpals and phalanges and enumerate the peculiarities of pisiform	153
AN8.6	Describe scaphoid fracture and explain the anatomical basis of avascular necrosis	162
AN9.1	Describe attachment, nerve supply and action of pectoralis major and pectoralis minor	176
AN9.2	Breast: Describe the location, extent, deep relations, structure, age changes, blood supply, lymphatic drainage, microanatomy and applied anatomy of breast	332
AN9.3	Describe development of breast	332
AN10.1	Identify and describe boundaries and contents of axilla	193
AN10.2	Identify, describe and demonstrate the origin, extent, course, parts, relations and branches of axillary artery and tributaries of vein	195, 198
AN10.3	Describe, identify and demonstrate formation, branches, relations, area of supply of branches, course and relations of terminal branches of brachial plexus	199
AN10.4	Describe the anatomical groups of axillary lymph nodes and specify their areas of drainage	198
AN10.5	Explain variations in formation of brachial plexus	209
AN10.6	Explain the anatomical basis of clinical features of Erb's palsy and Klumpke's paralysis	210
AN10.7	Explain anatomical basis of enlarged axillary lymph nodes	209
AN10.8	Describe, identify and demonstrate the position, attachment, nerve supply and actions of trapezius and latissimus dorsi	179, 180

Reference: National Medical Commission. Competency Based Undergraduate Curriculum for the Indian Medical Graduate, Vol. 1 (2018), pages 40 to 81. Available at https://www.nmc.org.in/wp-content/uploads/2020/01/UG-Curriculum-Vol-I.pdf

Number	Competencies	Page/s
AN10.9	Describe the arterial anastomosis around the scapula and mention the boundaries of triangle of auscultation	190, 207
AN10.10	Describe and identify the deltoid and rotator cuff muscles	183, 185
AN10.11	Describe and demonstrate attachment of serratus anterior with its action	178
AN10.12	Describe and demonstrate shoulder joint for–type, articular surfaces, capsule, synovial membrane, ligaments, relations, movements, muscles involved, blood supply, nerve supply and applied anatomy	279, 297
AN10.13	Explain anatomical basis of injury to axillary nerve during intramuscular injections	190
AN11.1	Describe and demonstrate muscle groups of upper arm with emphasis on biceps and triceps brachii	212
AN11.2	Identify and describe origin, course, relations, branches (or tributaries), termination of important nerves and vessels in arm	217, 218
AN11.3	Describe the anatomical basis of venepuncture of cubital veins	227
AN11.4	Describe the anatomical basis of saturday night paralysis	226
AN11.5	Identify and describe boundaries and contents of cubital fossa	220
AN11.6	Describe the anastomosis around the elbow joint	217
AN12.1	Describe and demonstrate important muscle groups of ventral forearm with attachments, nerve supply and actions	228
AN12.2	Identify and describe origin, course, relations, branches (or tributaries), termination of important nerves and vessels of forearm	241, 243, 244
AN12.3	Identify and describe flexor retinaculum with its attachments	228
AN12.4	Explain anatomical basis of carpal tunnel syndrome	251, 273
AN12.5	Identify and describe small muscles of hand. Also describe movements of thumb and muscles involved	256
AN12.6	Describe and demonstrate movements of thumb and muscles involved	256
AN12.7	Identify and describe course and branches of important blood vessels and nerves in hand	262, 265
AN12.8	Describe anatomical basis of claw hand	252, 274
AN12.9	Identify and describe fibrous flexor sheaths, ulnar bursa, radial bursa and digital synovial sheaths	262
AN12.10	Explain infection of fascial spaces of palm	272
AN12.11	Identify, describe and demonstrate important muscle groups of dorsal forearm with attachments, nerve supply and actions	233
AN12.12	Identify and describe origin, course, relations, branches (or tributaries), termination of important nerves and vessels of back of forearm	241, 243
AN12.13	Describe the anatomical basis of wrist drop	226, 253, 275
AN12.14	Identify and describe compartments deep to extensor retinaculum	235
AN12.15	Identify and describe extensor expansion formation	237
AN13.1	Describe and explain fascia of upper limb and compartments, veins of upper limb and its lymphatic drainage	164, 165, 167
AN13.2	Describe dermatomes of upper limb	169
AN13.3	Identify and describe the type, articular surfaces, capsule, synovial membrane, ligaments, relations, movements, blood and nerve supply of elbow joint, proximal and distal radio-ulnar joints, wrist joint and first carpometacarpal joint	284, 287, 291, 294
AN13.4	Describe sternoclavicular joint, acromioclavicular joint, carpometacarpal joints and metacarpophalangeal joint	277, 279
AN13.5	Identify the bones and joints of upper limb seen in anteroposterior and lateral view radiographs of shoulder region, arm, elbow, forearm and hand	196, 280, 285, 289, 290
AN13.6	Identify and demonstrate important bony landmarks of upper limb: Jugular notch, sternal angle, acromial angle, spine of the scapula, vertebral level of the medial end, Inferior angle of the scapula	156, 186
AN13.7	Identify and demonstrate surface projection of: Cephalic and basilic vein, palpation of brachial artery, radial artery, testing of muscles: Trapezius, pectoralis major, serratus anterior, latissimus dorsi, deltoid, biceps brachii, brachioradialis	176, 178, 179, 180, 183, 186, 214, 221, 235, 247
AN13.8	Describe development of upper limb	296
AN14.1	Identify the given bone, its side, important features and keep it in anatomical position	707
AN14.2	Identify and describe joints formed by the given bone	707
AN14.3	Describe the importance of ossification of lower end of femur and upper end of tibia	722, 724
AN14.4	Identify and name various bones in the articulated foot with individual muscle attachment	718, 814, 815, 816
AN15.1	Describe and demonstrate origin, course, relations, branches (or tributaries), termination of important nerves and vessels of anterior thigh	728, 731, 736, 752, 755
AN15.2	Describe and demonstrate major muscles with their attachment, nerve supply and actions	746, 749
AN15.3	Describe and demonstrate boundaries, floor, roof and contents of femoral triangle	752
AN15.4	Explain anatomical basis of Psoas abscess and femoral hernia	759, 762
AN15.5	Describe and demonstrate adductor canal with its content	757
AN16.1	Describe and demonstrate origin, course, relations, branches (or tributaries), termination of important nerves and vessels of gluteal region	773, 776, 778
AN16.2	Describe anatomical basis of sciatic nerve injury during gluteal intramuscular injections	784
AN16.3	Explain the anatomical basis of Trendelenburg sign	767, 783
AN16.4	Describe and demonstrate the hamstrings group of muscles with their attachment, nerve supply and actions	764, 770
AN16.5	Describe and demonstrate the origin, course, relations, branches (or tributaries), termination of important nerves and vessels on the back of thigh	737, 775, 776, 778
AN16.6	Describe and demonstrate the boundaries, roof, floor, contents and relations of popliteal fossa	785
AN17.1	Describe and demonstrate the type, articular surfaces, capsule, synovial membrane, ligaments, relations, movements and muscles involved, blood and nerve supply, bursae around the hip joint	828
AN17.2	Describe anatomical basis of complications of fracture neck of femur	722, 861
AN17.3	Describe dislocation of hip joint and surgical hip replacement	862
AN18.1	Describe and demonstrate major muscles of anterolateral compartment of leg with their attachment, nerve supply and actions	790, 794
AN18.2	Describe and demonstrate origin, course, relations, branches (or tributaries), termination of important nerves and vessels of anterior compartment of leg	737, 792
AN18.3	Explain the anatomical basis of foot drop	807
AN18.4	Describe and demonstrate the type, articular surfaces, capsule, synovial membrane, ligaments, relations, movements and muscles involved, blood and nerve supply, bursae around the knee joint	836

Number	Competencies	Page/s
AN18.5	Explain the anatomical basis of locking and unlocking of the knee joint	844
AN18.6	Describe knee joint injuries with its applied anatomy	864
AN18.7	Explain anatomical basis of osteoarthritis	863
AN19.1	Describe and demonstrate the major muscles of back of leg with their attachment, nerve supply and actions	798, 802
AN19.2	Describe and demonstrate the origin, course, relations, branches (or tributaries), termination of important nerves and vessels of back of leg	728, 731, 804
AN19.3	Explain the concept of "peripheral heart"	731, 809
AN19.4	Explain the anatomical basis of rupture of calcaneal tendon	809
AN19.5	Describe factors maintaining importance arches of the foot with its importance	857
AN19.6	Explain the anatomical basis of flat foot and club foot	870
AN19.7	Explain the anatomical basis of metatarsalgia and plantar fasciitis	826
AN20.1	Describe and demonstrate the type, articular surfaces, capsule, synovial membrane, ligaments, relations, movements and muscles involved, blood and nerve supply of tibiofibular and ankle joint	845, 849
AN20.2	Describe the subtalar and transverse tarsal joints	852, 853
AN20.3	Describe and demonstrate fascia lata, venous drainage, lymphatic drainage, retinacula and dermatomes of lower limb	728, 731, 733, 734, 778, 779, 789, 798, 822
AN20.4	Explain anatomical basis of enlarged inguinal lymph nodes	742
AN20.5	Explain anatomical basis of varicose veins and deep vein thrombosis	741
AN20.6	Identify the bones and joints of lower limb seen in anteroposterior and lateral view radiographs of various regions of lower limb	709, 715, 723, 727, 830, 835, 837, 840, 849, 850, 853, 859
AN20.7	Identify and demonstrate important bony landmarks of lower limb: • Vertebral levels of highest point of iliac crest, posterior superior iliac spines, iliac tubercle, pubic tubercle, ischial tuberosity, adductor tubercle, • Tibial tuberosity, head of fibula, • Medial and lateral malleoli, condyles of femur and tibia, sustentaculum tali, tuberosity of fifth metatarsal, tuberosity of the navicular	713, 714, 715, 717, 720, 721, 779, 859
AN20.8	Identify and demonstrate palpation of femoral, popliteal, post tibial, anti tibial and dorsalis pedis blood vessels in a simulated environment	730, 761, 806, 810, 827
AN20.9	Identify and demonstrate palpation of vessels (femoral, popliteal, dorsalis pedis, post tibial), mid inguinal point, surface projection of: femoral nerve, saphenous opening, sciatic, tibial, common peroneal and deep peroneal nerve, great and small saphenous veins	728, 730, 758, 780, 782, 806, 810, 827
AN20.10	Describe basic concept of development of lower limb	705
AN21.1	Identify and describe the salient features of sternum, typical rib, 1st rib and typical thoracic vertebra	310
AN21.2	Identify and describe the features of 2nd, 11th and 12th ribs, 1st, 11th and 12th thoracic vertebrae	310
AN21.3	Describe and demonstrate the boundaries of thoracic inlet, cavity and outlet	314
AN21.4	Describe and demonstrate extent, attachments, direction of fibres, nerve supply and actions of intercostal muscles	324
AN21.5	Describe and demonstrate origin, course, relations and branches of a typical intercostal nerve	327
AN21.6	Mention origin, course and branches/tributaries of: 1) anterior and posterior intercostal vessels 2) internal thoracic vessels	330
AN21.7	Mention the origin, course, relations and branches of: 1) atypical intercostal nerve 2) superior intercostal artery, subcostal artery	330
AN21.8	Describe and demonstrate type, articular surfaces and movements of manubriosternal, costovertebral, costotransverse and xiphisternal joints	315
AN21.9	Describe and demonstrate mechanics and types of respiration	317
AN21.10	Describe costochondral and interchondral joints	315
AN21.11	Mention boundaries and contents of the superior, anterior, middle and posterior mediastinum	367
AN22.1	Describe and demonstrate subdivisions, sinuses in pericardium, blood supply and nerve supply of pericardium	367
AN22.2	Describe and demonstrate external and internal features of each chamber of heart	375
AN22.3	Describe and demonstrate origin, course and branches of coronary arteries	384
AN22.4	Describe anatomical basis of ischaemic heart disease	396
AN22.5	Describe and demonstrate the formation, course, tributaries and termination of coronary sinus	388
AN22.6	Describe the fibrous skeleton of heart	376
AN22.7	Mention the parts, position and arterial supply of the conducting system of heart	389
AN23.1	Describe and demonstrate the external appearance, relations, blood supply, nerve supply, lymphatic drainage and applied anatomy of oesophagus	410, 477, 502
AN23.2	Describe and demonstrate the extent, relations tributaries of thoracic duct and enumerate its applied anatomy	411, 419
AN23.3	Describe and demonstrate origin, course, relations, tributaries and termination of superior venacava, azygos, hemiazygos and accessory hemiazygos veins	403, 413
AN23.4	Mention the extent, branches and relations of arch of aorta and descending thoracic aorta	403, 408
AN23.5	Identify and mention the location and extent of thoracic sympathetic chain	414
AN23.6	Describe the splanchnic nerves	414, 553
AN23.7	Mention the extent, relations and applied anatomy of lymphatic duct	411
AN24.1	Mention the blood supply, lymphatic drainage and nerve supply of pleura, extent of pleura and describe the pleural recesses and their applied anatomy	344, 353, 355, 358
AN24.2	Identify side, external features and relations of structures which form root of lung and bronchial tree and their clinical correlate	348, 350
AN24.3	Describe a bronchopulmonary segment	352
AN24.4	Identify phrenic nerve and describe its formation and distribution	406
AN24.5	Mention the blood supply, lymphatic drainage and nerve supply of lungs	353, 355
AN24.6	Describe the extent, length, relations, blood supply, lymphatic drainage and nerve supply of trachea	406
AN25.1	Identify, draw and label a slide of trachea and lung	356
AN25.2	Describe development of pleura, lung and heart	358, 391
AN25.3	Describe fetal circulation and changes occurring at birth	417

Number	Competencies	Page/s
AN25.4	Describe embryological basis of: 1) atrial septal defect, 2) ventricular septal defect, 3) Fallot's tetralogy and 4) tracheo-oesophageal fistula	391, 1114
AN25.5	Describe developmental basis of congenital anomalies, transposition of great vessels, dextrocardia, patent ductus arteriosus and coarctation of aorta	417
AN25.6	Mention development of aortic arch arteries, SVC, IVC and coronary sinus	417
AN25.8	Identify and describe in brief a barium swallow	410, 478
AN25.9	Demonstrate surface marking of lines of pleural reflection, lung borders and fissures, trachea, heart borders, apex beat and surface projection of valves of heart	344, 356, 414
AN26.1	Demonstrate anatomical position of skull, identify and locate individual skull bones in skull	879
AN26.2	Describe the features of norma frontalis, verticalis, occipitalis, lateralis and basalis	882, 886, 887
AN26.3	Describe cranial cavity, its subdivisions, foramina and structures passing through them	890
AN26.4	Describe morphological features of mandible	885
AN26.5	Describe features of typical and atypical cervical vertebrae (atlas and axis)	78, 1047, 1049
AN26.6	Explain the concept of bones that ossify in membrane	879, 896
AN26.7	Describe the features of the 7th cervical vertebra	80, 1049
AN27.1	Describe the layers of scalp, its blood supply, its nerve supply and surgical importance	900, 906, 912, 915, 917, 921
AN27.2	Describe emissary veins with its role in spread of infection from extracranial route to intracranial venous sinuses	917, 926
AN28.1	Describe and demonstrate muscles of facial expression and their nerve supply	901, 910
AN28.2	Describe sensory innervation of face	906
AN28.3	Describe and demonstrate origin/formation, course, branches/tributaries of facial vessels	912
AN28.4	Describe and demonstrate branches of facial nerve with distribution	910, 1138
AN28.5	Describe cervical lymph nodes and lymphatic drainage of head, face and neck	915
AN28.6	Identify superficial muscles of face, their nerve supply and actions	901, 910
AN28.7	Explain the anatomical basis of facial nerve palsy	918, 920, 1154
AN28.8	Explain surgical importance of deep facial vein	915, 932
AN28.9	Describe and demonstrate the parts, borders, surfaces, contents, relations and nerve supply of parotid gland with course of its duct and surgical importance	973, 974, 985
AN28.10	Explain the anatomical basis of Frey's syndrome	985
AN29.1	Describe and demonstrate attachments, nerve supply, relations and actions of sternocleidomastoid	1054, 1056
AN29.2	Explain anatomical basis of Erb's and Klumpke's palsy	210
AN29.3	Explain anatomical basis of wry neck	1072
AN29.4	Describe and demonstrate attachments of 1) inferior belly of omohyoid, 2) scalenus anterior, 3) scalenus medius and 4) levator scapulae	1067, 1077, 1078
AN30.1	Describe the cranial fossae and identify related structures	890
AN30.2	Describe and identify major foramina with structures passing through them	890
AN30.3	Describe and identify dural folds and dural venous sinuses	922, 924
AN30.4	Describe clinical importance of dural venous sinuses	933
AN30.5	Explain effect of pituitary tumours on visual pathway	1152
AN31.1	Describe and identify extra ocular muscles of eyeball	955
AN31.2	Describe and demonstrate nerves and vessels in the orbit	962, 963, 1129, 1132, 1135
AN31.3	Describe anatomical basis of Horner's syndrome	971, 1082
AN31.4	Enumerate components of lacrimal apparatus	949
AN31.5	Explain the anatomical basis of oculomotor, trochlear and abducent nerve palsies along with strabismus	972, 1152, 1153, 1154
AN32.1	Describe boundaries and subdivisions of anterior triangle	1055
AN32.2	Describe and demonstrate boundaries and contents of muscular, carotid, digastric and submental triangles	1055, 1064
AN33.1	Describe and demonstrate extent, boundaries and contents of temporal and infratemporal fossae	975
AN33.2	Describe and demonstrate attachments, direction of fibres, nerve supply and actions of muscles of mastication	980
AN33.3	Describe and demonstrate articulating surface, type and movements of temporomandibular joint	975
AN33.4	Explain the clinical significance of pterygoid venous plexus	926, 932, 980
AN33.5	Describe the features of dislocation of temporomandibular joint	986
AN34.1	Describe and demonstrate the morphology, relations and nerve supply of submandibular salivary gland and submandibular ganglion	1004, 1005, 1127
AN34.2	Describe the basis of formation of submandibular stones	1010
AN35.1	Describe the parts, extent, attachments, modifications of deep cervical fascia	1052
AN35.2	Describe and demonstrate location, parts, borders, surfaces, relations and blood supply of thyroid gland	1083
AN35.3	Demonstrate and describe the origin, parts, course and branches subclavian artery	1079
AN35.4	Describe and demonstrate origin, course, relations, tributaries and termination of internal jugular and brachiocephalic veins	403, 1060, 1069
AN35.5	Describe and demonstrate extent, drainage and applied anatomy of cervical lymph nodes	1062, 1105
AN35.6	Describe and demonstrate the extent, formation, relation and branches of cervical sympathetic chain	1082
AN35.7	Describe the course and branches of IX, X, XI and XII nerve in the neck	1060, 1070, 1080, 1142, 1143, 1146, 1148
AN35.8	Describe the anatomically relevant clinical features of thyroid swellings	1108
AN35.9	Describe the clinical features of compression of subclavian artery and lower trunk of brachial plexus by cervical rib	320, 321
AN35.10	Describe the fascial spaces of neck	1052
AN36.1	Describe the 1) morphology, relations, blood supply and applied anatomy of palatine tonsil 2) composition of soft palate	993, 1100
AN36.2	Describe the components and functions of Waldeyer's lymphatic ring	1103
AN36.3	Describe the boundaries and clinical significance of pyriform fossa	1101, 1113
AN36.4	Describe the anatomical basis of tonsillitis, tonsillectomy, adenoids and peri-tonsillar abscess	1113

Number	Competencies	Page/s
AN37.1	Describe and demonstrate features of nasal septum, lateral wall of nose, their blood supply and nerve supply	1015, 1016, 1019
AN37.2	Describe location and functional anatomy of paranasal sinuses	1020
AN37.3	Describe anatomical basis of sinusitis and maxillary sinus tumours	1024
AN38.1	Describe the morphology, identify structure of the wall, nerve supply, blood supply and actions of intrinsic and extrinsic muscles of the larynx	1087
AN38.3	Describe anatomical basis of recurrent laryngeal nerve injury	1109
AN39.1	Describe and demonstrate the morphology, nerve supply, embryological basis of nerve supply, blood supply, lymphatic drainage and actions of extrinsic and intrinsic muscles of tongue	997, 999, 1000
AN39.2	Explain the anatomical basis of hypoglossal nerve palsy	1009, 1156
AN40.1	Describe and identify the parts, blood supply and nerve supply of external ear	1026
AN40.2	Describe and demonstrate the boundaries, contents, relations and functional anatomy of middle ear and auditory tube	1027, 1030
AN40.3	Describe the features of internal ear	1033
AN40.4	Explain anatomical basis of otitis externa and otitis media	1038
AN40.5	Explain anatomical basis of myringotomy	1039
AN41.1	Describe and demonstrate parts and layers of eyeball	951
AN41.2	Describe the anatomical aspects of cataract, glaucoma and central retinal artery occlusion	970, 971, 972
AN41.3	Describe the position, nerve supply and actions of intraocular muscles	953
AN42.1	Describe the contents of the vertebral canal	130
AN42.2	Describe and demonstrate the boundaries and contents of suboccipital triangle	127
AN42.3	Describe the position, direction of fibres, relations, nerve supply, actions of semispinalis capitis and splenius capitis	120, 121, 123
AN43.1	Describe and demonstrate the movements with muscles producing the movements of atlantooccipital joint and atlantoaxial joint	128
AN43.2	Identify, describe and draw the microanatomy of pituitary gland, thyroid, parathyroid gland, tongue, salivary glands, tonsil, epiglottis, cornea, retina	951, 955, 975, 1002, 1005, 1006, 1085, 1086
AN43.3	Identify, describe and draw microanatomy of olfactory epithelium, eyelid, lip, sclero-corneal junction, optic nerve, cochlea- organ of corti, pineal gland	948, 951, 1016, 1037
AN43.4	Describe the development and developmental basis of congenital anomalies of face, palate, tongue, branchial apparatus, pituitary gland, thyroid gland and eye	917, 968, 996, 1002, 1009, 1107, 1113
AN43.5	Demonstrate- 1) Testing of muscles of facial expression, extraocular muscles, muscles of mastication, 2) Palpation of carotid arteries, facial artery, superficial temporal artery, 3) Location of internal and external jugular veins, 4) Location of hyoid bone, thyroid cartilage and cricoid cartilage with their vertebral levels	905, 920, 962, 1072, 1075, 1076, 1104
AN43.6	Demonstrate surface projection of- Thyroid gland, parotid gland and duct, pterion, common carotid artery, internal jugular vein, subclavian vein, external jugular vein, facial artery in the face and accessory nerve	913, 886, 1070, 1104
AN43.7	Identify the anatomical structures in 1) Plain x-ray skull, 2) AP view and lateral view 3) Plain x-ray cervical spine-AP and lateral view 4) Plain x- ray of paranasal sinuses	884, 1018, 1021, 1048

Number	Competencies	Page/s
AN43.8	Describe the anatomical route used for carotid angiogram and vertebral angiogram	941
AN43.9	Identify anatomical structures in carotid angiogram and vertebral angiogram	941
AN44.1	Describe and demonstrate the planes (transpyloric, transtubercular, subcostal, lateral vertical, linea alba, linea semilunaris), regions and quadrants of abdomen	432
AN44.2	Describe and identify the fascia, nerves and blood vessels of anterior abdominal wall	434, 441, 443
AN44.3	Describe the formation of rectus sheath and its contents	440
AN44.4	Describe and demonstrate extent, boundaries, contents of inguinal canal including Hesselbach's triangle	451
AN44.5	Explain the anatomical basis of inguinal hernia	453, 460
AN44.6	Describe and demonstrate attachments of muscles of anterior abdominal wall	435
AN44.7	Enumerate common abdominal incisions	446
AN45.1	Describe thoracolumbar fascia	563
AN45.2	Describe and demonstrate lumbar plexus for its root value, formation and branches	566
AN45.3	Mention the major subgroups of back muscles, nerve supply and action	565
AN46.1	Describe and demonstrate coverings, internal structure, side determination, blood supply, nerve supply, lymphatic drainage and descent of testis with its applied anatomy	453, 457, 459, 460
AN46.2	Describe parts of epididymis	458
AN46.3	Describe penis under following headings: (parts, components, blood supply and lymphatic drainage)	678
AN46.4	Explain the anatomical basis of varicocoele	463
AN46.5	Explain the anatomical basis of phimosis and circumcision	685
AN47.1	Describe and identify boundaries and recesses of lesser and greater sac	469
AN47.2	Name and identify various peritoneal folds and pouches with its explanation	467
AN47.3	Explain anatomical basis of ascites and peritonitis	471
AN47.4	Explain anatomical basis of subphrenic abscess	533
AN47.5	Describe and demonstrate major viscera of abdomen under following headings (anatomical position, external and internal features, important peritoneal and other relations, blood supply, nerve supply, lymphatic drainage and applied aspects)	478, 487, 491, 494, 503, 506, 507, 509, 513, 514, 517, 527, 531, 532, 533, 536, 542, 543, 545, 549, 550, 551
AN47.6	Explain the anatomical basis of splenic notch, accessory spleens, Kehr's sign, different types of vagotomy, liver biopsy (site of needle puncture), referred pain in cholecystitis, obstructive jaundice, referred pain around umbilicus, radiating pain of kidney to groin and lymphatic spread in carcinoma stomach	505, 506, 531, 536, 538, 551, 552
AN47.7	Mention the clinical importance of Calot's triangle	538
AN47.8	Describe and identify the formation, course relations and tributaries of portal vein, Inferior vena cava and renal vein	529, 546, 569
AN47.9	Describe and identify the origin, course, important relations and branches of abdominal aorta, coeliac trunk, superior mesenteric, inferior mesenteric and common iliac artery	484, 500, 567
AN47.10	Enumerate the sites of portosystemic anastomosis	530

Number	Competencies	Page/s
AN47.11	Explain the anatomic basis of hematemesisand caput medusae in portal hypertension	502, 538
AN47.12	Describe important nerve plexuses of posterior abdominal wall	553, 566
AN47.13	Describe and demonstrate the attachments, openings, nerve supply and action of the thoracoabdominal diaphragm	559
AN47.14	Describe the abnormal openings of thoracoabdominal diaphragm and diaphragmatic hernia	503, 571
AN48.1	Describe and identify the muscles of pelvic diaphragm	597
AN48.2	Describe and demonstrate the (position, features, important peritoneal and other relations, blood supply, nerve supply, lymphatic drainage and clinical aspects of) important male and female pelvic viscera	621, 622, 626, 631, 633, 636, 639, 640, 642, 646, 650, 654, 670, 675
AN48.3	Describe and demonstrate the origin, course, important relations and branches of internal iliac artery	607
AN48.4	Describe the branches of sacral plexus	615
AN48.5	Explain the anatomical basis of suprapubic cystostomy, urinary obstruction in benign prostatic hypertrophy, retroverted uterus, prolapse uterus, internal and external haemorrhoids, anal fistula, vasectomy, tubal pregnancy and tubal ligation	632, 639, 649, 650, 673, 676
AN48.6	Describe the neurological basis of automatic bladder	626
AN48.7	Mention the lobes involved in benign prostatic hypertrophy and prostatic cancer	639
AN48.8	Mention the structures palpable during vaginal and rectal examination	633, 652, 654
AN49.1	Describe and demonstrate the superficial and deep perineal pouch (boundaries and contents)	666
AN49.2	Describe and identify perineal body	664
AN49.3	Describe and demonstrate perineal membrane in male and female	663
AN49.4	Describe and demonstrate boundaries, content and applied anatomy of ischiorectal fossa	668
AN49.5	Explain the anatomical basis of perineal tear, episiotomy, perianal abscess and anal fissure	673, 675
AN50.1	Describe the curvatures of the vertebral column	104
AN50.2	Describe and demonstrate the type, articular ends, ligaments and movements of intervertebral joints, sacroiliac joints and pubic symphysis	97, 589, 591
AN50.3	Describe lumbar puncture (site, direction of the needle, structures pierced during the lumbar puncture)	140
AN50.4	Explain the anatomical basis of scoliosis, lordosis, prolapsed disc, spondylolisthesis and spina bifida	96, 112, 115
AN51.1	Describe and identify the cross-section at the level of T8, T10 and L1 (transpyloric plane)	577
AN51.2	Describe and identify the midsagittal section of male and female pelvis	623
AN52.1	Describe and identify the microanatomical features of gastro-intestinal system: Oesophagus, fundus of stomach, pylorus of stomach, duodenum, jejunum, ileum, large intestine, appendix, liver, gall bladder, pancreas and suprarenal gland	478, 482, 491, 494, 495, 502, 517, 527, 529, 545
AN52.2	Describe and identify the microanatomical features of: Urinary system: kidney, ureter and urinary bladder Male reproductive system: Testis, epididymis,vas deferens, prostate and penis Female reproductive system: Ovary, uterus, uterine tube, cervix, placenta and umbilical cord	458, 545, 622, 626, 635, 638, 642, 643, 646, 681
AN52.3	Describe and identify the microanatomical features of cardiooesophageal junction, corpus luteum	478, 642

Number	Competencies	Page/s
AN52.4	Describe the development of anterior abdominal wall	441
AN52.5	Describe the development and congenital anomalies of diaphragm	563
AN52.6	Describe the development and congenital anomalies of: Foregut, midgut and hindgut	478, 482, 491, 494, 495, 502, 507, 517, 527, 529, 629, 672
AN52.7	Describe the development of urinary system	545, 550, 621, 626, 677
AN52.8	Describe the development of male and female reproductive system	458, 635, 638, 640, 642, 643, 646, 681, 687
AN53.1	Identify and hold the bone in the anatomical position, describe the salient features, articulations and demonstrate the attachments of muscle groups	86, 585, 587
AN53.2	Demonstrate the anatomical position of bony pelvis and show boundaries of pelvic inlet, pelvic cavity, pelvic outlet	585
AN53.3	Define true pelvis and false pelvis and demonstrate sex determination in male and female bony pelvis	587, 588
AN53.4	Explain and demonstrate clinical importance of bones of abdominopelvic region (sacralization of lumbar vertebra, lumbarization of 1st sacral vertebra, types of bony pelvis and coccyx)	95, 592
AN54.1	Describe and identify features of plain X-ray abdomen	575
AN54.2	Describe and identify the special radiographs of abdominopelvic region (contrast X-ray barium swallow, barium meal, barium enema, cholecystography, intravenous pyelography and hysterosalpingography)	478, 481, 496, 545, 551, 649
AN54.3	Describe role of ERCP, CT abdomen, MRI, arteriography in radiodiagnosis of abdomen	493, 499, 515, 516, 518, 521, 530, 532, 550, 696
AN55.1	Demonstrate the surface marking of; regions and planes of abdomen, superficial inguinal ring, deep inguinal ring, McBurney's point, renal angle and Murphy's point	460, 509, 538
AN55.2	Demonstrate the surface projections of: Stomach, liver, fundus of gall bladder, spleen, duodenum, pancreas, ileocaecal junction, kidneys and root of mesentery	479, 491, 513, 518, 543
AN56.1	Describe and identify various layers of meninges with its extent and modifications	922
AN56.2	Describe circulation of CSF with its applied anatomy	938, 943
AN58.3	Enumerate cranial nerve nuclei in medulla oblongata with their functional group	1121
AN59.3	Enumerate cranial nerve nuclei in pons with their functional group	1121
AN62.1	Enumerate cranial nerve nuclei with its functional component	1124
AN62.6	Describe and identify formation, branches and major areas of distribution of circle of Willis	940
AN63.1	Describe and demonstrate parts, boundaries and features of IIIrd, IVth and lateral ventricle	935
AN63.2	Describe anatomical basis of congenital hydrocephalus	943
AN70.2	Identify the lymphoid tissue under the microscope and describe microanatomy of lymph node, spleen, thymus, tonsil and correlate the structure with function	514

Notes

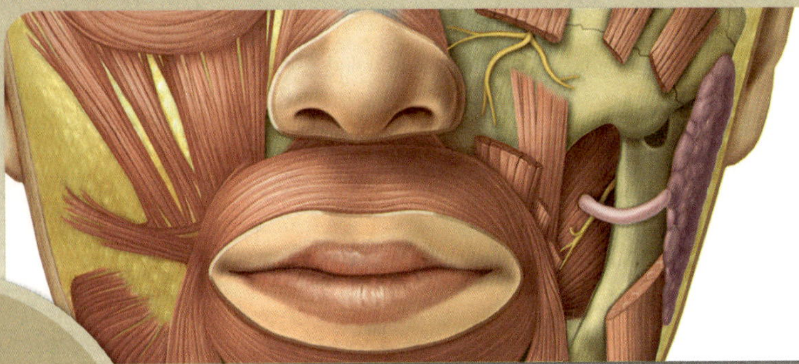

Head

8

OVERVIEW OF HEAD / 879

CRANIUM / 879

Facial Aspect of Cranium / 882

TABLE 8.1. Craniometric Points of Cranium / 885

Lateral Aspect of Cranium / 886

Occipital Aspect of Cranium / 886

Superior Aspect of Cranium / 887

External Surface of Cranial Base / 887

Internal Surface of Cranial Base / 890

TABLE 8.2. Foramina and Other Apertures of Cranial Fossae and Contents / 891

Walls of Cranial Cavity / 893

Regions of Head / 894

CLINICAL BOX: **Cranium** / 894

FACE AND SCALP / 900

Face / 900

Scalp / 900

Muscles of Face and Scalp / 901

TABLE 8.3. Muscles of Scalp and Face / 902

Nerves of Face and Scalp / 906

TABLE 8.4. Cutaneous Nerves of Face and Scalp / 908

Superficial Vasculature of Face and Scalp / 912

TABLE 8.5. Superficial Arteries of Face and Scalp / 913

TABLE 8.6. Veins of Face and Scalp / 914

Surface Anatomy of Face / 915

CLINICAL BOX: **Face and Scalp** / 917

CRANIAL MENINGES / 922

Dura Mater / 922

Arachnoid Mater and Pia Mater / 929

Meningeal Spaces / 929

CLINICAL BOX: **Cranial Cavity and Meninges** / 931

BRAIN / 935

Parts of Brain / 935

Ventricular System of Brain / 935

Arterial Blood Supply to Brain / 939

Venous Drainage of Brain / 940

TABLE 8.7. Arterial Blood Supply of Cerebral Hemispheres / 942

CLINICAL BOX: **Brain** / 942

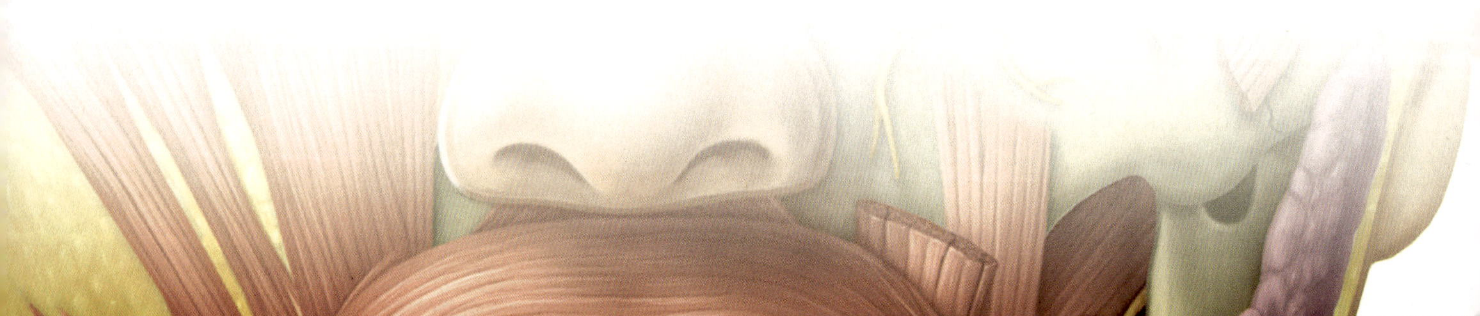

CLINICAL BOX KEY

Anatomical Variations | Diagnostic Procedures | Life Cycle | Surgical Procedures | Trauma | Pathology

EYE, ORBIT, ORBITAL REGION, AND EYEBALL / 946
Orbits / 946
Eyelids and Lacrimal Apparatus / 948
Eyeball / 951
Extra-Ocular Muscles of Orbit / 955
TABLE 8.8. Extra-Ocular Muscles of Orbit / 957
Nerves of Orbit / 962
Vasculature of Orbit / 963
TABLE 8.9. Arteries of Orbit / 965
Surface Anatomy of Eye and Lacrimal Apparatus / 965
CLINICAL BOX: **Orbital Region, Orbit, and Eyeball** / 968
PAROTID AND TEMPORAL REGIONS, INFRATEMPORAL FOSSA, AND TEMPOROMANDIBULAR JOINT / 973
Parotid Region / 973
Temporal Region / 975
Infratemporal Fossa / 975
TABLE 8.10. Movements of Temporomandibular Joint / 979
TABLE 8.11. Muscles Acting on Mandible/Temporomandibular Joint / 982
TABLE 8.12. Parts and Branches of Maxillary Artery / 983
CLINICAL BOX: **Parotid and Temporal Regions, Infratemporal Fossa, and Temporomandibular Joint** / 985
ORAL REGION / 987
Oral Cavity / 987
Lips, Cheeks, and Gingivae / 987
Teeth / 989
TABLE 8.13A. Deciduous Teeth / 992
TABLE 8.13B. Permanent Teeth / 992
Palate / 993
TABLE 8.14. Muscles of Soft Palate / 997
Tongue / 997
TABLE 8.15. Muscles of Tongue / 1001
Salivary Glands / 1002
CLINICAL BOX: **Oral Region** / 1006
PTERYGOPALATINE FOSSA / 1011
Pterygopalatine Part of Maxillary Artery / 1011
Maxillary Nerve / 1011
CLINICAL BOX: **Pterygopalatine Fossa** / 1014
NOSE / 1015
External Nose / 1015
Nasal Cavities / 1016
Vasculature and Innervation of Nose / 1019
Paranasal Sinuses / 1020
CLINICAL BOX: **The Nose** / 1023
EAR / 1026
External Ear / 1026
Middle Ear / 1027
Internal Ear / 1033
CLINICAL BOX: **Ear** / 1038
Multiple-Choice Questions / 1042

Competencies Covered in the Chapter

AN26.1 Demonstrate anatomical position of skull, and identify and locate individual skull bones in skull / 879
AN26.2 Describe the features of norma basalis / 887
AN26.2 Describe the features of norma frontalis / 882
AN26.2 Describe the features of norma lateralis / 886
AN26.2 Describe the features of norma occipitalis / 886
AN26.2 Describe the features of norma verticalis / 887
AN26.3 Describe cranial cavity, its subdivisions, foramina, and structures passing through them / 890
AN26.4 Describe morphological features of mandible / 885
AN26.6 Explain the concept of bones that ossify in membrane / 879, 896
AN27.1 Describe the arterial supply of scalp / 912
AN27.1 Describe the layers of scalp / 900
AN27.1 Describe the nerve supply of scalp / 906
AN27.1 Describe the surgical importance of scalp / 917, 921
AN27.1 Describe the veins of scalp / 915
AN27.2 Describe emissary veins with its role in spread of infection from extracranial route to intracranial venous sinuses / 917, 926
AN28.1 Describe and demonstrate muscles of facial expression and their nerve supply / 901, 910
AN28.2 Describe sensory innervation of face / 906
AN28.3 Describe and demonstrate formation, course and tributaries of facial veins / 912
AN28.3 Describe and demonstrate origin, course, branches of facial artery / 912
AN28.4 Describe and demonstrate branches of facial nerve with distribution / 910
AN28.5 Describe lymphatic drainage of head and face / 915
AN28.6 Identify superficial muscles of face, their nerve supply, and actions / 901, 910
AN28.7 Explain the anatomical basis of facial nerve palsy / 918, 920
AN28.8 Explain surgical importance of deep facial vein / 915, 932
AN28.9 Describe and demonstrate the parts, borders, surfaces, contents, and relations of parotid gland with course of its duct / 973
AN28.9 Describe the nerve supply of parotid gland / 974

AN28.9 Surgical significance of parotid gland and duct / 985
AN28.10 Explain the anatomical basis of Frey's syndrome / 985
AN30.1 Describe the cranial fossae and identify related structures / 890
AN30.2 Describe and identify major foramina with structures passing through them / 890
AN30.3 Describe and identify dural folds / 922
AN30.3 Describe and identify dural venous sinuses / 924
AN30.4 Describe clinical importance of dural venous sinuses / 933
AN31.1 Describe and identify extraocular muscles of eyeball / 955
AN31.2 Describe and demonstrate nerves in the orbit / 962
AN31.2 Describe and demonstrate vessels in the orbit / 963
AN31.3 Describe the anatomical basis of Horner's syndrome / 971
AN31.4 Enumerate the components of lacrimal apparatus / 949
AN31.5 Explain the anatomical basis of oculomotor, trochlear and abducent nerve palsies along with strabismus / 972
AN33.1 Describe and demonstrate extent, boundaries and contents of infratemporal fossa / 975
AN33.1 Describe and demonstrate extent, boundaries and contents of temporal fossa / 975
AN33.2 Describe and demonstrate attachments, direction of fibres, nerve supply and actions of muscles of mastication / 980
AN33.3 Describe and demonstrate articulating surface, type and movements of temporomandibular joint / 975
AN33.4 Explain the clinical significance of pterygoid venous plexus / 926, 932, 980
AN33.5 Describe the features of dislocation of temporomandibular joint / 986
AN34.1 Describe and demonstrate the morphology, relations and nerve supply of submandibular salivary gland / 1004
AN34.1 Describe submandibular ganglion / 1005
AN34.2 Describe the basis of formation of submandibular stones / 1010
AN36.1 Describe the composition of soft palate / 993
AN37.1 Describe and demonstrate blood supply and nerve supply of nasal septum and lateral wall of nose / 1019
AN37.1 Describe and demonstrate features of lateral wall of nose / 1016
AN37.1 Describe and demonstrate features of nasal septum / 1015
AN37.2 Describe location and functional anatomy of paranasal sinuses / 1020
AN37.3 Describe anatomical basis of sinusitis / 1024
AN39.1 Describe and demonstrate actions of extrinsic and intrinsic muscles of tongue / 999
AN39.1 Describe and demonstrate the morphology of tongue / 997
AN39.1 Describe the blood supply and lymphatic drainage of tongue / 1000
AN39.1 Describe the nerve supply and the embryological basis of nerve supply of tongue / 1000
AN39.2 Explain the anatomical basis of hypoglossal nerve palsy / 1009
AN40.1 Describe and identify the parts, blood supply and nerve supply of external ear / 1026
AN40.2 Describe and demonstrate the boundaries, contents, relations and functional anatomy of middle ear / 1027
AN40.2 Describe auditory tube / 1030
AN40.3 Describe the features of internal ear / 1033
AN40.4 Explain anatomical basis of otitis externa / 1038
AN40.4 Explain anatomical basis of otitis media / 1038
AN40.5 Explain anatomical basis of myringotomy / 1039
AN41.1 Describe and demonstrate parts and layers of eyeball / 951
AN41.2 Describe the anatomical aspects of cataract / 970
AN41.2 Describe the anatomical aspects of central retinal artery occlusion / 972
AN41.2 Describe the anatomical aspects of glaucoma / 971
AN41.3 Describe the position, nerve supply, and actions of intraocular muscles of eyeball / 953
AN43.2 & AN43.3 Identify, describe, and draw the microanatomy of cornea and sclerocorneal junction / 951
AN43.2 Identify, describe, and draw the microanatomy of mixed salivary glands / 1005
AN43.2 Identify, describe, and draw the microanatomy of mucous salivary glands / 1006
AN43.2 Identify, describe, and draw the microanatomy of retina / 955
AN43.2 Identify, describe, and draw the microanatomy of tongue / 1002
AN43.2 Identify, describe and draw the microanatomy of serous salivary gland / 975
AN43.3 Identify, describe, and draw microanatomy of olfactory epithelium / 1016
AN43.3 Identify, describe, and draw microantomy of cochlea-organ of corti / 1037
AN43.3 Identify, describe, and draw microantomy of eyelid, cochlea / 948
AN43.4 Describe the development and developmental anomalies of face / 917
AN43.4 Describe development and developmental basis of congenital anomalies of eye / 968
AN43.4 Describe development and developmental basis of congenital anomalies of palate / 996, 1009
AN43.4 Describe development and developmental basis of congenital anomalies of tongue / 1002
AN43.5 Demonstrate palpation of facial artery and superficial temporal artery / 920

AN43.5 Demonstrate testing of extraocular muscles / 962
AN43.5 Demonstrate testing of muscles of facial expression / 905
AN43.6 Demonstrate surface projection of facial artery in face / 913
AN43.6 Demonstrate surface projection of pterion / 886
AN43.7 Identify anatomical structures in plain X-ray of paranasal sinuses / 1018, 1021
AN43.7 Identify the anatomical structures in plain X-ray skull—lateral view / 884
AN43.8 Describe the anatomical route used for carotid angiogram / 941
AN43.9 Identify anatomical structures in carotid angiogram / 941
AN56.1 Describe and identify various layers of meninges with its extent and modifications / 922
AN56.2 Describe circulation of CSF with its applied anatomy / 938
AN56.2 Describe the applied anatomy of CSF / 943
AN62.6 Describe and identify formation, branches, and major areas of distribution of circle of Willis / 940
AN63.1 Describe and demonstrate parts, boundaries, and features of IIIrd, IVth, and lateral ventricles / 935
AN63.2 Describe anatomical basis of congenital hydrocephalus / 943

OVERVIEW OF HEAD

The **head** is the superior part of the body that is attached to the trunk by the neck. It is the control and communications center as well as the "loading dock" for the body. The head houses the brain; therefore, it is the site of our consciousness: ideas, creativity, imagination, responses, decision making, and memory. The head also includes special sensory receivers (eyes, ears, mouth, and nose), broadcast devices for voice and expression, and portals for the intake of fuel (food), water, and oxygen and the exhaust of carbon dioxide.

The head consists of the *brain* and its protective coverings (cranial vault and meninges), the *ears*, and the *face*. The face includes openings and passageways, with lubricating glands and valves (seals) to close some of them, the masticatory (chewing) devices, and the orbits that house the visual apparatus. The face also provides our identity as individuals. Disease, malformation, and trauma of structures in the head form the bases of many specialties, including dentistry, maxillofacial surgery, neurology, neuroradiology, neurosurgery, ophthalmology, oral surgery, otology, rhinology, and psychiatry.

CRANIUM

AN26.1 The **cranium** (skull[1]) is the skeleton of the head (Fig. 8.1A). It is composed of 22 named bones. A series of bones form its two parts, the neurocranium and viscerocranium (Fig. 8.1B). The **neurocranium** is the bony case of the brain and its membranous coverings, the cranial meninges. It also contains proximal parts of the cranial nerves and the vasculature of the brain. The neurocranium in adults is formed by a series of eight bones: four singular bones centered on the midline (*frontal*, *ethmoidal*, *sphenoidal*, and *occipital*), and two sets of bones occurring as bilateral pairs (*temporal* and *parietal*) (Figs. 8.1A, 8.2A, and 8.3).

The *neurocranium* has a dome-like roof, the **calvaria** (skullcap), and a floor or **cranial base** (**basicranium**). AN26.(The bones forming the *calvaria* are primarily flat bones (frontal, parietal, and occipital; see Fig. 8.8A) formed by intramembranous ossification of head mesenchyme from the neural crest. The bones contributing to the *cranial base* are primarily irregular bones with substantial flat portions (sphenoidal and temporal) formed by endochondral ossification of cartilage (*chondrocranium*) or from more than one type of ossification. The *ethmoid bone* is an irregular bone that makes a relatively minor midline contribution to the neurocranium but is primarily part of the viscerocranium (see Fig. 8.7A). The so-called flat bones and flat portions of the bones forming the neurocranium are actually curved, with convex external and concave internal surfaces.

Most calvarial bones are united by fibrous interlocking **sutures** (Fig. 8.1A, B; also see Chapter 1, Overview and Basic Concepts); however, during childhood, some bones (sphenoid and occipital) are united by hyaline cartilage (*synchondroses*—cartilaginous joints). The spinal cord is continuous with the brain through the *foramen magnum*, a large opening in the cranial base (Fig. 8.1C).

The **viscerocranium** (*facial skeleton*) comprises the facial bones that mainly develop in the mesenchyme of the embryonic pharyngeal arches (Moore et al., 2016). The viscerocranium forms the anterior part of the cranium, and it consists of the bones surrounding the mouth (upper and lower jaws), nose/nasal cavity, and most of the *orbits* (eye sockets or orbital cavities) (Figs. 8.2 and 8.3).

The *viscerocranium* consists of 15 irregular bones: 3 singular bones centered on or lying in the midline (*mandible*, *ethmoid*, and *vomer*), and 6 bones occurring as bilateral pairs (*maxillae; inferior nasal conchae*; and *zygomatic*, *palatine*, *nasal*, and *lacrimal bones*) (Figs. 8.1A and 8.4A). The maxillae and mandible house the teeth, that is, they provide the

(*continued on p.* 882)

[1]There is confusion about exactly what the term skull means. It may mean the cranium (which includes the mandible) or the part of the cranium excluding the mandible. There has also been confusion because some people have used the term cranium for only the neurocranium. The Federative International Committee on Anatomical Terminology (FICAT) has decided to follow the Latin term cranium for the skeleton of the head.

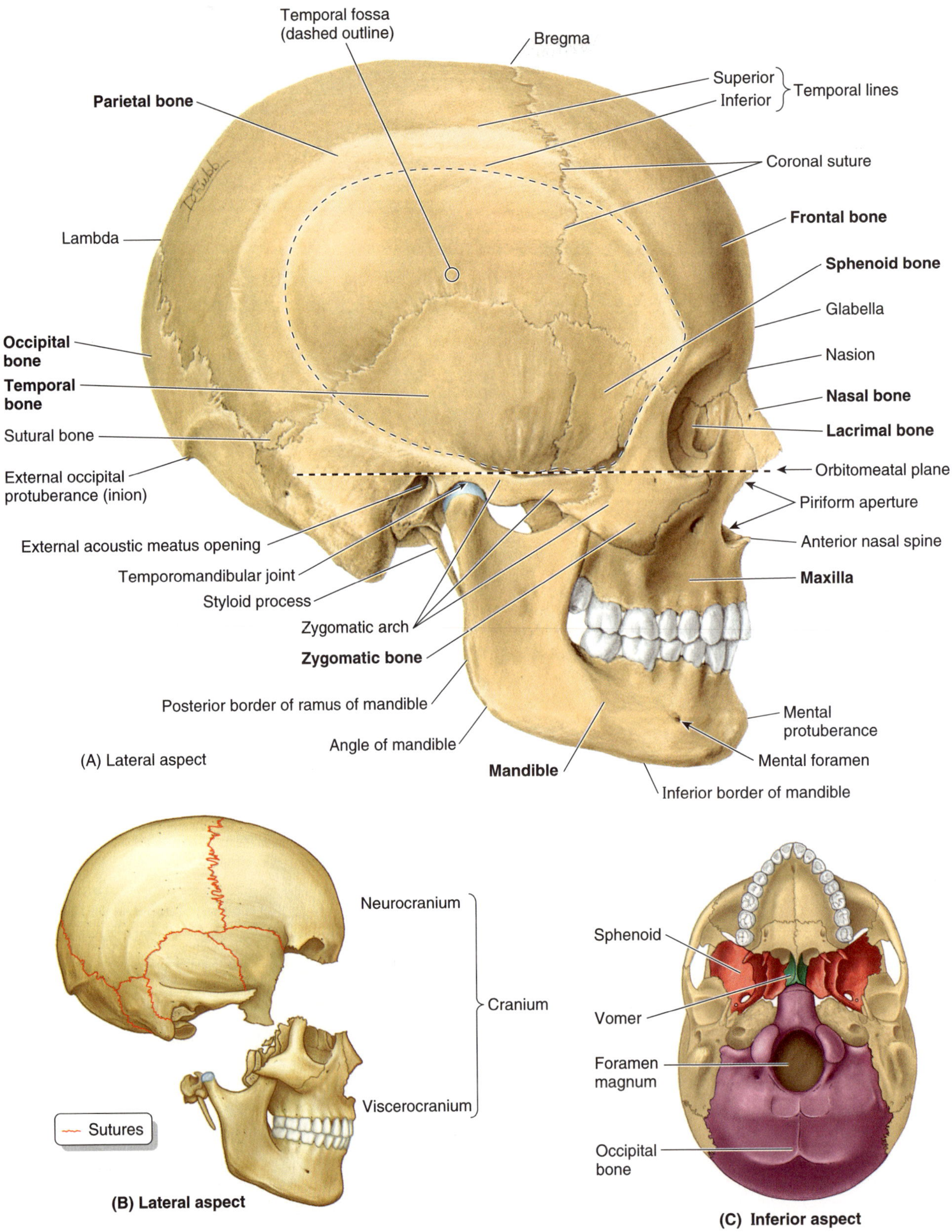

FIGURE 8.1. Adult cranium I. A. In the anatomical position, the inferior margin of the orbit and the superior margin of the external acoustic meatus lie in the same horizontal orbitomeatal (Frankfort horizontal) plane. **B.** The neurocranium and viscerocranium are the two primary functional parts of the cranium. From the lateral aspect, it is apparent that the volume of the neurocranium, housing the brain, is approximately double that of the viscerocranium. **C.** The unpaired sphenoid and occipital bones make substantial contributions to the cranial base. The spinal cord is continuous with the brain through the foramen magnum, the large opening in the basal part of the occipital bone.

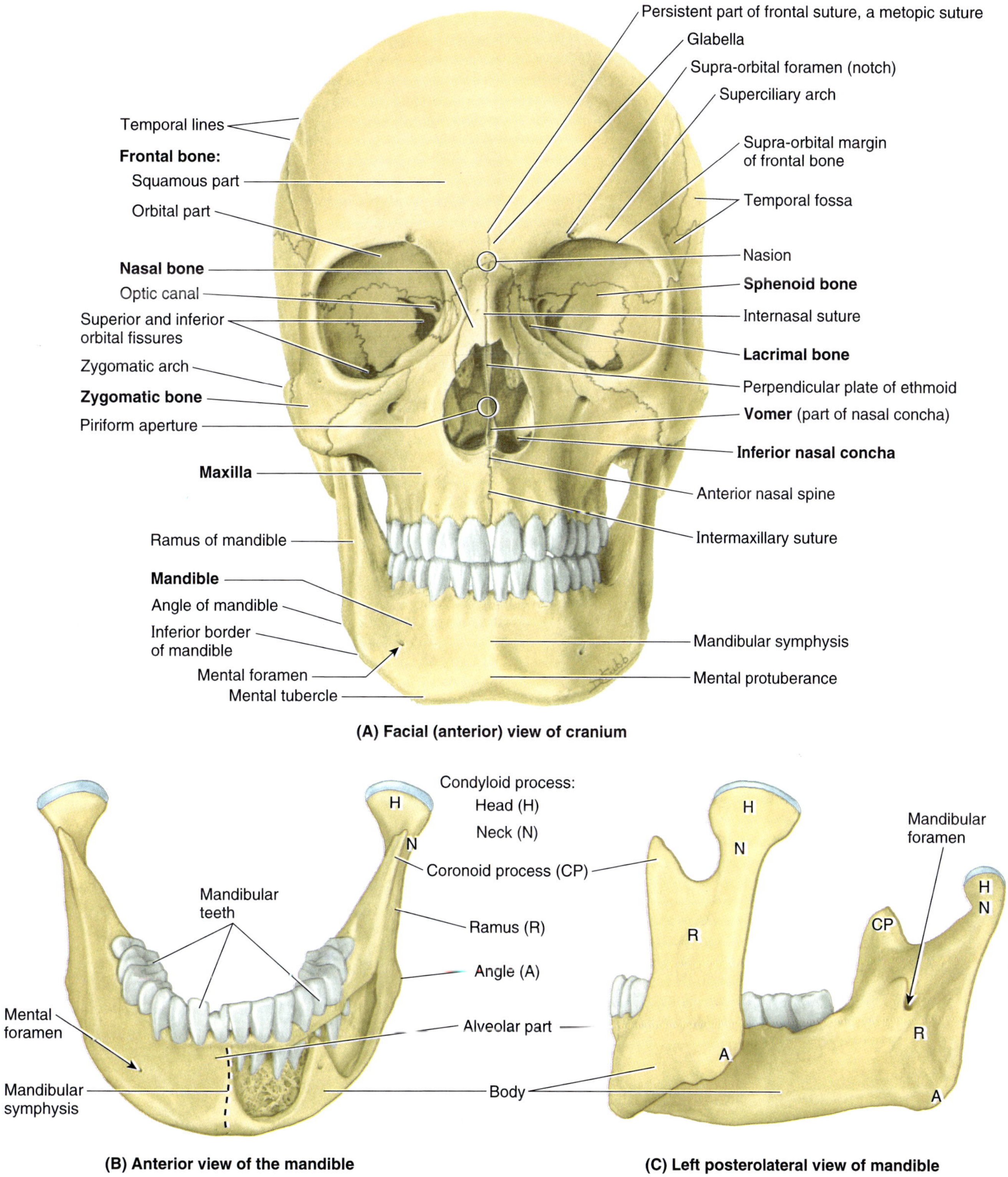

FIGURE 8.2. Adult cranium II. A. The viscerocranium, housing the optical apparatus, nasal cavity, paranasal sinuses, and oral cavity, dominates the facial aspect of the cranium. **B, C.** The mandible is a major component of the viscerocranium, articulating with the remainder of the cranium via the temporomandibular joint. The broad ramus and coronoid process of the mandible provide attachment for powerful muscles capable of generating great force in relationship to biting and chewing (mastication).

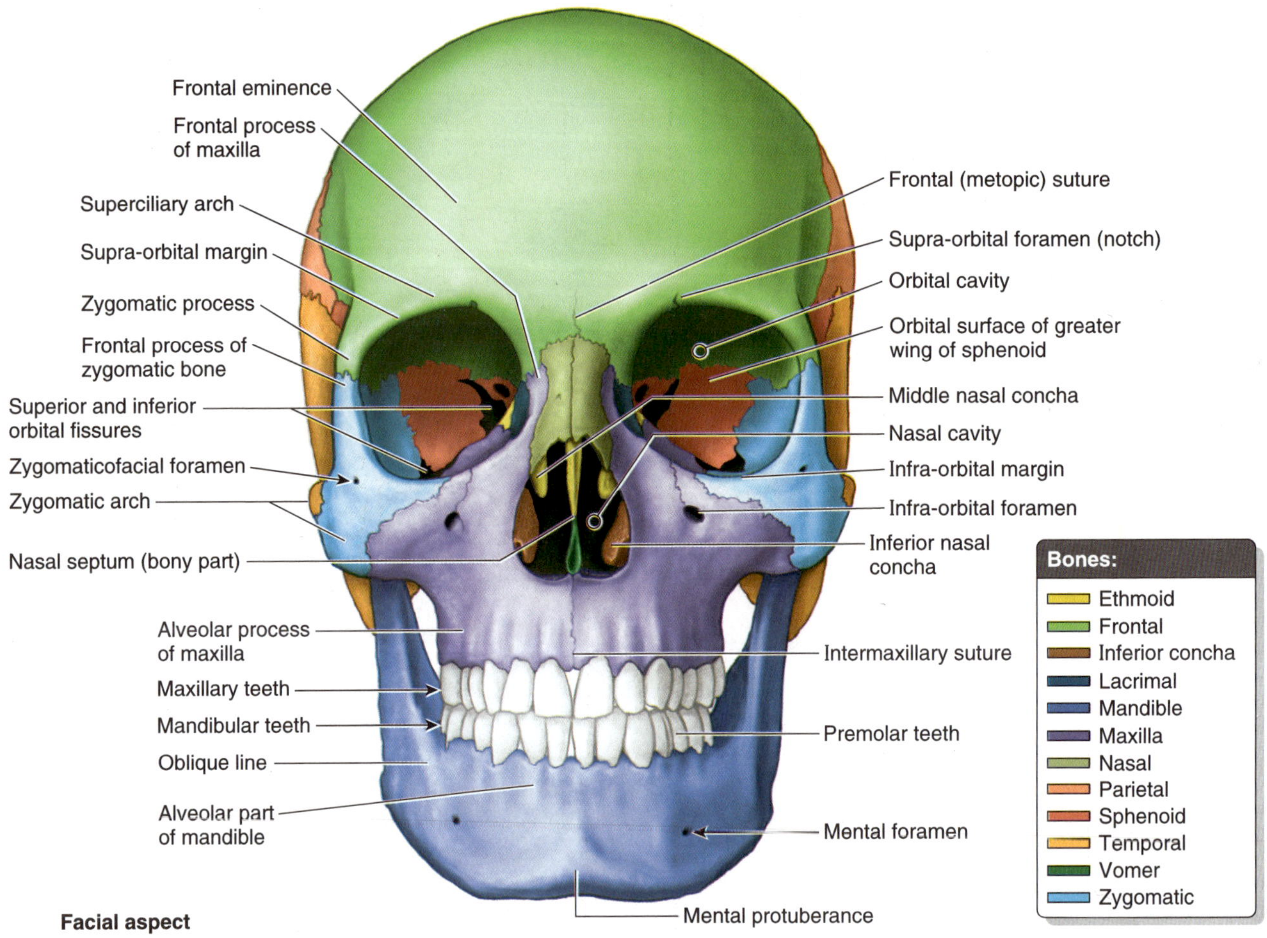

FIGURE 8.3. Adult cranium III. The individual bones of the cranium are color coded. The supra-orbital notch, the infra-orbital foramen, and the mental foramen, giving passage to major sensory nerves of the face, are approximately in a vertical line.

sockets and supporting bone for the maxillary and mandibular teeth. The *maxillae* contribute the greatest part of the upper facial skeleton, forming the skeleton of the upper jaw, which is fixed to the cranial base. The *mandible* forms the skeleton of the lower jaw, which is movable because it articulates with the cranial base at the *temporomandibular joints* (Figs. 8.1A and 8.2).

Several bones of the cranium (frontal, temporal, sphenoid, and ethmoid bones) are **pneumatized bones**, which contain **air spaces** (*air cells* or large *sinuses*), presumably to decrease their weight (Fig. 8.5). The total volume of the air spaces in these bones increases with age.

In the *anatomical position*, the cranium is oriented so that the inferior margin of the orbit and the superior margin of the external acoustic opening of the external acoustic meatus of both sides lie in the same horizontal plane (Fig. 8.1A). This standard craniometric reference is the **orbitomeatal plane** (Frankfort horizontal plane).

Facial Aspect of Cranium

Features of the anterior or **facial** (**frontal**) **aspect of the cranium** are the frontal and zygomatic bones, orbits, nasal region, maxillae, and mandible (Figs. 8.2 and 8.3). AN26.2

The **frontal bone**, specifically its **squamous** (flat) **part**, forms the skeleton of the forehead, articulating inferiorly with the nasal and zygomatic bones. In some adults, a *frontal suture* persists; this remnant is called a **metopic suture**. It is in the middle **glabella**, the smooth, slightly depressed area between the superciliary arches. The **frontal suture** divides the frontal bones of the fetal cranium (see the clinical box "Development of Cranium").

The intersection of the frontal and nasal bones is the **nasion** (L. *nasus*, nose), which in most people is related to a distinctly depressed area (bridge of the nose) (Figs. 8.1A and 8.2A). The nasion is one of many *craniometric points* that are used radiographically in medicine (or on dry crania in physical anthropology) to make cranial measurements, compare

(*continued on p. 884*)

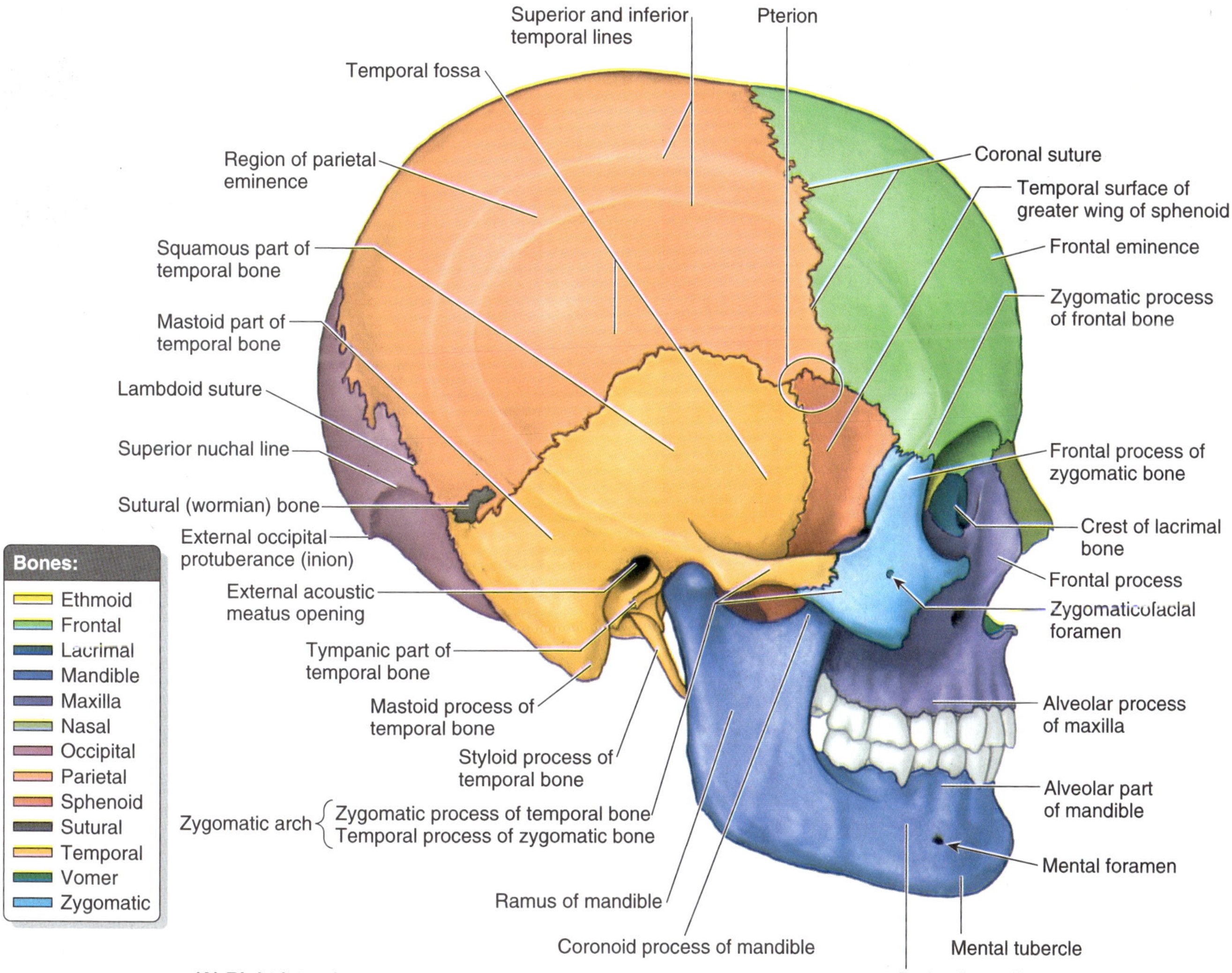

(A) Right lateral aspect

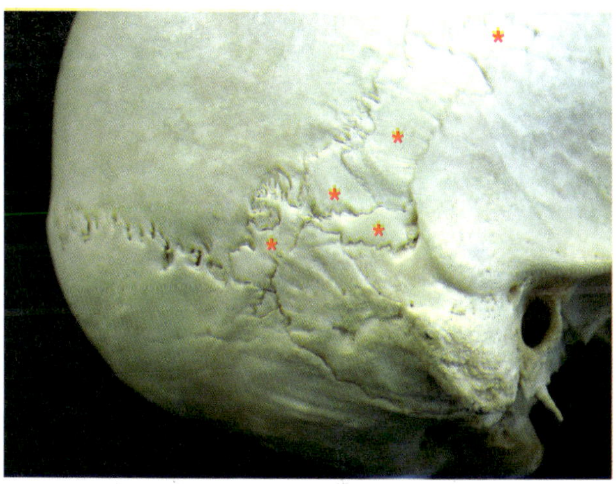

(B) Right lateral aspect * = sutural bones

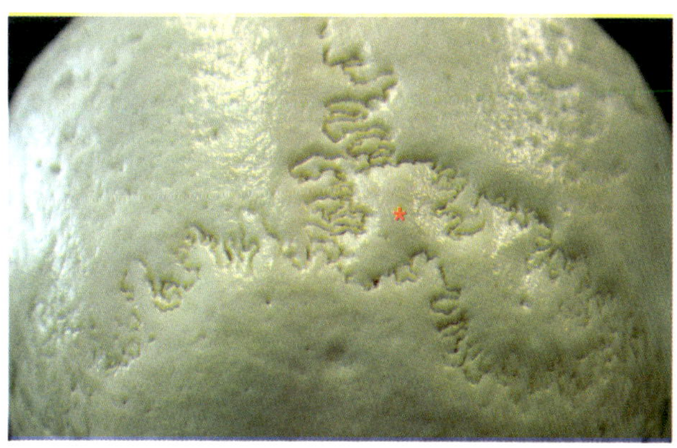

(C) Occipital aspect

FIGURE 8.4. Adult cranium IV. A. The individual bones of the cranium are color coded. Within the temporal fossa, the pterion is a craniometric point at the junction of the greater wing of the sphenoid, the squamous temporal bone, the frontal, and the parietal bones. **B, C.** Sutural bones occurring along the temporoparietal **(B)** and lambdoid **(C)** sutures are shown.

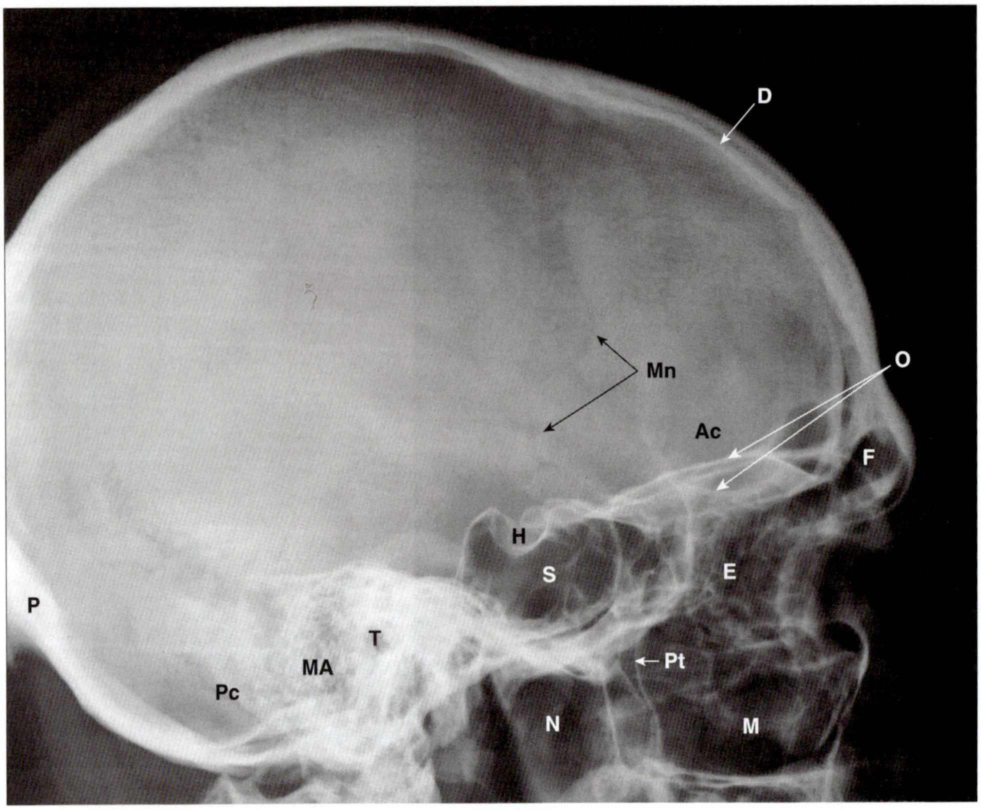

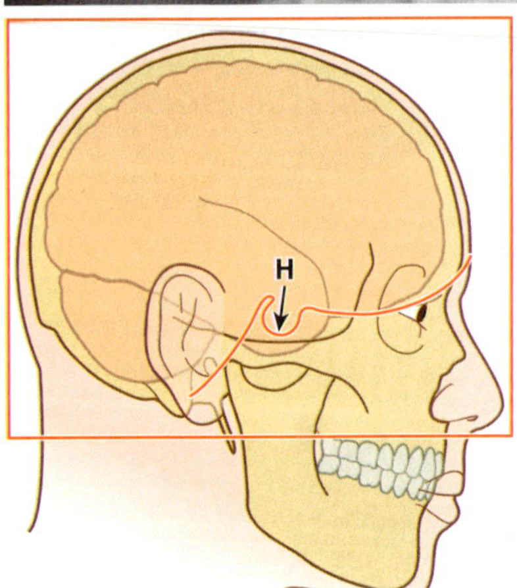

Lateral view

Ac	Anterior cranial fossa	O	Orbital plates of frontal bones
D	Diploë	P	Internal occipital protuberance
E	Ethmoid cells	Pc	Posterior cranial fossa
F	Frontal sinus	Pt	Pterygopalatine fossa
H	Hypophysial fossa	S	Sphenoidal sinus
M	Maxillary sinus	T	Petrous part of temporal bone
MA	Mastoid (air) cells		
Mn	Grooves for middle meningeal vessels		
N	Nasopharynx		

AN43.7 **FIGURE 8.5. Radiograph of cranium.** Pneumatized (air-filled) bones contain sinuses or cells that appear as radiolucencies (dark areas) and bear the name of the occupied bone. The right and left orbital parts of the frontal bone are not superimposed; therefore, the floor of the anterior cranial fossa appears as two lines (*P*). (Courtesy of Dr. E. Becker, Associate Professor of Medical Imaging, University of Toronto, Toronto, Ontario, Canada.)

and describe the topography of the cranium, and document abnormal variations (Fig. 8.6; Table 8.1). The frontal bone also articulates with the lacrimal, ethmoid, and sphenoids; a horizontal portion of bone (*orbital part*) forms both the roof of the orbit and part of the floor of the anterior part of the cranial cavity (Fig. 8.3).

The **supra-orbital margin** of the frontal bone, the angular boundary between the squamous and orbital parts, has a **supra-orbital foramen** (**notch**) in some crania for passage of the supra-orbital nerve and vessels. Just superior to the supra-orbital margin is a ridge, the **superciliary arch**, that extends laterally on each side from the glabella. The prominence of this ridge, deep to the eyebrows, is generally greater in males (Figs. 8.2A and 8.3).

The **zygomatic bones** (cheek bones, malar bones), forming the prominences of the cheeks, lie on the inferolateral sides of the orbits and rest on the maxillae. The anterolateral rims, walls, floor, and much of the infra-orbital margins of

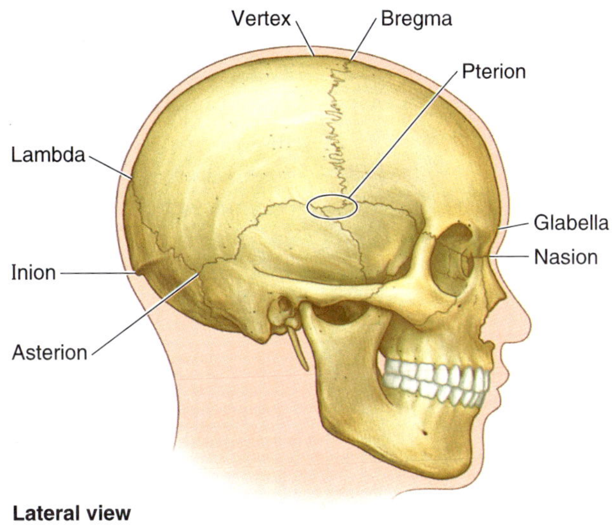

FIGURE 8.6. Craniometric points.

TABLE 8.1. CRANIOMETRIC POINTS OF CRANIUM

Landmark	Shape and Location
Pterion (G. wing)	Junction of greater wing of sphenoid, squamous temporal, frontal, and parietal bones; overlies course of anterior division of middle meningeal artery
Lambda (G. the letter *L*)	Point on calvaria at junction of lambdoid and sagittal sutures
Bregma (G. forepart of head)	Point on calvaria at junction of coronal and sagittal sutures
Vertex (L. whirl, whorl)	Superior point of neurocranium, in middle with cranium oriented in anatomical (orbitomeatal or Frankfort) plane
Asterion (G. *asterios*, starry)	Star shaped; located at junction of three sutures: parietomastoid, occipitomastoid, and lambdoid
Glabella (L. smooth, hairless)	Smooth prominence; most marked in males; on frontal bones superior to root of nose; most anterior projecting part of forehead
Inion (G. back of head)	Most prominent point of external occipital protuberance
Nasion (L. nose)	Point on cranium where frontonasal and internasal sutures meet

the orbits are formed by these quadrilateral bones. A small **zygomaticofacial foramen** pierces the lateral aspect of each bone (Figs. 8.3 and 8.4A). The zygomatic bones articulate with the frontal, sphenoid, and temporal bones and the maxillae.

Inferior to the nasal bones is the pear-shaped **piriform aperture**, the anterior nasal opening in the cranium (Figs. 8.1A and 8.2A). The **bony nasal septum** can be observed through this aperture, dividing the nasal cavity into right and left parts. On the lateral wall of each nasal cavity are curved bony plates, the **nasal conchae** (Figs. 8.2A and 8.3).

The **maxillae** form the upper jaw. Their **alveolar processes** include the tooth sockets (alveoli) and constitute the supporting bone for the **maxillary teeth**. The two maxillae are united at the **intermaxillary suture** in the median plane (Fig. 8.2A). The maxillae surround most of the piriform aperture and form the infra-orbital margins medially. They have a broad connection with the zygomatic bones laterally and an **infra-orbital foramen** inferior to each orbit for passage of the infra-orbital nerve and vessels (Fig. 8.3).

The **mandible** is a U-shaped bone with an alveolar part that supports the **mandibular teeth**. It consists of a horizontal part, the **body**, and a vertical part, the **ramus** (Fig. 8.2B, C). Inferior to the second premolar teeth are the **mental foramina** for the mental nerves and vessels (Figs. 8.1A, 8.2A, B, and 8.3). The **mental protuberance**, forming the prominence of the chin, is a triangular bony elevation inferior to the **mandibular symphysis** (L. *symphysis menti*), the osseous union where the halves of the infantile mandible fuse (Fig. 8.2A, B). AN26.

Lateral Aspect of Cranium

N26.2 The **lateral aspect of the cranium** is formed by both neurocranium and viscerocranium (Figs. 8.1A, B and 8.4A). The main features of the neurocranial part are the *temporal fossa*, the *external acoustic meatus opening*, and the *mastoid process of the temporal bone*. The main features of the viscerocranial part are the *infratemporal fossa*, *zygomatic arch*, and lateral aspects of the maxilla and mandible.

The **temporal fossa** is bounded superiorly and posteriorly by the **superior** and **inferior temporal lines**, anteriorly by the frontal and zygomatic bones, and inferiorly by the zygomatic arch (Figs. 8.1A and 8.4A). The superior border of this arch corresponds to the inferior limit of the cerebral hemisphere of the brain. The **zygomatic arch** is formed by the union of the **temporal process of the zygomatic bone** and the **zygomatic process of the temporal bone**.

N43.6 In the anterior part of the temporal fossa, 3–4 cm superior to the midpoint of the zygomatic arch, there is a clinically important area of bone junctions: the **pterion** (G. *pteron*, wing) (Figs. 8.4A and 8.6; Table 8.1). It is usually indicated by an H-shaped formation of sutures that unite the frontal, parietal, sphenoid (greater wing), and temporal bones. Less commonly, the frontal and temporal bones articulate. Sometimes all four bones meet at a point.

The **external acoustic meatus opening** (**pore**) is the entrance to the *external acoustic meatus* (canal), which leads to the tympanic membrane (eardrum) (Fig. 8.4A). The **mastoid process** of the temporal bone is postero-inferior to the external acoustic meatus opening. Anteromedial to the mastoid process is the *styloid process of the temporal bone*, a slender needle-like, pointed projection. The *infratemporal fossa* is an irregular space inferior and deep to the zygomatic arch and mandible and posterior to the maxilla (see Fig. 8.69B).

Occipital Aspect of Cranium

The posterior or **occipital aspect of the cranium** is com- AN26.2
posed of the **occiput** (L. back of head, the convex posterior protuberance of the **squamous part of the occipital bone**), parts of the parietal bones, and mastoid parts of the temporal bones (Fig. 8.7A).

The **external occipital protuberance** is usually easily palpable in the median plane. However, occasionally (especially in females), it may be inconspicuous. A craniometric point defined by the tip of the external protuberance is the **inion** (G. nape of neck) (Figs. 8.1A, 8.4A, and 8.6; Table 8.1). The **external occipital crest** descends from the external protuberance toward the *foramen magnum*,

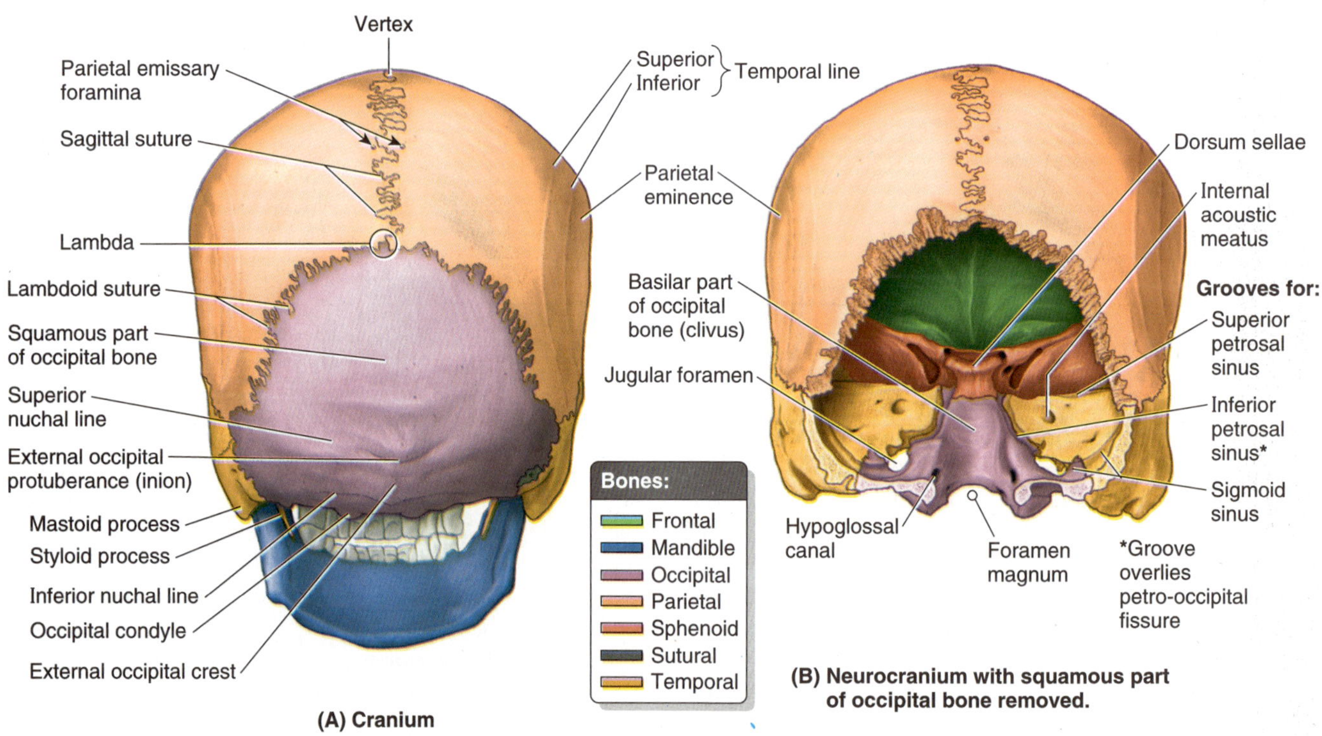

FIGURE 8.7. Adult cranium V: Occipital aspect. A. The posterior aspect of the neurocranium, or occiput, is composed of parts of the parietal bones, the occipital bone, and the mastoid parts of the temporal bones. The sagittal and lambdoid sutures meet at the lambda, which can often be felt as a depression in living persons. **B.** The squamous part of the occipital bone has been removed to expose the anterior part of the posterior cranial fossa.

the large opening in the basal part of the occipital bone (Figs. 8.1C, 8.7B, and 8.9).

The **superior nuchal line**, marking the superior limit of the neck, extends laterally from each side of the external protuberance. The **inferior nuchal line** is less distinct. In the center of the occiput, **lambda** indicates the junction of the sagittal and the lambdoid sutures (Figs. 8.1A, 8.6, and 8.7A; Table 8.1). Lambda can sometimes be felt as a depression. One or more **sutural bones** (accessory or wormian bones) may be located at lambda or near the mastoid process (Fig. 8.4B, C).

Superior Aspect of Cranium

AN26.2 The **superior** (**vertical**) **aspect of the cranium**, usually somewhat oval in form, broadens posterolaterally at the **parietal eminences** (Fig. 8.8A). In some people, **frontal eminences** are also visible, giving the calvaria a somewhat square appearance.

The **coronal suture** separates the frontal and parietal bones (Fig. 8.8A, B), the **sagittal suture** separates the parietal bones, and the **lambdoid suture** separates the parietal and temporal bones from the occipital bone (Fig. 8.8A, C). **Bregma** is the craniometric landmark formed by the intersection of the sagittal and coronal sutures (Figs. 8.6 and 8.8A; Table 8.1). **Vertex**, the most superior point of the calvaria, is near the midpoint of the sagittal suture (Figs. 8.6 and 8.7A).

The **parietal foramen** is a small, inconstant aperture located posteriorly in the parietal bone near the sagittal suture (Fig. 8.8A, C). Sometimes, paired parietal foramina are present. Most irregular, highly variable foramina that occur in the neurocranium are *emissary foramina* that transmit *emissary veins* connecting scalp veins to the venous sinuses of the dura mater (see "Scalp").

External Surface of Cranial Base

AN26.2 The *cranial base* (basicranium) is the inferior portion of the neurocranium (floor of the cranial cavity) and viscerocranium minus the mandible (Fig. 8.9). The **external surface of the cranial base** features the **alveolar arch of the maxillae** (the free border of the alveolar processes surrounding and supporting the maxillary teeth); the palatine processes of the maxillae; and the palatine, sphenoid, vomer, temporal, and occipital bones.

The **hard palate** (bony palate) is formed by the **palatal processes of the maxillae** anteriorly and the **horizontal plates of the palatine bones** posteriorly. The free posterior border of the hard palate projects posteriorly in the median plane as the **posterior nasal spine**. Posterior to the central incisor teeth is the **incisive foramen**, a depression in the midline of the bony palate into which the incisive canals open.

The right and left nasopalatine nerves pass from the nose through a variable number of incisive canals and foramina (they may be bilateral or merged into a single formation). Posterolaterally are the **greater** and **lesser palatine foramina**. Superior to the posterior edge of the palate are two large

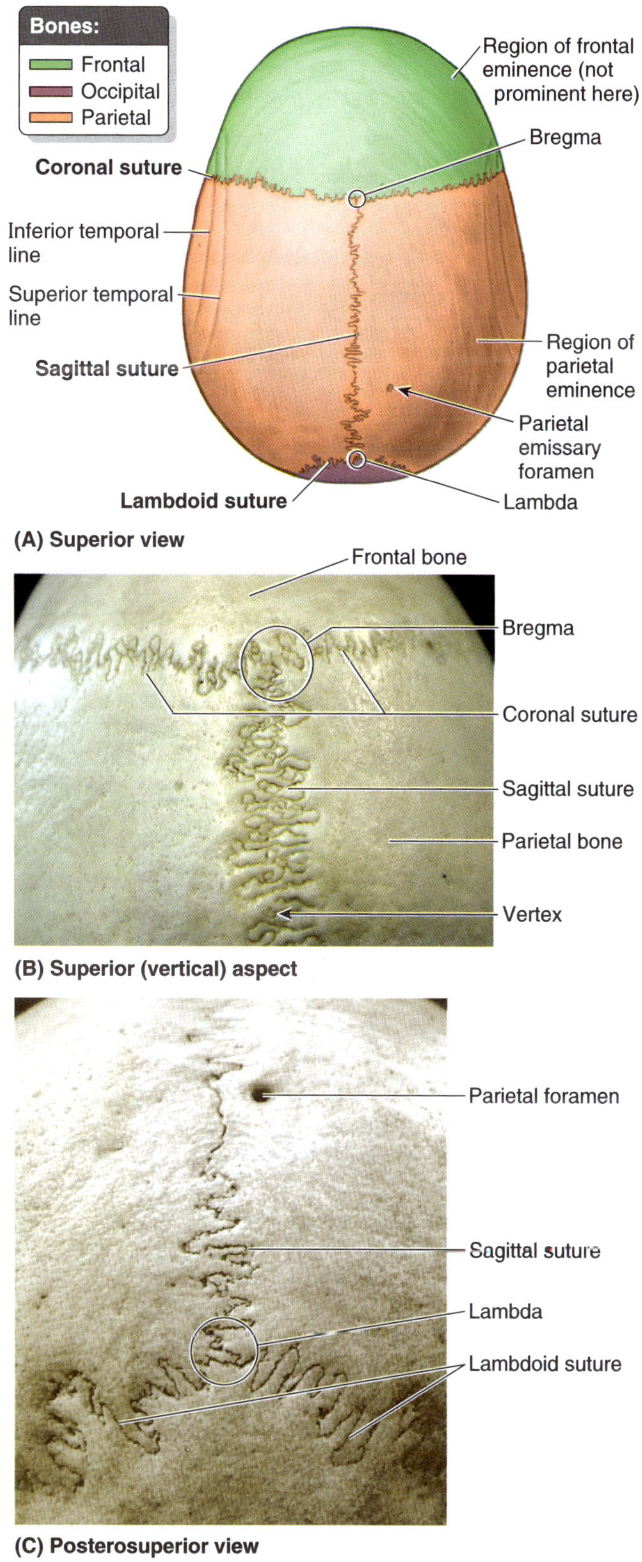

FIGURE 8.8. Adult cranium VI: Calvaria. A. The squamous parts of the frontal and occipital bones, and the paired parietal bones contribute to the calvaria. **B.** The external aspect of the anterior part of the calvaria demonstrates bregma, where the coronal and sagittal sutures meet, and vertex, the superior (topmost) point of the cranium. **C.** This external view demonstrates a prominent, unilateral parietal foramen. Although emissary foramina often occur in this general location, there is much variation.

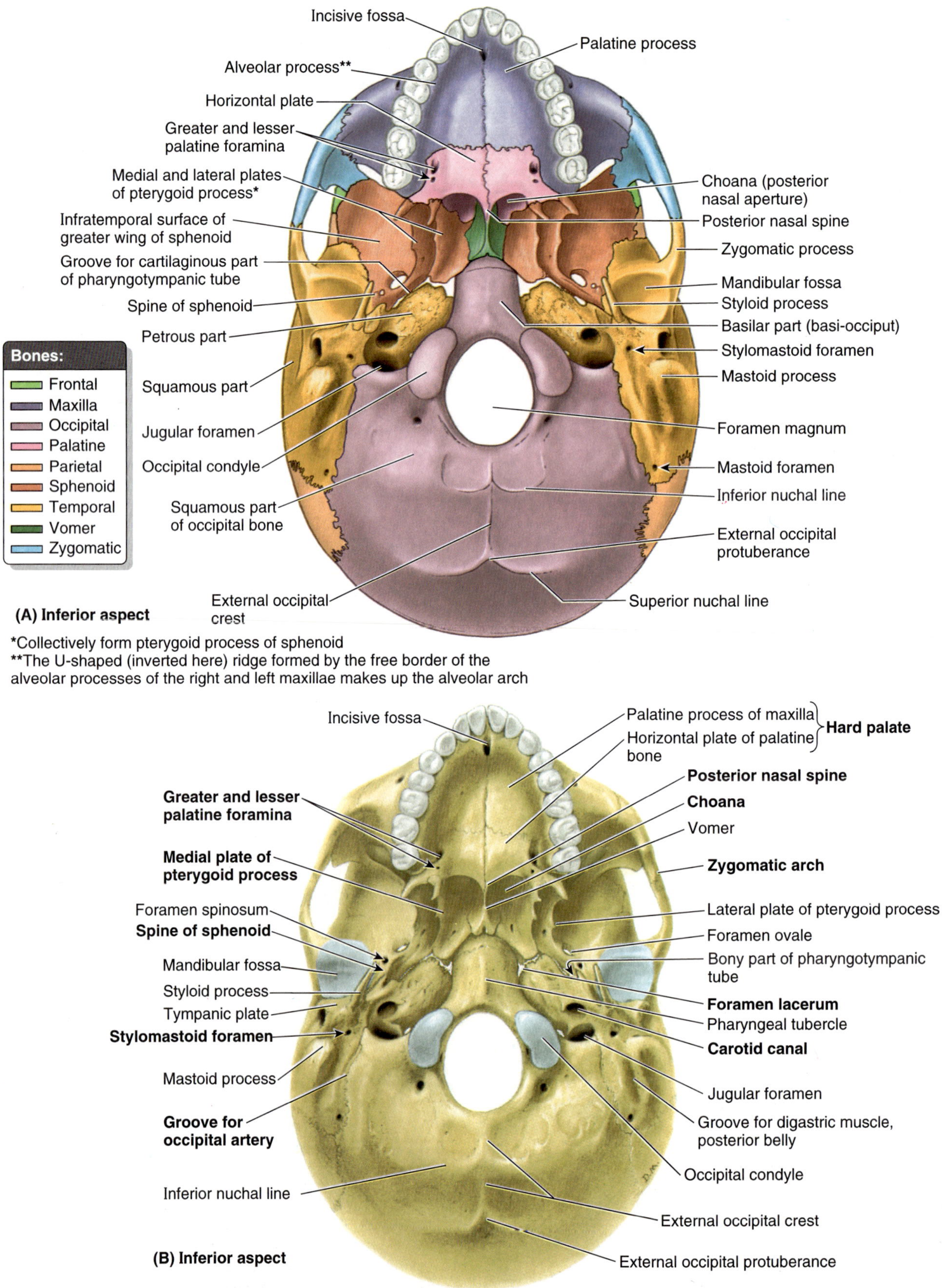

FIGURE 8.9. Adult cranium VII: External cranial base. A. The contributing bones are color coded. **B.** The foramen magnum is located midway between and on a level with the mastoid processes. The hard palate forms both a part of the roof of the mouth and the floor of the nasal cavity. The large choanae on each side of the vomer make up the posterior entrance to the nasal cavities.

openings: the **choanae** (posterior nasal apertures), which are separated from each other by the **vomer** (L. plowshare), a flat unpaired bone of trapezoidal shape that forms a major part of the bony nasal septum (Fig. 8.9B).

Wedged between the frontal, temporal, and occipital bones is the **sphenoid** (L. winged; *pterygoid* is an often-used synonym for sphenoid), an irregular unpaired bone that consists of a body and three pairs of processes: greater wings, lesser wings, and pterygoid processes (Fig. 8.10). The **greater** and **lesser wings of the sphenoid** spread laterally from the lateral aspects of the **body of the sphenoid**. The greater wings have orbital, temporal, and infratemporal surfaces apparent in facial, lateral, and inferior views of the exterior of the cranium (Figs. 8.3, 8.4A, and 8.9A). Their cerebral surfaces are seen in internal views of the cranial base (Fig. 8.11). The **pterygoid processes**, consisting of **lateral**

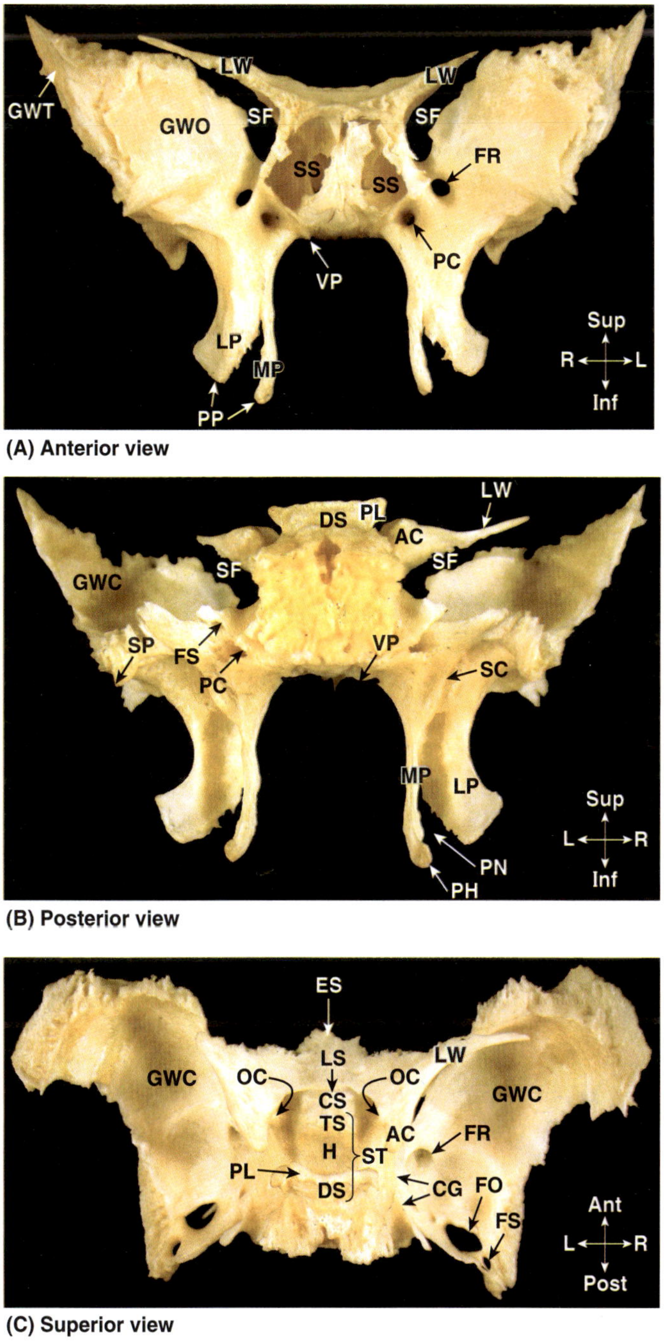

Key	
AC	Anterior clinoid process
CG	Carotid sulcus
CS	Prechiasmatic sulcus
DS	Dorsum sellae
ES	Ethmoidal spine
FO	Foramen ovale
FR	Foramen rotundum
FS	Foramen spinosum
GWC	Greater wing (cerebral surface)
GWO	Greater wing (orbital surface)
GWT	Greater wing (temporal surface)
H	Hypophysial fossa
LP	Lateral pterygoid plate
LS	Limbus of sphenoid
LW	Lesser wing
MP	Medial pterygoid plate
OC	Optic canal
PC	Pterygoid canal
PF	Pterygoid fossa
PH	Pterygoid hamulus
PL	Posterior clinoid process
PN	Pterygoid notch
PP	Pterygoid process
SC	Scaphoid fossa
SF	Superior orbital fissure
SP	Spine of sphenoid bone
SS	Sphenoidal sinus (in body of sphenoid)
ST	Sella turcica
TI	Greater wing of sphenoid (Infratemporal surface)
TS	Tuberculum sellae
VP	Vaginal process

FIGURE 8.10. Sphenoid. The unpaired, irregular sphenoid is a pneumatic (air-filled) bone. **A.** Parts of the thin anterior wall of the body of the sphenoid have been chipped off revealing the interior of the sphenoid sinus, which typically is unevenly divided into separate right and left cavities. **B.** The superior orbital fissure is a gap between the lesser and greater wings of the sphenoid. The medial and lateral pterygoid plates are components of the pterygoid processes. **C.** Details of the sella turcica, the midline formation that surrounds the hypophysial fossa, are shown.

and **medial pterygoid plates**, extend inferiorly on each side of the sphenoid from the junction of the body and greater wings (Figs. 8.9A and 8.10A, B).

The **groove for the cartilaginous part of the pharyngotympanic (auditory) tube** lies medial to the **spine of the sphenoid**, inferior to the junction of the greater wing of the sphenoid and the **petrous** (L. rock-like) **part of the temporal bone** (Fig. 8.9B). Depressions in the **squamous** (L. flat) **part of the temporal bone**, called the **mandibular fossae**, accommodate the mandibular condyles when the mouth is closed.

The **occipital bone** articulates with the sphenoid anteriorly, forming the posterior part of the cranial base. The four parts of the occipital bone are arranged around the *foramen magnum*, the most conspicuous feature of the cranial base. The major structures passing through this large foramen are the *spinal cord* (where it becomes continuous with the medulla oblongata of the brain); the *meninges* (coverings) of the brain and spinal cord; the *vertebral arteries*; the anterior and posterior *spinal arteries*; and the *spinal accessory nerve* (CN XI). On the lateral parts of the occipital bone are two large protuberances, the **occipital condyles**, by which the cranium articulates with the vertebral column.

The large opening between the occipital bone and the petrous part of the temporal bone is the **jugular foramen**, from which the internal jugular vein (IJV) and several cranial nerves (CN IX–CN XI) emerge from the cranium (Figs. 8.9A and 8.11; Table 8.2). The entrance to the *carotid canal* for the internal carotid artery is just anterior to the jugular foramen (Fig. 8.9B). The *mastoid processes* provide for muscle attachments. The **stylomastoid foramen**, transmitting the facial nerve (CN VII) and stylomastoid artery, lies posterior to the base of the styloid process.

Internal Surface of Cranial Base

AN26.3 AN30.1 AN30.2 The **internal surface of the cranial base** (L. *basis cranii interna*) has three large depressions that lie at different levels: the *anterior*, *middle*, and *posterior cranial fossae*, which form the bowl-shaped floor of the **cranial cavity**, the space enclosed within the neurocranium occupied by the brain (Fig. 8.12). The anterior cranial fossa is at the highest level, and the posterior cranial fossa is at the lowest level.

ANTERIOR CRANIAL FOSSA

The inferior and anterior parts of the frontal lobes of the brain occupy the **anterior cranial fossa**, the shallowest of the three cranial fossae (Fig. 8.12B). The fossa is formed by the frontal bone anteriorly, the ethmoid bone in the middle, and the body and lesser wings of the sphenoid posteriorly. The greater part of the fossa is formed by the **orbital parts of the frontal bone**, which support the frontal lobes of the brain and form the roofs of the orbits. This surface shows sinuous impressions (*brain markings*) of the orbital gyri (ridges) of the frontal lobes (Fig. 8.11).

The **frontal crest** is a median bony extension of the frontal bone (Fig. 8.12A). At its base is the **foramen cecum** of the frontal bone, which gives passage to vessels during fetal development, but is insignificant postnatally. The **crista galli** (L. cock's comb) is a thick, median ridge of bone posterior to the foramen cecum, which projects superiorly from the ethmoid. On each side of this ridge is the sieve-like cribriform plate of ethmoid bone. Its numerous tiny foramina transmit the olfactory nerves (CN I) from the olfactory areas of the nasal cavities to the olfactory bulbs of the brain, which lie on this plate (Fig. 8.12A; Table 8.2).

MIDDLE CRANIAL FOSSA

The butterfly-shaped **middle cranial fossa** has a central part composed of the *sella turcica* on the body of the sphenoid and large, depressed *lateral parts* on each side (Fig. 8.12). The middle cranial fossa is postero-inferior to the anterior cranial fossa, separated from it by the sharp *sphenoidal crests* laterally and the *limbus of the sphenoid* centrally. The **sphenoidal crests** are formed mostly by the sharp posterior borders of the *lesser wings of the sphenoid bones*, which overhang the lateral parts of the fossae anteriorly. The sphenoidal crests end medially in two sharp bony projections, the *anterior clinoid processes*.

A variably prominent ridge, the **limbus of the sphenoid** forms the anterior boundary of the transversely oriented **prechiasmatic sulcus** extending between the right and the left *optic canals*. The bones forming the lateral parts of the fossa are the greater wings of the sphenoid, the squamous parts of the temporal bones laterally, and the petrous parts of the temporal bones posteriorly. The lateral parts of the middle cranial fossa support the temporal lobes of the brain. The boundary between the middle and the posterior cranial fossae is the **superior border (crest) of the petrous part of the temporal bone** laterally, and a flat plate of bone, the *dorsum sellae of the sphenoid*, medially.

The **sella turcica** (L. Turkish saddle) is the saddle-like bony formation on the upper surface of the body of the sphenoid, which is surrounded by the **anterior** and **posterior clinoid processes** (Figs. 8.10C and 8.12A). *Clinoid* means "bedpost," and the four processes (two anterior and two posterior) surround the hypophysial fossa, the "bed" of the pituitary gland, like the posts of a four-poster bed. The sella turcica is composed of three parts:

1. The **tuberculum sellae** (horn of saddle): a variable slight to prominent median elevation forming the posterior boundary of the *prechiasmatic sulcus* and the anterior boundary of the hypophysial fossa.
2. The **hypophysial fossa** (pituitary fossa): a median depression (seat of saddle) in the body of the sphenoid that accommodates the *pituitary gland* (L. *hypophysis*).
3. The **dorsum sellae** (back of saddle): a square plate of bone projecting superiorly from the *body of the sphenoid*. It forms the posterior boundary of the sella turcica, and its prominent superolateral angles make up the *posterior clinoid processes*.

(*continued on p.* 892)

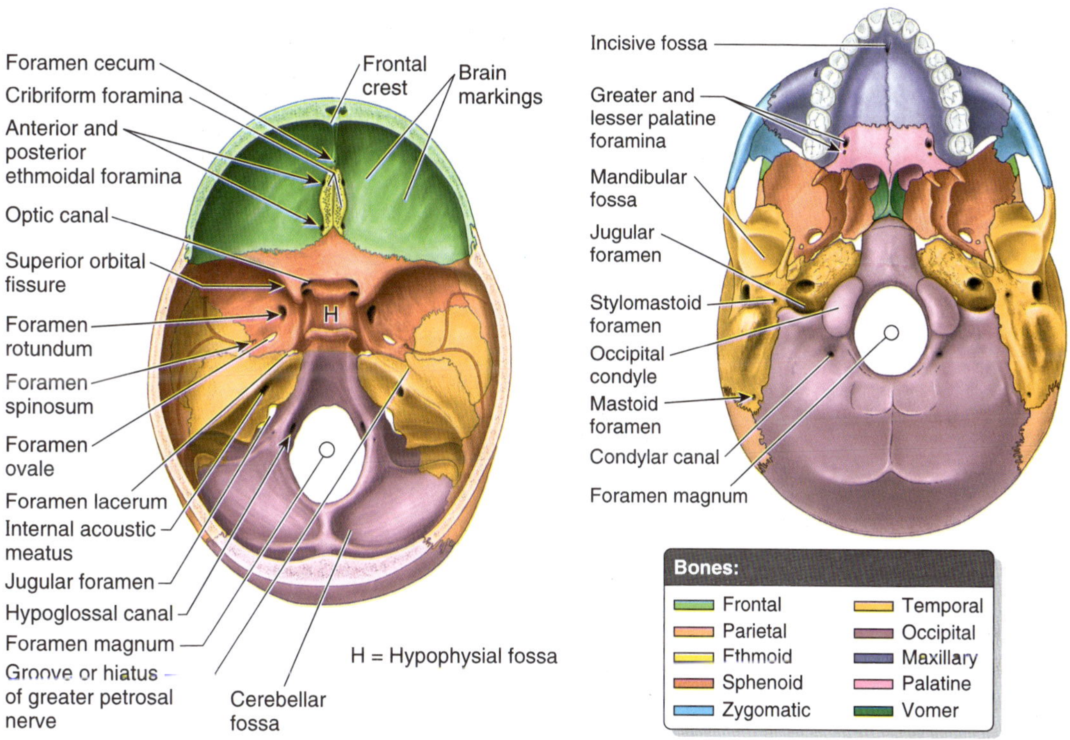

FIGURE 8.11. Adult cranium VIII: Cranial foramina.

TABLE 8.2. FORAMINA AND OTHER APERTURES OF CRANIAL FOSSAE AND CONTENTS

Foramina/Apertures	Contents
Anterior cranial fossa	
Foramen cecum	Nasal emissary vein (1% of population)
Cribriform foramina in cribriform plate	Axons of olfactory cells in olfactory epithelium that form olfactory nerves
Anterior and posterior ethmoidal foramina	Vessels and nerves with same names
Middle cranial fossa	
Optic canals	Optic nerves (CN II) and ophthalmic arteries
Superior orbital fissure	Ophthalmic veins; ophthalmic nerve (CN V_1); CN III, IV, and VI; and sympathetic fibers
Foramen rotundum	Maxillary nerve (CN V_2)
Foramen ovale	Mandibular nerve (CN V_3) and accessory meningeal artery
Foramen spinosum	Middle meningeal artery and vein and meningeal branch of CN V_3
Foramen lacerum[a]	Deep petrosal nerve and some meningeal arterial branches and small veins
Groove or hiatus of greater petrosal nerve	Greater petrosal nerve and petrosal branch of middle meningeal artery
Posterior cranial fossa	
Foramen magnum	Medulla and meninges, vertebral arteries, CN XI, dural veins, anterior and posterior spinal arteries
Jugular foramen	CN IX, X, and XI; superior bulb of internal jugular vein; inferior petrosal and sigmoid sinuses; and meningeal branches of ascending pharyngeal and occipital arteries
Hypoglossal canal	Hypoglossal nerve (CN XII)
Condylar canal	Emissary vein that passes from sigmoid sinus to vertebral veins in neck
Mastoid foramen	Mastoid emissary vein from sigmoid sinus and meningeal branch of occipital artery

[a]The internal carotid artery and its accompanying sympathetic and venous plexuses actually pass horizontally *across* (rather than vertically through) the area of the foramen lacerum, an artifact of dry crania, which is closed by cartilage in life.

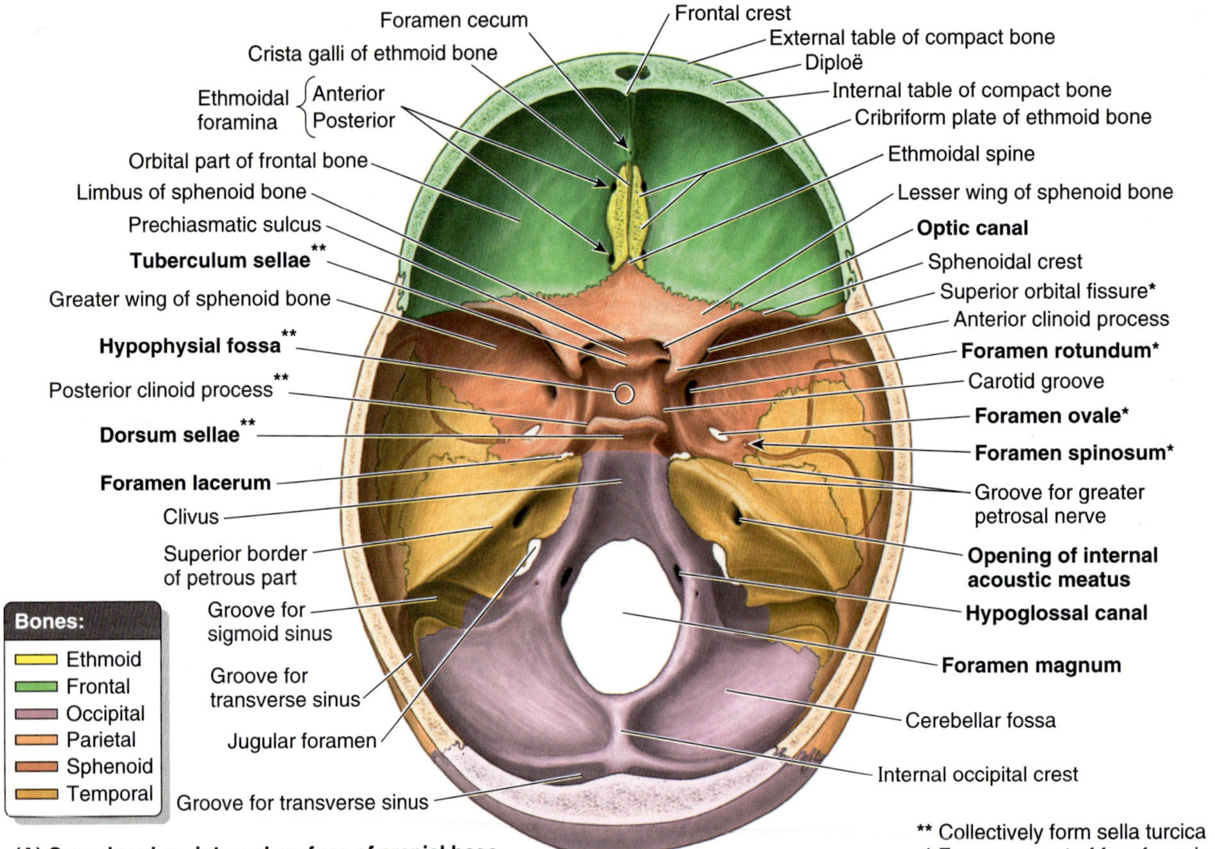

(A) Superior view, internal surface of cranial base

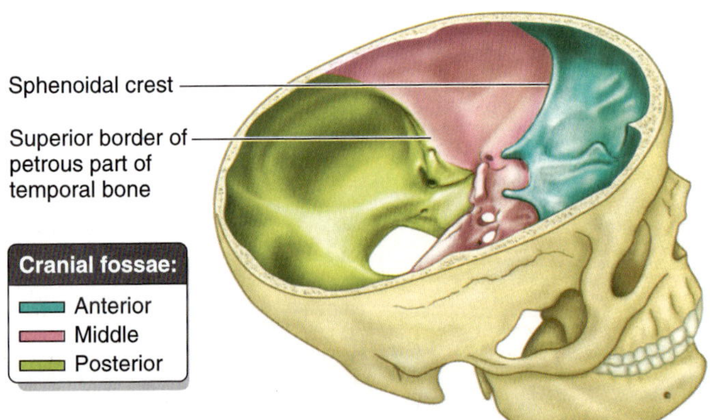

(B) Superolateral view of cranial base

FIGURE 8.12. Adult cranium IX: Internal cranial base. A. The internal aspect demonstrates the contributing bones and features. **B.** The floor of the cranial cavity is divisible into three levels (steps): anterior, middle, and posterior cranial fossae.

On each side of the body of the sphenoid, a *crescent of four foramina* perforates the roots of the cerebral surfaces of the greater wings of the sphenoids (Figs. 8.10C, 8.11, and 8.12A); structures transmitted by the foramina are listed in Table 8.2:

1. **Superior orbital fissure**: Located between the greater and the lesser wings, it opens anteriorly into the orbit (Fig. 8.2A).
2. **Foramen rotundum** (round foramen): Located posterior to the medial end of the superior orbital fissure, it runs a horizontal course to an opening on the anterior aspect of the root of the greater wing of the sphenoid (Figs. 8.10A and 8.11A) into a bony formation between the sphenoid, the maxilla, and the palatine bones, the *pterygopalatine fossa*.
3. **Foramen ovale** (oval foramen): A large foramen posterolateral to the foramen rotundum; it opens inferiorly into the infratemporal fossa (Fig. 8.9B).

4. **Foramen spinosum** (spinous foramen): Located posterolateral to the foramen ovale and opens into the infratemporal fossa in relationship to the *spine of the sphenoid* (Fig. 8.11).

The **foramen lacerum** (lacerated or torn foramen) is not part of the crescent of foramina. This ragged foramen lies posterolateral to the hypophysial fossa and is an artifact of a dried cranium (Fig. 8.12A). In life, it is closed by a cartilage plate. Only some meningeal arterial branches and small veins are transmitted vertically through the cartilage, completely traversing this foramen. The internal carotid artery and its accompanying sympathetic and venous plexuses pass across the superior aspect of the cartilage (i.e., pass over the foramen), and some nerves traverse it horizontally, passing to a foramen in its anterior boundary.

Extending posteriorly and laterally from the foramen lacerum is a narrow **groove for the greater petrosal nerve** on the anterosuperior surface of the petrous part of the temporal bone. There is also a small **groove for the lesser petrosal nerve**.

POSTERIOR CRANIAL FOSSA

The **posterior cranial fossa**, the largest and deepest of the three cranial fossae, lodges the cerebellum, pons, and medulla oblongata (Fig. 8.12B). The posterior cranial fossa is formed mostly by the occipital bone, but the *dorsum sellae of the sphenoid* marks its anterior boundary centrally (Fig. 8.12A), and the petrous and mastoid parts of the temporal bones contribute its anterolateral "walls."

From the dorsum sellae, there is a marked incline, the **clivus**, in the center of the anterior part of the fossa leading to the *foramen magnum*. Posterior to this large opening, the posterior cranial fossa is partly divided by the **internal occipital crest** into bilateral large concave impressions, the **cerebellar fossae**. The internal occipital crest ends in the **internal occipital protuberance** formed in relationship to the *confluence of the sinuses*, a merging of dural venous sinuses.

Broad grooves show the horizontal course of the *transverse sinus* and the S-shaped *sigmoid sinus*. At the base of the petrous ridge of the temporal bone is the *jugular foramen*, which transmits several cranial nerves in addition to the sigmoid sinus that exits the cranium as the internal jugular vein (IJV) (Fig. 8.11; Table 8.2). Anterosuperior to the jugular foramen is the *internal acoustic meatus* for the facial (CN VII) and vestibulocochlear nerves (CN VIII) and the labyrinthine artery. The **hypoglossal canal** for the hypoglossal nerve (CN XII) is superior to the anterolateral margin of the foramen magnum.

Walls of Cranial Cavity

The walls of the cranial cavity vary in thickness in different regions. They are usually thinner in females than in males and are thinner in children and elderly people. The bones tend to be thinnest in areas that are well covered with muscles, such as the squamous part of the temporal bone (Fig. 8.11). Thin areas of bone can be seen radiographically (Fig. 8.5) or by holding a dried cranium up to a bright light.

Most bones of the calvaria consist of **internal** and **external tables of compact bone**, separated by diploë (Figs. 8.5 and 8.11). The **diploë** is cancellous bone containing red bone marrow during life, through which run canals formed by diploic veins. The diploë in a dried calvaria is not red because the protein was removed during preparation of the cranium. The internal table of bone is thinner than the external table, and in some areas, there is only a thin plate of compact bone with no diploë.

The bony substance of the cranium is unequally distributed. Relatively thin (but mostly curved) flat bones provide the necessary strength to maintain cavities and protect their contents. However, in addition to housing the brain, the bones of the neurocranium (and processes from them) provide proximal attachment for the strong muscles of mastication that attach distally to the mandible. Consequently, high traction forces occur across the nasal cavity and orbits that are sandwiched between. Therefore, thickened portions of the cranial bones form stronger pillars or *buttresses* that transmit forces, bypassing the orbits and nasal cavity (Fig. 8.13). The main buttresses are the **frontonasal buttress**, extending from the region of the canine teeth between the nasal and the orbital cavities to the central frontal bone, and the **zygomatic arch–lateral orbital margin buttress** from the region of the molars to the lateral frontal and temporal bones. Similarly, **occipital buttresses** transmit forces received lateral to the foramen magnum from the vertebral column. Perhaps to compensate for the denser bone required for these buttresses, some areas of the cranium not as mechanically stressed become pneumatized (air filled).

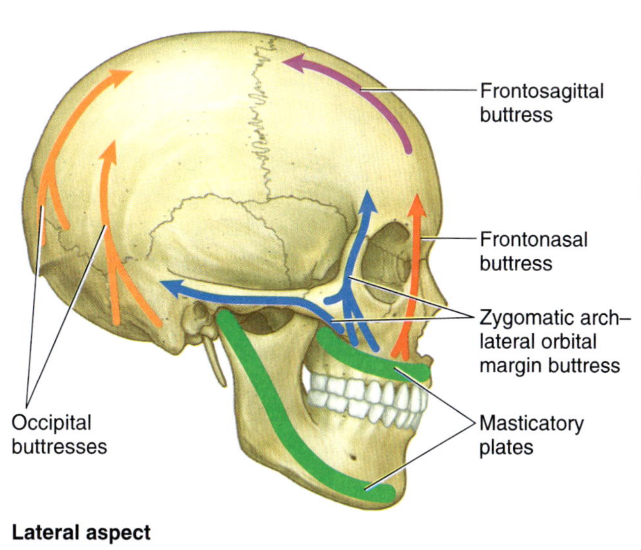

FIGURE 8.13. Buttresses of cranium. The buttresses are thicker portions of cranial bone that transmit forces around weaker regions of the cranium.

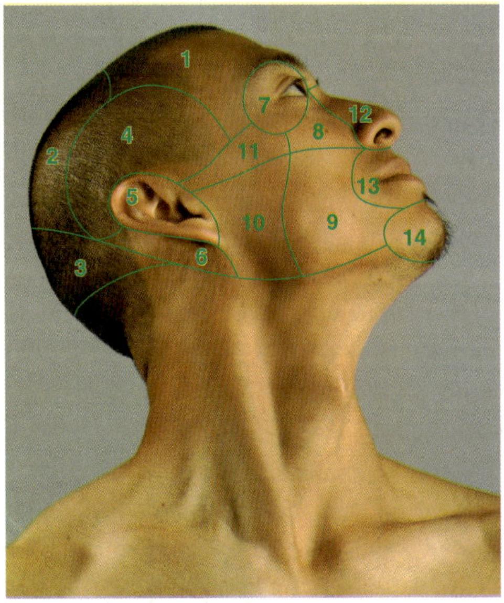

Regions of the head:

1 Frontal region
2 Parietal region
3 Occipital region
4 Temporal region
5 Auricular region
6 Mastoid region

Facial region:

7 Orbital region
8 Infra-orbital region
9 Buccal region
10 Parotid region
11 Zygomatic region
12 Nasal region
13 Oral region
14 Mental region

FIGURE 8.14. Regions of head.

Regions of Head

To allow clear communications regarding the location of structures, injuries, or pathologies, the head is divided into regions (Fig. 8.14). The large number of regions into which the relatively small area of the face is divided (eight) reflects its functional complexity and personal importance, as do annual expenditures for elective aesthetic surgery. Except for the auricular region, which includes the external ear, the names of the regions of the *neurocranial portion of the head* correspond to the underlying bones or bony features: frontal, parietal, occipital, temporal, and mastoid regions.

The *viscerocranial portion of the head* includes the facial region, which is divided into five bilateral and three median regions related to superficial features (oral and buccal regions), to deeper soft tissue formations (parotid region), and to skeletal features (orbital, infra-orbital, nasal, zygomatic, and mental regions). The remainder of this chapter discusses several of these regions in detail, as well as some deep regions not represented on the surface (e.g., the infratemporal region and pterygopalatine fossa). The surface anatomy of these regions will be discussed with the description of each region.

CLINICAL BOX

CRANIUM

Head Injuries

Head injuries are a major cause of death and disability. The complications of head injuries include hemorrhage, infection, and injury to the brain (e.g., concussion) and cranial nerves. Disturbance in the level of consciousness is the most common symptom of head injury. Almost 10% of all deaths in the United States are caused by injury, and approximately half of traumatic deaths involve the brain (Louis et al., 2016). Head injuries occur mostly in young persons between the ages of 15 and 24 years. The major cause of brain injury varies; however, motor vehicle and motorcycle accidents are prominent.

Headaches and Facial Pain

Few complaints are more common than *headaches* and *facial pain*. Although usually benign and frequently associated with tension, fatigue, or mild fever, headaches may indicate a serious intracranial problem such as a brain tumor, subarachnoid hemorrhage, or meningitis. *Neuralgias* (G. *algos*, pain) are characterized by severe throbbing or stabbing pain along the course of a nerve caused by a demyelinating lesion. They are a common cause of facial pain. Terms such as *facial neuralgia* describe diffuse painful sensations. Localized aches have specific names, such as *earache* (otalgia) and *toothache* (odontalgia). A sound knowledge of the clinical anatomy of the head helps in understanding the causes of headaches and facial pain.

Injury to Superciliary Arches

The superciliary arches are relatively sharp bony ridges (see Fig. 8.3). Consequently, a blow to them (e.g., during boxing) may lacerate the skin and cause bleeding. Bruising of the skin surrounding the orbit causes tissue fluid and blood to accumulate in the surrounding connective tissue, which gravitates into the superior (upper) eyelid and around the eye ("black eye"; see Fig. B8.12).

Malar Flush

The zygomatic bone was once called the malar bone; consequently, you are likely to hear the clinical term *malar flush*. This redness of the skin covering the zygomatic process (malar eminence) is associated with a rise in temperature in various fevers occurring with certain diseases, such as *tuberculosis* and *systemic lupus erythematosus disease*.

Fractures of Maxillae and Associated Bones

Dr. Léon-Clement Le Fort (a Paris surgeon and gynecologist, 1829–1893) classified three common variants of fractures of the maxillae (Fig. B8.1):

- **Le Fort I fracture:** wide variety of horizontal fractures of the maxillae, passing superior to the maxillary alveolar process (i.e., to the roots of the teeth), crossing the bony nasal septum and possibly the pterygoid plates of the sphenoid.
- **Le Fort II fracture:** passes from the posterolateral parts of the maxillary sinuses (cavities in the maxillae) superomedially through the infra-orbital foramina, lacrimals, or ethmoids to the bridge of the nose. As a result, the entire central part of the face, including the hard palate and alveolar processes, is separated from the rest of the cranium.
- **Le Fort III fracture:** horizontal fracture that passes through the superior orbital fissures and the ethmoid and nasal bones and extends laterally through the greater wings of the sphenoid and the frontozygomatic sutures. Concurrent fracturing of the zygomatic arches causes the maxillae and zygomatic bones to separate from the rest of the cranium.

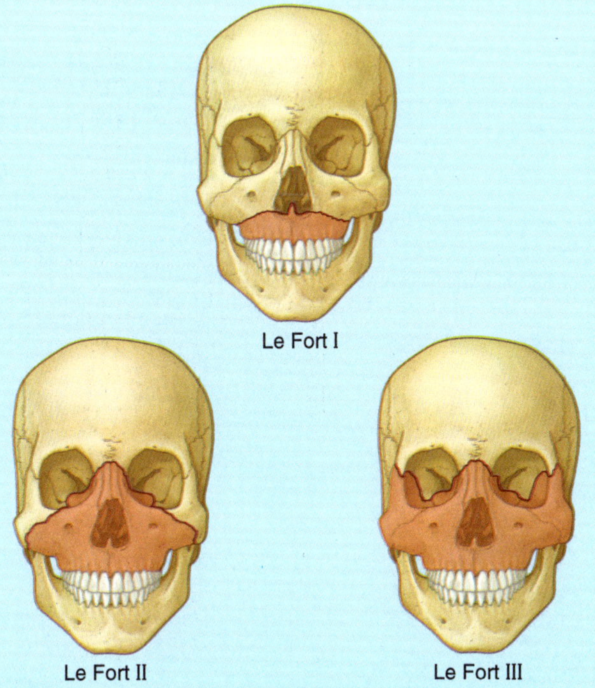

FIGURE B8.1. **Le Fort fractures.**

Fractures of Mandible

A broken mandible usually involves two fractures, which frequently occur on opposite sides of the mandible. Therefore, if one fracture is observed, a search should be made for another (e.g., a hard blow to the jaw often fractures the neck and body of the mandible in the region of the opposite canine tooth).

Fractures of the coronoid process of the mandible are uncommon and usually single (Fig. B8.2). *Fractures of the neck of the mandible* are often transverse and may be associated with dislocation of the temporomandibular joint (TMJ) on the same side. *Fractures of the angle of the mandible* are usually oblique and may involve the bony socket or alveolus of the 3rd molar tooth (Fig. B8.2, *line C*). *Fractures of the body of the mandible* frequently pass through the socket of a canine tooth (Fig. B8.2, *line D*).

Resorption of Alveolar Bone

Extraction of teeth causes the alveolar bone to resorb in the affected region(s) (Fig. B8.3). Following complete loss or extraction of maxillary teeth, the tooth sockets begin to fill in with bone, and the alveolar process begins to resorb. Similarly, extraction of mandibular teeth causes the bone of the alveolar part to resorb. Gradually, the mental foramen lies near the superior border of the body of the mandible (Fig. B8.3A–C). In some cases, the mental foramina disappear, exposing the mental nerves to injury. *Pressure from a dental prosthesis*

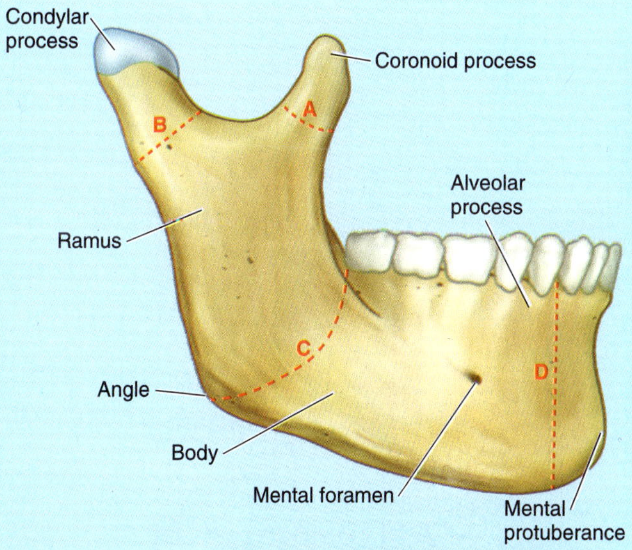

FIGURE B8.2. **Fractures of mandible.** *Line A*, fracture of the coronoid process; *line B*, fracture of the neck of the mandible; *line C*, fracture of the angle of the mandible; *line D*, fracture of the body of the mandible.

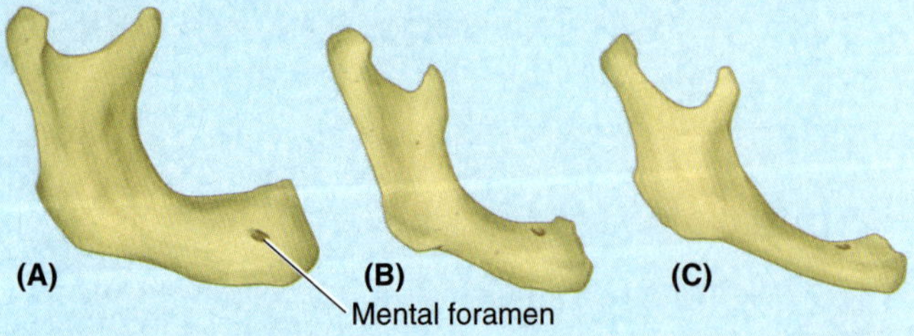

FIGURE B8.3. Stages of resorption of edentulous (toothless) alveolar bone.

(e.g., a denture resting on an exposed mental nerve) may produce pain during eating. Loss of all the teeth results in a decrease in the vertical facial dimension and *mandibular prognathism* (overclosure). Deep creases in the facial skin also appear that pass posteriorly from the corners of the mouth.

Fractures of Calvaria

The convexity of the calvaria distributes and thereby usually minimizes the effects of a blow to the head. However, hard blows in thin areas of the calvaria are likely to produce *depressed fractures*, in which a bone fragment is depressed inward, compressing and/or injuring the brain (Fig. B8.4). *Linear calvarial fractures*, the most frequent type, usually occur at the point of impact, but fracture lines often radiate away from it in two or more directions. In *comminuted fractures*, the bone is broken into several pieces. If the area of the calvaria is thick at the site of impact, the bone may bend inward without fracturing. However, a fracture may occur some distance from the site of direct trauma where the calvaria is thinner. In a *contrecoup (counterblow) fracture*, no fracture occurs at the point of impact, but one occurs on the opposite side of the cranium.

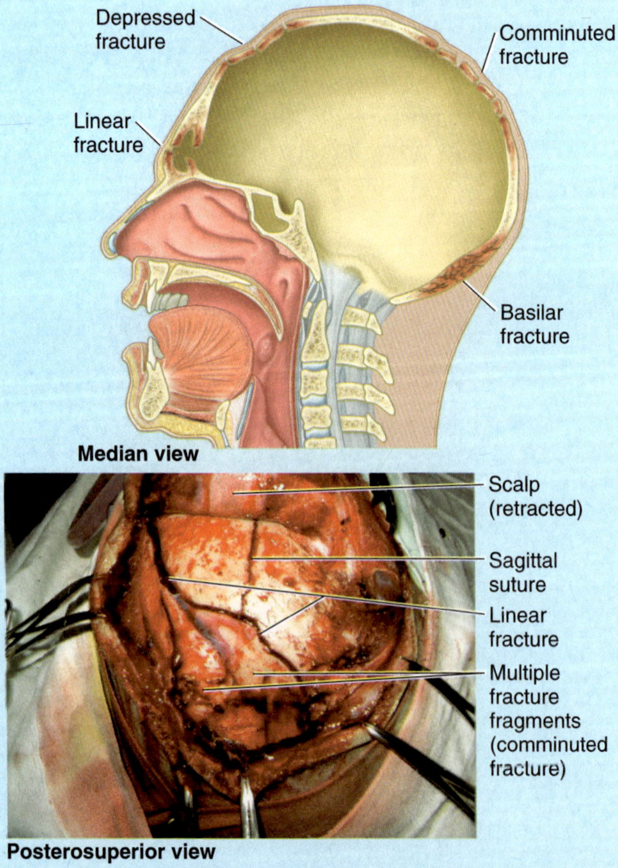

FIGURE B8.4. Fractures of calvaria.

Surgical Access to Cranial Cavity: Bone Flaps

Surgeons access the cranial cavity and brain by performing a *craniotomy*, in which a section of the neurocranium, called a bone flap, is elevated or removed (Fig. B8.5). Because the adult pericranium (periosteum of cranium) has poor osteogenic (bone-forming) properties, little regeneration occurs after bone loss (e.g., when pieces of bone are removed during repair of a comminuted cranial fracture). Surgically produced bone flaps are put back into place and wired to other parts of the calvaria or held in place temporarily with metal plates. Reintegration is most successful when the bone is reflected with its overlying muscle and skin, so that it retains its own blood supply during the procedure and after repositioning. If the bone flap is not replaced (i.e., a permanent plastic or metal plate replaces the flap), the procedure is called a *craniectomy*.

Development of Cranium AN26.6

The bones of the calvaria and some parts of the cranial base develop by *intramembranous ossification*. Most parts of the cranial base develop by

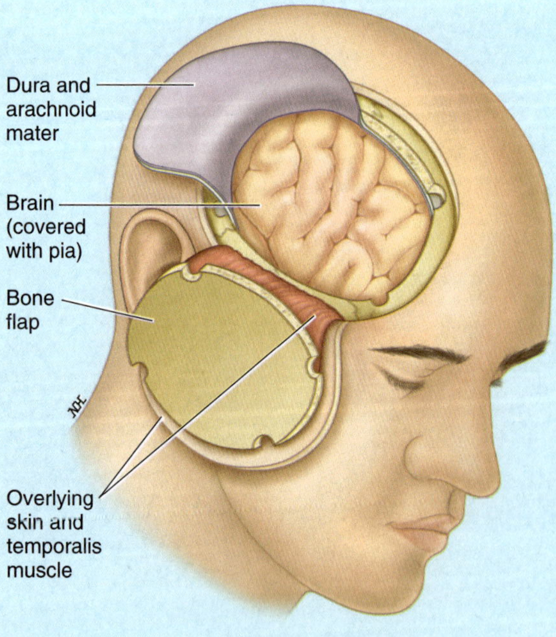

FIGURE B8.5. Craniotomy.

endochondral ossification. At birth, the bones of the calvaria are smooth and unilaminar; no diploë is present. The frontal and parietal eminences are especially prominent (Fig. B8.6). The cranium of a neonate is disproportionately large compared to other parts of the skeleton; however, the facial aspect is small compared to the *calvaria*, which forms approximately one eighth of the cranium. In the adult, the facial skeleton forms one third of the cranium. The large size of the calvaria in infants results from precocious growth and development of the brain and eyes.

The rudimentary development of the face makes the orbits appear relatively large (Fig. B8.6A). The smallness of the face results from the rudimentary development of the maxillae, mandible, and paranasal sinuses (air-filled bone cavities), the absence of erupted teeth, and the small size of the nasal cavities.

The halves of the frontal bone in the neonate are separated by the *frontal suture*, the frontal and parietal bones are separated by the *coronal suture*, and the maxillae and mandibles are separated by the *intermaxillary suture* and *mandibular symphysis* (secondary cartilaginous joint), respectively. There are no mastoid and styloid processes (Fig. B8.6A, B). Because there are no mastoid processes at birth, the facial nerves are close to the surface when they emerge from the stylomastoid foramina. Thus, the facial nerves may be injured by forceps during a difficult delivery or later by an incision posterior to the auricle of the external ear (e.g., for the surgical treatment of mastoiditis or middle ear problems). The mastoid processes form gradually during the 1st year as the sternocleidomastoid muscles complete their development and pull on the petromastoid parts of the temporal bones.

The bones of the calvaria of neonates are separated by **fontanelles** (fibrous membranes; palpable deep to the scalp, these are perceived as "soft spots"). The largest occur between the angles (corners) of the flat bones (Fig. B8.6A, B). They include the *anterior* and *posterior fontanelles* and the paired *sphenoidal* and *mastoid fontanelles*. Palpation of the fontanelles during infancy, especially the anterior and posterior ones, enables physicians to determine the following:

- Progress of growth of the frontal and parietal bones.
- Degree of hydration of an infant (a depressed fontanelle indicates dehydration).
- Level of intracranial pressure (a bulging fontanelle indicates increased pressure on the brain).

The **anterior fontanelle**, the largest one, is diamond or star shaped. It is bounded by the halves of the frontal bone anteriorly and the parietal bones posteriorly (Fig. B8.6). Therefore, it is located at the junction of the sagittal, coronal, and frontal sutures, the future site of *bregma* (Fig. 8.6; Table 8.1). By 18 months of age, the surrounding bones have fused, and the anterior fontanelle is no longer clinically palpable.

At birth, the frontal bone consists of two halves. Union of the halves begins in the 2nd year. In most cases, the

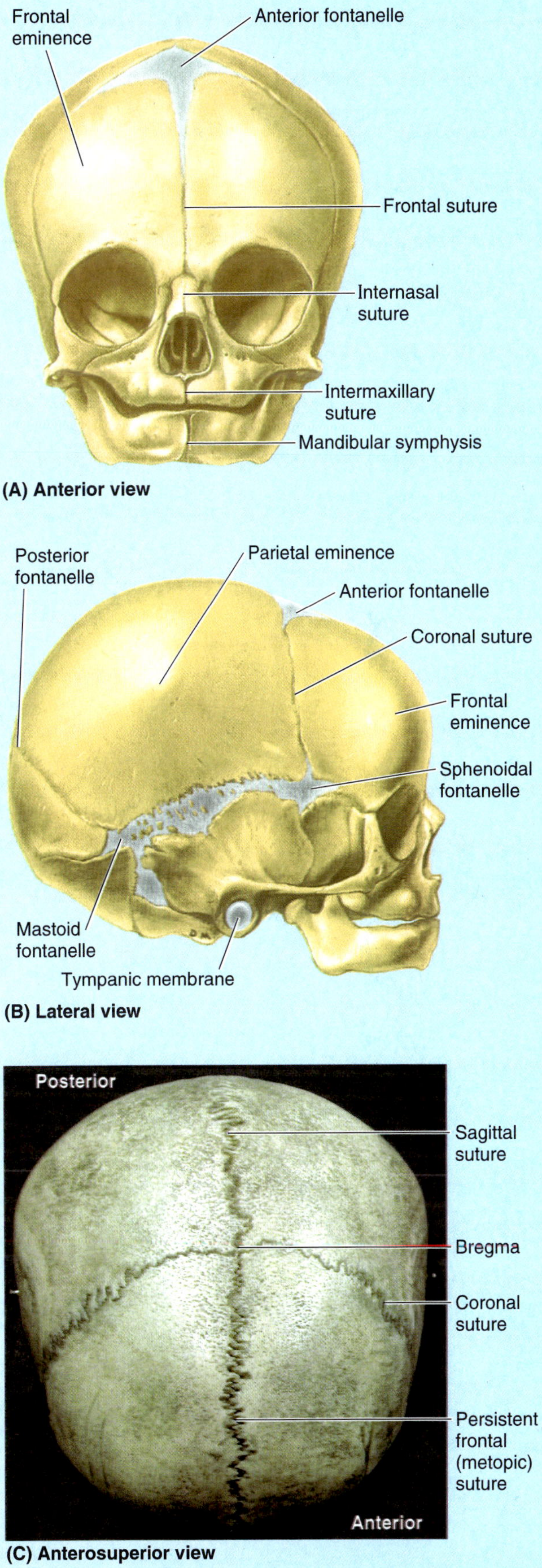

FIGURE B8.6. Cranial development.

frontal suture is obliterated by the 8th year. However, in approximately 8% of people, a remnant of the frontal suture, the **metopic suture**, persists (Figs. 8.2A and 8.3). Much less frequently, the entire suture remains (Fig. B8.6C). A persistent suture must not be interpreted as a fracture in a radiograph or another medical image (e.g., a CT scan).

The **posterior fontanelle** is triangular and bounded by the parietal bones anteriorly and the occipital bone posteriorly. It is located at the junction of the lambdoid and sagittal sutures, the future site of *lambda* (Figs. 8.7A and 8.8C). The posterior fontanelle begins to close during the first few months after birth, and by the end of the 1st year, it is small and no longer clinically palpable. The **sphenoidal** and **mastoid fontanelles**, overlain by the temporalis muscle (Fig. 8.16A), fuse during infancy and are less important clinically than the midline fontanelles. The halves of the mandible fuse early in the 2nd year. The two maxillae and nasal bones usually do not fuse.

The softness of the cranial bones in fetuses and their loose connections at the sutures and fontanelles enable the shape of the cranium to be molded during birth (Fig. B8.7). During passage of the fetus through the birth canal, the halves of the frontal bone become flat, the occipital bone is drawn out, and one parietal bone slightly overrides the other. Within a few days after birth, the shape of the neonatal cranium returns to normal. The resilience of the cranial bones of infants allows them to resist forces that would produce fractures in adults. The fibrous sutures of the calvaria also permit the cranium to enlarge during infancy and childhood. The increase in the size of the calvaria is greatest during the first 2 years, the period of most rapid brain development. The calvaria normally increases in capacity for 15–16 years. After this, the calvaria usually increases slightly in size for 3–4 years due to bone thickening.

Age Changes in Face

The mandible is the most dynamic of our bones; its size and shape and the number of teeth it normally bears undergo considerable change with age. In the neonate, the mandible consists of two halves united in the median plane by a cartilaginous joint, the *mandibular symphysis*. Union between the halves of the mandible is effected by means of fibrocartilage. This union begins during the 1st year, and the halves are fused by the end of the 2nd year. The body of the mandible in neonates is a mere shell lacking an alveolar part with each half enclosing five deciduous teeth. These teeth usually begin to erupt in infants at approximately 6 months of age. The body of the mandible elongates, particularly posterior to the mental foramen (Fig. B8.2), to accommodate this development. Later, eight permanent teeth begin to erupt during the 6th year of life (Fig. B8.8). Eruption of the permanent teeth is not complete until early adulthood.

Rapid growth of the face during infancy and early childhood coincides with the eruption of deciduous teeth. Vertical growth of the upper face results mainly from dentoalveolar development of alveolar bone. These changes are more marked after the permanent teeth erupt. Concurrent enlargement of the frontal and facial regions is associated with the increase in the size of the *paranasal sinuses*, the air-filled extensions of the nasal cavities in certain cranial bones (Fig. B8.9). Most paranasal sinuses are rudimentary or absent at birth. Growth of the paranasal sinuses is important in altering the shape of the face and in adding resonance to the voice.

Obliteration of Cranial Sutures

The obliteration of sutures between the bones of the calvaria usually begins between the ages of 30 and 40 years on the internal surface. Approximately

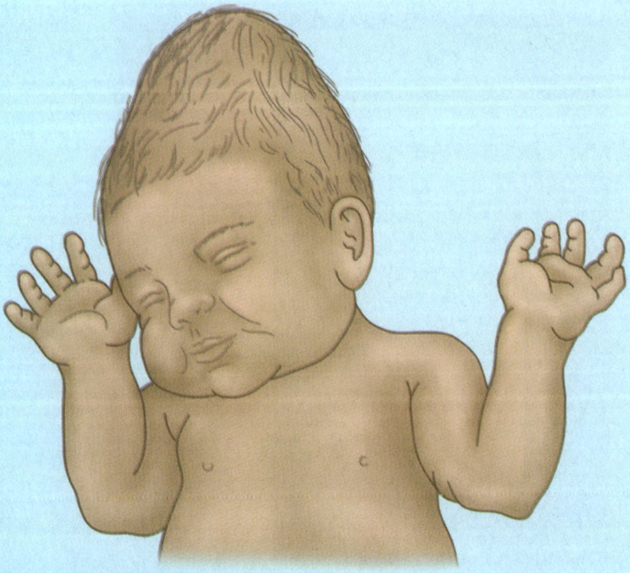

FIGURE B8.7. Molding of calvaria.

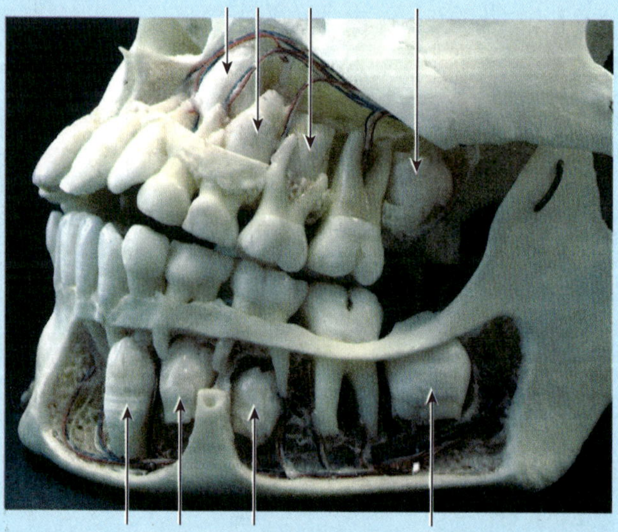

FIGURE B8.8. Left lateral view of dentition. *Arrows*, unerupted permanent teeth.

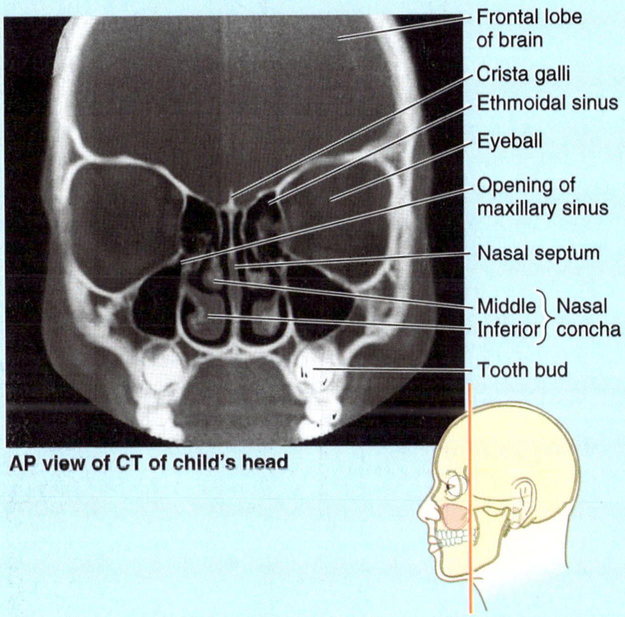

FIGURE B8.9. Paranasal sinuses in a child cranium.

10 years later, the sutures on the external surface obliterate (Fig. B8.10; cf. Fig. 8.8B). Obliteration of sutures usually begins at the bregma and continues sequentially in the sagittal, coronal, and lambdoid sutures. Closure times vary considerably.

Age Changes in Cranium

As people age, the cranial bones normally become progressively thinner and lighter, and the diploë gradually becomes filled with a gray gelatinous material. In these individuals, the bone marrow has lost its blood cells and fat, giving it a gelatinous appearance.

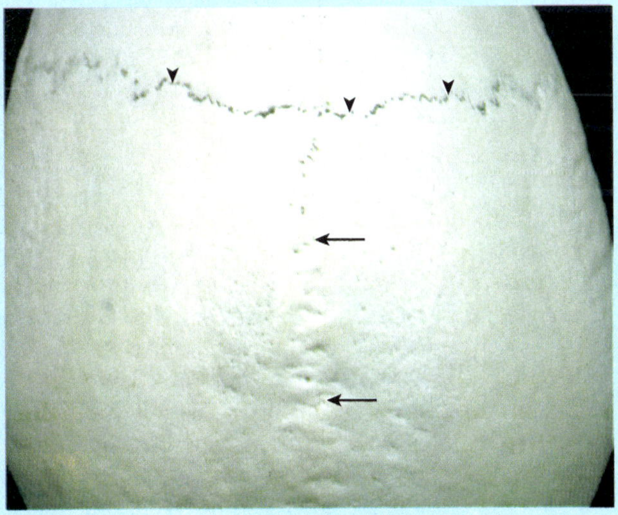

FIGURE B8.10. Obliteration (synostosis) of cranial sutures. *Arrows*, sagittal; *arrowheads*, coronal.

Craniosynostosis and Cranial Malformations

Premature closure of the cranial sutures (*primary craniosynostosis*) results in several cranial malformations (Fig. B8.11). The incidence of primary craniosynostosis is approximately 1 per 2,000 births (Kliegman et al., 2016). The cause of craniosynostosis is unknown, but genetic factors appear to be important. The prevailing hypothesis is that abnormal development of the cranial base creates exaggerated forces on the *dura mater* (outer covering membrane of the brain) that disrupt normal cranial sutural development. These malformations are more common in males than in females and are often associated with other skeletal anomalies. The type of malformed cranium that forms depends on which sutures close prematurely.

Premature closure of the sagittal suture, in which the anterior fontanelle is small or absent, results in a long, narrow, wedge-shaped cranium, a condition called *scaphocephaly* (Fig. B8.11A). When *premature closure of the coronal or the lambdoid suture* occurs on one side only, the cranium is twisted and asymmetrical, a condition known as *plagiocephaly* (Fig. B8.11B). *Premature closure of the coronal suture* results in a high, tower-like cranium, called *oxycephaly* or *turricephaly* (Fig. B8.11C). The latter type of cranial malformation is more common in females. Premature closure of sutures usually does not affect brain development.

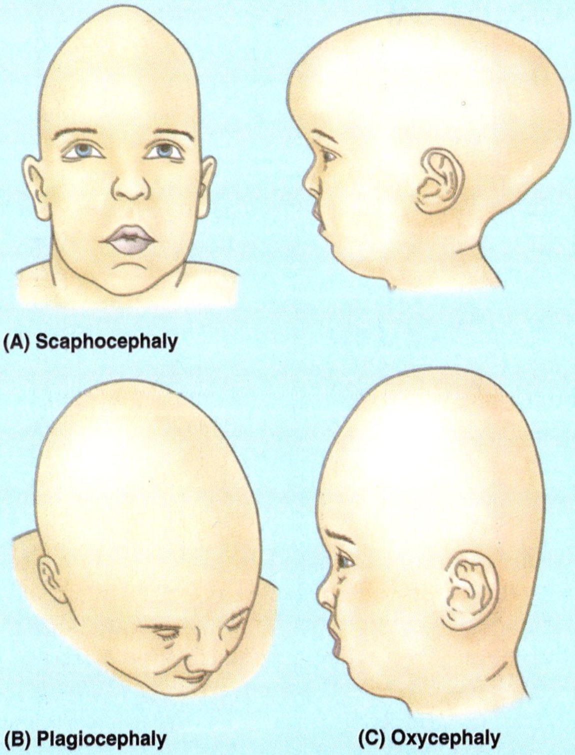

FIGURE B8.11. Cranial malformations.

The Bottom Line: Cranium

The cranium is the skeleton of the head, an amalgamation of functional components united to form a single skeletal formation. • The basic functional components include the *neurocranium*, the container of the brain and internal ears, and *viscerocranium*, providing paired orbits, nasal cavities, and teeth-bearing plates (alveolar processes) of the oral cavity. • Although some mobility between cranial bones is advantageous during birth, they become fixed together by essentially immovable joints (sutures), allowing independent movement of only the mandible. • Abundant fissures and foramina facilitate communication and passage of neurovascular structures between functional components. • The bony substance of the cranium is unequally distributed. Relatively thin (but mostly curved) flat bones provide the necessary strength to maintain cavities and protect contents. • However, the bones and processes of the neurocranium also provide proximal attachment for the strong muscles of mastication (chewing) that attach distally to the mandible. • The high traction forces generated across the nasal cavity and orbits, sandwiched between the muscle attachments, are resisted by thickened portions of the bones forming stronger pillars or buttresses. • The mostly superficial surface of the cranium provides both visible and palpable landmarks.

Internal features of the cranial base reflect the major formations of the brain that rest on it. • Bony ridges radiating from the centrally located sella turcica divide it into three cranial fossae. • The frontal lobes of the brain lie in the anterior cranial fossa. • The temporal lobes lie in the middle cranial fossa. • The hindbrain, consisting of the pons, cerebellum, and medulla, occupies the posterior cranial fossa, with the medulla continuing through the foramen magnum where it is continuous with the spinal cord.

FACE AND SCALP

Face

The **face** is the anterior aspect of the head from the forehead to the chin and from one ear to the other. The face provides our identity as an individual human. Thus, birth defects, scarring, or other alterations resulting from pathology or trauma have marked consequences beyond their physical effects.

The basic shape of the face is determined by the underlying bones. The individuality of the face results primarily from anatomical variations in the shape and relative prominence of the features of the underlying cranium; in the deposition of fatty tissue; in the color and effects of aging on the overlying skin; and in the abundance, nature, and placement of hair on the face and scalp. The relatively large size of the **buccal fat-pads** in infants prevents collapse of the cheeks during sucking and produces their chubby-cheeked appearance. Growth of the facial bones takes longer than those of the calvaria. The ethmoid bone, orbital cavities, and superior parts of the nasal cavities have nearly completed their growth by the 7th year. Expansion of the orbits and growth of the nasal septum carry the maxillae infero-anteriorly. Considerable facial growth occurs during childhood as the paranasal sinuses develop and permanent teeth erupt.

The face plays an important role in communication. Our interactions with others take place largely via the face (including the ears) and thus the term *interface* for a site of interactions. Whereas the shape and features of the face provide our identity, much of our effect on others and their perceptions about us result from the way we use facial muscles to make the slight alterations in the features that constitute facial expression.

Scalp

The **scalp** consists of skin (normally hair bearing) and subcutaneous tissue that cover the neurocranium from the superior nuchal lines on the occipital bone to the supra-orbital margins of the frontal bone (Figs. 8.3 and 8.4A). Laterally, the scalp extends over the temporal fascia to the zygomatic arches. AN27.1

The scalp is composed of five layers, the first three of which are connected intimately and move as a unit (e.g., when wrinkling the forehead and moving the scalp). Each letter in the word *scalp* serves as a memory key for one of its five layers (Fig. 8.15A):

1. Skin: thin, except in the occipital region, contains many sweat and sebaceous glands and hair follicles. It has an abundant arterial supply and good venous and lymphatic drainage.
2. Connective tissue: forms the thick, dense, richly vascularized subcutaneous layer that is well supplied with cutaneous nerves.
3. Aponeurosis (**epicranial aponeurosis**): the broad, strong, tendinous sheet that covers the calvaria and serves as the attachment for muscle bellies converging from the forehead and occiput (**occipitofrontalis muscle**) (Fig. 8.15B) and from the temporal bones on each side (**temporoparietalis** and **superior auricular muscles**). Collectively, these structures constitute the musculo-aponeurotic **epicranius**. The *frontal belly of the occipitofrontalis* pulls the scalp anteriorly, wrinkles the forehead, and elevates the eyebrows. The *occipital belly of the occipitofrontalis* pulls the scalp posteriorly, smoothing the skin of the forehead. The superior auricular muscle (a specialized posterior part of the temporoparietalis)

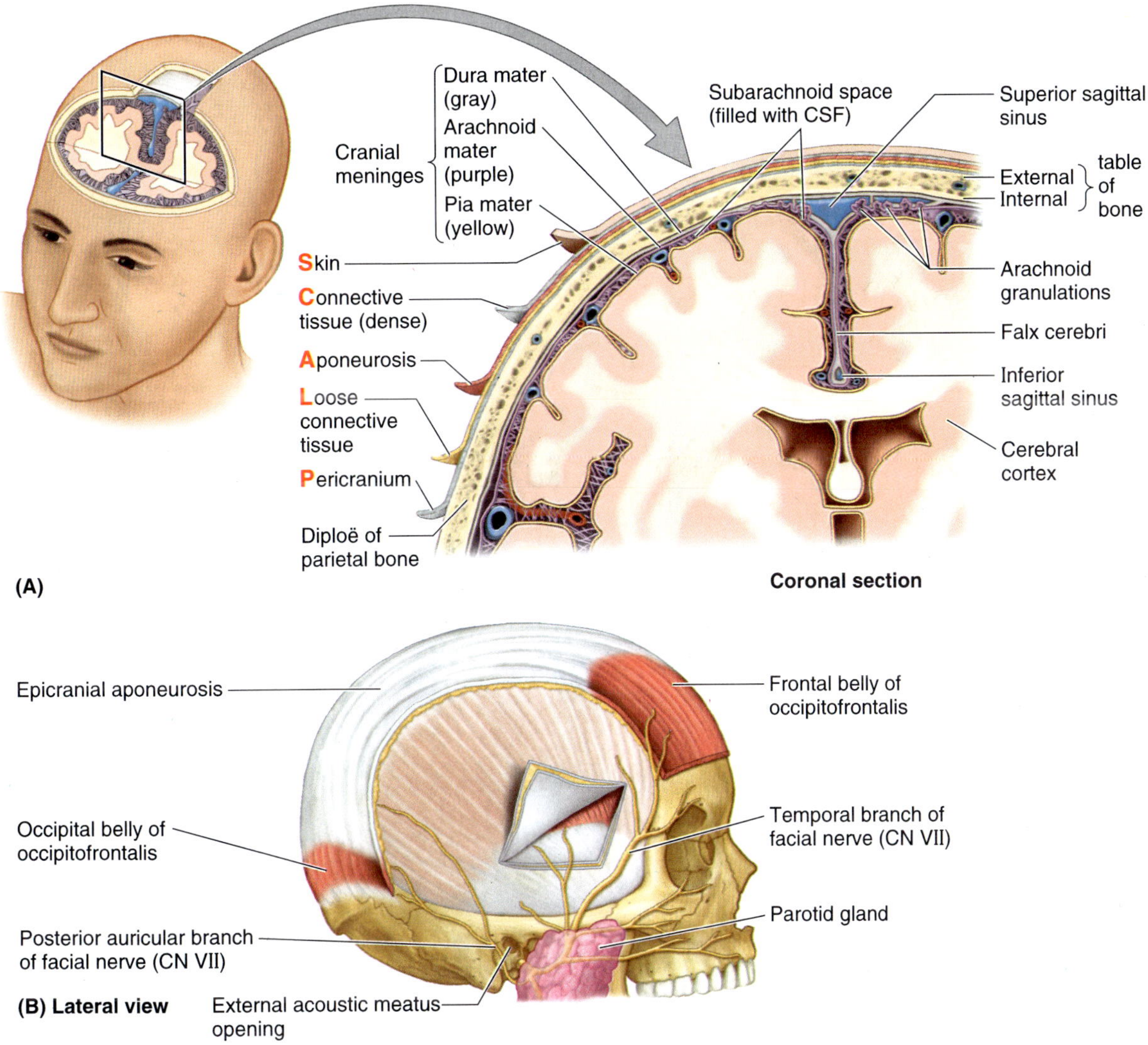

FIGURE 8.15. Layers of scalp, cranium, and meninges. A. The skin is bound tightly to the epicranial aponeurosis, which moves freely over the pericranium and cranium because of the intervening loose connective tissue. *Aponeurosis* refers to the epicranial aponeurosis, the flat intermediate tendon of the occipitofrontalis muscle. The cranial meninges and the subarachnoid (leptomeningeal) space are shown. *CSF*, cerebrospinal fluid. **B.** The occipitofrontalis muscle. Innervation of the two bellies by the posterior auricular and temporal branches of the facial nerve is demonstrated.

elevates the auricle of the external ear. All parts of the epicranius (muscle and aponeurosis) are innervated by the facial nerve.

4. **Loose** areolar tissue: a sponge-like layer including potential spaces that may distend with fluid as a result of injury or infection. This layer allows free movement of the **scalp proper** (the first three layers—skin, connective tissue, and epicranial aponeurosis) over the underlying calvaria.
5. **Pericranium**: a dense layer of connective tissue that forms the external periosteum of the neurocranium. It is firmly attached but can be stripped from the crania of living persons, except where the pericranium is continuous with the fibrous tissue in the cranial sutures.

AN28.1 Muscles of Face and Scalp

AN28.6 The facial muscles (muscles of facial expression) are in the
AN43.5 subcutaneous tissue of the anterior and posterior scalp, face, and neck. They move the skin and change facial expressions to convey mood. Most muscles attach to bone or fascia and produce their effects by pulling the skin. The muscles of the scalp and face are illustrated in Figure 8.16, and their attachments and actions are provided in Table 8.3. Certain muscles and/or muscle groups will be discussed in further detail.

All muscles of facial expression develop from mesoderm in the second pharyngeal arches. A subcutaneous muscular sheet forms during embryonic development that spreads over the neck and face, carrying branches of the nerve of the arch (the facial nerve, CN VII) with it to supply all the muscles formed from the arch (Moore et al., 2016). The muscular sheet differentiates into muscles that surround the facial orifices (mouth, eyes, and nose), serving as sphincter and dilator mechanisms that also produce many facial expressions (Fig. 8.17). Because of their common embryological origin, the platysma and facial muscles are often fused, and their fibers are frequently intermingled.

(*continued on p.* 903)

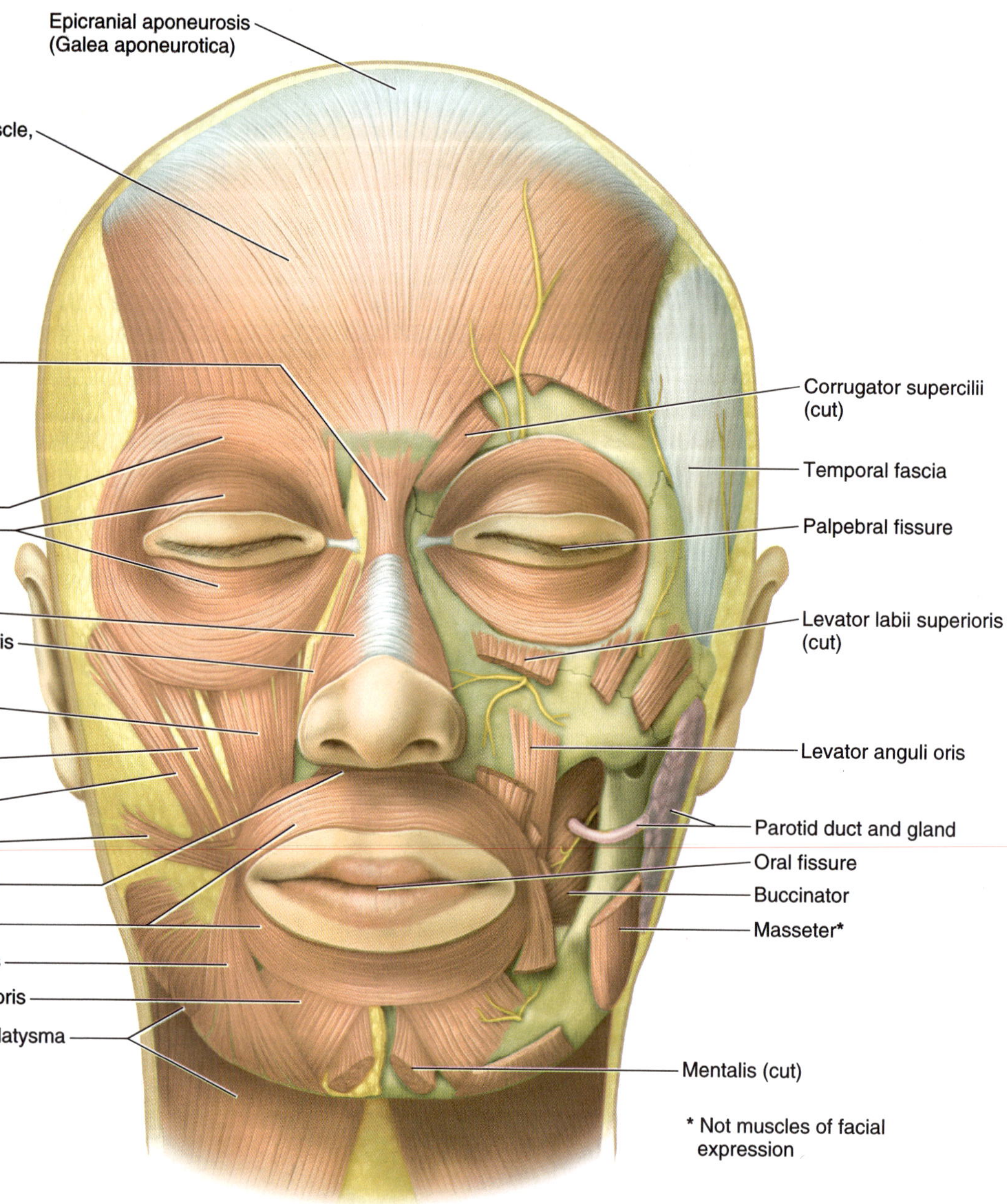

FIGURE 8.16. Muscles of scalp and face.

TABLE 8.3. MUSCLES OF SCALP AND FACE

Muscle[a]	Origin	Insertion	Main Action(s)
Occipitofrontalis			
Front belly[2]	Epicranial aponeurosis	Skin and subcutaneous tissue of eyebrows and forehead	Elevates eyebrows and wrinkles skin of forehead; protracts scalp (indicating surprise or curiosity)
Occipital belly[1]	Lateral two thirds of superior nuchal line	Epicranial aponeurosis	Retracts scalp; increasing effectiveness of frontal belly
Orbicularis oculi (orbital sphincter)[2,3]	Medial orbital margin; medial palpebral ligament; lacrimal bone	Skin around margin of orbit; superior and inferior tarsal plates	Closes eyelids: palpebral part does so gently; orbital part tightly (winking)
Corrugator supercilii[2]	Medial end of superciliary arch	Skin superior to middle of supra-orbital margin and superciliary arch	Draws eyebrow medially and inferiorly, creating vertical wrinkles above nose (demonstrating concern or worry)

(Continued)

TABLE 8.3. MUSCLES OF SCALP AND FACE (Continued)

Muscle[a]	Origin	Insertion	Main Action(s)
Procerus plus **transverse part of nasalis**[4]	Fascia aponeurosis covering nasal bone and lateral nasal cartilage	Skin of inferior forehead, between eyebrows	Depresses medial end of eyebrow; wrinkles skin over dorsum of nose (conveying disdain or dislike)
Alar part of nasalis plus **levator labii superioris alaeque nasii**[4]	Frontal process of maxilla (inferomedial margin of orbit)	Major alar cartilage	Depresses ala laterally, dilating anterior nasal aperture (i.e., "flaring nostrils," as during anger or exertion)
Orbicularis oris (oral sphincter)[4]	Medial maxilla and mandible; deep surface of peri-oral skin; angle of mouth (modiolus)	Mucous membrane of lips	Tonus closes oral fissure; phasic contraction compresses and protrudes lips (kissing) or resists distension (when blowing)
Levator labii superioris[4]	Infra-orbital margin (maxilla)	Skin of upper lip	Part of dilators of mouth; retract (elevate) and/or evert upper lip; deepen nasolabial sulcus (showing sadness)
Zygomaticus minor[4]	Anterior aspect, zygomatic bone		
Buccinator (cheek muscle)[4]	Mandible, alveolar process of maxilla and alveolar part of mandible, pterygomandibular raphe	Angle of mouth (modiolus); orbicularis oris	Presses cheek against molar teeth; works with tongue to keep food between occlusal surfaces and out of oral vestibule; resists distension (when blowing)
Zygomaticus major[4]	Lateral aspect of zygomatic bone	Angle of mouth (modiolus)	Part of dilators of mouth; elevate labial commissure—bilaterally to smile (happiness); unilaterally to sneer (disdain)
Levator anguli oris[4]	Infra-orbital maxilla (canine fossa)		Part of dilators of mouth; widens oral fissure, as when grinning or grimacing
Risorius[4]	Parotid fascia and buccal skin (highly variable)		Part of dilators of mouth; depresses labial commissure bilaterally to frown (sadness)
Depressor anguli oris[5]	Anterolateral base of mandible		
Depressor labii inferioris[5]	Platysma and anterolateral body of mandible	Skin of lower lip	Part of dilators of mouth; retracts (depresses) and/or everts lower lip (pouting, sadness)
Mentalis[5]	Body of mandible (anterior to roots of inferior incisors)	Skin of chin (mentolabial sulcus)	Elevates and protrudes lower lip; elevates skin of chin (showing doubt)
Platysma[6]	Subcutaneous tissue of infraclavicular and supraclavicular regions	Base of mandible; skin of cheek and lower lip; angle of mouth (modiolus); orbicularis oris	Depresses mandible (against resistance); tenses skin of inferior face and neck (conveying tension and stress)

[a]All facial muscles are innervated by the facial nerve (CN VII) via its posterior auricular branch (*1*) or via the temporal (2), zygomatic (3), buccal (4), marginal mandibular (5), or cervical (6) branches of the parotid plexus.

MUSCLES OF SCALP, FOREHEAD, AND EYEBROWS

The **occipitofrontalis** is a flat digastric muscle, with **occipital** and **frontal bellies** that share a common tendon, the **epicranial aponeurosis** (Figs. 8.15 and 8.16A, B; Table 8.3). Because the aponeurosis is a layer of the scalp, independent contraction of the occipital belly retracts the scalp and contraction of the frontal belly protracts it. Acting simultaneously, the occipital belly, with bony attachments, works as a synergist with the frontal belly, which has no bony attachments, to elevate the eyebrows and produce transverse wrinkles across the forehead. This gives the face a surprised look.

MUSCLES OF MOUTH, LIPS, AND CHEEKS

The lips, shape, and degree of opening of the mouth are important for clear speech. In addition, we add emphasis to our vocal communication with our facial expressions. Several muscles alter the shape of the mouth and lips during speaking as well as during such activities as singing, whistling, and mimicry. The shape of the mouth and lips is controlled by a complex three-dimensional group of muscular slips, which include the following (Fig. 8.16B, C; Table 8.3):

- Elevators, retractors, and evertors of the upper lip.
- Depressors, retractors, and evertors of the lower lip.
- The orbicularis oris, the sphincter around the mouth.
- The buccinator in the cheek.

At rest, the lips are in gentle contact and the teeth are close together.

The **orbicularis oris**, the first of the series of sphincters associated with the alimentary system (digestive tract), encircles the mouth within the lips, controlling entry and exit through the **oral fissure** (L. *rima oris*, the opening between the lips). The orbicularis oris is important during articulation (speech).

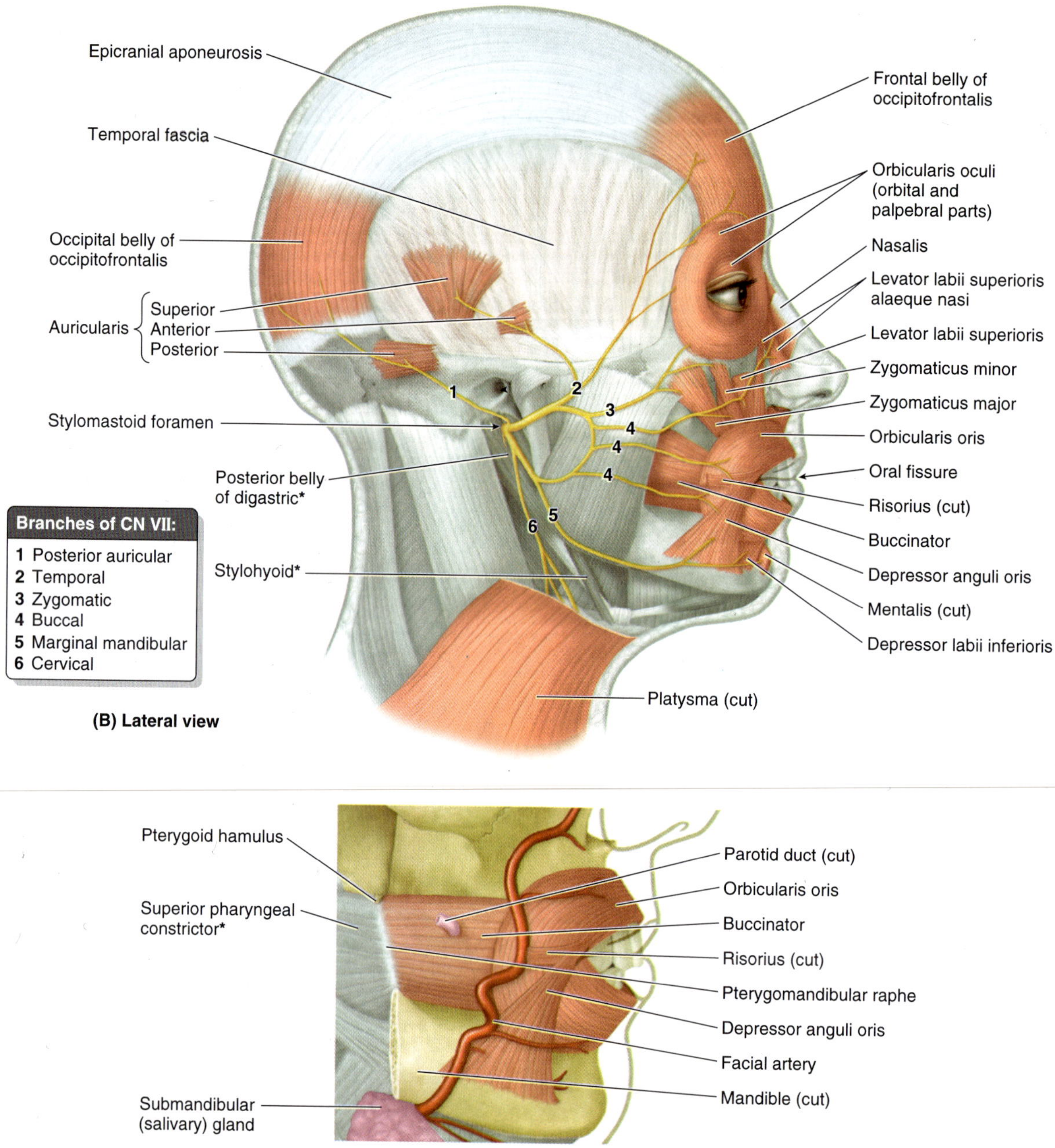

(B) Lateral view

(C) Lateral view of oral and buccal regions

*Not muscles of facial expression

FIGURE 8.16. (Continued)

The **buccinator** (L. trumpeter) is a thin, flat, rectangular muscle that attaches laterally to the alveolar process of the maxillae and alveolar part of the mandible, opposite the molar teeth. It also attaches to the **pterygomandibular raphe**, a tendinous thickening of the buccopharyngeal fascia separating and giving origin to the superior pharyngeal constrictor posteriorly. The buccinator occupies a deeper, more medially placed plane than the other facial muscles, passing deep to the mandible so that it is more closely related to the buccal mucosa than to the skin of the face. The buccinator, active in smiling, also keeps the cheek taut, thereby preventing it from folding and being injured during chewing.

Anteriorly, the fibers of the buccinator mingle medially with those of the orbicularis oris, and the tonus of the two muscles compresses the cheeks and lips against the teeth and gums. The tonic contraction of the buccinator, and especially of the orbicularis oris, provides a gentle but continual resistance to the tendency of the teeth to tilt in an outward direction. In the presence of a short upper lip, or retractors that remove this force, crooked or protrusive ("buck") teeth develop.

The orbicularis oris (from the labial aspect) and buccinator (from the buccal aspect) work with the tongue (from the lingual aspect) to keep food between the occlusal surfaces of the teeth during mastication (chewing) and to prevent food

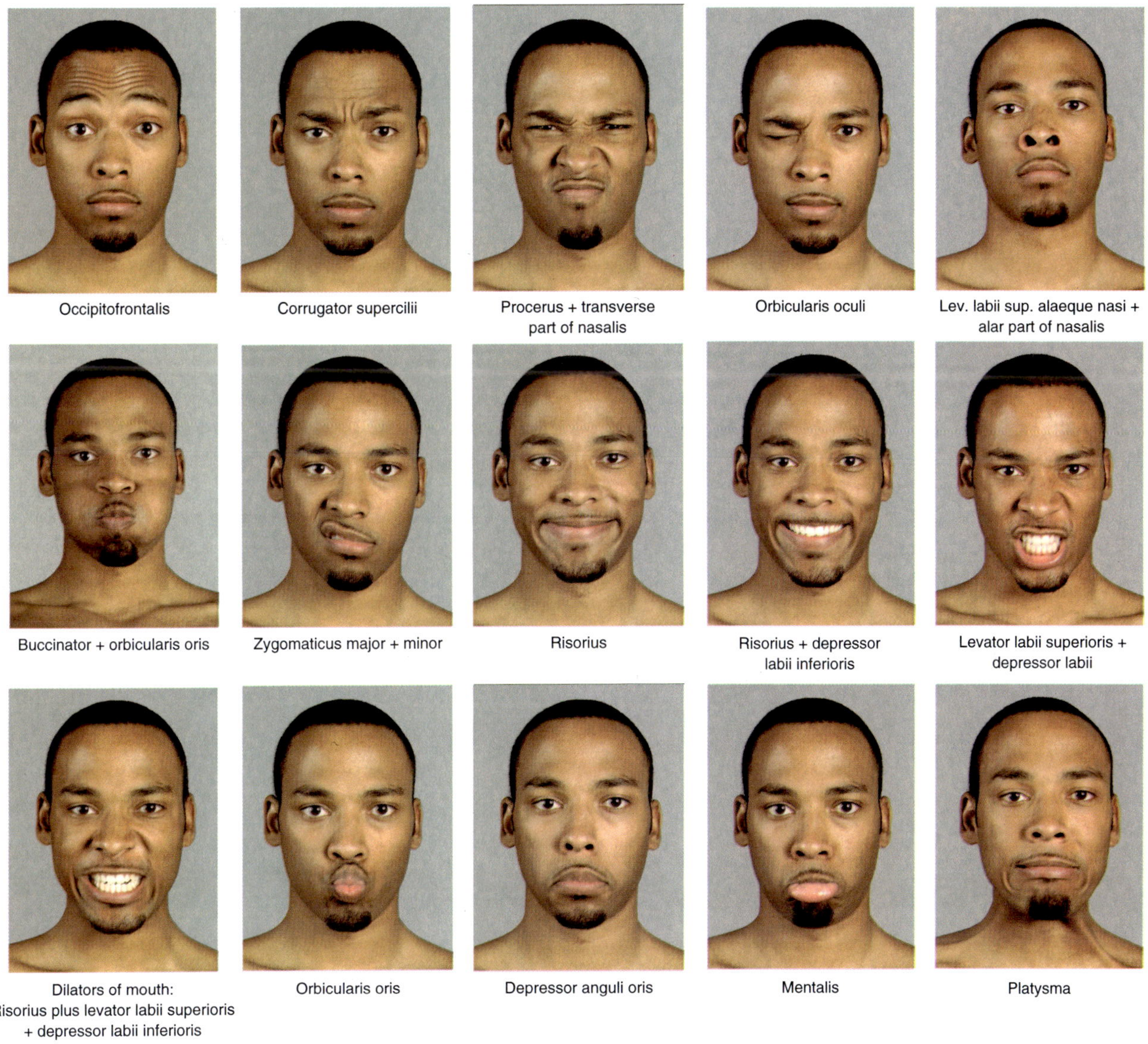

AN43.5 **FIGURE 8.17. Muscles of facial expression in action.** These muscles are superficial sphincters and dilators of the orifices of the head. The facial muscles, supplied by the facial nerve (CN VII), are attached to and move the skin of the face, producing many facial expressions.

from accumulating in the oral vestibule. The buccinator also helps the cheeks resist the forces generated by whistling and sucking. The buccinator was given its name because it compresses the cheeks (L. *buccae*) during blowing (e.g., when a musician plays a wind instrument). Some trumpeters (notably the late Dizzy Gillespie) stretch their buccinators and other cheek muscles so much that their cheeks balloon out when they blow forcibly on their instruments.

Several dilator muscles radiate from the lips and angles of the mouth, somewhat like the spokes of a wheel, retracting the various borders of the *oral fissure* collectively, in groups, or individually. Lateral to the angles of the mouth or **commissures of the lips** (the junctions of the upper and lower lips), fibers of as many as nine facial muscles interlace or merge in a highly variable and multiplanar formation called the **modiolus**, which is largely responsible for the occurrence of dimples in many people.

The **platysma** (G. flat plate) is a broad, thin sheet of muscle in the subcutaneous tissue of the neck (Fig. 8.16A, B; Table 8.3). The anterior borders of the two muscles decussate over the chin and blend with the facial muscles. Acting from its superior attachment, the platysma tenses the skin, producing vertical skin ridges, conveying great stress, and releasing pressure on the superficial veins. Acting from its inferior attachment, the platysma helps depress the mandible and draw the corners of the mouth inferiorly, as in a grimace.

MUSCLES OF ORBITAL OPENING

The function of the eyelids (L. *palpebrae*) is to protect the eyeballs from injury and excessive light. The eyelids also keep the cornea moist by spreading the tears.

The **orbicularis oculi** closes the eyelids and wrinkles the forehead vertically (Figs. 8.16A, B and 8.18; Table 8.3).

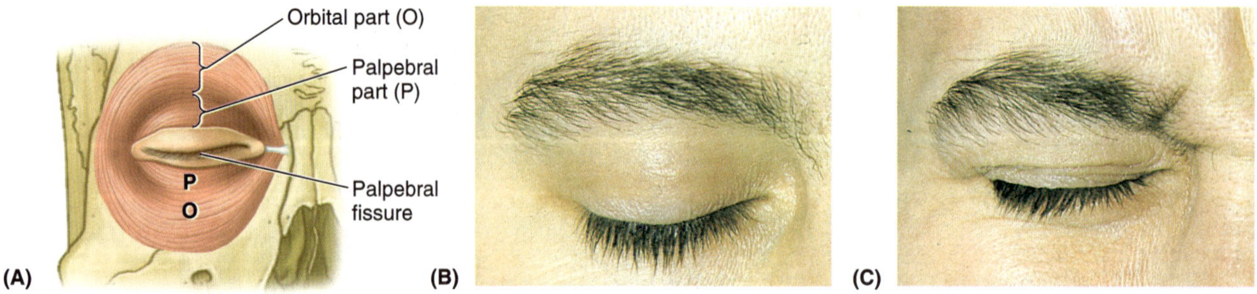

FIGURE 8.18. Disposition and actions of orbicularis oculi muscle. A. The orbital and palpebral parts of the orbicularis oculi are demonstrated. **B.** The palpebral part gently closes the eyelids. **C.** The orbital part tightly closes the eyelids.

Its fibers sweep in concentric circles around the orbital margin and eyelids. Contraction of these fibers narrows the **palpebral fissure** (aperture between the eyelids) and assists the flow of lacrimal fluid (tears) by bringing the lids together laterally first, closing the palpebral fissure in a lateral to medial direction. The orbicularis oculi muscle consists of three parts:

1. *Palpebral part*: arising from the **medial palpebral ligament** and mostly located within the eyelids, gently closes the eyelids (as in blinking or sleep) to keep the cornea from drying.
2. *Lacrimal part*: passing posterior to the *lacrimal sac*, draws the eyelids medially, aiding drainage of tears.
3. *Orbital part*: overlying the orbital rim and attached to the frontal bone and maxilla medially, tightly closes the eyelids (as in winking or squinting) to protect the eyeballs against glare and dust.

When all three parts of the orbicularis oculi contract, the eyes are firmly closed (Figs. 8.17 and 8.18C).

MUSCLES OF NOSE AND EARS

As demonstrated in the clinical box "Flaring of Nostrils," the muscles of the nose may provide evidence of breathing behaviors. Otherwise, although these muscles are functionally important in certain mammals (elephants, tapirs, rabbits, and some diving mammals), they are relatively unimportant in humans, except in terms of facial expression and in the specialized field of aesthetic plastic surgery. The muscles of the ears, important in animals capable of cocking or directing the ears toward the sources of sounds, are even less critical in humans.

Nerves of Face and Scalp

Cutaneous (sensory) innervation of the face and anterosuperior part of the scalp is provided primarily by the *trigeminal nerve* (CN V), whereas motor innervation to the facial muscles is provided by the *facial nerve* (CN VII).

CUTANEOUS NERVES OF FACE AND SCALP

N27.1 The **trigeminal nerve** (CN V) originates from the lateral
N28.2 surface of the pons of the midbrain by two roots: motor and sensory. These roots are comparable to the motor (anterior) and sensory (posterior) roots of spinal nerves. The sensory root of CN V consists of the central processes of pseudounipolar neurons located in a sensory ganglion (**trigeminal ganglion**) at the distal end of the root, which is bypassed by the multipolar neuronal axons making up the motor root. CN V is the sensory nerve for the face and the motor nerve for the muscles of mastication and several small muscles (Fig. 8.19).

The peripheral processes of the neurons of the trigeminal ganglion constitute three divisions of the nerve: the *ophthalmic nerve* (CN V_1), the *maxillary nerve* (CN V_2), and the sensory component of the *mandibular nerve* (CN V_3). These nerves are named according to their main areas of termination: the eye, maxilla, and mandible, respectively. The first two divisions (ophthalmic and maxillary nerves) are wholly sensory. The mandibular nerve is largely sensory, but it also receives the motor fibers (axons) from the motor root of CN V that mainly supply the muscles of mastication. The cutaneous nerves derived from each division of CN V are illustrated in Figure 8.20, and the origin, course, and distribution of each nerve are listed and described in Table 8.4.

The cutaneous nerves of the neck overlap those of the face. Cutaneous branches of cervical nerves from the *cervical plexus* extend over the posterior aspect of the neck and scalp. The **great auricular nerve** innervates the inferior aspect of the auricle (external ear) and much of the parotid region of the face (the area overlying the angle of the jaw).

OPHTHALMIC NERVE

The **ophthalmic nerve** (CN V_1), the superior division of the trigeminal nerve, is the smallest of the three divisions of CN V. It arises from the trigeminal ganglion as a wholly sensory nerve and supplies the area of skin derived from the embryonic *frontonasal prominence* (Moore et al., 2016). As CN V_1 enters the orbit through the *superior orbital fissure*, it trifurcates into the frontal, nasociliary, and lacrimal nerves (Fig. 8.19). Except for the external nasal nerve, the cutaneous branches of CN V_1 reach the skin of the face via the orbital opening (Fig. 8.21).

The **frontal nerve**, the largest branch produced by the trifurcation of CN V_1, runs along the roof of the orbit toward the orbital opening, bifurcating approximately midway into the cutaneous **supra-orbital** and **supratrochlear nerves**, distributed to the forehead and scalp (Figs. 8.21 and 8.22).

(*continued on p.* 910)

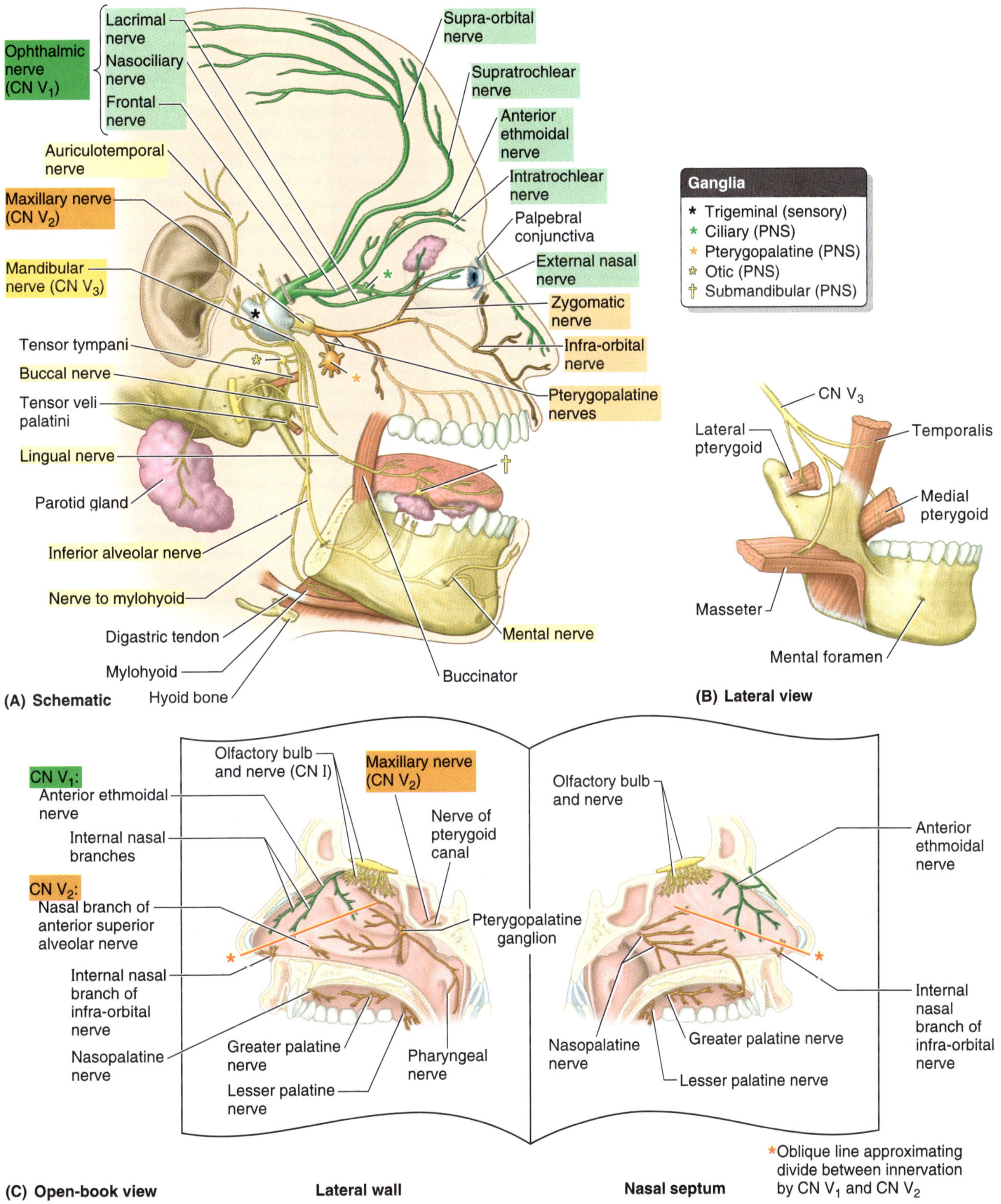

FIGURE 8.19. Distribution of trigeminal nerve (CN V). A. The three divisions of CN V arise from the trigeminal ganglion. In addition to the trigeminal ganglion, a sensory ganglion (similar to the sensory or dorsal root ganglia of spinal nerves) and four parasympathetic ganglia (three of which are shown here) are associated with the branches of the trigeminal nerve. **B.** Branches of the mandibular nerve (CN V_3) pass to the muscles of mastication. **C.** This "opened book" view of the lateral wall and septum of the right nasal cavity demonstrates superficial and deep distribution of CN V_1, and CN V_2 (and, incidentally, CN I) to the nasal and upper oral cavity, in and near the midline of the head.

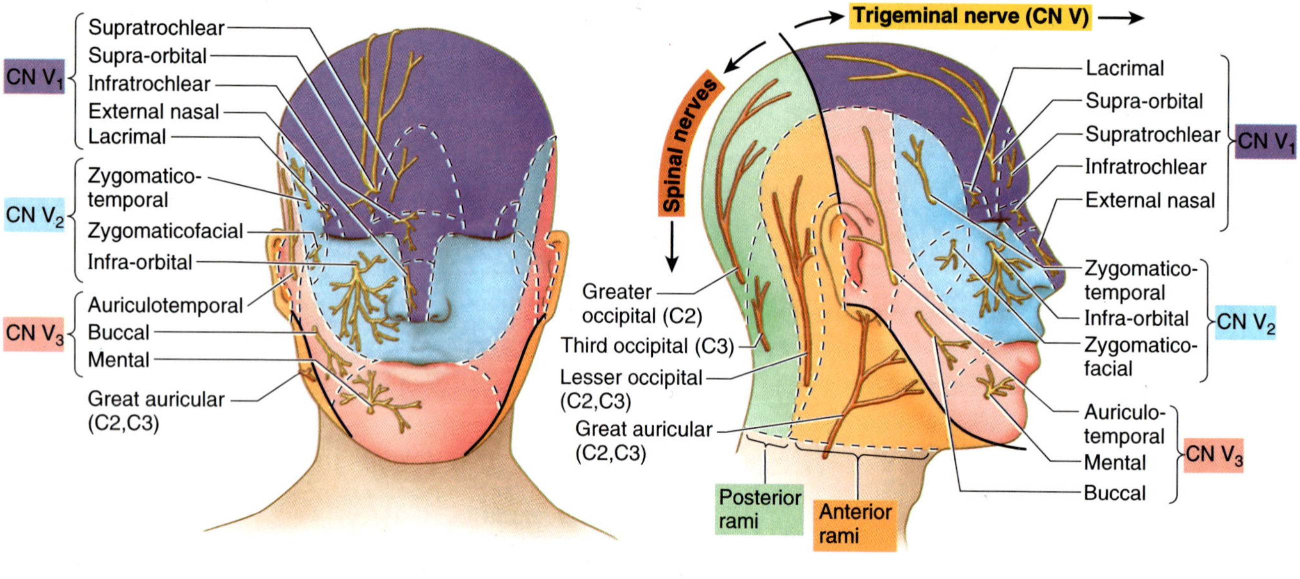

(A) Anterior view **(B) Lateral view**

FIGURE 8.20. Cutaneous nerves of face and scalp.

TABLE 8.4. CUTANEOUS NERVES OF FACE AND SCALP

Nerve	Origin	Course	Distribution
Cutaneous nerves derived from ophthalmic nerve (CN V_1)			
Supra-orbital	Largest branch from bifurcation of *frontal nerve*, approximately in middle of orbital roof	Continues anteriorly along roof of orbit, emerging via supra-orbital notch or foramen; ascends forehead, breaking into branches	Mucosa of *frontal sinus;* skin and conjunctiva of middle of *superior eyelid;* skin and pericranium of *anterolateral forehead* and *scalp* to vertex (interauricular line)
Supratrochlear	Smaller branch from bifurcation of *frontal nerve*, approximately in middle of orbital roof	Continues anteromedially along roof of orbit, passing lateral to trochlea and ascending forehead	Skin and conjunctive of medical aspect of *superior eyelid;* skin and pericranium of *anteromedial forehead*
Lacrimal	Smallest branch from trifurcation of *CN V_1* proximal to superior orbital fissure	Runs superolaterally through orbit, receiving secretomotor fibers via a communicating branch from the zygomaticotemporal nerve	*Lacrimal gland* (secretomotor fibers); small area of skin and conjunctive of *lateral part of superior eyelid*
Infratrochlear	Terminal branch (with anterior ethmoidal nerve) of *nasociliary nerve*	Follows medial wall of orbit, passing inferior to trochlea	Skin lateral to *root of nose;* skin and conjunctiva of *eyelids adjacent to medial canthus*, *lacrimal sac*, and *lacrimal caruncle*
External nasal	Terminal branch of *anterior ethmoidal nerve*	Emerges from nasal cavity by passing between nasal bone and lateral nasal cartilage	Skin of nasal *ala*, *vestibule*, and *dorsum of nose*, including *apex*
Cutaneous nerves derived from maxillary nerve (CN V_2)			
Infra-orbital	Continuation of *CN V_2* distal to its entrance into the orbit via the inferior orbital fissure	Traverses infra-orbital groove and canal in orbital floor, giving rise to superior alveolar branches; then emerges via infra-orbital foramen, immediately dividing into inferior palpebral, internal and external nasal, and superior labial branches	Mucosa of *maxillary sinus;* premolar, canine, and incisor *maxillary teeth;* skin and conjunctiva of *inferior eyelid;* skin of *cheek*, *lateral nose*, and antero-inferior *nasal septum*; skin and oral mucosa of *superior lip*
Zygomaticofacial	Smaller terminal branch (with zygomaticotemporal nerve) of *zygomatic nerve*	Traverses zygomaticofacial canal in zygomatic bone at inferolateral angle of orbit	Skin on prominence of *cheek*
Zygomaticotemporal	Larger terminal branch (with zygomaticofacial nerve) of *zygomatic nerve*	Sends communicating branch to lacrimal nerve in orbit; then passes to temporal fossa via zygomaticotemporal canal in zygomatic bone	Hairless skin *anterior part of temporal fossa*

(Continued)

TABLE 8.4. CUTANEOUS NERVES OF FACE AND SCALP (Continued)

Nerve	Origin	Course	Distribution
Cutaneous nerves derived from mandibular nerve (CN V_3)			
Auriculotemporal	In infratemporal fossa via two roots from *posterior trunk of* CN V_3 *that encircle middle meningeal artery*	Passes posteriorly deep to ramus of mandible and superior deep part of parotid gland, emerging posterior to temporomandibular joint	Skin anterior to auricle and posterior two thirds of *temporal region;* skin of tragus and adjacent helix of *auricle;* skin of roof of *external acoustic meatus;* and skin of superior *tympanic membrane*
Buccal	In infratemporal fossa as sensory branch of *anterior trunk of* CN V_3	Passes between two parts of lateral pterygoid muscle, emerging anteriorly from cover of ramus of mandible and masseter, uniting with buccal branches of facial nerve	Skin and oral mucosa of *cheek* (overlying and deep to anterior part of buccinator); *buccal gingivae* (gums) adjacent to second and third molars
Mental	Terminal branch of *inferior alveolar nerve* (CN V_3)	Emerges from mandibular canal via mental foramen in anterolateral aspect of body of mandible	Skin of *chin* and skin; oral mucosa of *inferior lip*
Cutaneous nerves derived from anterior rami of cervical spinal nerves			
Great auricular	Spinal nerves C2 and C3 via cervical plexus	Ascends vertically across sternocleidomastoid, posterior to external jugular vein	Skin overlying angle of mandible and inferior lobe of auricle; parotid sheath
Lesser occipital		Follows posterior border of sternocleidomastoid; then ascends posterior to auricle	Scalp posterior to auricle
Cutaneous nerves derived from posterior rami of cervical spinal nerves			
Greater occipital nerve	As medial branch of posterior ramus of spinal nerve C2	Emerges between axis and obliquus capitis inferior; then pierces trapezius	Scalp of occipital region
Third occipital nerve	As lateral branch of posterior ramus of spinal nerve C3	Pierces trapezius	Scalp of lower occipital and suboccipital regions

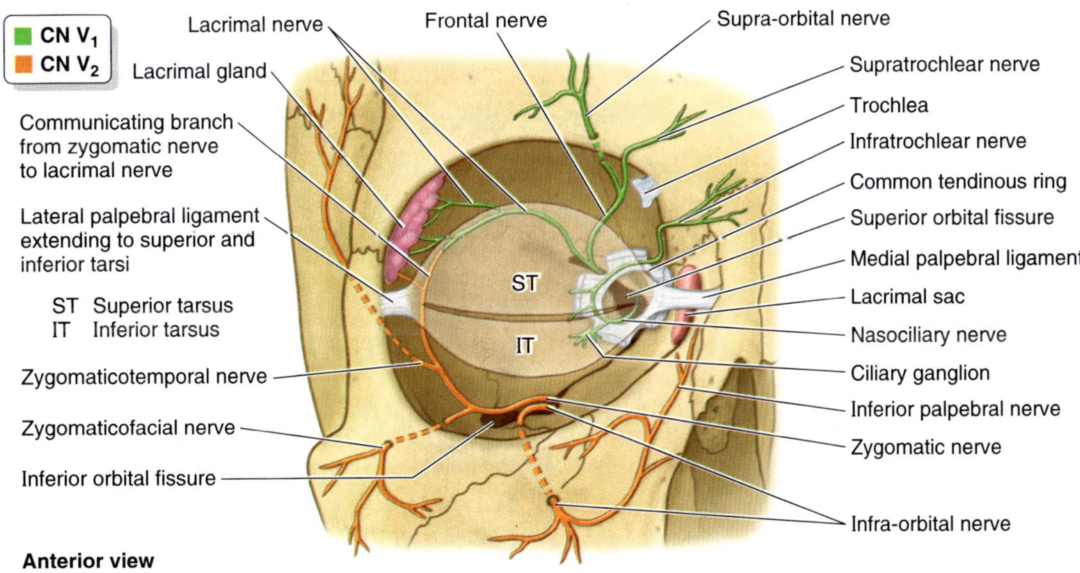

FIGURE 8.21. Cutaneous nerves of orbital/periorbital region. Cutaneous nerves are shown in relation to the orbital walls and rim and the fibrous skeleton of the eyelids. The skin of the superior eyelid is supplied by branches of the ophthalmic nerve (CN V_1), whereas the inferior eyelid is supplied mainly by branches of the maxillary nerve (CN V_2).

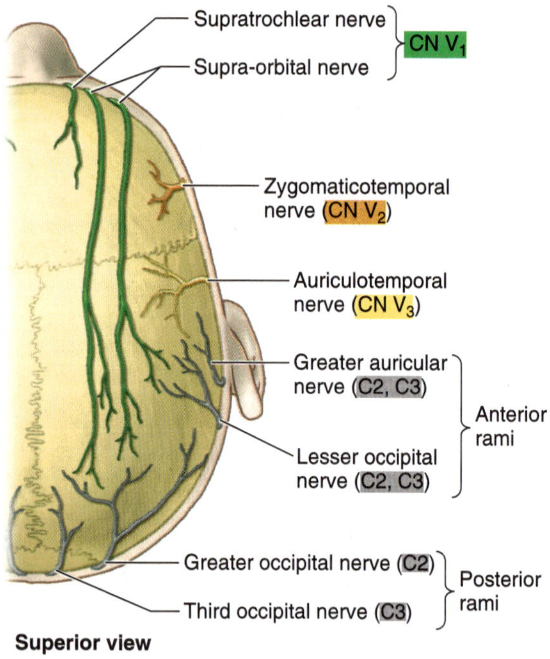

FIGURE 8.22. Nerves of scalp. The nerves appear in sequence: CN V_1, CN V_2, CN V_3, anterior rami of C2 and C3, and posterior rami of C2 and C3.

The **nasociliary nerve**, the intermediate branch of the CN V_1 trifurcation, supplies branches to the eyeball and divides within the orbit into the posterior ethmoidal, anterior ethmoidal, and infratrochlear nerves (Fig. 8.19). The *posterior* and *anterior ethmoidal nerves* leave the orbit, the latter running a circuitous course passing through the cranial and nasal cavities. Its terminal branch, the **external nasal nerve**, is a cutaneous nerve supplying the external nose. The **infratrochlear nerve** is a terminal branch of the nasociliary nerve and its main cutaneous branch.

The **lacrimal nerve**, the smallest branch from the trifurcation of CN V_1, is primarily a cutaneous branch, but it also conveys some secretomotor fibers, sent via a communicating branch, from a ganglion associated with the maxillary nerve for innervation of the lacrimal gland (Figs. 8.20 and 8.21).

MAXILLARY NERVE

The **maxillary nerve** (CN V_2), the intermediate division of the trigeminal nerve, also arises as a wholly sensory nerve (Fig. 8.19A). CN V_2 passes anteriorly from the *trigeminal ganglion* and leaves the cranium through the *foramen rotundum* in the base of the greater wing of the sphenoid. The maxillary nerve enters the *pterygopalatine fossa*, where it gives off branches to the *pterygopalatine ganglion* and continues anteriorly, entering the orbit through the *inferior orbital fissure* (Fig. 8.19). It gives off the zygomatic nerve and passes anteriorly into the *infra-orbital groove and foramen* as the infra-orbital nerve (Fig. 8.21).

The **zygomatic nerve** runs to the lateral wall of the orbit, giving rise to two of the three cutaneous branches of CN V_2, the **zygomaticofacial** and **zygomaticotemporal nerves**. The zygomatic nerve then continues as a communicating branch conveying secretomotor fibers to the lacrimal nerve. En route to the face, the **infra-orbital** nerve gives off palatine branches, branches to the mucosa of the maxillary sinus, and branches to the middle and anterior upper teeth. It reaches the skin of the face by traversing the *infra-orbital foramen* on the infra-orbital surface of the maxilla. The three cutaneous branches of the maxillary nerve supply the area of skin derived from the embryonic *maxillary prominences* (Moore et al., 2016).

MANDIBULAR NERVE

The **mandibular nerve** (CN V_3) is the inferior and largest division of the trigeminal nerve (Fig. 8.19A). It is formed by the union of sensory fibers from the sensory ganglion and the motor root of CN V in the *foramen ovale* in the greater wing of the sphenoid, through which CN V_3 emerges from the cranium. CN V_3 has three sensory branches that supply the area of skin derived from the embryonic *mandibular prominence*. It also supplies motor fibers to the muscles of mastication (Fig. 8.19B). CN V_3 is the only division of CN V that carries motor fibers. The major cutaneous branches of CN V_3 are the **auriculotemporal**, **buccal**, and **mental nerves**. En route to the skin, the auriculotemporal nerve passes deep to the parotid gland, conveying secretomotor fibers to it from a ganglion associated with this division of CN V.

NERVES OF SCALP

Innervation of the scalp anterior to the auricles of the external ears is through branches of all three divisions of CN V, the *trigeminal nerve* (Figs. 8.22 and 8.20B; Table 8.4). Posterior to the auricles, the nerve supply is from spinal cutaneous nerves (C2 and C3).

MOTOR NERVES OF FACE AN28.1

The motor nerves of the face are the *facial nerve* to the mus- AN28.6
cles of facial expression and the *motor root of the trigeminal nerve/mandibular nerve* to the muscles of mastication (masseter, temporal, medial, and lateral pterygoids). These nerves also supply some more deeply placed muscles (described later in this chapter in relation to the mouth, middle ear, and neck) (Fig. 8.19A).

FACIAL NERVE

CN VII, the **facial nerve**, has a motor root and a sensory/ AN28.4
parasympathetic root (the latter being the *intermediate nerve*). The **motor root of CN VII** supplies the muscles of facial expression, including the superficial muscle of the neck (platysma), auricular muscles, scalp muscles,

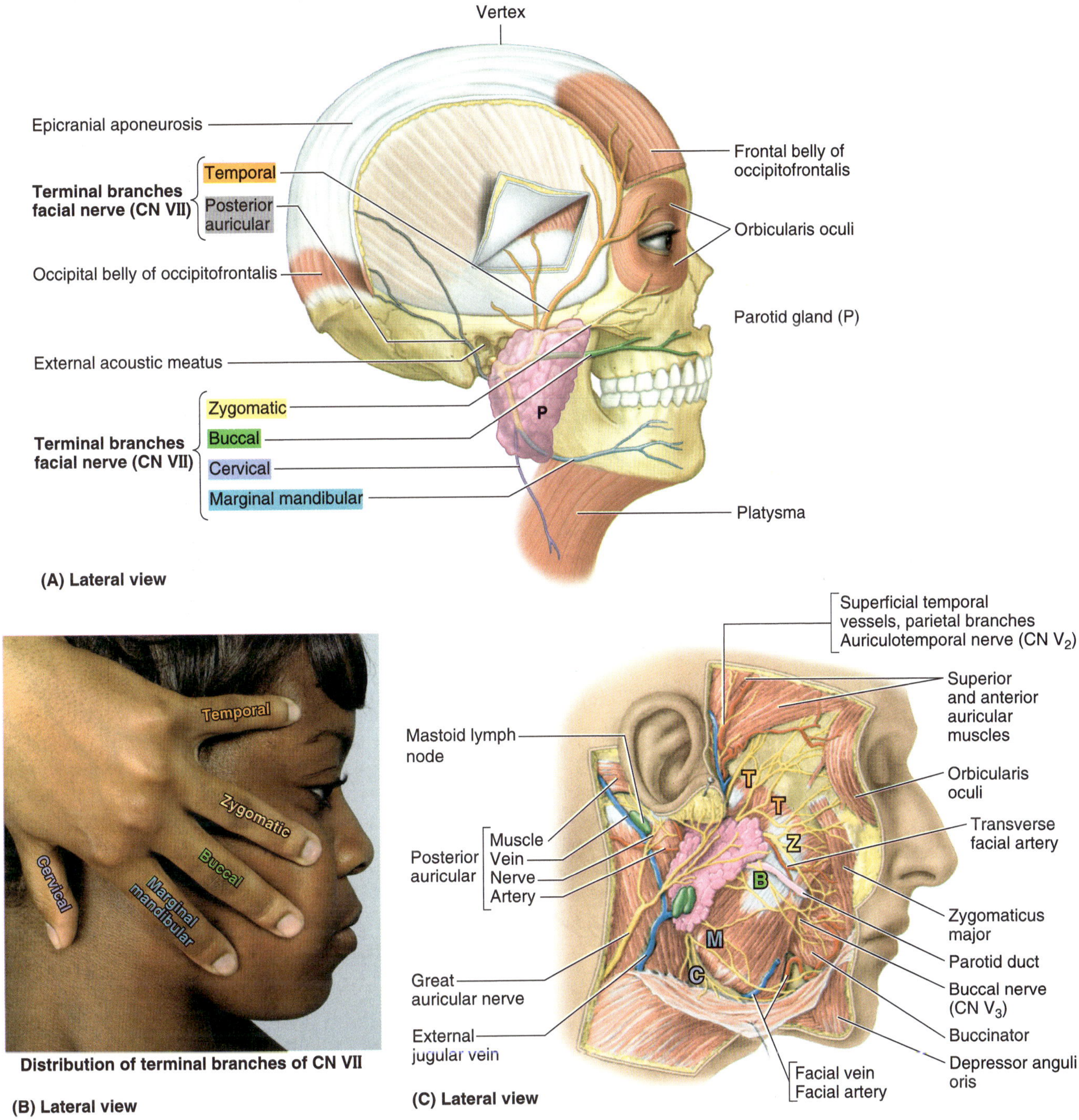

FIGURE 8.23. Branches of facial nerve (CN VII). A. The terminal branches of CN VII arise from the parotid plexus within the parotid gland. They emerge from the gland under cover of its lateral surface and radiate in a generally anterior direction across the face. Although intimately related to the parotid gland (and often contacting the submandibular gland via one or more of its lower branches), CN VII does not send nerve fibers to the salivary glands. Two muscles representing the extremes of the distribution of CN VII, the occipitofrontalis and platysma, are also shown. **B.** A simple method for demonstrating and remembering the general course of the five terminal branches of CN VII to the face and neck. **C.** Dissection of the right side of the head showing the great auricular nerve (C2 and C3), which supplies the parotid sheath and skin over the angle of the mandible, and terminal branches of the facial nerve, which supply the muscles of facial expression: *B*, buccal; *C*, cervical; *M*, marginal mandibular; *T*, temporal; *Z*, zygomatic.

and certain other muscles derived from mesoderm in the embryonic second pharyngeal arch (Fig. 8.23). Following a circuitous route through the temporal bone, CN VII emerges from the cranium through the *stylomastoid foramen* located between the mastoid and styloid processes (Figs. 8.9B and 8.11). It immediately gives off the **posterior auricular nerve**, which passes posterosuperior to the auricle of the ear to supply the auricularis posterior and occipital belly of the occipitofrontalis muscle (Fig. 8.23A, C).

The main trunk of CN VII runs anteriorly and is engulfed by the parotid gland, in which it forms the **parotid plexus**. This plexus gives rise to the five terminal branches of the facial nerve: *temporal*, *zygomatic*, *buccal*, *marginal mandibular*, and *cervical*. The names of the branches refer to the regions they supply. Specific muscles supplied by each branch are identified in Table 8.3.

The **temporal branch of CN VII** emerges from the superior border of the parotid gland and crosses the zygomatic arch to supply the auricularis superior and auricularis anterior; the frontal belly of the occipitofrontalis; and, most important, the superior part of the orbicularis oculi.

The **zygomatic branch of CN VII** passes via two or three branches superior and mainly inferior to the eye to supply the inferior part of the orbicularis oculi and other facial muscles inferior to the orbit.

The **buccal branch of CN VII** passes external to the buccinator to supply this muscle and the muscles of the upper lip (upper parts of orbicularis oris and inferior fibers of levator labii superioris).

The **marginal mandibular branch of CN VII** supplies the risorius and muscles of the lower lip and chin. It emerges from the inferior border of the parotid gland and crosses the inferior border of the mandible deep to the platysma to reach the face. In approximately 20% of people, this branch passes inferior to the angle of the mandible.

The **cervical branch of CN VII** passes inferiorly from the inferior border of the parotid gland and runs posterior to the mandible to supply the platysma (Fig. 8.23).

Cutaneous branches from the geniculate ganglion accompany the auricular branch of the vagus nerve to skin on both sides of the auricle, in the region of the concha. Although not evident anatomically, their existence is most evident through clinical manifestations.

Superficial Vasculature of Face and Scalp

The face is richly supplied by with superficial arteries and external veins, as is evident in blushing and blanching (e.g., becoming pale due to cold). The terminal branches of both arteries and veins anastomose freely, including anastomoses across the midline with contralateral partners.

SUPERFICIAL ARTERIES OF FACE

AN28.3 Most superficial arteries of the face are branches or deriva-
AN43.6 tives of *branches of the external carotid artery*, as illustrated in Figure 8.24. The origin, course, and distribution of these arteries are presented in Table 8.5. The **facial artery** provides the major arterial supply to the face. It arises from the external carotid artery and winds its way to the inferior border of the mandible, just anterior to the masseter (Figs. 8.23C and 8.24B). The artery lies superficially here, immediately deep to the platysma. The facial artery crosses the mandible, buccinator, and maxilla as it courses over the face to the medial angle (canthus) of the eye, where the superior and inferior eyelids meet (Fig. 8.24B). The facial artery lies deep to the zygomaticus major and levator labii superioris muscles. Near the termination of its sinuous course through the face, the facial artery passes approximately a finger's breadth lateral to the angle of the mouth. The facial artery sends branches to the upper and lower lips (**superior** and **inferior labial arteries**), ascends along the side of the nose, and anastomoses with the dorsal nasal branch of the ophthalmic artery. Distal to the **lateral nasal artery** at the side of the nose, the terminal part of the facial artery is called the **angular artery**.

The **superficial temporal artery** is the smaller terminal branch of the external carotid artery; the other branch is the *maxillary artery*. The superficial temporal artery emerges on the face between the temporomandibular joint (TMJ) and the auricle, enters the temporal fossa, and ends in the scalp by dividing into *frontal* and *parietal branches*. These arterial branches accompany or run in close proximity to the corresponding branches of the auriculotemporal nerve.

The **transverse facial artery** arises from the superficial temporal artery within the parotid gland and crosses the face superficial to the masseter (Figs. 8.23C and 8.24B), approximately a finger's breadth inferior to the zygomatic arch. It divides into numerous branches that supply the parotid gland and duct, the masseter, and the skin of the face. It anastomoses with branches of the facial artery.

In addition to the superficial temporal arteries, several other arteries accompany cutaneous nerves in the face. **Supra-orbital** and **supratrochlear arteries**, branches of the ophthalmic artery, accompany nerves of the same name across the eyebrows and forehead (Fig. 8.24; Table 8.5). The supra-orbital artery continues and supplies the anterior scalp to the vertex. The **mental artery**, the only superficial branch derived from the maxillary artery, accompanies the nerve of the same name in the chin.

ARTERIES OF SCALP

The scalp has a rich blood supply (Fig. 8.24A; Table 8.5). AN27.1
The arteries course within layer two of the scalp, the subcutaneous connective tissue layer between the skin and the epicranial aponeurosis. The arteries anastomose freely with adjacent arteries and across the midline with the contralateral artery. The arterial walls are firmly attached to the dense connective tissue in which the arteries are embedded, limiting their ability to constrict when cut. Consequently, bleeding from scalp wounds is profuse.

The arterial supply is from the **external carotid arteries** through the *occipital*, *posterior auricular*, and *superficial temporal arteries* and from the *internal carotid arteries* through the *supratrochlear* and *supra-orbital arteries*. The arteries of the scalp supply little blood to the neurocranium, which is supplied primarily by the middle meningeal artery.

EXTERNAL VEINS OF FACE

Most external facial veins are drained by veins that accom- AN28.3
pany the arteries of the face. As with most superficial veins, they are subject to many variations; a common pattern is shown in Figure 8.25, and Table 8.6 provides details.

(*continued on p.* 915)

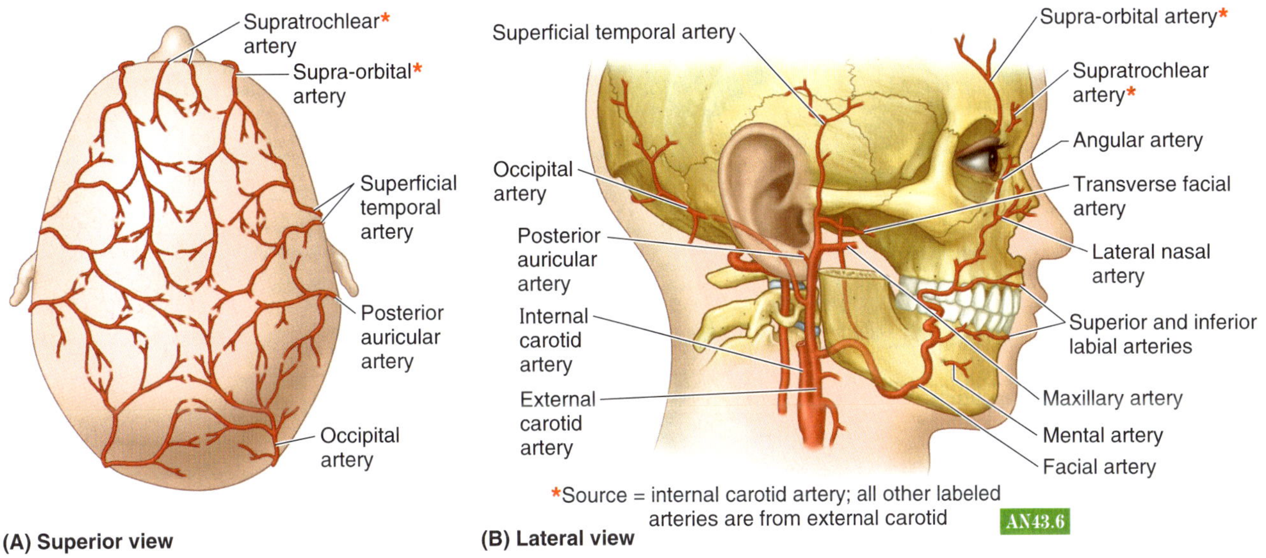

FIGURE 8.24. Superficial arteries of face and scalp.

TABLE 8.5. SUPERFICIAL ARTERIES OF FACE AND SCALP

Artery	Origin	Course	Distribution
Facial	External carotid artery	Ascends deep to submandibular gland; winds around inferior border of mandible and enters face	Muscles of facial expression and face
Inferior labial	Facial artery near angle of mouth	Runs medially in lower lip	Lower lip
Superior labial		Runs medially in upper lip	Upper lip and ala (side) and septum of nose
Lateral nasal	Facial artery as it ascends alongside nose	Passes to ala of nose	Skin on ala and dorsum of nose
Angular	Terminal branch of facial artery	Passes to medial angle (canthus) of eye	Superior part of cheek and inferior eyelid
Occipital	External carotid artery	Passes medial to posterior belly of digastric and mastoid process; accompanies occipital nerve in occipital region	Scalp of back of head, as far as vertex
Posterior auricular	External carotid artery	Passes posteriorly, deep to parotid gland, along styloid process between mastoid process and ear	Auricle of ear and scalp posterior to auricle
Superficial temporal	Smaller terminal branch of external carotid artery	Ascends anterior to ear to region and ends in scalp	Facial muscles and skin of temporal frontal and temporal regions
Transverse facial	Superficial temporal artery within parotid gland	Crosses face superficial to masseter and inferior to zygomatic arch	Parotid gland and duct, muscles and skin of face
Mental	Terminal branch of inferior alveolar artery	Emerges from mental foramen and passes to chin	Facial muscles and skin of chin
Supra-orbital[a]	Terminal branches of ophthalmic artery	Passes superiorly from supra-orbital foramen	Muscles and skin of forehead and scalp and superior conjunctiva
Supratrochlear[a]		Passes superiorly from supratrochlear notch	

[a]Source is internal carotid artery.

8

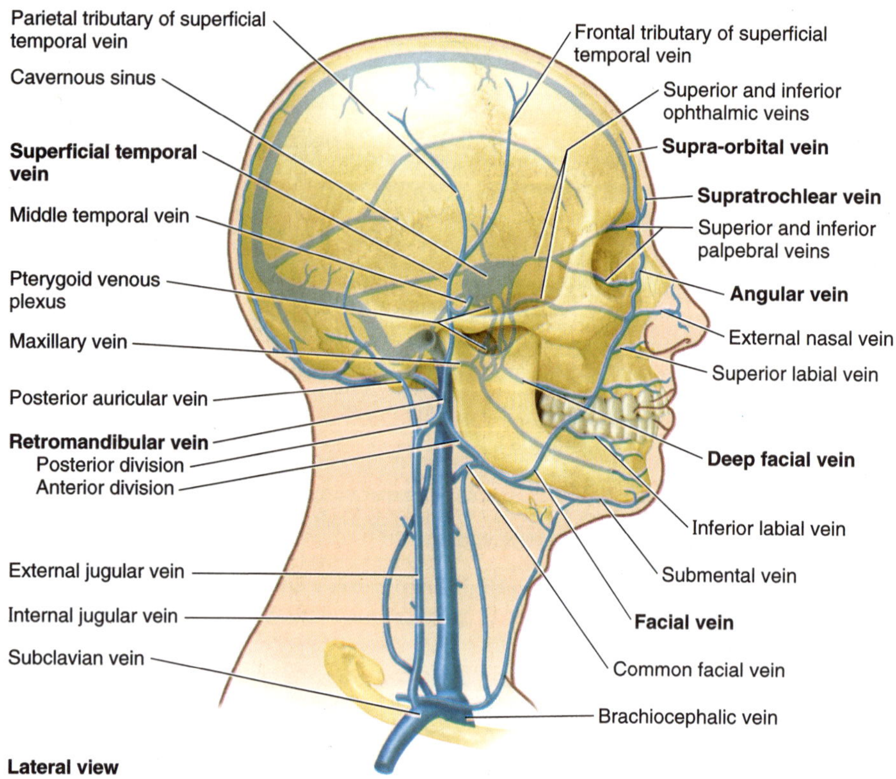

FIGURE 8.25. Veins of face and scalp.

TABLE 8.6. VEINS OF FACE AND SCALP

Vein	Origin	Course	Termination	Area Drained
Supratrochlear	Begins from venous plexus on forehead and scalp, through which it communicates with frontal branch of superficial temporal vein, its contralateral partner, and supra-orbital vein	Descends near midline of forehead to root of nose, where it joins supra-orbital vein	Angular vein at root of nose	Anterior part of scalp and forehead
Supra-orbital	Begins in forehead by anastomosing with frontal tributary of superficial temporal vein	Passes medially superior to orbit; joins supratrochlear vein; a branch passes through supra-orbital notch and joins with superior ophthalmic vein		
Angular	Begins at root of nose by union of supratrochlear and supra-orbital veins	Descends obliquely along root and side of nose to inferior orbital margin	Becomes facial vein at inferior margin of orbit	Anterior part of scalp and forehead; superior and inferior eyelids and conjunctiva; may receive drainage from cavernous sinus
Facial	Continuation of angular vein past inferior margin of orbit	Descends along lateral border of nose, receiving external nasal and inferior palpebral veins; then passes obliquely across face to cross inferior border of mandible; receives communication from retromandibular vein (after which, it is sometimes called common facial vein)	Internal jugular vein opposite or inferior to level of hyoid bone	Anterior scalp and forehead; eyelids; external nose; anterior cheek; lips; chin; and submandibular gland
Deep facial	Pterygoid venous plexus	Runs anteriorly on maxilla superior to buccinator and deep to masseter, emerging medial to anterior border of masseter onto face	Enters posterior aspect of facial vein	Infratemporal fossa (most areas supplied by maxillary artery)

(*Continued*)

TABLE 8.6. VEINS OF FACE AND SCALP (Continued)

Vein	Origin	Course	Termination	Area Drained
Superficial temporal	Begins from widespread plexus of veins on side of scalp and along zygomatic arch	Frontal and parietal tributaries unite anterior to the auricle; crosses temporal root of zygomatic arch to pass from temporal region and enter substance of the parotid gland	Joins maxillary vein posterior to neck of mandible to form retromandibular vein	Side of scalp; superficial aspect of temporal muscle; and external ear
Retromandibular	Formed anterior to ear by union of superficial temporal and maxillary veins	Runs posterior and deep to ramus of mandible through substance of parotid gland; communicates at inferior end with facial vein	Unites with posterior auricular vein to form external jugular vein	Parotid gland and masseter muscle

Like veins elsewhere, they have abundant anastomoses that allow drainage to occur by alternate routes during periods of temporary compression. The alternate routes include both superficial pathways (via the facial and retromandibular/external jugular veins) and deep drainage (via the anastomoses with the cavernous sinus, pterygoid venous plexus, and the internal jugular vein).

AN28.8 The **facial veins**, coursing with or parallel to the facial arteries, are *valveless veins* that provide the primary superficial drainage of the face. Tributaries of the facial vein include the **deep facial vein**, which drains the *pterygoid venous plexus* of the infratemporal fossa. Inferior to the margin of the mandible, the facial vein is joined by the anterior (communicating) branch of the retromandibular vein. The facial vein drains directly or indirectly into the internal jugular vein (IJV). At the medial angle of the eye, the facial vein communicates with the *superior ophthalmic vein*, which drains into the *cavernous sinus*.

The **retromandibular vein** is a deep vessel of the face formed by the union of the superficial temporal vein and the maxillary vein, the latter draining the pterygoid venous plexus. The retromandibular vein runs posterior to the ramus of the mandible within the substance of the parotid gland, superficial to the external carotid artery and deep to the facial nerve. As it emerges from the inferior pole of the parotid gland, the retromandibular vein divides into an anterior branch that unites with the facial vein and a posterior branch that joins the posterior auricular vein inferior to the parotid gland to form the **external jugular vein**. This vein passes inferiorly and superficially in the neck to empty into the subclavian vein.

VEINS OF SCALP

AN27.1 The venous drainage of the superficial parts of the scalp is through the accompanying veins of the scalp arteries, the **supra-orbital** and **supratrochlear veins**. The **superficial temporal veins** and **posterior auricular veins** drain the scalp anterior and posterior to the auricles, respectively. The posterior auricular vein often receives a *mastoid emissary vein* from the sigmoid sinus, a dural venous sinus (see Fig. 8.33). The **occipital veins** drain the occipital region of the scalp. Venous drainage of deep parts of the scalp in the temporal region is through **deep temporal veins**, which are tributaries of the pterygoid venous plexus.

LYMPHATIC DRAINAGE OF FACE AND SCALP

There are no lymph nodes in the scalp, and except for the parotid/buccal region, there are no lymph nodes in the face. Lymph from the scalp, face, and neck drains into the *superficial ring* (pericervical collar) of *lymph nodes*—submental, submandibular, parotid, mastoid, and occipital—located at the junction of the head and neck (Fig. 8.26A). The lymphatic vessels of the face accompany other facial vessels. Superficial lymphatic vessels accompany veins, and deep lymphatics accompany arteries. All lymphatic vessels from the head and neck drain directly or indirectly into the *deep cervical lymph nodes* (Fig. 8.26B), a chain of nodes mainly located along the IJV in the neck. Lymph from these deep nodes passes to the **jugular lymphatic trunk**, which joins the *thoracic duct* on the left side and the IJV or **brachiocephalic vein** on the right side. A summary of the lymphatic drainage of the face follows: AN28.

- Lymph from the lateral part of the face and scalp, including the eyelids, drains to the superficial **parotid lymph nodes**.
- Lymph from the deep parotid nodes drains to the **deep cervical lymph nodes**.
- Lymph from the upper lip and lateral parts of the lower lip drains to the **submandibular lymph nodes**.
- Lymph from the chin and central part of the lower lip drains to the **submental lymph nodes**.

Surface Anatomy of Face

Despite the apparently infinite variations that enable people to be identified as individuals, the features of the human face are constant (Fig. 8.27). The **eyebrows** (L. *supercilia*) are linear growths of hair overlying the **supra-orbital margin**. The hairless region between the eyebrows overlies the *glabella*, and the prominent ridges that extend laterally on each side above the eyebrows are the *superciliary arches*.

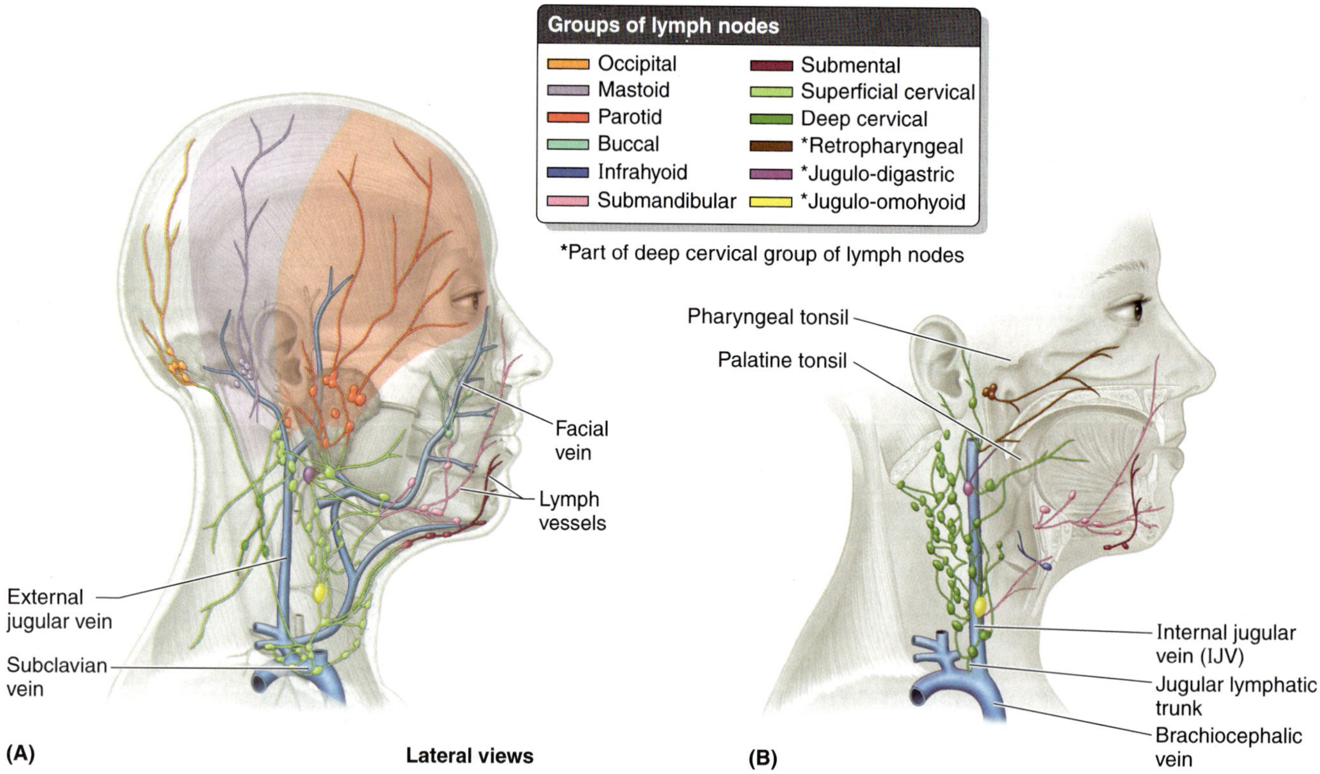

FIGURE 8.26. Lymphatic drainage of face and scalp. A. Superficial drainage. A pericervical collar of superficial lymph nodes is formed at the junction of the head and neck by the submental, submandibular, parotid, mastoid, and occipital nodes. These nodes initially receive most of the lymph drainage from the face and scalp. **B.** Deep drainage. All lymphatic vessels from the head and neck ultimately drain into the deep cervical lymph nodes, either directly from the tissues or indirectly after passing through an outlying group of nodes.

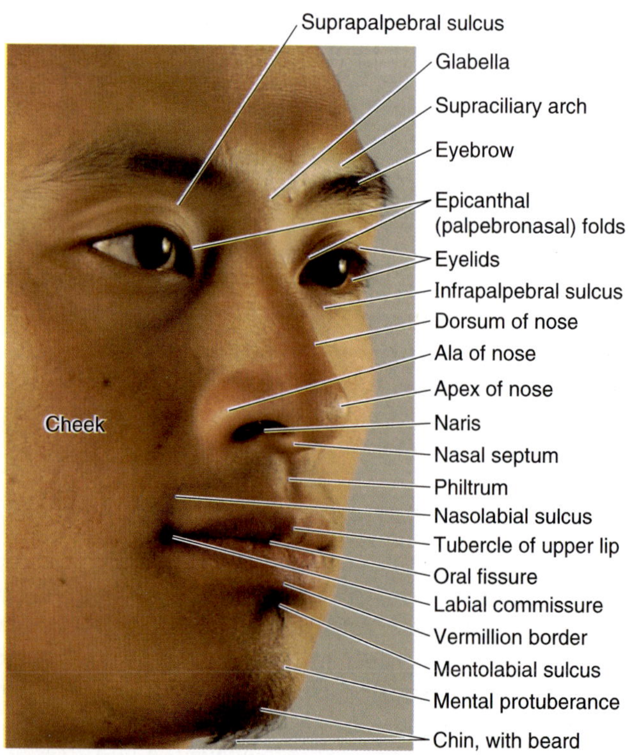

FIGURE 8.27. Surface anatomy of face.

The **eyelids** (L. *palpebrae*) are mobile, musculofibrous folds that overlie the eyeball. They are joined at each end of the **palpebral fissure** between the eyelids at the **medial** and **lateral angles** (canthi) of the eye. The **epicanthal fold** (**epicanthus**) is a fold of skin that covers the medial angle of the eye in some people, chiefly Asians. The depressions superior and inferior to the eyelids are the **suprapalpebral** and **infrapalpebral** sulci.

The shape of the nose varies remarkably. The external nose presents a prominent *apex* and is continuous with the forehead at the *root of the nose* (bridge). The rounded anterior border between the root and apex is the *dorsum of the nose*. Inferior to the apex, the nasal cavity of each side opens anteriorly by a *naris* (plural = nares), bounded medially by the *nasal septum* and laterally by an *ala* (wing) *of the nose*.

The lips surround the opening of the mouth, the *oral fissure*. The **vermillion border of the lip** marks the beginning of the *transitional zone* (commonly referred to as the lip) between the skin and mucous membrane of the lip. The skin of the **transitional zone** is hairless and thin, increasing its sensitivity and causing its color to be different (because of underlying capillary beds) from that of the adjacent skin of the face. The lateral junction of the lips is the **labial commissure**; the angle between the lips, medial to the commissure, that increases as the mouth opens and decreases as it closes is the **angle of the mouth**.

The median part of the upper lip features a **tubercle**, superior to which is a shallow groove, the **philtrum** (G. love charm), extending to the nasal septum. The musculofibrous folds of the lips continue laterally as the **cheek**, which also contains the buccinator muscle and buccal fat-pad. The cheek is separated from the lips by the **nasolabial sulcus**, which runs obliquely between the ala of the nose and the angle of the mouth. These grooves are easiest to observe during smiling. The lower lip is separated from the **mental protuberance** (chin) by the **mentolabial sulcus**. The lips, cheeks, and chin of the mature male grow hair as part of the secondary sex characteristics, the **beard**.

For development and developmental basis of congenital anomalies of face, refer *Langman's Medical Embryology*, South Asian Edition, Chapter 17, Head and Neck, pp. 308–316. AN43.

CLINICAL BOX

FACE AND SCALP

Facial Lacerations and Incisions

Because the face has no distinct deep fascia and the subcutaneous tissue between the cutaneous attachments of the facial muscles is loose, *facial lacerations* tend to gape (part widely). Consequently, the skin must be carefully sutured to prevent scarring. The looseness of the subcutaneous tissue also enables fluid and blood to accumulate in the loose connective tissue following bruising of the face.

Similarly, facial inflammation causes considerable swelling (e.g., a beesting on the root of the nose may close both eyes). As a person ages, the skin loses its resiliency (elasticity) resulting in ridges and wrinkles in the skin perpendicular to the direction of the facial muscle fibers. Skin incisions along these cleavage or wrinkle lines (Langer lines) heal with minimal scarring (see the clinical box "Skin Incisions and Scarring," in Chapter 1, Overview and Basic Concepts).

Scalp Injuries

AN27.1 Because the scalp arteries arising at the sides of the head are well protected by dense connective tissue and anastomose freely, a *partially detached scalp* may be replaced with a reasonable chance of healing as long as one of the vessels supplying the scalp remains intact. During an *attached craniotomy* (surgical removal of a segment of the calvaria with a soft tissue scalp flap to expose the cranial cavity), the incisions are usually made convex and upward, and the superficial temporal artery is included in the tissue flap.

The *scalp proper*, the first three layers of the scalp (see Fig. 8.15A), is often regarded clinically as a single layer because they remain together when a scalp flap is made during a craniotomy and when part of the scalp is torn off (e.g., during an industrial accident). Nerves and vessels of the scalp enter inferiorly and ascend through layer two to the skin. Consequently, surgical pedicle scalp flaps are made so that they remain attached inferiorly to preserve the nerves and vessels, thereby promoting good healing.

The arteries of the scalp supply little blood to the calvaria, which is supplied by the middle meningeal arteries. Therefore, loss of the scalp does not produce necrosis (death) of the calvarial bones.

Scalp Wounds

The epicranial aponeurosis is clinically important. Because of the strength of this aponeurosis, *superficial scalp wounds* do not gape, and the margins of the wound are held together. Furthermore, deep sutures are not necessary when suturing superficial wounds because the epicranial aponeurosis does not allow wide separation of the skin. *Deep scalp wounds* gape widely when the epicranial aponeurosis is lacerated in the coronal plane because of the pull of the frontal and occipital bellies of the occipitofrontalis muscle in opposite directions (anteriorly and posteriorly).

Scalp Infections

The loose connective tissue layer (layer four) of the scalp is the *danger area of the scalp* because pus or blood spreads easily in it. Infection in this layer can also pass into the cranial cavity through small *emissary veins*, which pass through parietal foramina in the calvaria, and reach intracranial structures such as the meninges (Fig. 8.8A, C). An infection cannot pass into the neck because the occipital bellies of the occipitofrontalis muscle attach to the occipital bone and mastoid parts of the temporal bones (Fig. 8.16A). Neither can a scalp infection spread laterally beyond the zygomatic arches because the epicranial aponeurosis is continuous with the temporal fascia that attaches to these arches. AN27.

An infection or fluid (e.g., pus or blood) can enter the eyelids and the root of the nose because the occipitofrontalis inserts into the skin and subcutaneous tissue and does not attach to the bone (Fig. 8.16B). The skin of the eyelid is the thinnest of the body and is delicate and sensitive. Because of the loose nature of the subcutaneous tissue within the eyelids, even a relatively slight injury or inflammation may result in an accumulation of fluid, causing the eyelids to swell. Blows to the periorbital region usually produce soft tissue damage because the tissues are crushed against the strong and relatively sharp margin. Consequently, "black eyes" (*periorbital ecchymosis*) can result from an injury to the scalp and/or the forehead (Fig. B8.12). **Ecchymoses** (purple patches) develop as a result of extravasation of blood into the subcutaneous tissue and skin of the eyelids and surrounding regions.

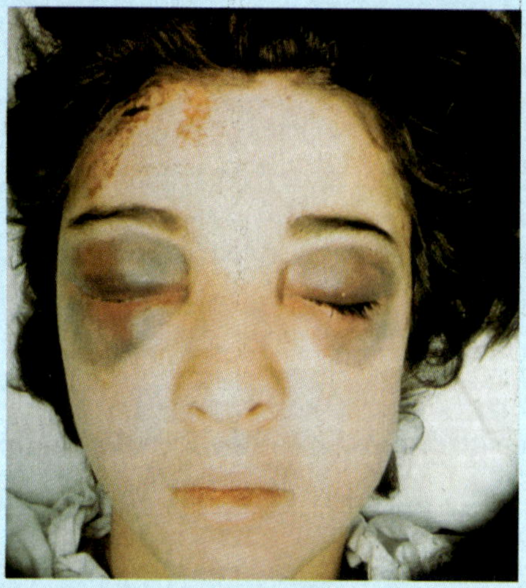

FIGURE B8.12. Ecchymosis (extravasation of blood under the skin).

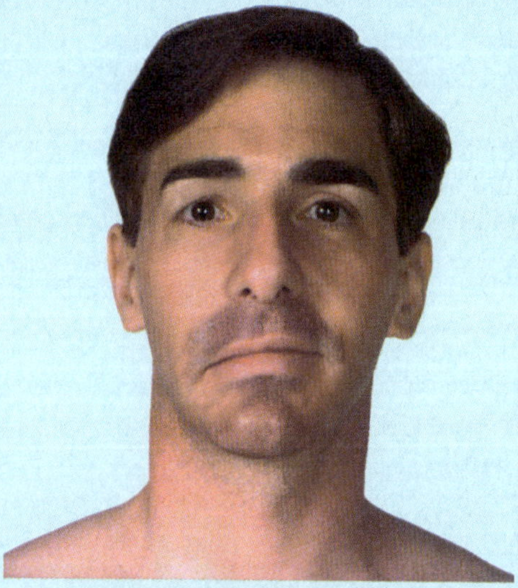

FIGURE B8.13. Bell palsy.

Sebaceous Cysts

The ducts of sebaceous glands associated with hair follicles in the scalp may become obstructed, resulting in the retention of secretions and the formation of *sebaceous cysts* (pilar cysts). Because they are in the skin, sebaceous cysts move with the scalp.

Cephalohematoma

Sometimes after a difficult birth, bleeding occurs between the baby's pericranium (layer 5 of scalp; see Fig. 8.15A) and calvaria, usually over one parietal bone. Blood becomes trapped in this area, forming a *cephalohematoma*. This benign condition frequently seen in neonates results from birth trauma that ruptures multiple, minute periosteal arteries that nourish the bones of the calvaria.

Flaring of Nostrils

The actions of the nasalis muscles (Fig. 8.17, center top row) have generally been held as insignificant. However, observant clinicians study their action because of their diagnostic value (e.g., true *nasal breathers* can flare their nostrils distinctly). Habitual mouth breathing, caused by chronic nasal obstruction, for example, diminishes and sometimes eliminates the ability to flare the nostrils. Children who are *chronic mouth breathers* often develop dental malocclusion (improper bite) because the alignment of the teeth is maintained to a large degree by normal periods of occlusion and labial closure. *Antisnoring devices* have been developed that attach to the nose to flare the nostrils and maintain a more patent air passageway.

Paralysis of Facial Muscles

N28.7 *Injury to the facial nerve* (CN VII) or its branches produces paralysis of some or all facial muscles on the affected side (*Bell palsy*). The affected area sags, and facial expression is distorted, making it appear passive or sad (Fig. B8.13). The loss of tonus of the orbicularis oculi causes the inferior eyelid to evert (fall away from the surface of the eyeball). Thus, lacrimal fluid is not spread over the cornea, preventing adequate lubrication, hydration, and flushing of the surface of the cornea.

This makes the cornea vulnerable to ulceration. A resulting corneal scar can impair vision. If the injury weakens or paralyzes the buccinator and orbicularis oris, food will accumulate in the oral vestibule during chewing, usually requiring continual removal with a finger. When the sphincters or dilators of the mouth are affected, displacement of the mouth (drooping of its corner) is produced by contraction of unopposed contralateral facial muscles and gravity, resulting in food and saliva dribbling out of the side of the mouth. Weakened lip muscles affect speech as a result of an impaired ability to produce labial (*B*, *M*, *P*, or *W*) sounds. Affected persons cannot whistle or blow a wind instrument. They frequently dab their eyes and mouth with a handkerchief to wipe the fluid (tears and saliva), which runs from the drooping lid and mouth. The fluid and constant wiping may result in localized skin irritation.

Infra-Orbital Nerve Block

For treating wounds of the upper lip and cheek or, more commonly, for repairing the maxillary incisor teeth, local anesthesia of the inferior part of the face is achieved by infiltration of the infra-orbital nerve with an anesthetic agent. The injection is made in the region of the infra-orbital foramen, by elevating the upper lip and passing the needle through the junction of the oral mucosa and gingiva at the superior aspect of the oral vestibule.

To determine where the infra-orbital nerve emerges, pressure is exerted on the maxilla in the region of the infra-orbital foramen. Too much pressure on the nerve causes considerable pain. Because companion infra-orbital vessels leave the infra-orbital foramen with the nerve, aspiration of the syringe during injection prevents inadvertent injection of anesthetic fluid into a blood vessel. Because the orbit is located just superior to the injection site, a careless injection could result in passage of anesthetic fluid into the orbit, causing temporary paralysis of the extra-ocular muscles.

Mental and Incisive Nerve Blocks

Occasionally, it is desirable to anesthetize one side of the skin and mucous membrane of the lower lip and the skin of the chin (e.g., to suture a severe laceration of the lip or chin). Injection of an anesthetic agent into the mental foramen blocks the mental nerve that supplies the skin and mucous membrane of the lower lip from the mental foramen to the midline, including the skin of the chin.

Buccal Nerve Block

To anesthetize the skin and mucous membrane of the cheek (e.g., to suture a knife wound), an anesthetic injection can be made into the mucosa covering the *retromolar fossa*, a triangular depression posterior to the 3rd mandibular molar tooth between the anterior border of the ramus and the temporal crest.

Trigeminal Neuralgia

Trigeminal neuralgia or *tic douloureux* is a sensory disorder of the sensory root of CN V that occurs most often in middle-aged and elderly persons. It is characterized by sudden attacks of excruciating, lightening-like jabs of facial pain. A *paroxysm* (sudden sharp pain) can last for 15 minutes or more. The pain may be so intense that the person winces, thus the common term *tic* (twitch). In some cases, the pain may be so severe that psychological changes occur, leading to depression and even suicide attempts.

CN V_2 is most frequently involved, then CN V_3, and least frequently, CN V_1. The paroxysms are often set off by touching the face, brushing the teeth, shaving, drinking, or chewing. The pain is often initiated by touching an especially sensitive *trigger zone*, frequently located around the tip of the nose or the cheek (Haines, 2013). In trigeminal neuralgia, demyelination of axons in the sensory root occurs. In most cases, this is caused by pressure of a small aberrant artery (Kiernan, 2013). Often, when the aberrant artery is moved away from the sensory root of CN V, the symptoms disappear. Other scientists believe the condition is caused by a pathological process affecting neurons in the trigeminal ganglion.

Medical or surgical treatment or both are used to alleviate the pain. In cases involving the CN V_2, attempts have been made to block the infra-orbital nerve at the infra-orbital foramen using alcohol. This treatment usually relieves pain temporarily. The simplest surgical procedure is avulsion or cutting of the branches of the nerve at the infra-orbital foramen.

Other treatments have used *radiofrequency selective ablation of parts of the trigeminal ganglion* by a needle electrode passing through the cheek and foramen ovale. In some cases, it is necessary to section the sensory root for relief of the pain. To prevent regeneration of nerve fibers, the sensory root of the trigeminal nerve may be partially cut between the ganglion and the brainstem (*rhizotomy*). Although the axons may regenerate, they do not do so within the brainstem. Surgeons attempt to differentiate and cut only the sensory fibers to the division of CN V involved.

The same result may be achieved by sectioning the spinal tract of CN V (*tractotomy*). After this operation, the sensation of pain, temperature, and simple (light) touch is lost over the area of skin and mucous membrane supplied by the affected component of the CN V. This loss of sensation may annoy the patient, who may not recognize the presence of food on the lip and cheek or feel it within the mouth on the side of the nerve section. However, these disabilities are usually preferable to excruciating pain.

Lesions of Trigeminal Nerve

Lesions of the entire trigeminal nerve cause widespread anesthesia involving the:

- Corresponding anterior half of the scalp.
- Face (except for skin over the angle of the mandible) and the cornea and conjunctiva.
- Mucous membranes of the nose, mouth, and anterior part of the tongue.

Paralysis of the muscles of mastication also occurs.

Herpes Zoster Infection of Trigeminal Ganglion

A *herpes zoster virus infection* may produce a lesion in the cranial ganglia. Involvement of the trigeminal ganglion occurs in approximately 20% of cases (Mukerji et al., 2016). The infection is characterized by an eruption of groups of vesicles following the course of the affected nerve (e.g., *ophthalmic herpes zoster*). Any division of CN V may be involved, but the ophthalmic division is most commonly affected. Usually, the cornea is involved, often resulting in painful *corneal ulceration* and subsequent *scarring of the cornea*.

Testing Sensory Function of CN V

The sensory function of the trigeminal nerve is tested by asking the person to close his or her eyes and respond when types of touch are felt (e.g., a piece of dry gauze is gently stroked across the skin of one side of the face and then to the corresponding position on the other side). The test is then repeated until the skin of the forehead (CN V_1), cheek (CN V_2), and lower jaw (CN V_3) has been tested. The person is asked if one side feels the same as or different from the other side. The testing may then be repeated using warm or cold instruments and the gentle touch of a sharp pin, again alternating sides (Fig. B8.14).

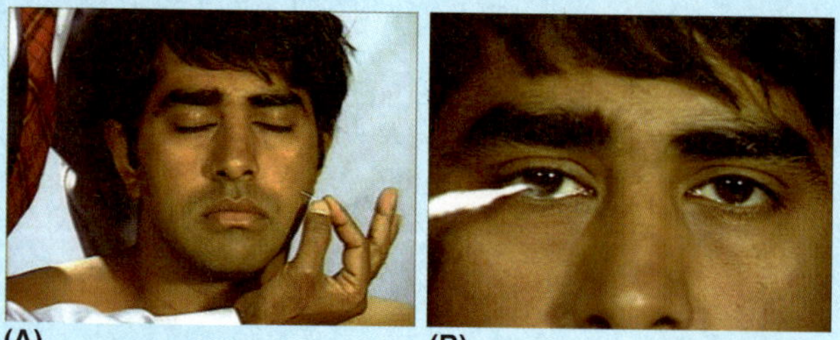

(A) (B)

FIGURE B8.14. Testing sensory function of CN V.

Injuries to Facial Nerve

AN28.7 Injury to branches of the facial nerve causes paralysis of the facial muscles (Bell palsy), with or without loss of taste on the anterior two thirds of the tongue or altered secretion of the lacrimal and salivary glands (see the clinical box "Paralysis of Facial Muscles,"). Lesions near the origin of CN VII from the pons of the brain, or proximal to the origin of the greater petrosal nerve (in the region of the geniculate ganglion), result in loss of motor, gustatory (taste), and autonomic functions. Lesions distal to the geniculate ganglion, but proximal to the origin of the chorda tympani nerve, produce the same dysfunction, except that lacrimal secretion is not affected. Lesions near the stylomastoid foramen result in loss of motor function only (i.e., facial paralysis).

Facial nerve palsy has many causes. The most common nontraumatic cause of facial paralysis is *inflammation of the facial nerve* near the stylomastoid foramen (see Fig. 8.9A), often as a result of a viral infection. This produces edema (swelling) and compression of the nerve in the facial canal. Injury of the facial nerve may result from *fracture of the temporal bone*. Facial paralysis is evident soon after the injury. If the nerve is completely sectioned, the chances of complete or even partial recovery are remote. Muscular movement usually improves when the nerve damage is associated with blunt head trauma; however, recovery may not be complete (Russo et al., 2016). Facial nerve palsy may be idiopathic (occurring without a known cause). However, it often follows exposure to cold, as occurs when riding in a car with a window open.

Facial paralysis may be a complication of surgery; consequently, identification of the facial nerve and its branches is essential during surgery (e.g., *parotidectomy*, removal of a parotid gland). The facial nerve is most distinct as it emerges from the stylomastoid foramen. If necessary, electrical stimulation may be used for confirmation. Facial nerve palsy may also be associated with dental manipulation, vaccination, pregnancy, HIV infection, Lyme disease (inflammatory disorder causing headache and stiff neck), and infections of the middle ear (otitis media). Because the branches of the facial nerve are superficial, they are subject to injury by stab and gunshot wounds, cuts, and injury at birth (Fig. 8.23):

- A *lesion of the zygomatic branch* of CN VII causes paralysis, including loss of tonus of the orbicularis oculi in the inferior eyelid.
- *Paralysis of the buccal branch* of CN VII causes paralysis of the buccinator and superior portion of the orbicularis oris and upper lip muscles.
- *Paralysis of the marginal mandibular branch* of CN VII may occur when an incision is made along the inferior border of the mandible. Injury to this branch (e.g., during a surgical approach to the submandibular gland) causes paralysis of the inferior portion of the orbicularis oris and lower lip muscles.

The consequences of such paralyses are discussed in the clinical box "Paralysis of Facial Muscles."

Compression of Facial Artery

The facial artery can be occluded by pressure against the mandible where the vessel crosses it. Because of the numerous anastomoses between the branches of the facial artery and the other arteries of the face, compression of the facial artery on one side does not stop all bleeding from a lacerated facial artery or one of its branches. In lacerations of the lip, pressure must be applied on both sides of the cut to stop the bleeding. In general, facial wounds bleed freely and heal quickly.

Pulses of Arteries of Face and Scalp

The pulses of the superficial temporal and facial AN43.5 arteries may be used for taking the pulse. For example, anesthesiologists at the head of the operating table often take the *temporal pulse* where the superficial temporal artery crosses the zygomatic process just anterior to the auricle (Fig. B8.15A). Clench your teeth and palpate the *facial pulse* as the facial artery crosses the inferior border of the mandible immediately anterior to the masseter muscle (Fig. B8.15B).

Stenosis of Internal Carotid Artery

At the medial angle of the eye, an anastomosis occurs between the facial artery, a branch of the external carotid artery, and cutaneous branches of the internal carotid artery. With advancing age, the inter-

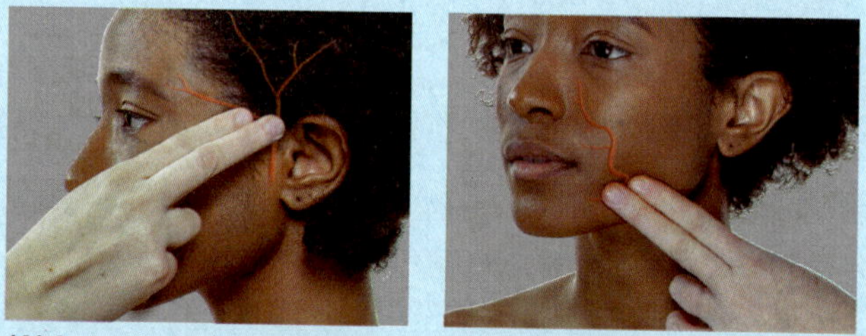

(A) Lateral view, superficial temporal artery pulse **(B) Anterolateral view, facial artery pulse**

FIGURE B8.15. Face and scalp pulses.

nal carotid artery may become narrow (stenotic) owing to atherosclerotic thickening of the intima (innermost coat) of the arteries. Because of the arterial anastomosis, intracranial structures such as the brain can receive blood from the connection of the facial artery to the dorsal nasal branch of the ophthalmic artery.

Scalp Lacerations

AN27.1 *Scalp lacerations* are the most common type of head injury requiring surgical care. These wounds bleed profusely because the arteries entering the periphery of the scalp bleed from both ends owing to abundant anastomoses. The arteries do not retract when lacerated because they are held open by the dense connective tissue in layer two of the scalp. Spasms of the occipitofrontalis muscle can increase gaping of scalp wounds. Bleeding from scalp lacerations can be fatal if not controlled (e.g., by sutures).

Squamous Cell Carcinoma of Lip

Squamous cell carcinoma (cancer) of the lip usually involves the lower lip (Fig. B8.16). Overexposure to sunshine over many years is a common factor in these cases. Chronic irritation from pipe smoking is also a contributing cause. Cancer cells from the central part of the lower lip, the floor of the mouth, and the apex of the tongue spread to the *submental lymph nodes*, whereas cancer cells from lateral parts of the lower lip drain to the *submandibular lymph nodes*.

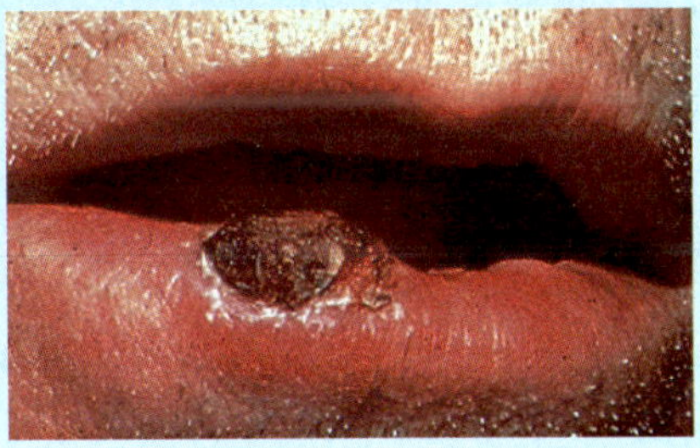

FIGURE B8.16. Carcinoma of lip.

The Bottom Line: Face and Scalp

The face provides our identity as an individual human. Thus, birth or acquired defects have consequences beyond their physical effects. • The individuality of the face results primarily from anatomical variation. • The way in which the facial muscles alter the basic features is critical to communication. • Lips and the shape and degree of opening of the mouth are important components of speech, but emphasis and subtleties of meaning are provided by our facial expressions.

Structure of scalp: The scalp is a somewhat mobile soft tissue mantle covering the calvaria. • The primary subcutaneous component of the scalp is the musculo-aponeurotic epicranius to which the overlying skin is firmly attached, but it is separated from the outer periosteum (pericranium) of the cranium by loose areolar tissue. • The areolar layer enables the mobility of the scalp over the calvaria and permits traumatic separation of the scalp from the cranium. • Attachment of the skin to the epicranial aponeurosis keeps the edges of superficial wounds together, but a wound that also penetrates the epicranial aponeurosis gaps widely. • Blood may collect in the areolar space deep to the aponeurosis after a head injury.

Muscles of face and scalp: The facial muscles play important roles as the dilators and sphincters of the portals of the alimentary (digestive), respiratory, and visual systems (oral and palpebral fissures and nostrils), controlling what enters and some of what exits from our bodies. • Other facial muscles assist the muscles of mastication by keeping food between the teeth during chewing. • Fleshy portions of the face (eyelids and cheeks) form dynamic containing walls for the orbits and oral cavity. • Facial muscles are all derived from the second pharyngeal arch and are therefore supplied by the nerve of this arch, the facial nerve (CN VII). • Facial muscles are subcutaneous, most having a skeletal origin and a cutaneous insertion. • The face lacks the deep fascia present elsewhere in the body.

Innervation of face and scalp: The face is highly sensitive. It receives sensory innervation from the three divisions of the trigeminal nerve (CN V). • The major terminal branches of each division reach the subcutaneous tissue of each side of the face via three foramina that are aligned vertically. • Each division supplies a distinct sensory zone, similar to a dermatome, but without the overlapping of adjacent nerves; therefore, injuries result in distinct and defined areas of paresthesia. • The divisions of CN V supply sensation not only to the superficial skin of the face but also to deep mucosal surfaces of the conjunctival sacs, cornea, nasal cavity, and paranasal sinuses and to the oral cavity and vestibule. • The skin covering the angle of the mandible is innervated by the great auricular nerve, a branch of the cervical plexus. • Eight nerves supply sensation to the scalp via branches arising from all three divisions of CN V, anterior to the auricle of the external ear and branches of cervical spinal nerves posterior to the auricle. • The facial nerve (CN VII) is the motor nerve of the face, supplying all the muscles of facial expression, including the platysma, occipital belly of occipitofrontalis, and auricular muscles that are not part of the face per se. • These muscles receive innervation from CN VII primarily via five branches of the parotid (nerve) plexus.

Vasculature of face and scalp: The face and scalp are highly vascular. The terminal branches of the arteries of the face

continued on next page

The Bottom Line (continued)

anastomose freely (including anastomoses across the midline with their contralateral partners). Thus, bleeding from facial lacerations may be diffuse, with the lacerated vessel bleeding from both ends. • Most arteries of the face are branches or derivatives of branches of the external carotid artery; the arteries arising from the internal carotid that supply the forehead are exceptions. • The main artery to the face is the facial artery. • The arteries of the scalp are firmly embedded in the dense connective tissue overlying the epicranial aponeurosis. Thus, when lacerated, these arteries bleed from both ends, like those of the face, but are less able to constrict or retract than other superficial vessels; therefore, profuse bleeding results.

The veins of the face and scalp generally accompany arteries, providing a primarily superficial venous drainage. • However, they also anastomose with the pterygoid venous plexus and with dural venous sinuses via emissary veins, which provide a potentially dangerous route for the spread of infection. • Most nerves and vessels of the scalp run vertically toward the vertex; thus, a horizontal laceration may produce more neurovascular damage than a vertical one.

The lymphatic drainage of most of the face follows the venous drainage to lymph nodes around the base of the anterior part of the head (submandibular, parotid, and superficial cervical nodes). • An exception to this pattern is the lymph drainage of the central part of the lip and chin, which initially drains to the submental lymph nodes. All nodes of the face drain in turn to the deep cervical lymph nodes.

CRANIAL MENINGES

N56.1 The **cranial meninges** are membranous coverings of the brain that lie immediately internal to the cranium (Figs. 8.15A and 8.28). The cranial meninges

- protect the brain.
- form the supporting framework for arteries, veins, and venous sinuses.
- enclose a fluid-filled cavity, the subarachnoid space, which is vital to the normal function of the brain.

The meninges are composed of three membranous connective tissue layers (Fig. 8.28A, B, D):

1. *Dura mater (dura)*: tough, thick external fibrous layer.
2. *Arachnoid mater (arachnoid)*: thin intermediate layer.
3. *Pia mater (pia)*: delicate internal vasculated layer.

The intermediate and internal layers (arachnoid and pia) are continuous membranes that collectively make up the **leptomeninx** (G. slender membrane) (Fig. 8.28B). The arachnoid is separated from the pia by the **subarachnoid (leptomeningeal) space**, which contains **cerebrospinal fluid** (CSF). This fluid-filled space helps maintain the balance of extracellular fluid in the brain. CSF is a clear liquid similar to blood plasma in constitution. It provides nutrients but it has less protein and a different ion concentration. CSF is formed by the choroid plexuses of the four ventricles of the brain (Fig. 8.28A). This fluid leaves the ventricular system and enters the subarachnoid space between the arachnoid and pia mater, where it cushions and nourishes the brain.

Dura Mater

The **cranial dura mater** (dura), a thick, dense, bilaminar membrane, is also called the *pachymeninx* (G. *pachy*, thick + G. *menix*, membrane) (Fig. 8.28A). It is adherent to the internal table of the calvaria. The two layers of the cranial dura are an *external periosteal layer*, formed by the periosteum covering the internal surface of the calvaria, and an *internal meningeal layer*, a strong fibrous membrane that is continuous at the foramen magnum with the spinal dura covering the spinal cord.

The external periosteal layer of dura adheres to the internal surface of the cranium. Its attachment is tenacious along the suture lines and in the cranial base (Haines, 2013). The external periosteal layer is continuous at the cranial foramina with the periosteum on the external surface of the calvaria (Fig. 8.28C). This outer layer is not continuous with the dura mater of the spinal cord, which consists of only a meningeal layer.

Except where the dural sinuses and infoldings occur (Fig. 8.28B), *the internal meningeal layer is intimately fused with the periosteal layer* and cannot be separated from it (Fig. 8.28B, C). The fused external and internal layers of dura over the calvaria can be easily stripped from the cranial bones (e.g., when the calvaria is removed at autopsy). In the cranial base, the two dural layers are firmly attached and difficult to separate from the bones. In life, such separation at the dural–cranial interface occurs only pathologically, creating an actual (blood- or fluid-filled) epidural space.

DURAL INFOLDINGS OR REFLECTIONS

The internal **meningeal layer of dura mater** is a supporting layer that reflects away from the external periosteal layer of dura to form dural infoldings (reflections) (Figs. 8.28B and 8.29). The dural infoldings divide the cranial cavity into compartments, forming partial partitions (dural septa) between certain parts of the brain and providing support for other parts. The dural infoldings include the following: AN30.3

- *Falx cerebri* (cerebral falx).
- *Tentorium cerebelli* (cerebellar tentorium).
- *Falx cerebelli* (cerebellar falx).
- *Diaphragma sellae* (sellar diaphragm).

(*continued on p.* 924)

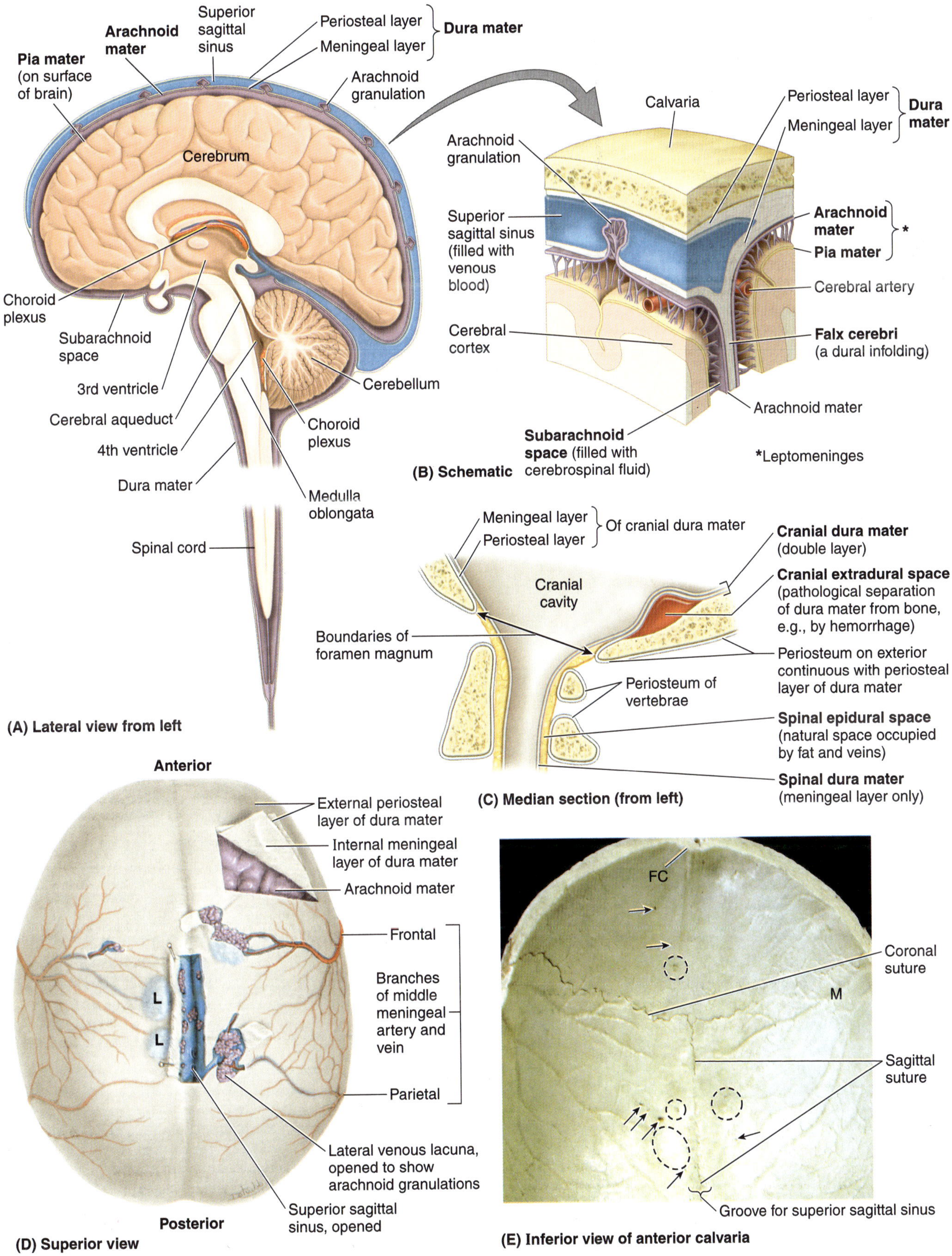
Pia mater (on surface of brain)
Arachnoid mater
Superior sagittal sinus
Periosteal layer
Meningeal layer
Dura mater
Arachnoid granulation
Cerebrum
Choroid plexus
Subarachnoid space
3rd ventricle
Cerebral aqueduct
4th ventricle
Dura mater
Cerebellum
Choroid plexus
Medulla oblongata
Spinal cord
(A) Lateral view from left
Calvaria
Periosteal layer
Meningeal layer
Dura mater
Arachnoid granulation
Superior sagittal sinus (filled with venous blood)
Arachnoid mater
Pia mater
*
Cerebral artery
Cerebral cortex
Falx cerebri (a dural infolding)
Arachnoid mater
Subarachnoid space (filled with cerebrospinal fluid)
*Leptomeninges
(B) Schematic
Meningeal layer
Periosteal layer
Of cranial dura mater
Cranial dura mater (double layer)
Cranial cavity
Cranial extradural space (pathological separation of dura mater from bone, e.g., by hemorrhage)
Boundaries of foramen magnum
Periosteum on exterior continuous with periosteal layer of dura mater
Periosteum of vertebrae
Spinal epidural space (natural space occupied by fat and veins)
Spinal dura mater (meningeal layer only)
(C) Median section (from left)
Anterior
External periosteal layer of dura mater
Internal meningeal layer of dura mater
Arachnoid mater
Frontal
Branches of middle meningeal artery and vein
Parietal
L
L
Lateral venous lacuna, opened to show arachnoid granulations
Superior sagittal sinus, opened
Posterior
(D) Superior view
FC
Coronal suture
M
Sagittal suture
Groove for superior sagittal sinus
(E) Inferior view of anterior calvaria

The **falx cerebri** (L. *falx*, sickle shaped), the largest dural infolding, lies in the **longitudinal cerebral fissure** that separates the right and the left *cerebral hemispheres*. The falx cerebri attaches in the median plane to the internal surface of the calvaria, from the *frontal crest of the frontal bone* and *crista galli of the ethmoid bone* anteriorly to the *internal occipital protuberance* posteriorly (Figs. 8.29A and 8.30). It ends by becoming continuous with the tentorium cerebelli.

The **tentorium cerebelli**, the second largest dural infolding, is a wide crescentic septum that separates the occipital lobes of the cerebral hemispheres from the cerebellum (Fig. 8.29A, B). The tentorium cerebelli attaches rostrally to the clinoid processes of the sphenoid, rostrolaterally to the petrous part of the temporal bone, and posterolaterally to the internal surface of the occipital bone and part of the parietal bone.

The falx cerebri attaches to the tentorium cerebelli and holds it up, giving it a tent-like appearance (L. *tentorium*, tent). The tentorium cerebelli divides the cranial cavity into *supratentorial* and *infratentorial compartments*. The supratentorial compartment is divided into right and left halves by the falx cerebri. The concave anteromedial border of the tentorium cerebelli is free, producing a gap called the **tentorial notch** through which the brainstem (midbrain, pons, and medulla oblongata) extends from the posterior into the middle cranial fossa (Fig. 8.31A, B).

The **falx cerebelli** is a vertical dural infolding that lies inferior to the tentorium cerebelli in the posterior part of the posterior cranial fossa (Figs. 8.29 and 8.30). It is attached to the internal occipital crest and partially separates the cerebellar hemispheres.

The **diaphragma sellae**, the smallest dural infolding, is a circular sheet of dura that is suspended between the clinoid processes forming a partial roof over the hypophysial fossa in the sphenoid (Fig. 8.29A). The diaphragma sellae covers the pituitary gland in this fossa and has an aperture for passage of the infundibulum and hypophysial veins.

DURAL VENOUS SINUSES

AN30.3 The **dural venous sinuses** are endothelium-lined spaces between the periosteal and meningeal layers of the dura. They form where the dural septa attach along the free edge of the falx cerebri and in relation to formations of the cranial floor (Figs. 8.29, 8.31, and 8.32). Large veins from the surface of the brain empty into these sinuses and most of the blood from the brain ultimately drains through them into the internal jugular veins (IJVs). The **superior sagittal sinus** lies in the convex attached border of the falx cerebri (Fig. 8.29). This sinus begins at the crista galli and ends near the internal occipital protuberance (Fig. 8.30) at the confluence of sinuses, a meeting place of the superior sagittal, straight, occipital, and transverse sinuses (Fig. 8.32). The superior sagittal sinus receives the superior cerebral veins and communicates on each side through slit-like openings with the **lateral venous lacunae** (L, small lakes), lateral expansions of the superior sagittal sinus (Fig. 8.28D).

Arachnoid granulations (collections of arachnoid villi) are tufted prolongations of the arachnoid that protrude through the meningeal layer of the dura mater into the dural venous sinuses, especially the lateral lacunae and affect transfer of CSF to the venous system (Figs. 8.29B, D and 8.35). Enlarged arachnoid granulations (*pacchionian bodies*) may erode bone, forming pits called **granular foveolae** in the calvaria (Fig. 8.28E). They are usually observed especially in the vicinity of the superior sagittal sinus, but may also occur in the transverse, superior petrosal and straight dural venous sinuses. Arachnoid granulations are structurally adapted for the transport of CSF from the subarachnoid space to the venous system.

The **inferior sagittal sinus** is much smaller than the superior sagittal sinus (Fig. 8.29). It runs in the inferior concave free border of the falx cerebri and ends in the straight sinus. The **straight sinus** (L. *sinus rectus*) is formed by the union of the inferior sagittal sinus with the *great cerebral vein*. It runs inferoposteriorly along the line of attachment of the falx cerebri to the tentorium cerebelli, where it joins the confluence of sinuses.

The **transverse sinuses** pass laterally from the confluence of sinuses, forming a groove in the occipital bones and the postero-inferior angles of the parietal bones (Figs. 8.30 to 8.32). The transverse sinuses course along the posterolateral attached margins of the tentorium cerebelli and then become the sigmoid sinuses as they approach the posterior aspect of the petrous temporal bones. Blood received by the *confluence of sinuses* is drained by the transverse sinuses, but rarely equally. Usually, the left sinus is dominant (larger).

The **sigmoid sinuses** follow S-shaped courses in the posterior cranial fossa, forming deep grooves in the temporal and occipital bones. Each sigmoid sinus turns anteriorly and then continues inferiorly as the IJV after traversing the

FIGURE 8.28. Meninges and their relationship to calvaria, brain, and spinal cord. A. The dura mater and subarachnoid space (purple) surround the brain and are continuous with that around the spinal cord. **B.** The two layers of dura separate to form dural venous sinuses, such as the superior sagittal sinus. Arachnoid granulations protrude through the meningeal layer of the dura into the dural venous sinuses and effect transfer of cerebrospinal fluid (CSF) to the venous system. **C.** The normal fat- and vein-filled spinal epidural (extradural) space is not continuous with the potential or pathological cranial epidural space. Cranial dura mater has two layers, whereas spinal dura mater consists of a single layer. **D.** The calvaria has been removed to reveal the external (periosteal layer) of the dura mater. In the median plane, a part of the thick roof of the superior sagittal sinus has been incised and retracted; laterally, parts of the thin roof of two lateral lacunae (*L*) are reflected to demonstrate the abundant arachnoid granulations, which are responsible for absorption of CSF. On the right, an angular flap of dura has been turned anteriorly; the convolutions of the cerebral cortex are visible through the arachnoid mater. **E.** The internal aspect of the calvaria reveals pits (*dotted lines*, granular foveolae) in the frontal and parietal bones, which are produced by enlarged arachnoid granulations or clusters of smaller ones (as in **D**). Multiple small emissary veins pass between the superior sagittal sinus and the veins in the diploë and scalp through small emissary foramina (*arrows*) located on each side of the sagittal suture. The sinuous vascular groove (*M*) on the lateral wall is formed by the frontal branch of the middle meningeal artery. The falx cerebri attaches anteriorly to the frontal crest (*FC*).

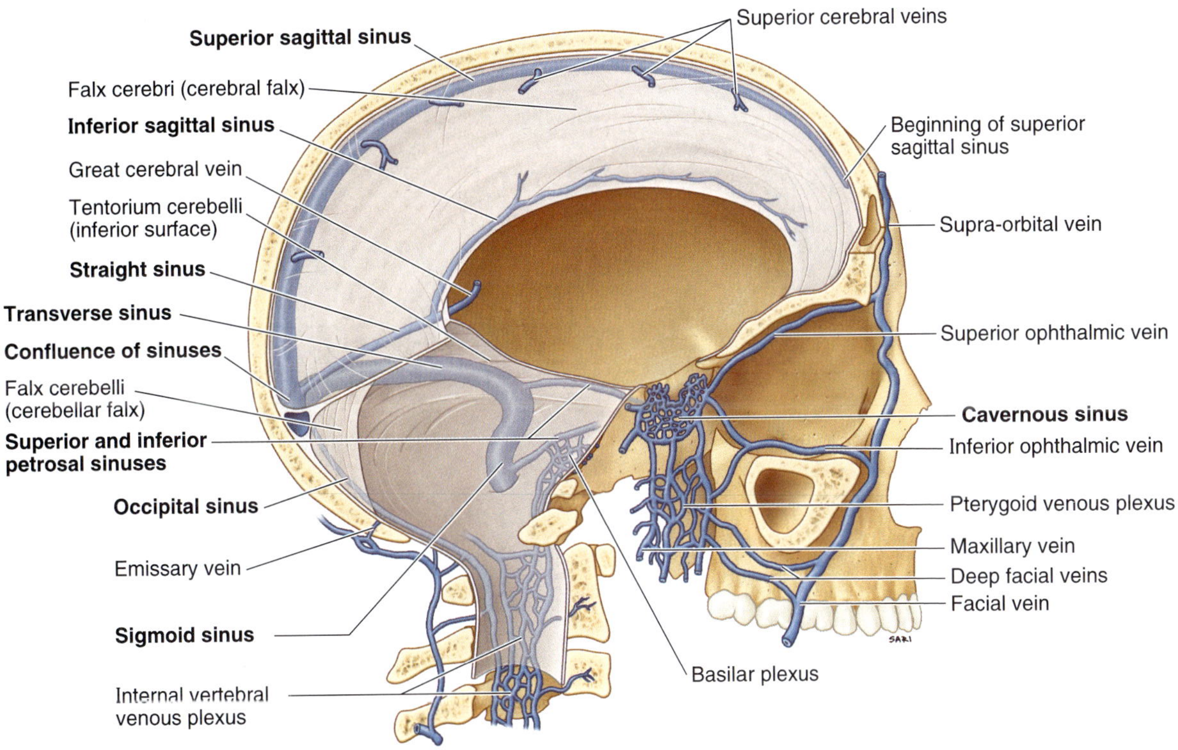

(A) Medial view

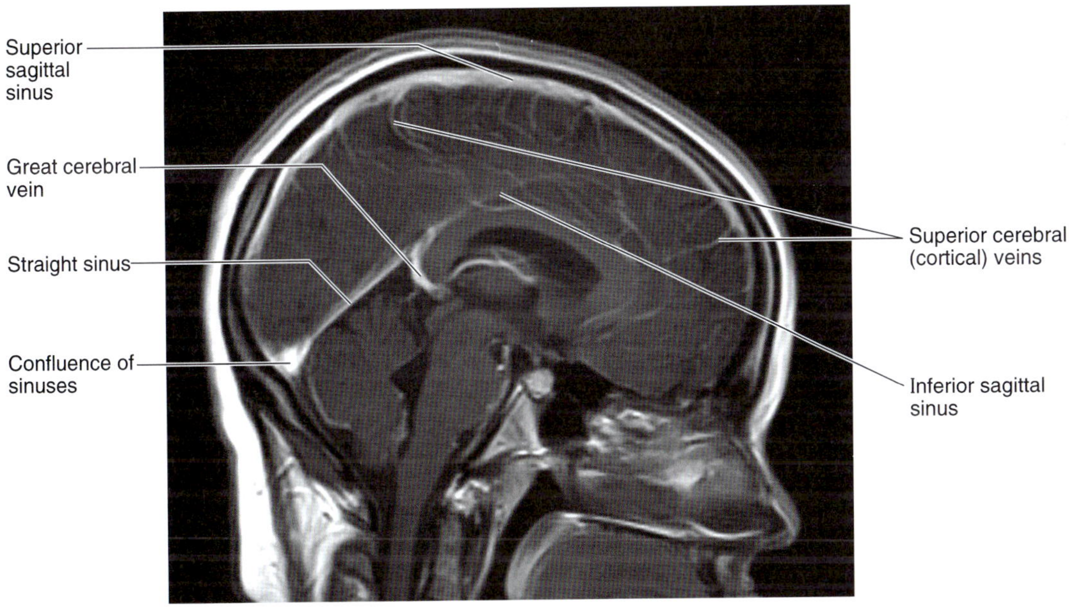

(B) Median (contrast enhanced) MRI of brain

FIGURE 8.29. Dural infoldings and dural venous sinuses. The left side of the bisected head is shown. **A.** Two sickle-shaped dural folds (septae), the falx cerebri and falx cerebelli, are vertically oriented in the median plane; two roof-like folds, the tentorium cerebelli and the small diaphragma sellae, lie horizontally. **B.** Venous sinuses of the dura mater and their communications are demonstrated in the midline vicinity.

jugular foramen. The **occipital sinus** lies in the attached border of the falx cerebelli and ends superiorly in the confluence of sinuses (Fig. 8.29A, B). The occipital sinus communicates inferiorly with the *internal vertebral venous plexus* (Figs. 8.29A and 8.33).

The **cavernous sinuses**, large venous plexuses, are located on each side of the sella turcica on the upper surface of the body of the sphenoid, which contains the sphenoidal (air) sinus (Figs. 8.29A and 8.31). The cavernous sinus consists of a venous plexus of extremely thin-walled veins that extends

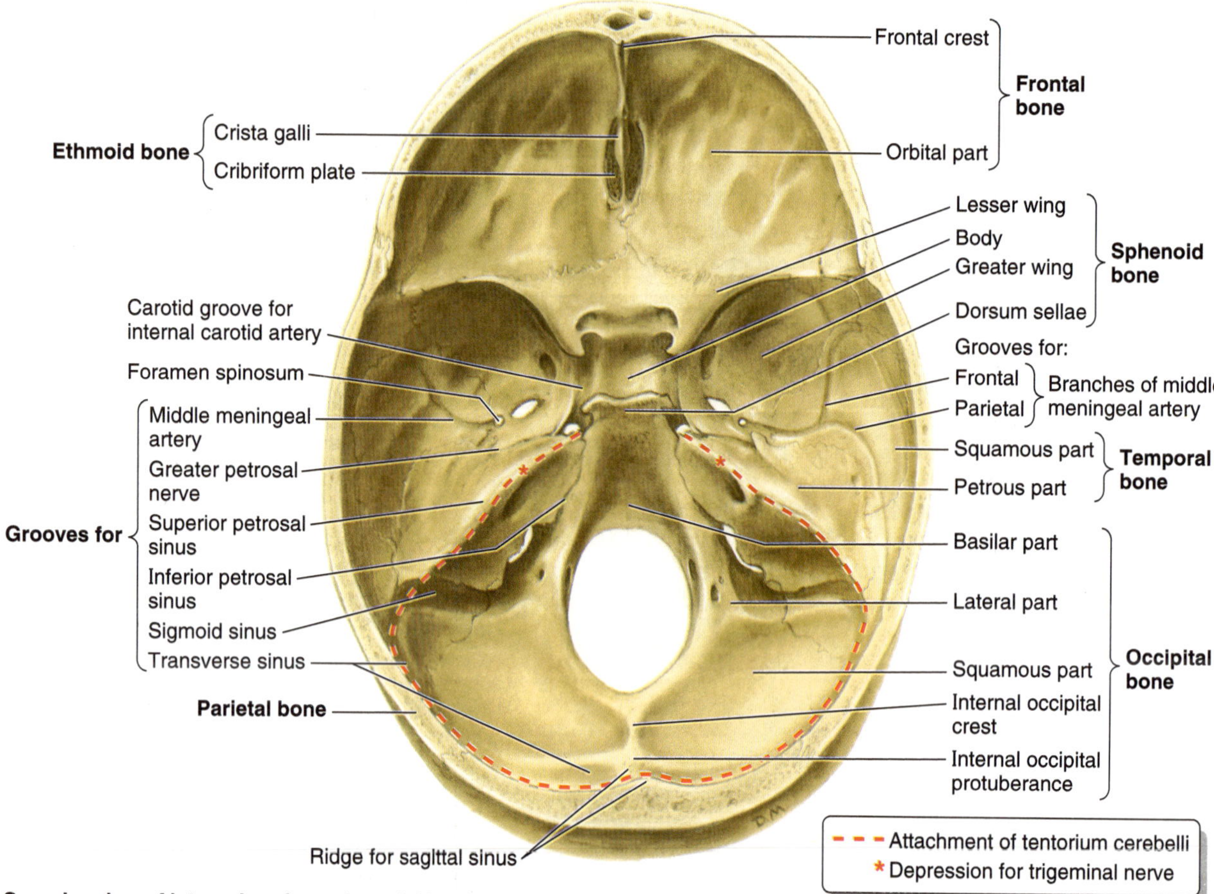

Superior view of internal surface of cranial base

FIGURE 8.30. Interior of base of cranium. The internal occipital protuberance is formed in relationship to the confluence of sinuses (Fig. 8.31*A*), and grooves are formed in the cranial base by the dural venous sinuses (e.g., the sigmoid sinus). The tentorium cerebelli is attached along the lengths of the transverse and superior petrosal sinuses (*dashed line*).

from the superior orbital fissure anteriorly to the apex of the petrous part of the temporal bone posteriorly. The sinus receives blood from the superior and inferior ophthalmic veins, superficial middle cerebral vein, and sphenoparietal sinus. The venous channels in these sinuses communicate with each other through venous channels anterior and posterior to the stalk of the pituitary gland—the **intercavernous sinuses** (Fig. 8.31A, B)—and sometimes through veins inferior to the pituitary gland. The cavernous sinuses drain postero-inferiorly through the superior and inferior petrosal sinuses and emissary veins to the *basilar* and *pterygoid plexuses* (Fig. 8.29A).

Inside each cavernous sinus is the **internal carotid artery** with its small branches, surrounded by the carotid plexus of sympathetic nerve(s), and the abducent nerve (CN VI) (Fig. 8.31C). The oculomotor (CN III) and trochlear (CN IV) nerves, plus two of the three divisions of the trigeminal nerve (CN V), are embedded in the lateral wall of the sinus. The artery, carrying warm blood from the body's core, traverses the sinus filled with cooler blood returning from the capillaries of the body's periphery, allowing for heat exchange to conserve energy or cool the arterial blood. This does not appear to be as important in humans as it is in running animals (e.g., horses and cheetahs) in which the carotid artery runs a longer, more tortuous course through the cavernous sinuses, allowing cooling of blood before it enters the brain. Pulsations of the artery within the cavernous sinus are said to promote propulsion of venous blood from the sinus, as does gravity (Standring, 2016).

The **superior petrosal sinuses** run from the posterior ends of the veins making up the cavernous sinus to the transverse sinuses at the site where these sinuses curve inferiorly to form the sigmoid sinuses (Fig. 8.32B). Each superior petrosal sinus lies in the anterolateral attached margin of the tentorium cerebelli, which attaches to the superior border (crest) of the petrous part of the temporal bone (Fig. 8.30).

The **inferior petrosal sinuses** also commence at the posterior end of the cavernous sinus (Fig. 8.31A, B). Each inferior petrosal sinus runs in a groove between the petrous part of the temporal bone and the basilar part of the occipital bone (Fig. 8.30). The inferior petrosal sinuses drain the cavernous sinus directly into the transition of the sigmoid sinus to the IJV at the jugular foramen (Fig. 8.31B). The **basilar plexus** connects the inferior petrosal sinuses and communicates inferiorly with the *internal vertebral venous plexus* (Figs. 8.29B and 8.33). **Emissary veins** connect the dural AN27.2
venous sinuses with veins outside the cranium. Although AN33.4
they are valveless and blood may flow in both directions,

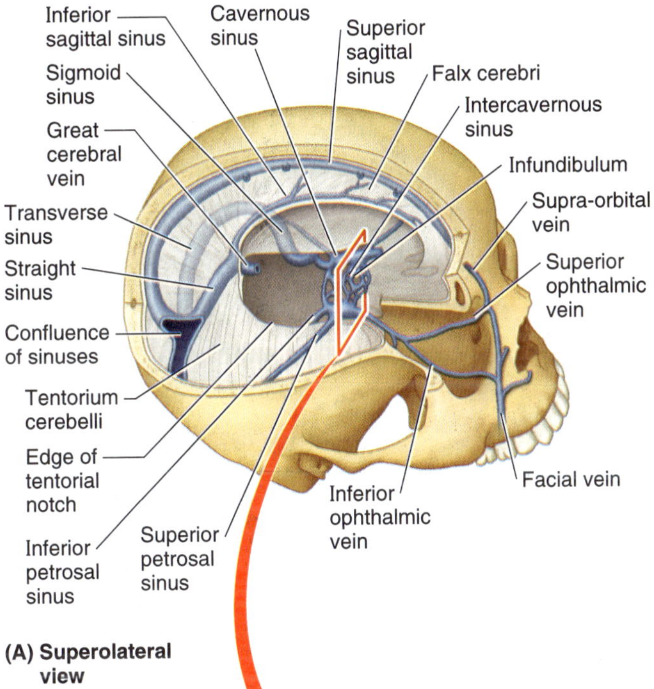

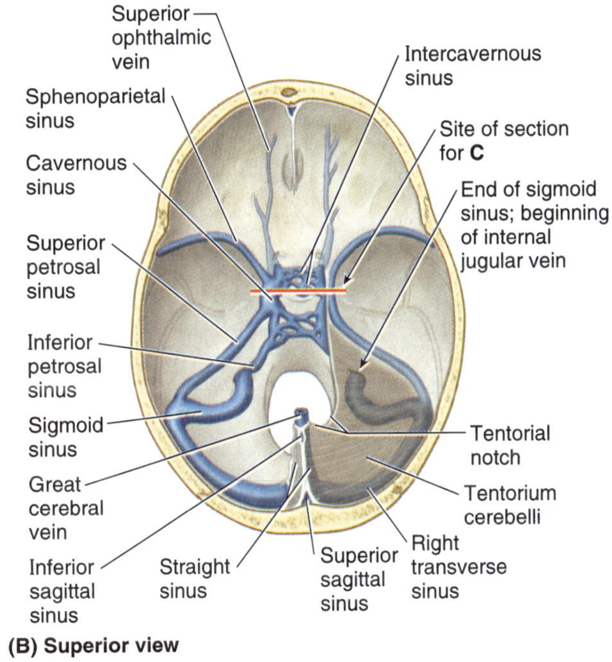

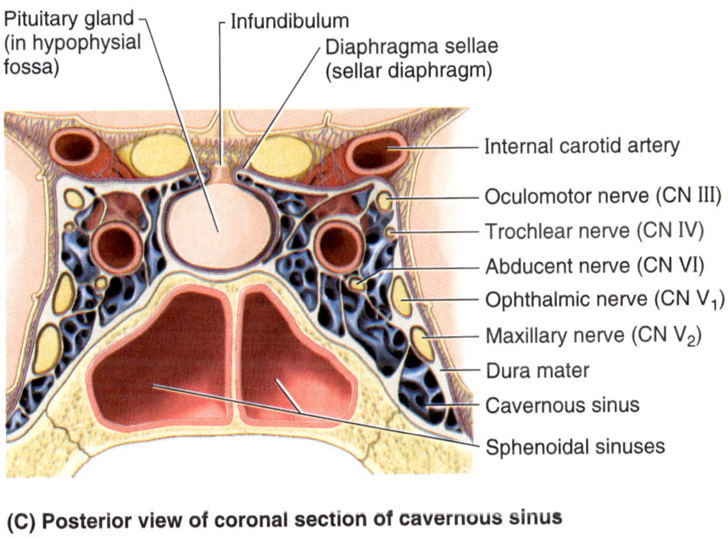

FIGURE 8.31. Venous sinuses of dura mater. Blood from the brain drains into the sinuses within the dura. **A.** The brain and part of the calvaria are removed to demonstrate the sinuses related to the falx cerebri and tentorium cerebelli. **B.** This view of the interior of the base of the cranium demonstrates most communications of the cavernous sinuses (the inferior communication with the pterygoid venous plexus is a notable exception) and drainage of the confluence of sinuses. The ophthalmic veins drain into the cavernous sinus. **C.** The orientation and placement of this section of the cavernous sinuses and the body of the sphenoid are indicated in parts **A** and **B**. The cavernous sinus is situated bilaterally at the lateral aspect of the hollow body of the sphenoid and the hypophysial fossa. The internal carotid arteries, having made acute bends, are cut twice. Inferiorly, the cavernous parts of the arteries are sectioned as they pass anteriorly along the carotid groove toward the acute bend of the artery (some radiologists refer to the bend as the "carotid siphon"). Superiorly, the cerebral parts of the arteries are sectioned as they pass posteriorly from the bend to join the cerebral arterial circle.

flow in the emissary veins is usually away from the brain. The size and number of emissary veins vary; many small ones are unnamed. A **frontal emissary vein** is present in children and some adults. It passes through the foramen cecum of the cranium, connecting the superior sagittal sinus with veins of the frontal sinus and nasal cavities. A **parietal emissary vein**, which may be paired bilaterally, passes through the *parietal foramen* in the calvaria, connecting the superior sagittal sinus with the veins external to it, particularly those in the scalp (see Fig. 8.8A, C). A **mastoid emissary vein** passes through the *mastoid foramen* and connects each sigmoid sinus with the *occipital* or *posterior auricular vein* (Fig. 8.33). A **posterior condylar emissary vein** may also be present, passing through the condylar canal, connecting the sigmoid sinus with the *suboccipital venous plexus*.

VASCULATURE OF DURA MATER

The **arteries of the dura** supply more blood to the calvaria than to the dura. The largest of these vessels, the **middle meningeal artery**, is a branch of the maxillary artery (Fig. 8.28D). It enters the floor of the middle cranial fossa through the *foramen spinosum* (Fig. 8.30), runs laterally in the fossa, and turns supero-anteriorly on the greater wing of the sphenoid, where it divides into anterior and posterior branches (Fig. 8.28D). The **frontal branch of the middle meningeal artery** runs superiorly to the pterion and then curves posteriorly to ascend toward the vertex of the cranium. The **parietal branch of the middle meningeal artery** runs posterosuperiorly and ramifies (breaks up into distributing branches) over the posterior aspect of the cranium.

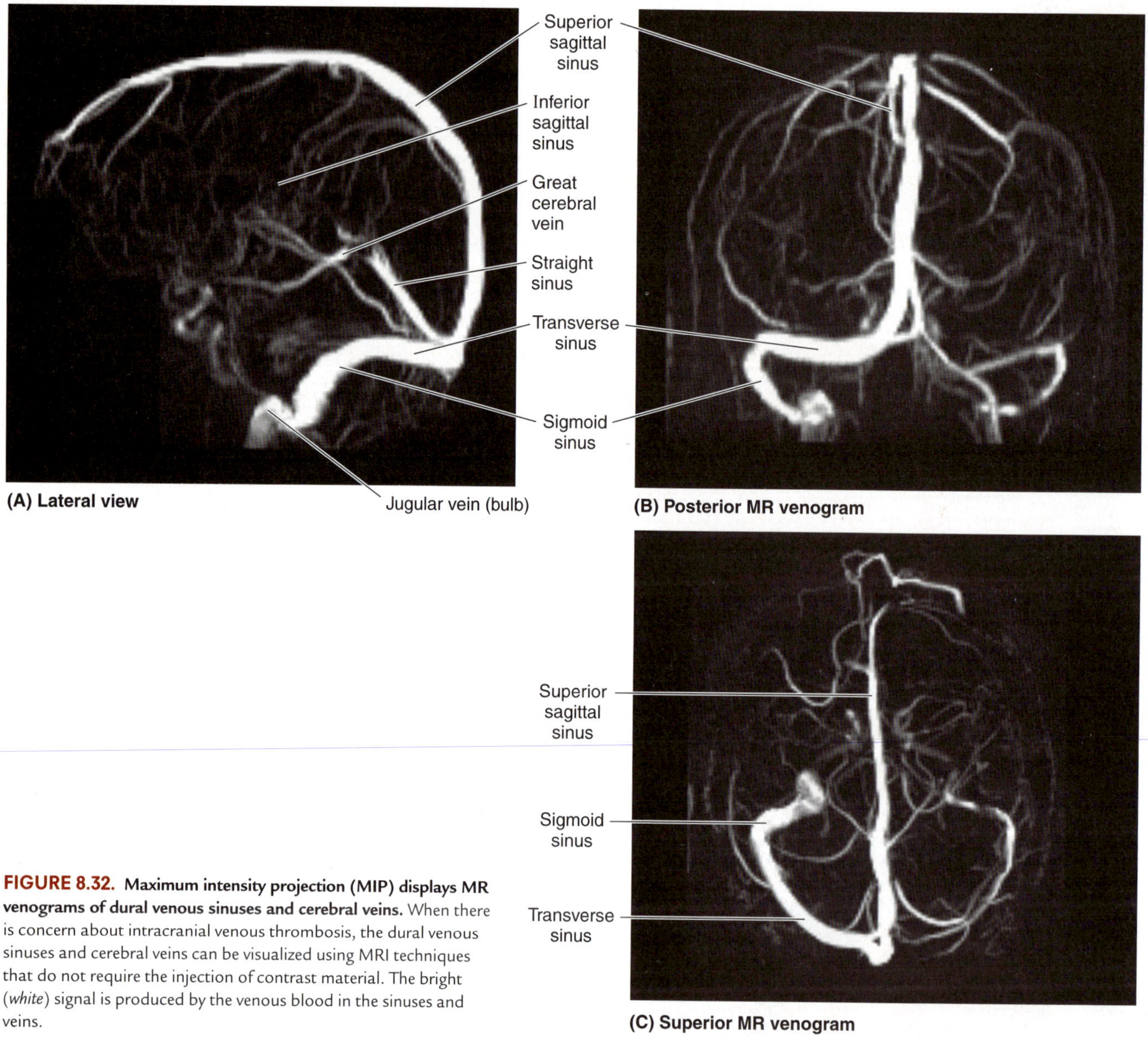

FIGURE 8.32. Maximum intensity projection (MIP) displays MR venograms of dural venous sinuses and cerebral veins. When there is concern about intracranial venous thrombosis, the dural venous sinuses and cerebral veins can be visualized using MRI techniques that do not require the injection of contrast material. The bright (*white*) signal is produced by the venous blood in the sinuses and veins.

Small areas of dura are supplied by other arteries: meningeal branches of the ophthalmic arteries, branches of the occipital arteries, and small branches of the vertebral arteries.

The **veins of the dura** accompany the meningeal arteries, often in pairs. The **middle meningeal veins** accompany the middle meningeal artery, leave the cranial cavity through the foramen spinosum or foramen ovale, and drain into the *pterygoid venous plexus* (Fig. 8.29B).

NERVE SUPPLY OF DURA MATER

The dura on the floors of the anterior and middle cranial fossa and the roof of the posterior cranial fossa is innervated by meningeal branches arising directly or indirectly from the trigeminal nerve (CN V) (Fig. 8.34). There are three divisions of CN V (CN V_1, CN V_2, and CN V_3), each of which contributes a meningeal branch or branches. The **anterior meningeal branches of the ethmoidal nerves** (CN V_1) and the **meningeal branches of the maxillary** (CN V_2) and **mandibular** (CN V_3) **nerves** supply the dura of the anterior cranial fossa. The latter two nerves also supply the dura of the middle cranial fossa (Fig. 8.34B). The meningeal branches of CN V_2 and CN V_3 are distributed as peri-arterial plexuses, accompanying the branches of the middle meningeal artery (Fig. 8.34A, *inset*).

The dura forming the roof of the posterior cranial fossa (tentorium cerebelli) and posterior part of the falx cerebri is supplied by the **tentorial nerve** (a branch of the ophthalmic nerve), whereas the anterior falx cerebri is innervated by ascending branches of the anterior meningeal branches (Fig. 8.34A). The dura of the floor of the posterior cranial fossa receives sensory fibers from the spinal

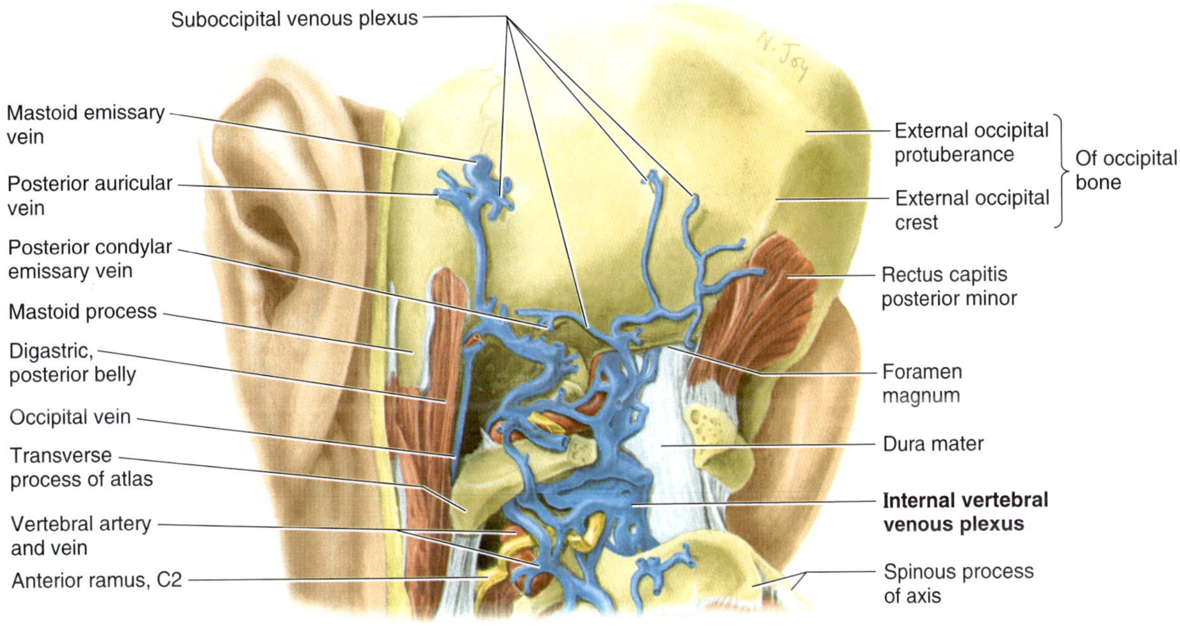

FIGURE 8.33. Deep dissection of suboccipital region. The external vertebral venous system has numerous intercommunications and connections, some of which are shown here. Superiorly, the system communicates with the veins of the scalp and the intracranial venous sinuses via the foramen magnum, the mastoid foramina, and the condylar canals. Anteromedially, it passes between the laminae and through the intervertebral foramina to communicate with the internal vertebral venous plexus and veins around the vertebral artery.

ganglia of C2 and C3 carried by those spinal nerves or by fibers transferred to and traveling centrally with the vagus (CN X) and hypoglossal (CN XII) nerves. Sensory endings are more numerous in the dura along each side of the superior sagittal sinus and in the tentorium cerebelli than they are in the floor of the cranium.

Pain fibers are most numerous where arteries and veins course in the dura. Pain arising from the dura is generally referred, perceived as a headache arising in cutaneous or mucosal regions supplied by the involved cervical nerve or division of the trigeminal nerve.

Arachnoid Mater and Pia Mater

The *arachnoid mater* and *pia mater* (or simply *arachnoid* and *pia*; together the leptomeninges) develop from a single layer of mesenchyme surrounding the embryonic brain, becoming the parietal part (arachnoid) and visceral part (pia) of the *leptomeninx* (Fig. 8.35). The derivation of the arachnoid–pia from a single embryonic layer is indicated in the adult by the numerous web-like *arachnoid trabeculae* passing between the arachnoid and pia, which give the arachnoid its name (G. *arachne*–, spider, cobweb + G. *eidos*, resemblance). The trabeculae are composed of flattened, irregularly shaped fibroblasts that bridge the subarachnoid space (Haines, 2013). The arachnoid and pia are in continuity immediately proximal to the exit of each cranial nerve from the dura mater. The **cranial arachnoid mater** contains fibroblasts, collagen fibers, and some elastic fibers. Although thin, the arachnoid is thick enough to be manipulated with forceps. The avascular arachnoid, although closely applied to the meningeal layer of the dura, is not attached to the dura. It is held against the inner surface of the dura by the pressure of the CSF in the subarachnoid space.

The **cranial pia mater** is an even thinner membrane than the arachnoid. It is highly vascularized by a network of fine blood vessels. The pia is difficult to see, but it gives the surface of the brain a shiny appearance. *The pia adheres to the surface of the brain and follows all its contours.* When the cerebral arteries penetrate the cerebral cortex, the pia follows them for a short distance, forming a **pial coat** and a **peri-arterial space** (Fig. 8.35).

Meningeal Spaces

Of the three meningeal "spaces" commonly mentioned in relation to the cranial meninges, only one exists as a space in the absence of pathology:

- The **dura–cranial interface** (extradural or epidural "space") is not a natural space between the cranium and the external periosteal layer of the dura because the dura is attached to the bones. It becomes an **extradural space** only pathologically (e.g., when blood from torn meningeal vessels pushes the periosteum away from the cranium) (Fig. 8.28C). The potential or pathological cranial epidural space is not continuous with the **spinal epidural space** (a natural space occupied by epidural fat and a venous plexus) because the former is external to the periosteum

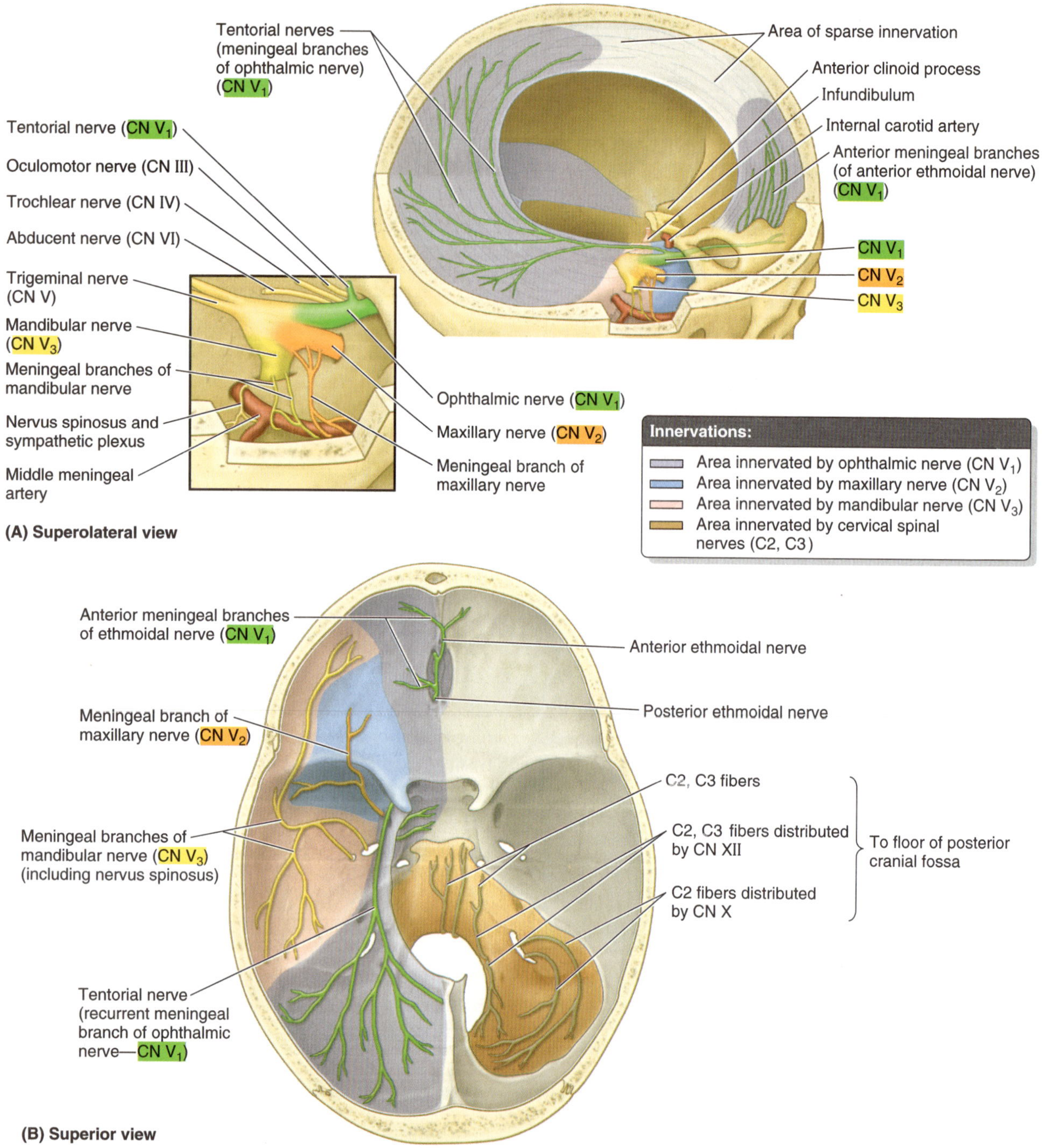

FIGURE 8.34. Innervation of dura mater. A. The right side of the calvaria and brain is removed, and CN V is dissected. The meningeal branches of the maxillary (CN V_2) and mandibular (CN V_3) nerves are distributed to the dura of the lateral part of the anterior and the middle cranial fossae as peri-arterial plexuses that accompany the branches of the middle meningeal artery along with vasomotor sympathetic nerve fibers from the superior cervical ganglion (**inset**). **B.** The internal aspect of the cranial base shows innervation of the dura by branches of the trigeminal and sensory fibers of cervical spinal nerves (C2, C3) passing directly from those nerves or via meningeal branches of the vagus (CN X) and hypoglossal (CN XII) nerves.

lining the cranium, and the latter is internal to the periosteum covering the vertebrae.

- The *dura–arachnoid interface* or junction ("subdural space") is likewise not a natural space between the dura and arachnoid. A space may develop in the dural border cell layer as the result of trauma, such as a hard blow to the head (Haines, 1993, 2013).
- The *subarachnoid space*, between the arachnoid and pia, is a real space that contains CSF, trabecular cells, arteries, and veins.

Although it is commonly stated that the brain "floats" in CSF, the brain is suspended in the CSF-filled subarachnoid space by the arachnoid trabeculae.

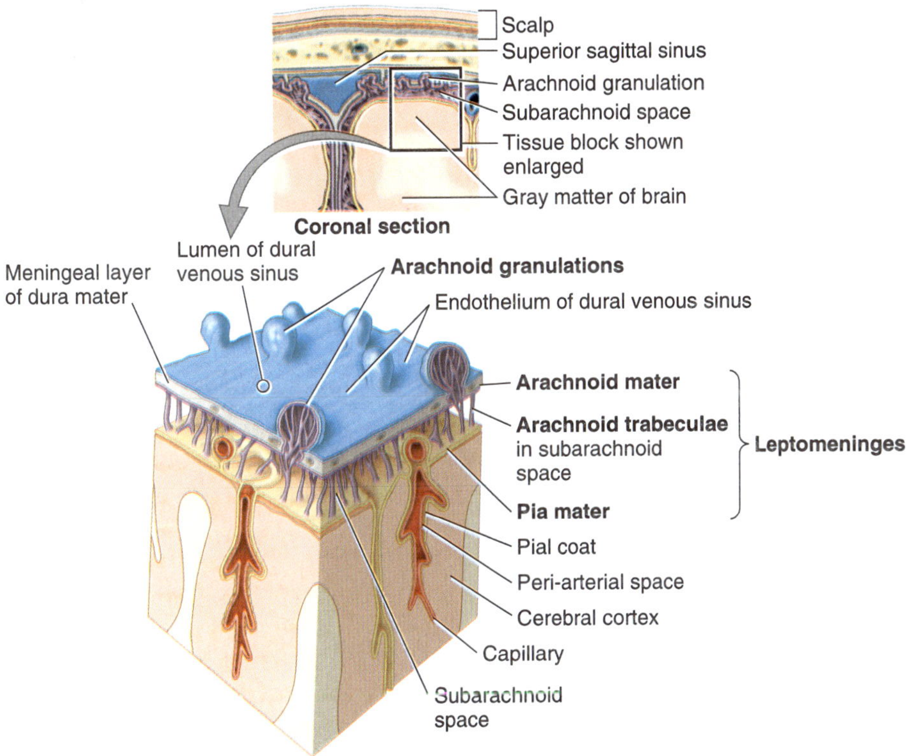

FIGURE 8.35. Leptomeninges. The coronal section (*above*) indicates the site of the tissue block (*below*). The subarachnoid space separates the two layers of the leptomeninges, the arachnoid and pia. CSF pressure keeps the arachnoid apposed to the meningeal layer of dura, and in the region of the superior sagittal sinus and adjacent venous lacunae (Fig. 8.28D), arachnoid granulations project through the dura into the blood-filled dural venous sinus.

CLINICAL BOX

CRANIAL CAVITY AND MENINGES

Fracture of Pterion

Fracture of the pterion can be life threatening because it overlies the frontal branches of the middle meningeal vessels, which lie in grooves on the internal aspect of the lateral wall of the calvaria (Fig. 8.30). The pterion is two fingers' breadth superior to the zygomatic arch and a thumb's breadth posterior to the frontal process of the zygomatic bone (Fig. B8.17A). A hard blow to the side of the head (e.g., during boxing) may fracture the thin bones forming the pterion (Fig. 8.4A), producing a rupture of the frontal branch of the middle meningeal artery or vein crossing

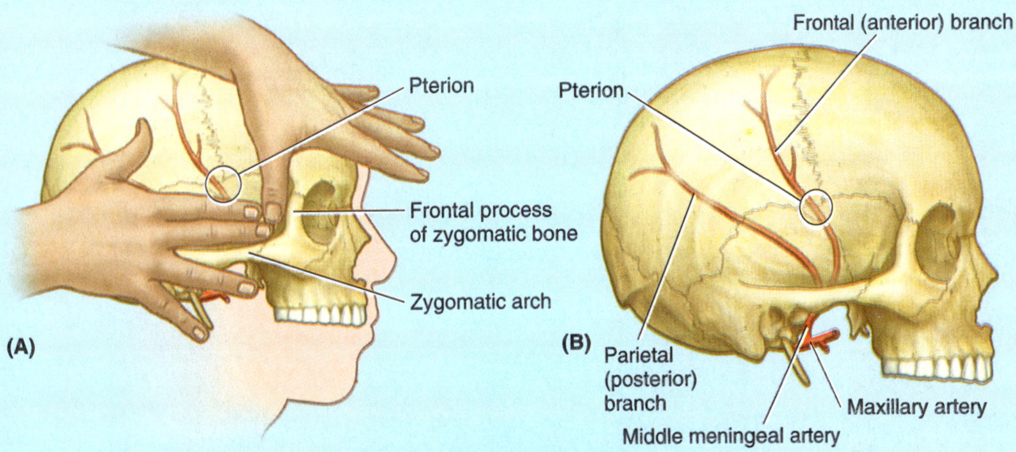

FIGURE B8.17. Location and relationships of pterion.

the pterion (Fig. B8.17B). The resulting hematoma exerts pressure on the underlying cerebral cortex (Fig. 8.19A). An untreated *middle meningeal vessel hemorrhage* may cause death in a few hours.

Thrombophlebitis of Facial Vein

AN28.8 AN33.4

The facial vein makes clinically important connections with the cavernous sinus through the superior ophthalmic vein, and the pterygoid venous plexus through the inferior ophthalmic and deep facial veins (Figs. 8.25 and 8.29A; Table 8.6). Because of these connections, an infection of the face may spread to the cavernous sinus and pterygoid venous plexus.

Blood from the medial angle of the eye, nose, and lips usually drains inferiorly through the facial vein, especially when a person is erect. Because the facial vein has no valves, blood may pass through it in the opposite direction. Consequently, venous blood from the face may enter the cavernous sinus. In individuals with *thrombophlebitis of the facial vein*—inflammation of the facial vein with secondary thrombus (clot) formation—pieces of an infected clot may extend into the intracranial venous system and produce *thrombophlebitis of the cavernous sinus*. Infection of the facial veins spreading to the dural venous sinuses may result from lacerations of the nose or be initiated by squeezing pustules (pimples) on the side of the nose and upper lip. Consequently, the triangular area from the upper lip to the bridge of the nose is considered the *danger triangle of the face* (Fig. B8.18).

Blunt Trauma to Head

A substantial blow to the head can detach the periosteal layer of dura mater from the calvaria without fracturing the cranial bones. In the cranial base, the two dural layers are firmly attached and difficult to separate from the bones. Consequently, a fracture of the cranial base usually tears the dura and results in leakage of CSF. The innermost part of the dura, *the dural border cell layer*, is composed of flattened fibroblasts that are separated by large extracellular spaces. This layer constitutes a plane of structural weakness at the dura–arachnoid junction (Haines, 2013).

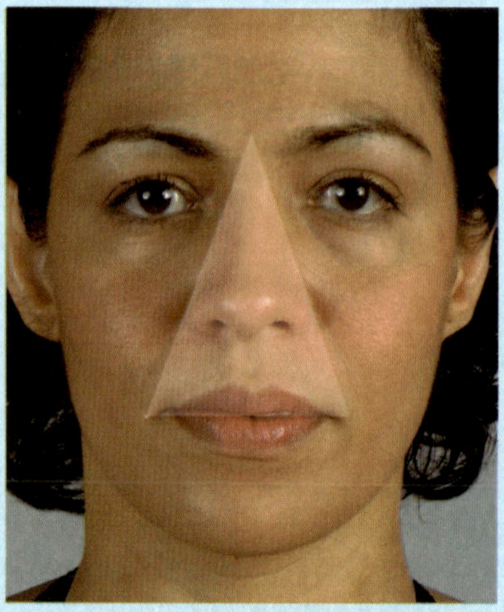

FIGURE B8.18. Danger triangle of face.

Tentorial Herniation

The tentorial notch is the opening in the tentorium cerebelli for the brainstem, which is slightly larger than is necessary to accommodate the midbrain (Fig. B8.19). Hence, *space-occupying lesions*, such as tumors in the supratentorial compartment, produce increased intracranial pressure, and may cause part of the adjacent temporal lobe of the brain to herniate through the tentorial notch. During *tentorial herniation*, the temporal lobe may be lacerated by the tough tentorium cerebelli, and the oculomotor nerve (CN III) may be stretched, compressed, or both. *Oculomotor lesions* may produce paralysis of the extrinsic eye muscles supplied by CN III.

Bulging of Diaphragma Sellae

Pituitary tumors may extend superiorly through the aperture in the diaphragma sellae or cause it to bulge. These tumors often expand the diaphragma sellae, producing disturbances in endocrine function early or late (i.e., before or after enlargement of the diaphragma sellae). Superior extension of a tumor may cause visual

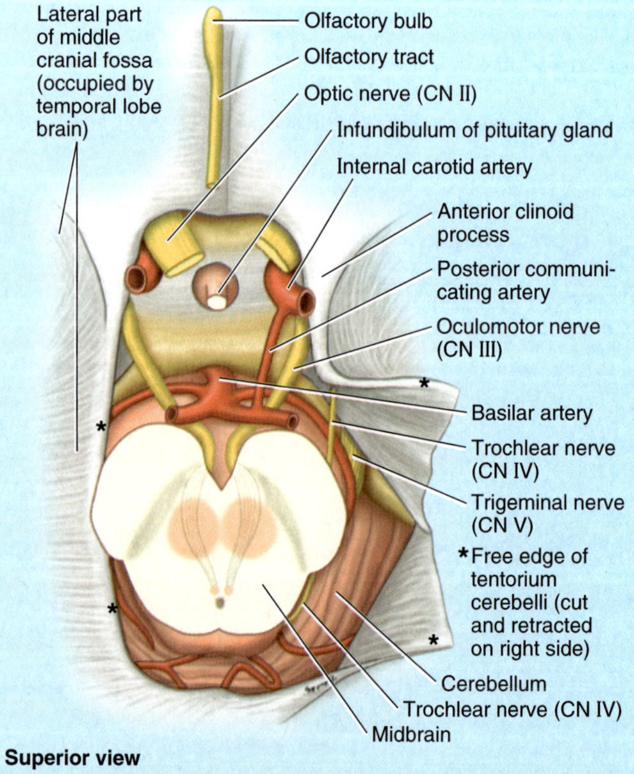

FIGURE B8.19. Structures and relationships in vicinity of tentorial notch.

symptoms owing to pressure on the optic chiasm, the place where the optic nerve fibers cross (Fig. 8.37B).

AN30.4 Occlusion of Cerebral Veins and Dural Venous Sinuses

Occlusion of cerebral veins and dural venous sinuses may result from thrombi (clots), thrombophlebitis (venous inflammation), or tumors (e.g., meningiomas). The dural venous sinuses most frequently thrombosed are the transverse, cavernous, and superior sagittal sinuses (Organek, 2016).

The facial veins make clinically important connections with the cavernous sinus through the superior ophthalmic veins (Fig. 8.29A). *Cavernous sinus thrombosis* usually results from infections in the orbit, nasal sinuses, and superior part of the face (the danger triangle, Fig. B8.18). In persons with *thrombophlebitis of the facial vein*, pieces of an infected thrombus may extend into the cavernous sinus, producing *thrombophlebitis of the cavernous sinus*. The infection usually involves only one sinus initially, but it may spread to the opposite side through the intercavernous sinuses. Thrombophlebitis of the cavernous sinus may affect the abducent nerve as it traverses the sinus (see Chapter 10, Summary of Cranial Nerves, Fig. 10.3, p. 1122) and may also effect the nerves embedded within the lateral wall of the sinus (Fig. 8.31C; see Chapter 10, Summary of Cranial Nerves, Fig. 10.3, p. 1122). Septic thrombosis of the cavernous sinus often results in the development of *acute meningitis*.

Metastasis of Tumor Cells to Dural Venous Sinuses

The basilar and occipital sinuses communicate through the foramen magnum with the internal vertebral venous plexuses (Figs. 8.29A and 8.33). Because these venous channels are valveless, compression of the thorax, abdomen, or pelvis, as occurs during heavy coughing and straining, may force venous blood from these regions into the internal vertebral venous system and from it into the dural venous sinuses. As a result, pus in abscesses and tumor cells in these regions may spread to the vertebrae and brain.

Fractures of Cranial Base

In fractures of the cranial base, the internal carotid artery may be torn, producing an *arteriovenous fistula* within the cavernous sinus. Arterial blood rushes into the cavernous sinus, enlarging it and forcing retrograde blood flow into its venous tributaries, especially the ophthalmic veins. As a result, the eyeball protrudes (*exophthalmos*) and the conjunctiva becomes engorged (*chemosis*). The protruding eyeball pulsates in synchrony with the radial pulse, a phenomenon known as *pulsating exophthalmos*. Because CN III, CN IV, CN V_1, CN V_2, and CN VI lie in or close to the lateral wall of the cavernous sinus, these nerves may also be affected when the sinus is injured (Fig. 8.31C).

Dural Origin of Headaches

The cranial dura mater is sensitive to pain, especially where it is related to the dural venous sinuses and meningeal arteries (Fig. 8.31A). Consequently, pulling on arteries at the cranial base or veins near the vertex, where they pierce the dura, causes pain. Distension of the scalp or meningeal vessels (or both) is believed to be one cause of headache (Chou, 2016).

Many headaches appear to be dural in origin, such as the headache occurring after a lumbar spinal puncture for removal of CSF (see Chapter 2, Back). These headaches are thought to result from stimulation of sensory nerve endings in the dura. When CSF is removed, the brain sags slightly, pulling on the dura; this may also cause a headache. For this reason, patients are asked to keep their heads down after a lumbar puncture to minimize the pull on the dura, reducing the chances of getting a headache.

Leptomeningitis

Leptomeningitis is an inflammation of the leptomeninges (arachnoid and pia) resulting from pathogenic microorganisms. The infection and inflammation are usually confined to the subarachnoid space and the arachnoid–pia (Jubelt, 2016). The bacteria may enter the subarachnoid space through the blood (*septicemia*, or "blood poisoning") or spread from an infection of the heart, lungs, or other viscera. Microorganisms may also enter the subarachnoid space from a compound cranial fracture or a fracture of the nasal sinuses. *Acute purulent meningitis* can result from infection with almost any pathogenic bacteria (e.g., *meningococcal meningitis*).

Head Injuries and Intracranial Hemorrhage

Extradural (epidural) hemorrhage is arterial in origin. Blood from torn branches of a middle meningeal artery collects between the external periosteal layer of the dura and the calvaria. The extravasated blood strips the dura from the cranium. Usually this follows a hard blow to the head, and forms an *extradural (epidural) hematoma* (Fig. B8.20A, B). Typically, a brief *concussion* (loss of consciousness) occurs, followed by a lucid interval of some hours. Later, drowsiness and coma (profound unconsciousness) occur. Compression of the brain occurs as the blood mass increases, necessitating evacuation of the blood and occlusion of the bleeding vessel(s).

A *dural border hematoma* is commonly called a *subdural hematoma* (Fig. B8.20B). However, this term is a misnomer because there is no actual "subdural space" at the dura–arachnoid junction—only a potential one. *Hematomas* at this junction are usually caused by extravasated blood that splits

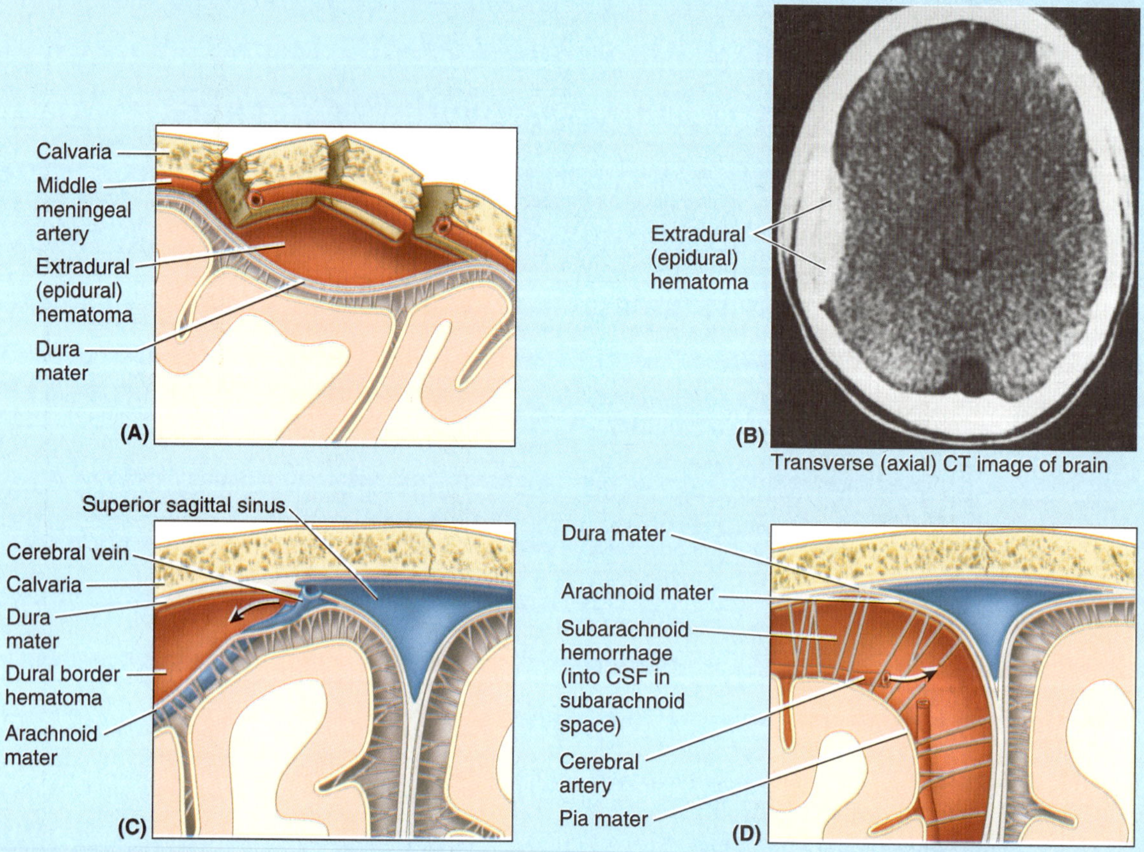

FIGURE B8.20. Intracranial hemorrhages. A, B. Extradural (epidural) hemorrhage. **C.** Dural border (subdural) hematoma. **D.** Subarachnoid hemorrhage.

open the dural border cell layer (Haines, 2013). The blood does not collect within a preexisting space, but rather creates a space at the dura–arachnoid junction. *Dural border hemorrhage* usually follows a hard blow to the head that jerks the brain inside the cranium and injures it (e.g., hitting the dashboard or windshield in a motor vehicle accident). Sometimes the precipitating trauma may be trivial or forgotten. Dural border hemorrhage is typically venous in origin and commonly results from tearing a superior cerebral vein as it enters the superior sagittal sinus (Fig. 8.29A, B) (Haines et al., 2013).

Subarachnoid hemorrhage is an extravasation of blood, usually arterial, into the subarachnoid space (Fig. B8.20C). Most of these hemorrhages result from *rupture of a saccular aneurysm* (sac-like dilation on the side of an artery), such as an aneurysm of the internal carotid artery (see the clinical box "Strokes").

Some subarachnoid hemorrhages are associated with head trauma involving cranial fractures and cerebral lacerations. Bleeding into the subarachnoid space results in meningeal irritation, severe headache, stiff neck, and often loss of consciousness.

The Bottom Line: Cranial Meninges

The cranial meninges consist of three intracranial layers: a substantial, fibrous bilaminar outer layer—the dura—and two continuous, delicate, membranous inner layers—the arachnoid and pia.

Dura mater: The outer (periosteal) lamina of the dura is continuous with the periosteum on the external surface of the cranium and is intimately applied to the internal surface of the cranial cavity. • The inner (meningeal) lamina is a sustentacular (supporting) layer that more closely reflects the contours of the brain. • This inner layer separates from the outer layer in certain locations to form dural folds or reflections that penetrate the large fissures between parts of the brain, partially subdividing the cranial cavity into smaller compartments that prevent inertial brain movement. • In separating from the periosteal lamina, intralaminar spaces are created that accommodate the dural venous sinuses, which receive the venous drainage of the brain and mainly drain, in turn, to the internal jugular vein.

Leptomeninx: The arachnoid and pia are continuous parietal and visceral layers, respectively, of the leptomeninx

continued on next page

The Bottom Line (continued)

that surround the CSF-filled subarachnoid space. • The arachnoid and pia are connected by fine trabeculae that traverse the subarachnoid space. • The subarachnoid space of the cranial cavity is continuous with that of the vertebral canal. • The arachnoid is normally applied to the internal surface of the dura by CSF pressure. • The pia intimately invests the neural tissue and its surface vasculature, coursing deeply along the vessels as they enter or exit the central nervous system.

Neurovasculature of meninges: The cranial meninges receive blood primarily from the middle meningeal branches of the maxillary arteries. • The dura receives sensory innervation from meningeal branches of all three divisions of the trigeminal nerve and fibers from the C2 spinal ganglion.

BRAIN

The brain is the body's controller and coordinator of almost all of its functions. It is the organ that raised mankind to the summit of the animal world. It is a delicate structure that is enclosed in a rigid cranium; however, it can be damaged by a blow to the head, compressed by a tumor, or deprived of oxygen by a leak or clot of blood in one of the cerebral arteries.

Because the brain is usually studied in detail in a separate neuroanatomy course, the brain is covered by only a superficial survey of its gross structure in the typical anatomy course, with attention primarily concerned with the relationship between the brain and its environment, that is, its meningeal coverings, the CSF-filled subarachnoid space, and internal features of its bony encasement (neurocranium).

Because of their role in the production of CSF (cerebrospinal fluid), the ventricles of the brain and the CSF-producing choroid plexuses found there are also covered. Furthermore, 11 of 12 cranial nerves arise from the brain (see Chapter 10, Summary of Cranial Nerves, Table 10.2, p. 1124).

Parts of Brain

The **brain** (contained by the neurocranium) is composed of the cerebrum, cerebellum, and brainstem (Fig. 8.36). When the calvaria and dura are removed, **gyri** (folds), **sulci** (grooves), and **fissures** (clefts) of the cerebral cortex are visible through the delicate arachnoid–pia layer. Whereas the gyri and sulci demonstrate much variation, the other features of the brain, including overall brain size, are remarkably consistent from individual to individual.

- The **cerebrum** (L. *brain*) includes the cerebral hemispheres and basal ganglia. The **cerebral hemispheres**, separated by the falx cerebri within the **longitudinal cerebral fissure**, are the dominant features of the brain (Fig. 8.36A–C). Each cerebral hemisphere is divided for descriptive purposes into four lobes, each of which is related to, but the boundaries of which do not correspond to, the overlying bones of the same name. From a superior view, the cerebrum is essentially divided into quarters by the median longitudinal cerebral fissure and the coronal **central sulcus** (Fig. 8.36A). The central sulcus separates the **frontal lobes** (anteriorly) from the **parietal lobes** (posteriorly). In a lateral view, these lobes lie superior to the transverse **lateral sulcus** and the temporal lobe inferior to it. The posteriorly placed **occipital lobes** are separated from the parietal and temporal lobes by the plane of the **parieto-occipital sulcus**, visible on the medial surface of the cerebrum in a hemisected brain (Fig. 8.36C). The anteriormost points of the anteriorly projecting frontal and temporal lobes are the **frontal** and **temporal poles**. The posteriormost point of the posteriorly projecting occipital lobe is the **occipital pole**. The hemispheres occupy the entire supratentorial cranial cavity (Fig. 8.31A, B). The frontal lobes occupy the anterior cranial fossae, the temporal lobes occupy the lateral parts of the middle cranial fossae, and the occipital lobes extend posteriorly over the tentorium cerebelli.
- The **diencephalon** is composed of the epithalamus, thalamus, and hypothalamus and forms the central core of the brain (Fig. 8.36D).
- The **midbrain**, the rostral part of the brainstem, lies at the junction of the middle and posterior cranial fossae. CN III and IV are associated with the midbrain.
- The **pons** is the part of the brainstem between the midbrain rostrally and the medulla oblongata caudally. The pons lies in the anterior part of the posterior cranial fossa. CN V is associated with the pons (Fig. 8.36A, C, D).
- The **medulla oblongata** (medulla) is the most caudal subdivision of the brainstem that is continuous with the spinal cord. The medulla lies in the posterior cranial fossa. CN IX, X, and XII are associated with the medulla, whereas CN VI–VIII are associated with the junction of the pons and medulla.
- The **cerebellum** is the large brain mass lying posterior to the pons and medulla and inferior to the posterior part of the cerebrum (Fig. 8.36A, C, D). It lies beneath the tentorium cerebelli in the posterior cranial fossa. It consists of two lateral hemispheres that are united by a narrow middle part, the **vermis**.

Ventricular System of Brain

The ventricular system of the brain consists of two lateral ventricles and the midline 3rd and 4th ventricles connected by the cerebral aqueduct (Figs. 8.37 and 8.38). CSF, largely secreted by the choroid plexuses of the ventricles, fills these brain cavities and the subarachnoid space of the brain and spinal cord.

VENTRICLES OF BRAIN

The **lateral ventricles**, the 1st and 2nd ventricles, are the largest cavities of the ventricular system and occupy large

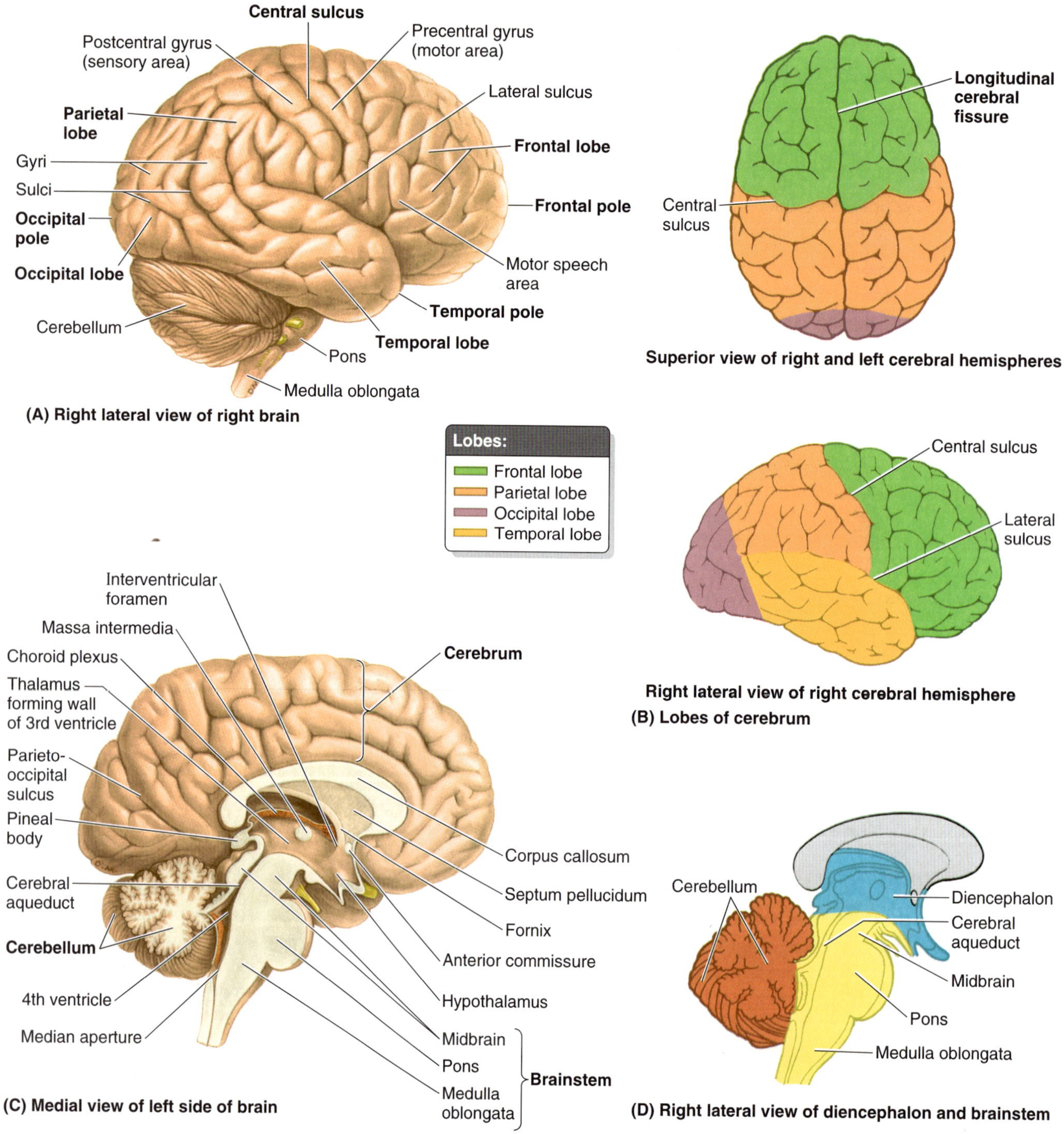

FIGURE 8.36. Structure of brain. A. The cerebral surface features the gyri (folds) and sulci (grooves) of the cerebral cortex. **B.** The lobes of the cerebrum are color coded. Whereas distinct central and lateral sulci demarcate the frontal lobe and anterior boundaries of the parietal and temporal lobes of the cerebrum, the demarcation of the posterior boundaries of the latter and the occipital lobe is less distinct externally. **C.** The medial surface of the cerebrum and deeper parts of the brain (diencephalon and brainstem) are shown after bisection of the brain. The parieto-occipital sulcus demarcating the parietal and occipital lobes is seen on the medial aspect of the cerebrum. **D.** The parts of the brainstem are identified.

areas of the cerebral hemispheres. Each lateral ventricle opens through an **interventricular foramen** into the **3rd ventricle**. The 3rd ventricle, a slit-like cavity between the right and the left halves of the diencephalon (Fig. 8.36D), is continuous postero-inferiorly with the **cerebral aqueduct**, a narrow channel in the midbrain connecting the 3rd and 4th ventricles (Figs. 8.36C and 8.37A, B).

The pyramid-shaped **4th ventricle** in the posterior part of the pons and medulla extends inferoposteriorly. Inferiorly, it tapers to a narrow channel that continues into the cervical region of the spinal cord as the central canal (Fig. 8.37A). CSF drains into the subarachnoid space from the 4th ventricle through a single **median aperture** and paired **lateral apertures**. These apertures are the only means by which CSF

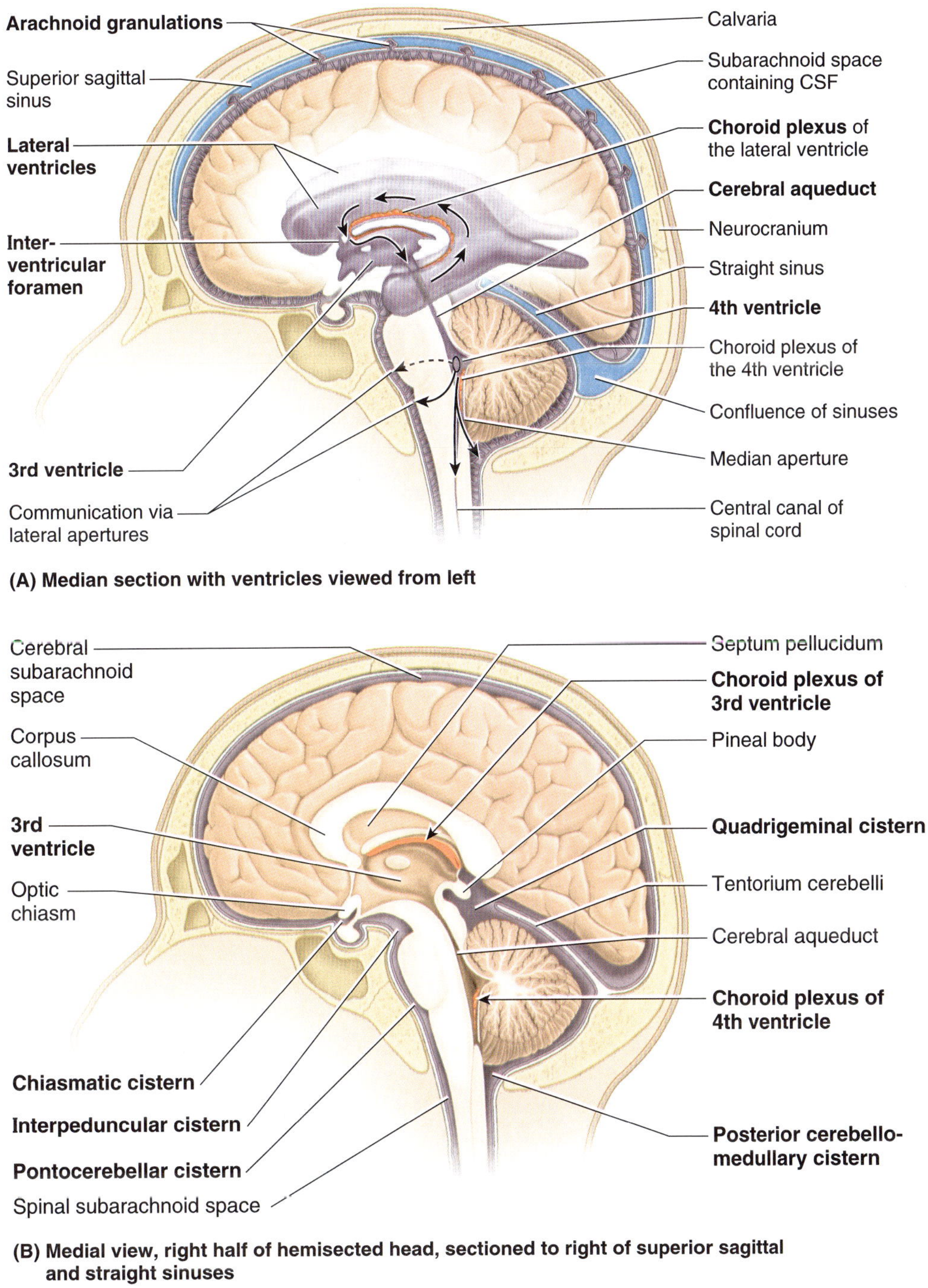

FIGURE 8.37. Ventricles, subarachnoid spaces, and cisterns. A. The ventricular system and circulation of the CSF are shown. The production of CSF is mainly by the choroid plexuses of the lateral, 3rd, and 4th ventricles. The plexuses of the lateral ventricles are the largest and most important. **B.** Subarachnoid cisterns, expanded regions of the subarachnoid space, contain more substantial amounts of CSF.

enters the subarachnoid space. If they are blocked, CSF accumulates and the ventricles distend, producing compression of the substance of the cerebral hemispheres.

SUBARACHNOID CISTERNS

Although it is not accurate to say that the brain "floats" in the CSF, the brain actually has minimal attachment to the neurocranium. At certain areas on the base of the brain, the arachnoid and pia are widely separated by subarachnoid cisterns (Fig. 8.37B), which contain CSF, and soft tissue structures that "anchor" the brain, such as the arachnoid trabeculae, vasculature, and, in some cases, cranial nerve roots. The cisterns are usually named according to the structures related to them.

Major intracranial subarachnoid cisterns include the following:

- **Cerebellomedullary cistern**: the largest of the subarachnoid cisterns, located between the cerebellum and the medulla; receives CSF from the apertures

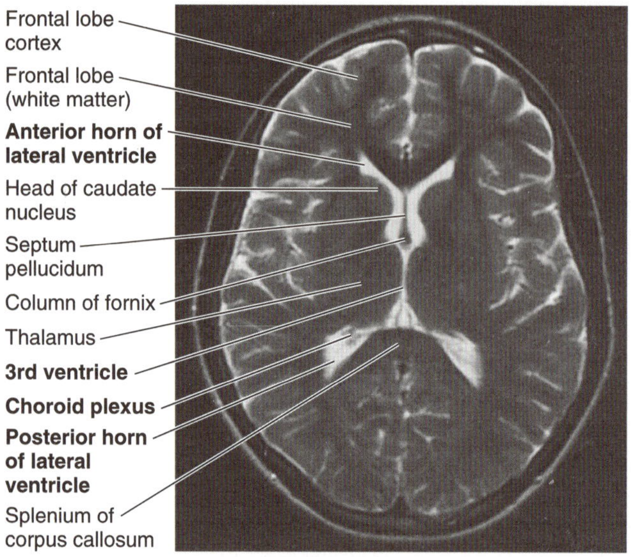

FIGURE 8.38. Transverse MRI of brain. CSF surrounding the brain, extending into the sulci and fissures, and occupying the ventricles, appears bright white.

of the 4th ventricle. It is divided into the **posterior cerebellomedullary cistern** (cisterna magna) and the **lateral cerebellomedullary cistern**.

- **Pontocerebellar cistern** (pontine cistern): an extensive space ventral to the pons, continuous inferiorly with the spinal subarachnoid space.
- **Interpeduncular cistern** (basal cistern): located in the interpeduncular fossa between the cerebral peduncles of the midbrain.
- **Chiasmatic cistern** (cistern of optic chiasma): inferior and anterior to the *optic chiasm*, the point of crossing or decussation of optic nerve fibers.
- **Quadrigeminal cistern** (cistern of great cerebral vein): located between the posterior part of the corpus callosum and the superior surface of the cerebellum; contains parts of the great cerebral vein (Figs. 8.29 and 8.31A, B).
- **Cisterna ambiens** (ambient cistern): located on the lateral aspect of the midbrain and continuous posteriorly with the quadrigeminal cistern (not illustrated).

SECRETION OF CEREBROSPINAL FLUID

Cerebrospinal fluid (CSF) is secreted (at the rate of 400–500 mL/d) mainly by choroidal epithelial cells (modified ependymal cells) of the **choroid plexuses** in the lateral, 3rd, and 4th ventricles (Figs. 8.36C, 8.37, and 8.38). The choroid plexuses consist of fringes of vascular pia mater (tela choroidea) covered by cuboidal epithelial cells. They are invaginated into the roofs of the 3rd and 4th ventricles and on the floors of the bodies and inferior horns of the lateral ventricles.

CIRCULATION OF CEREBROSPINAL FLUID

N56.2 CSF leaves the lateral ventricles through the *interventricular foramina* and enters the 3rd ventricle (Fig. 8.37A). From here, CSF passes through the *cerebral aqueduct* into the 4th ventricle. Some CSF leaves this ventricle through its *median* and *lateral apertures* and enters the *subarachnoid space*, which is continuous around the spinal cord and posterosuperiorly over the cerebellum. However, most CSF flows into the interpeduncular and quadrigeminal cisterns. CSF from the various subarachnoid cisterns flows superiorly through the sulci and fissures on the medial and superolateral surfaces of the cerebral hemispheres. CSF also passes into the extensions of the subarachnoid space around the cranial nerves, the most important of which are the subarachnoid space extensions surrounding the optic nerves (CN II).

ABSORPTION OF CEREBROSPINAL FLUID

The main site of CSF absorption into the venous system is through the **arachnoid granulations** (Figs. 8.35 and 8.37A), especially those that protrude into the superior sagittal sinus and its lateral lacunae (Figs. 8.28D and 8.37A). The subarachnoid space containing CSF extends into the cores of the arachnoid granulations. CSF enters the venous system through two routes: (1) most CSF enters the venous system by transport through the cells of the arachnoid granulations into the dural venous sinuses, and (2) some CSF moves between the cells making up the arachnoid granulations (Corbett et al., 2013).

FUNCTIONS OF CEREBROSPINAL FLUID

Along with the meninges and calvaria, CSF protects the brain by providing a cushion against blows to the head. The CSF in the subarachnoid space provides the buoyancy that prevents the weight of the brain from compressing the cranial nerve roots and blood vessels against the internal surface of the cranium. Because the brain is slightly heavier than the CSF, the gyri on the basal surface of the brain (see Fig. 8.42) are in contact with the floor of the cranial cavity when a person is standing erect. In many places at the base of the brain, only the cranial meninges intervene between the brain and cranial bones. In the erect position, the CSF is in the subarachnoid cisterns and sulci on the superior and lateral parts of the brain; therefore, CSF and dura normally separate the superior part of the brain from the calvaria (Fig. 8.37A).

Small, rapidly recurring changes take place in **intracranial pressure** owing to the beating heart; slow recurring changes result from unknown causes. Momentarily large changes in pressure occur during coughing and straining and during changes in position (erect vs. supine). Any change in the volume of the intracranial contents, for example, a brain tumor, an accumulation of ventricular fluid caused by blockage of the cerebral aqueduct (see Fig. B8.21B), or blood from a ruptured aneurysm (a pathologically bulging artery) will be reflected by a change in intracranial pressure. This rule is called the **Monro-Kellie doctrine**, which states that the cranial cavity is a closed rigid box and that a change in the quantity of intracranial blood can occur only through the displacement or replacement of CSF.

Arterial Blood Supply to Brain

Although it accounts for only about 2.5% of body weight, the brain receives about one sixth of the cardiac output and one fifth of the oxygen consumed by the body at rest. The *blood supply to the brain* is derived from the internal carotid and vertebral arteries (Fig. 8.39), the terminal branches of which lie in the subarachnoid space. *Venous drainage from the brain* occurs via cerebral and cerebellar veins that drain to the adjacent dural venous sinuses (Fig. 8.29A, B). See also "Venous Drainage of Brain" later in this chapter.

INTERNAL CAROTID ARTERIES

The **internal carotid arteries** arise in the neck from the common carotid arteries (Fig. 8.39). The cervical part of each artery ascends vertically through the neck, without branching, to the cranial base. Each internal carotid artery enters the cranial cavity through the **carotid canal** in the petrous part of the temporal bone. The intracranial course of the internal carotid artery is illustrated and described in Figure 8.40 and demonstrated radiographically in Figure 8.41. In addition to the carotid arteries, the carotid canals contain venous plexuses and *carotid plexuses of sympathetic nerves* (Fig. 8.40). The internal carotid arteries course anteriorly through the *cavernous sinuses* with the abducent nerves (CN VI) and in close proximity to the oculomotor (CN III) and trochlear (CN IV) nerves. The arteries run in the carotid groove located on the side of the body of the sphenoid (Figs. 8.31C and 8.40). The terminal branches of the internal carotid arteries are the **anterior** and **middle cerebral arteries** (Figs. 8.41 and 8.42).

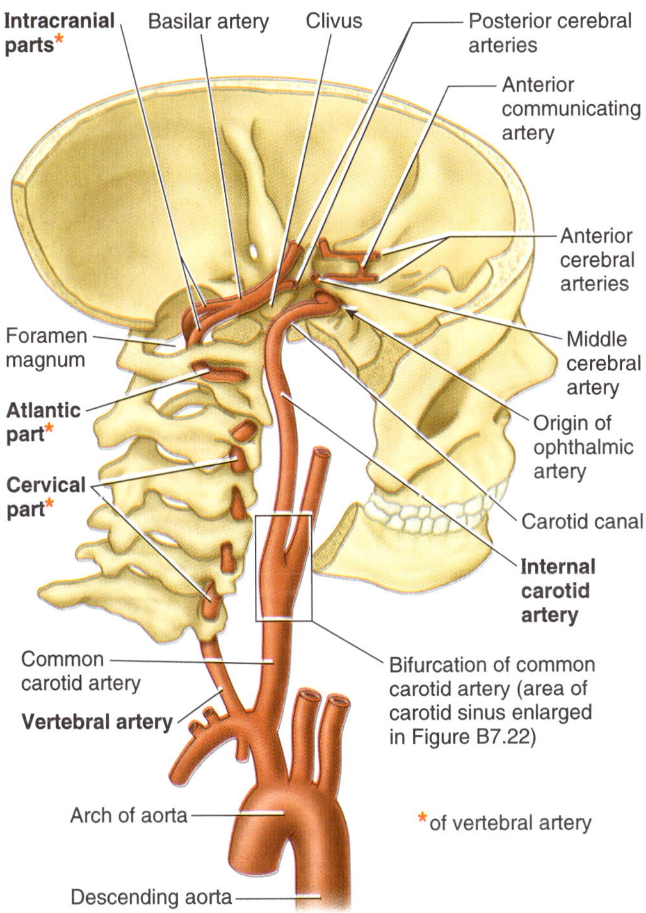

FIGURE 8.39. Arterial supply to brain. The bilaterally paired internal carotid and vertebral arteries deliver an abundant supply of oxygen-rich blood.

Clinically, the internal carotid arteries and their branches are often referred to as the *anterior circulation of the brain*. The anterior cerebral arteries are connected by the **anterior communicating artery**. Near their termination, the internal carotid arteries are joined to the **posterior cerebral arteries** by the posterior communicating arteries, completing the *cerebral arterial circle* around the *interpeduncular fossa*, the deep depression on the inferior surface of the midbrain between the cerebral peduncles (Figs. 8.42 and 8.43).

VERTEBRAL ARTERIES

The **vertebral arteries** begin in the root of the neck (the prevertebral parts of the vertebral arteries) as the first branches of the first part of the subclavian arteries (Fig. 8.39). The two vertebral arteries are usually unequal in size, the left being larger than the right. The **cervical parts of the vertebral arteries** ascend through the *transverse foramina* of the first six cervical vertebrae. The **atlantic parts of the vertebral arteries** (parts related to the atlas, vertebra C1) perforate the dura and arachnoid and pass through the foramen magnum. The **intracranial parts of the vertebral arteries** unite at the caudal border of the pons to form the *basilar artery* (Figs. 8.39, 8.42, and 8.43C). The vertebrobasilar arterial system and its branches are often referred to clinically as the *posterior circulation of the brain*.

The **basilar artery**, so-named because of its close relationship to the *cranial base*, ascends the *clivus*, the sloping surface from the dorsum sellae to the foramen magnum, through the pontocerebellar cistern to the superior border of the pons. It ends by dividing into the two **posterior cerebral arteries**.

CEREBRAL ARTERIES

In addition to supplying branches to deeper parts of the brain, the cortical branches of each cerebral artery supply a surface and a pole of the cerebrum (Figs. 8.41 and 8.43A, B; Table 8.7). The cortical branches of the

- **anterior cerebral artery** supply most of the medial and superior surfaces of the brain and the *frontal pole*.
- **middle cerebral artery** supply the lateral surface of the brain and the *temporal pole*.
- **posterior cerebral artery** supply the inferior surface of the brain and the *occipital pole*.

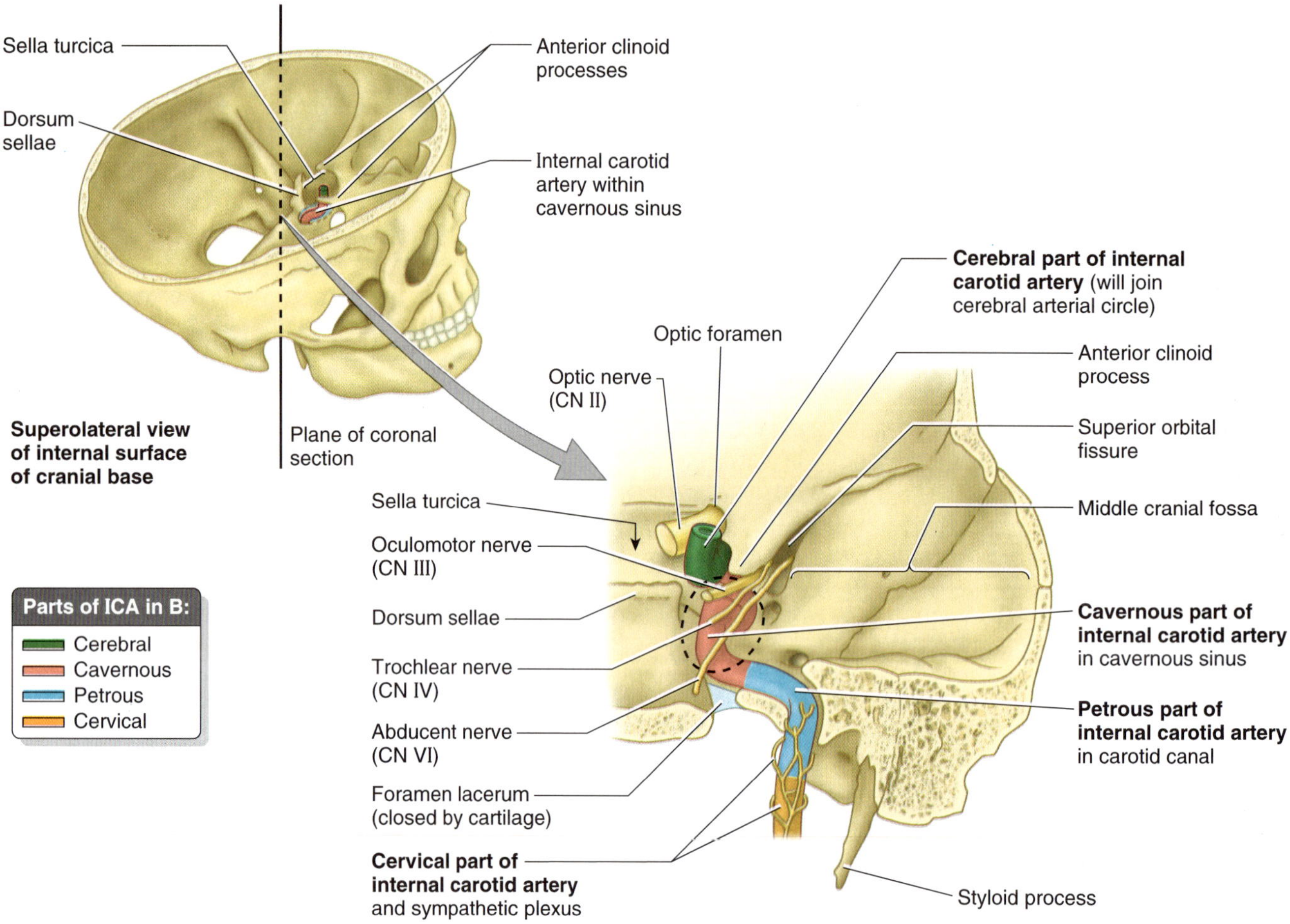

Posterior view (of right side of anterior portion following bisection in coronal plane)

FIGURE 8.40. Course of internal carotid artery. The orientation drawing (*left*) indicates the plane of the coronal section that intersects the carotid canal (*right*). The cervical part of the internal carotid artery ascends vertically in the neck to the entrance of the carotid canal in the petrous temporal bone. The petrous part of the artery turns horizontally and medially in the carotid canal, toward the apex of the petrous temporal bone. It emerges from the canal superior to the foramen lacerum, closed in life by cartilage, and enters the cranial cavity. The artery runs anteriorly across the cartilage; then the cavernous part of the artery runs along the carotid grooves on the lateral side of the body of the sphenoid, traversing the cavernous sinus. Inferior to the anterior clinoid process, the artery makes a 180° turn, its cerebral part heading posteriorly to join the cerebral arterial circle (Figs. 8.42 and 8.43C).

CEREBRAL ARTERIAL CIRCLE

AN62.6 The **cerebral arterial circle** (of Willis) is a roughly pentagon-shaped circle of vessels on the ventral surface of the brain. It is an important anastomosis at the base of the brain between four arteries (two vertebral and two internal carotid arteries) that supply the brain (Figs. 8.42 and 8.43C; Table 8.7). The arterial circle is formed sequentially in an anterior to posterior direction by the following arteries:

- Anterior communicating artery.
- Anterior cerebral arteries.
- Internal carotid arteries.
- Posterior communicating arteries.
- Posterior cerebral arteries.

The various components of the cerebral arterial circle give numerous small branches to the brain.

Venous Drainage of Brain

The thin-walled, valveless veins draining the brain pierce the arachnoid and meningeal layers of dura mater to end in the nearest dural venous sinuses (Figs. 8.28A, 8.29A, B to 8.32), which ultimately drain for the most part into the IJVs. The **superior cerebral veins** on the superolateral surface of the brain drain into the superior sagittal sinus; **inferior** and **superficial middle cerebral veins** from the inferior, postero-inferior, and deep aspects of the cerebral hemispheres drain into the straight, transverse, and superior petrosal sinuses. The **great cerebral vein** (of Galen) is a single, midline vein formed inside the brain by the union of two internal cerebral veins. The great cerebral vein ends by merging with the inferior sagittal sinus to form the straight sinus (Fig. 8.29A, B). The cerebellum is drained by **superior** and **inferior cerebellar veins**, draining the respective aspect of the cerebellum into the transverse and sigmoid sinuses (Fig. 8.32).

(*continued on p.* 946)

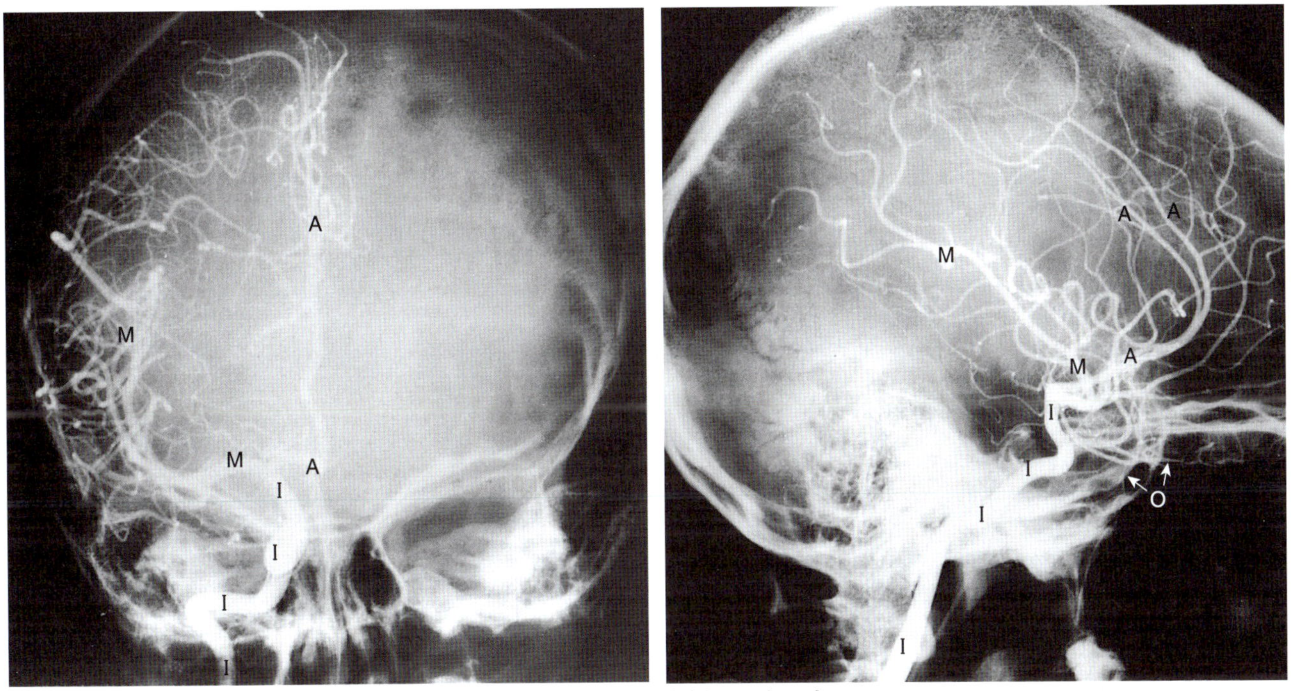

(A) Anteroposterior angiogram

(B) Lateral angiogram

AN43.8 AN43.9 **FIGURE 8.41. Carotid arteriograms. A, B.** Radiopaque dye injected into the carotid arterial system demonstrates unilateral distribution to the brain from the internal carotid artery. *A*, anterior cerebral artery and its branches; *I*, the four parts of the internal carotid artery; *M*, middle cerebral artery and its branches; *O*, ophthalmic artery. (Courtesy of Dr. D. Armstrong, Associate Professor of Medical Imaging, University of Toronto, Ontario, Canada.) Also refer *Snell's Neuroanatomy*, South Asian Edition, Chapter 17, Blood Supply of the Brain and Spinal Cord, Figures 7.9–7.12, pp. 493–495.

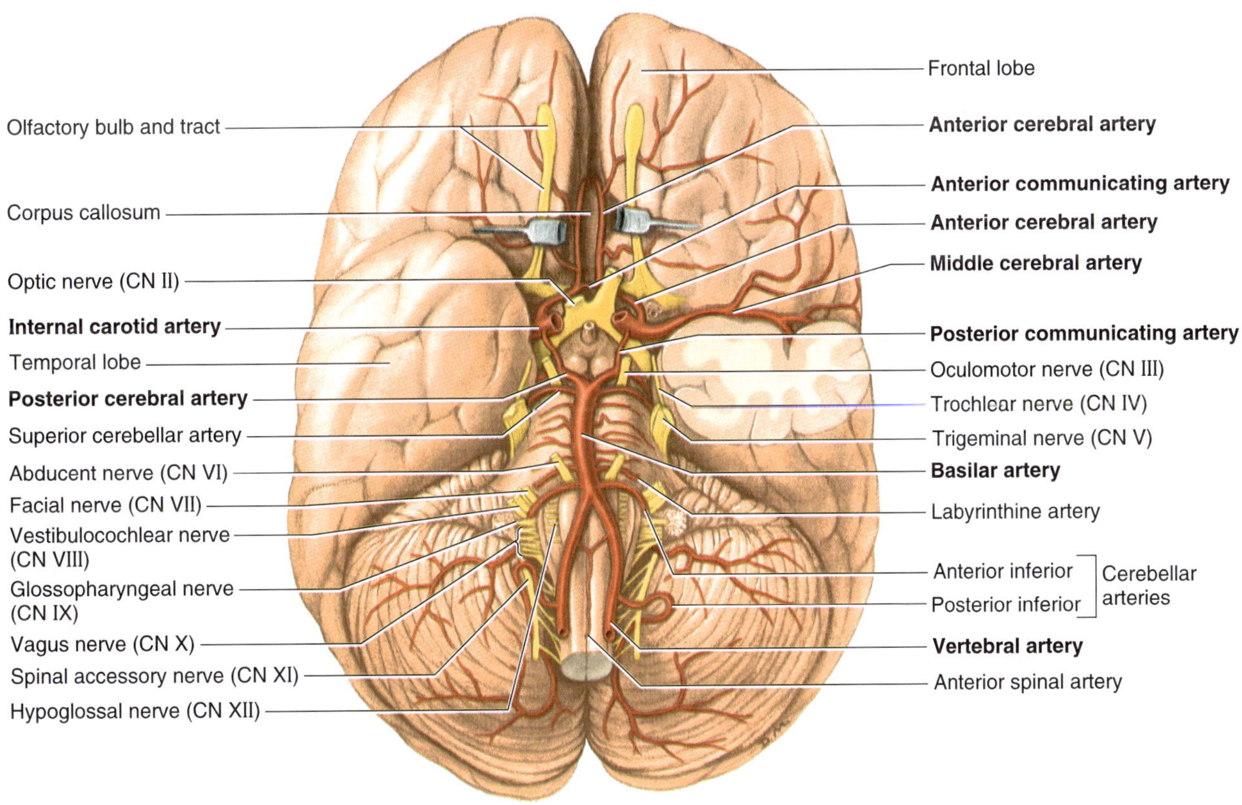

Inferior view

FIGURE 8.42. Base of brain with cerebral arterial circle. The internal carotid and basilar arteries converge, divide, and anastomose to form the cerebral arterial circle (of Willis). The left temporal pole is removed to show the middle cerebral artery in the lateral sulcus of the brain. The frontal lobes are separated to expose the anterior cerebral arteries.

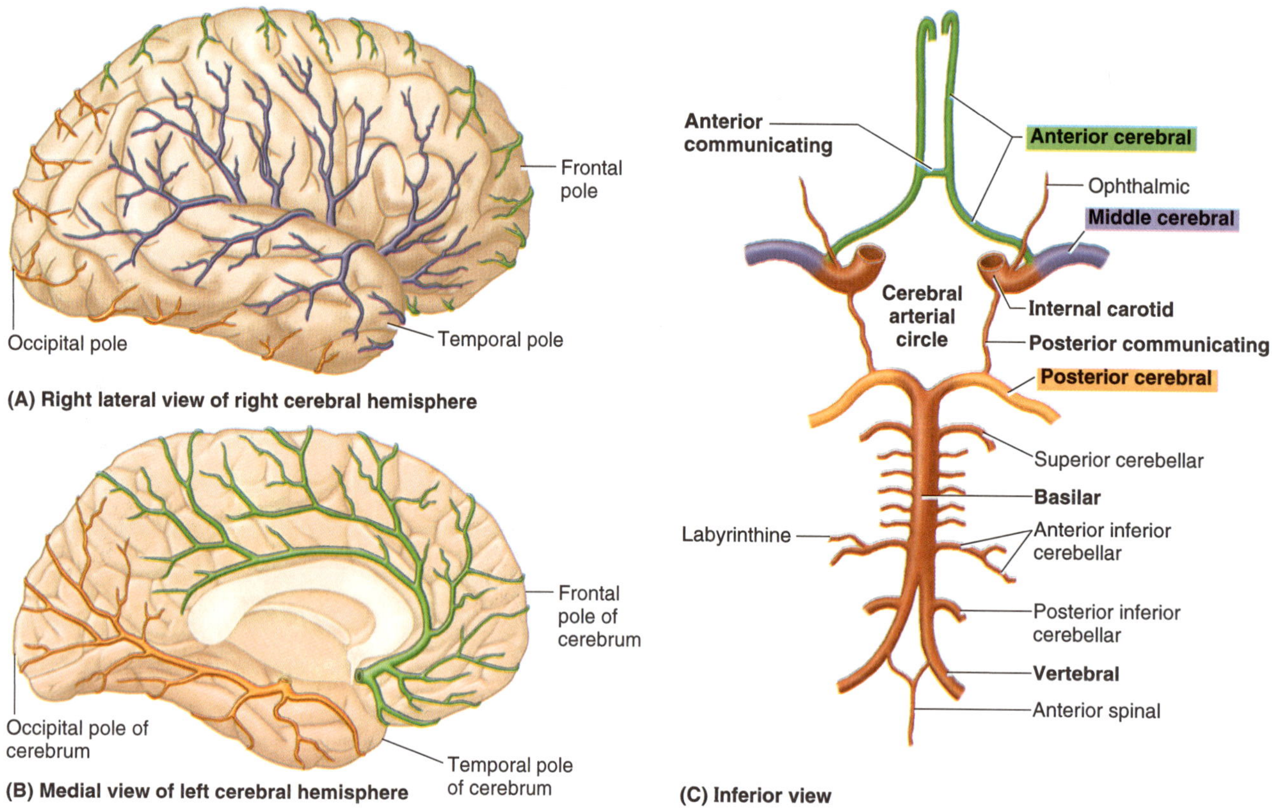

FIGURE 8.43. Arterial blood supply of cerebrum.

TABLE 8.7. ARTERIAL BLOOD SUPPLY OF CEREBRAL HEMISPHERES

Artery	Origin	Distribution
Internal carotid:	Common carotid artery at superior border of thyroid cartilage	Gives branches to walls of cavernous sinus, pituitary gland, and trigeminal ganglion; provides primary supply to brain
Anterior cerebral	Internal carotid artery	Cerebral hemispheres, except for occipital lobes
Anterior communicating	Anterior cerebral artery	Cerebral arterial circle (of Willis)
Middle cerebral	Continuation of internal carotid artery distal to anterior cerebral artery	Most of lateral surface of cerebral hemispheres
Vertebral:	Subclavian artery	Cranial meninges and cerebellum
Basilar	Formed by union of vertebral arteries	Brainstem, cerebellum, and cerebrum
Posterior cerebral	Terminal branch of basilar artery	Inferior aspect of cerebral hemisphere and occipital lobe
Posterior communicating	Posterior cerebral artery	Optic tract, cerebral peduncle, internal capsule, and thalamus

CLINICAL BOX

BRAIN

Cerebral Injuries

Cerebral concussion is an abrupt, brief loss of consciousness immediately after a severe head injury. Consciousness may be lost for only 10 seconds, as occurs in most knockdowns during boxing. With a more severe injury, such as that resulting from an automobile accident, consciousness may be lost for hours and even days. If a person recovers consciousness within 6 hours, the long-term outcome is excellent (Louis, 2016). If the coma lasts longer than 6 hours, brain tissue injury usually occurs.

Professional boxers are especially at risk for *chronic traumatic encephalopathy*, or *"punchdrunk syndrome,"* a brain injury characterized by weakness in the lower limbs, unsteady gait, slowness of muscular movements, tremors of the hands, hesitancy of speech, and slow cerebration (use of one's brain). Brain injuries result from acceleration and deceleration of the head that shears or stretches axons (*diffuse axonal injury*). The sudden stopping of the moving head results in the brain hitting the suddenly stationary cranium. Sometimes concussion occurs without loss of consciousness. The absence of loss of consciousness does not mean that the concussion is any less serious. Over 90% of head injuries are referred to as minor traumatic brain injuries.

Cerebral contusion results from brain trauma in which the pia is stripped from the injured surface of the brain and may be torn, allowing blood to enter the subarachnoid space. The bruising results either from the sudden impact of the still-moving brain against the suddenly stationary cranium or from the suddenly moving cranium against the still-stationary brain. Cerebral contusion may result in an extended loss of consciousness, but if there is no diffuse axonal injury, brain swelling, or secondary hemorrhage, recovery from a contusion may be excellent (Louis, 2016).

Cerebral lacerations are often associated with depressed cranial fractures (Fig. B8.4) or gunshot wounds. Lacerations result in rupture of blood vessels and bleeding into the brain and subarachnoid space, causing increased intracranial pressure and cerebral compression.

Cerebral compression may be produced by:

- intracranial collections of blood.
- obstruction of CSF circulation or absorption.
- intracranial tumors or abscesses.
- brain swelling caused by *brain edema*, an increase in brain volume resulting from an increase in water and sodium content (Mayer, 2016).

Cisternal Puncture

AN56.2

CSF may be obtained from the posterior cerebellomedullary cistern through a *cisternal puncture* for diagnostic or therapeutic purposes. The cerebellomedullary cistern is the site of choice in infants and young children. The lumbar cistern is used most frequently in adults (see Chapter 2, Back, Fig. B2.19, p. 140). The needle is carefully inserted through the posterior atlanto-occipital membrane into the cerebellomedullary cistern. The subarachnoid space or the ventricular system may also be entered for measuring or monitoring CSF pressure, injecting antibiotics, or administering contrast media for medical imaging.

Hydrocephalus

AN63.2

Overproduction of CSF, obstruction of CSF flow, or interference with CSF absorption results in excess fluid in the cerebral ventricles and enlargement of the head, a condition called *obstructive hydrocephalus* (Fig. B8.21A). The excess CSF dilates the ventricles, thins the cerebral cortex, and separates the bones of the calvaria in infants. Although an obstruction can occur any place, the blockage usually occurs in the cerebral aqueduct (Fig. B8.21B) or an interventricular foramen. *Aqueductal stenosis* (narrow aqueduct) may be caused by a nearby tumor in the midbrain or by cellular debris following intraventricular hemorrhage or bacterial and fungal infections of the central nervous system (Corbett et al., 2013).

Blockage of CSF circulation results in dilation of the ventricles superior to the point of obstruction and increased pressure on the cerebral hemispheres. This condition squeezes the brain between the ventricular fluid and the calvarial bones. In infants, the internal pressure results in expansion of the brain and calvaria because the sutures and fontanelles are still open. It is possible to produce an artificial drainage system to bypass the blockage and allow CSF to escape, thereby lessening damage to the brain.

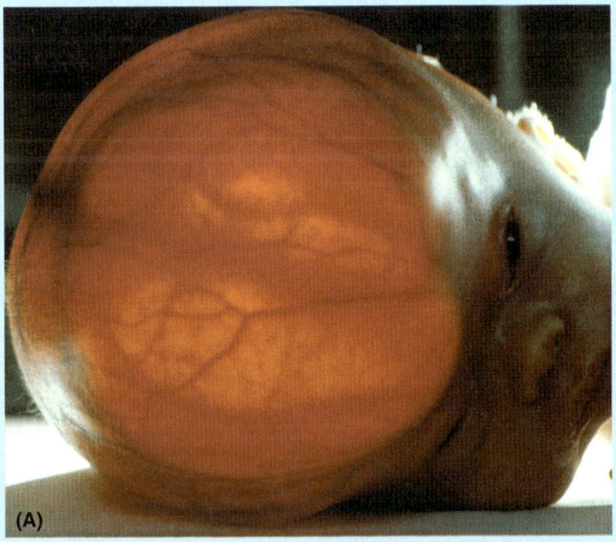

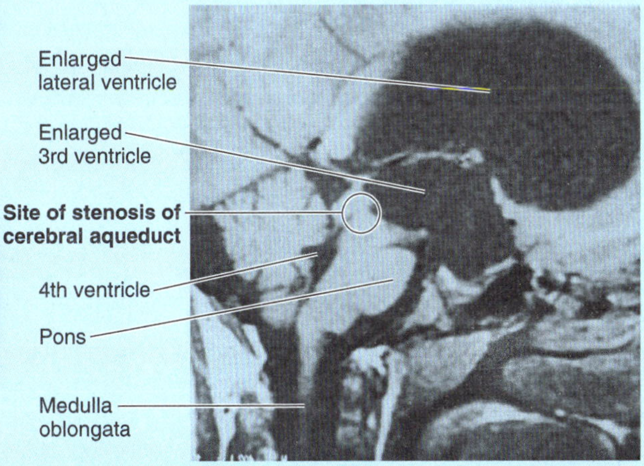

(B) Right sagittal MRI (compare to Fig. 8.37)

FIGURE B8.21. **Obstruction of CSF flow. A.** Hydrocephalus **B.** Aqueductal stenosis.

In *communicating hydrocephalus*, the flow of CSF through the ventricles and into the subarachnoid space is not impaired. However, movement of CSF from this space into the venous system is partly or completely blocked. The blockage may be caused by the congenital absence of arachnoid granulations, or the granulations may be blocked by red blood cells as the result of a subarachnoid hemorrhage (Corbett et al., 2013).

Leakage of Cerebrospinal Fluid

Fractures in the floor of the middle cranial fossa may result in CSF leakage from the external acoustic meatus (*CSF otorrhea*) if the meninges superior to the middle ear are torn and the tympanic membrane is ruptured. Fractures in the floor of the anterior cranial fossa may involve the cribriform plate of the ethmoid (see Fig. 8.12A), resulting in CSF leakage through the nose (*CSF rhinorrhea*). CSF can be distinguished from mucus by testing its glucose level. The glucose level of the CSF reflects that of the blood. CSF otorrhea and rhinorrhea may be the primary indications of a cranial base fracture and increased risk of meningitis because an infection could spread to the meninges from the ear or nose (Louis, 2016).

Anastomoses of Cerebral Arteries and Cerebral Embolism

Branches of the three cerebral arteries anastomose with each other on the surface of the brain; however, if a cerebral artery is obstructed by a *cerebral embolism* (e.g., a blood clot), these microscopic anastomoses are not capable of providing enough blood for the area of cerebral cortex concerned. Consequently, *cerebral ischemia* and *infarction* occur and an area of necrosis (dead tissue) results. Large cerebral emboli occluding major cerebral vessels may cause severe neurologic problems and death.

Variations of Cerebral Arterial Circle

Variations in the size of the vessels forming the cerebral arterial circle are common. The posterior communicating arteries are absent in some individuals; in others, there may be two anterior communicating arteries. In approximately 1 in 3 persons, one posterior cerebral artery is a major branch of the internal carotid artery. One of the anterior cerebral arteries is often small in the proximal part of its course; the anterior communicating artery is larger than usual in these individuals. These variations may become clinically significant if emboli or arterial disease occur.

Strokes

A stroke is an acute disruption of the normal blood flow (hypoperfusion) of the brain that results in the death of brain cells producing brain malfunction. Strokes are the most common neurologic disorders affecting adults in the United States. Worldwide, stroke accounts for approximately 10% of all deaths (Sevusch-Garcy, 2016); they are more often disabling than fatal. The cardinal feature of a stroke is the sudden onset of neurological symptoms. There are two main types of stroke: *ischemic*, due to impaired cerebral blood flow, and *hemorrhagic*, due to bleeding.

Ischemic strokes account for the great majority of strokes. In this type of stroke, focal neurological deficits develop due to occlusive *atherosclerotic disease* (see "Brain Infarction" given on next page) or *thromboembolism* in a cerebral artery. A *thrombus* is a clot developing within a blood vessel, and an *embolus* a clot or plug formed elsewhere that travels to and becomes lodged in a blood vessel.

The cerebral arterial circle is an important means of collateral circulation in the event of gradual obstruction of one of the major arteries forming the circle. Sudden occlusion, even if only partial, results in neurological deficits. In elderly persons, the anastomoses of the arterial circle are often inadequate when a large artery (e.g., the internal carotid) is occluded, even if the occlusion is gradual (in which case function is impaired at least to some degree).

Hemorrhagic stroke follows leakage or rupture of an intracerebral artery or a *saccular aneurysm* of a subarachnoid artery, a sac-like dilation on a weak part of the arterial wall (Fig. B8.22A). The most common type of saccular

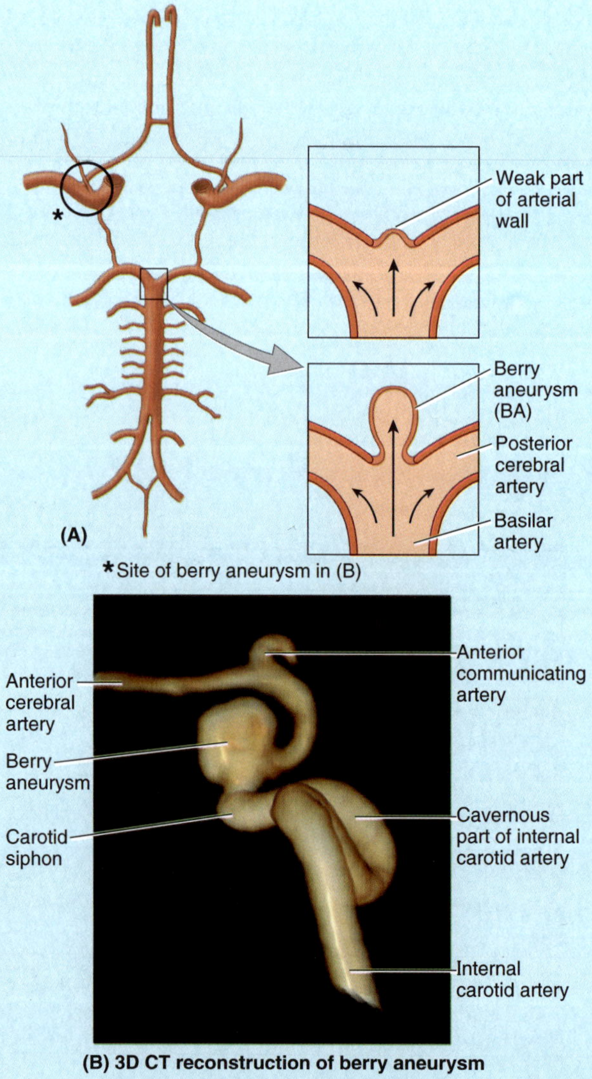

FIGURE B8.22. Berry aneurysm.

aneurysm is a *berry aneurysm*, occurring in the vessels of or near the cerebral arterial circle and the medium arteries at the base of the brain (Fig. B8.22B). Aneurysms also occur at the bifurcation of the basilar artery into the posterior cerebral arteries.

In time, especially in individuals with *hypertension* (high blood pressure), the weak part of the wall of the aneurysm expands and may rupture (Fig. B8.22C), allowing blood to enter the subarachnoid space. Sudden *rupture of an aneurysm* usually produces a severe, almost unbearable headache and a stiff neck. These symptoms result from gross bleeding into the subarachnoid space.

Prevention of or recovery from stroke involves lifestyle changes, such as controlling blood pressure, smoking cessation, healthy dietary changes, control of weight and diabetes, exercise, and use of anticlotting drugs if indicated.

Brain Infarction

An *atheromatous plaque* at a bend of an artery (e.g., at the bifurcation of a common carotid artery) results in progressive narrowing (*stenosis*) of the artery, producing increasingly severe neurologic deficits (Fig. B8.23). An embolus may separate from the plaque and be carried in the blood until it lodges in an artery, usually an intracranial branch that is too small to allow its passage. This event usually results in *acute cortical infarction*, a sudden insufficiency of arterial blood to the brain (e.g., of the left parietal lobes). An interruption of blood supply for 30 seconds alters a person's brain metabolism. After 1–2 minutes, neural function may be lost; after 5 minutes, lack of oxygen (*anoxia*) can result in cerebral infarction.

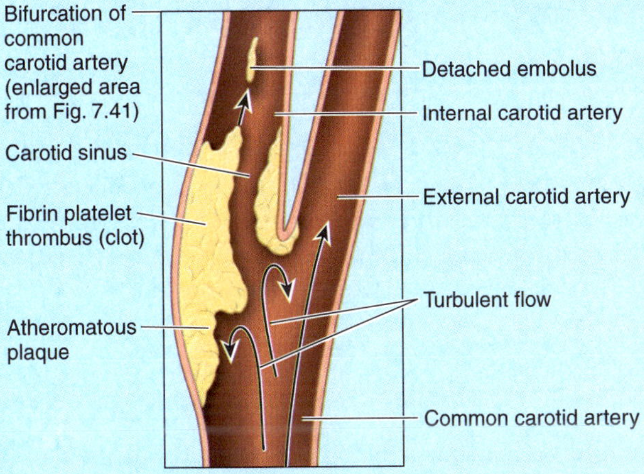

FIGURE B8.23. Atheromatous plaque.

Quickly restoring oxygen to the blood supply may reverse the brain damage (Esenwa et al., 2016).

Transient Ischemic Attacks

Transient ischemic attacks (TIAs) refer to temporary neurologic symptoms resulting from ischemia lasting <24 hours. Most TIAs last only a few minutes to an hour. With major *carotid* or *vertebrobasilar stenosis* (narrowing of the arterial lumen), the TIA tends to last longer, as a result of transient occlusion of distal intracranial arteries before spontaneous dissolution of the embolus. The symptoms of TIA may be ambiguous: staggering, dizziness, light-headedness, fainting, and *paresthesias*. Persons with TIAs are at increased risk for subsequent ischemic stroke and myocardial infarction (Marshall, 2016).

The Bottom Line: Brain

Parts of brain: The two hemispheres of the cerebral cortex, separated by the falx cerebri, are the dominant features of the human brain. • Although the pattern of gyri and sulci are highly variable, other features of the brain, including overall brain size, are remarkably consistent from individual to individual. • Each cerebral hemisphere is divided for descriptive purposes into four lobes that are related to, but the boundaries of which do not correspond to, the overlying bones of the same name. • The diencephalon forms the central core of the brain, with the midbrain, pons, and medulla oblongata making the brainstem; the medulla is continuous with the spinal cord. • The cerebellum is the subtentorial brain mass occupying the posterior cranial fossa.

Ventricles of brain: Each cerebral hemisphere includes a lateral ventricle in its core; otherwise, the ventricular system of the brain is an unpaired, median formation that communicates with the subarachnoid space surrounding the brain and spinal cord. • Choroid plexuses secrete CSF into the ventricles, which flows out of them into the subarachnoid space. • CSF is absorbed into the venous system, normally at the same rate at which it is produced, by the arachnoid granulations related to the superior sagittal sinus.

Arterial supply and venous drainage of brain: A continuous supply of oxygen and nutrients is essential for brain function. • The brain receives a dual blood supply from the cerebral branches of the bilaterally paired internal carotid and vertebral arteries. • Anastomoses between these arteries form the cerebral arterial circle. • Anastomoses also occur between the branches of the three cerebral arteries on the surface of the brain. • In adults, if one of the four arteries delivering blood to the brain is blocked, the remaining three are not usually capable of providing adequate collateral circulation; consequently, impaired cerebral blood flow (ischemia) and an ischemic stroke result. • Venous drainage from the brain occurs via the dural venous sinuses and internal jugular veins.

EYE, ORBIT, ORBITAL REGION, AND EYEBALL

The eye is the organ of vision and consists of the eyeball and the optic nerve. The *orbit* contains the eyeball and its *accessory visual structures* (L., adnexa oculi). The **orbital region** is the area of the face overlying the orbit and eyeball and includes the upper and lower eyelids and lacrimal apparatus.

Orbits

The **orbits** are bilateral bony cavities in the facial skeleton that resemble hollow, quadrangular pyramids with their bases directed anterolaterally and their apices, posteromedially (Fig. 8.44A). The medial walls of the two orbits, separated by the ethmoidal sinuses and the upper parts of the nasal cavity, are nearly parallel, whereas their lateral walls are approximately at a right (90°) angle.

Consequently, the axes of the orbits (*orbital axes*) diverge at approximately 45°. The *optical axes* (axes of gaze, the direction or line of sight) for the two eyeballs are parallel and, in the anatomical position, run directly anteriorly ("looking straight ahead"). This position of the eyeballs is referred to as the *primary position*. The orbits and orbital region anterior to them contain and protect the **eyeballs** and **accessory visual structures** (Fig. 8.45), which include the

- *eyelids*, which bound the orbits anteriorly, controlling exposure of the anterior eyeball.

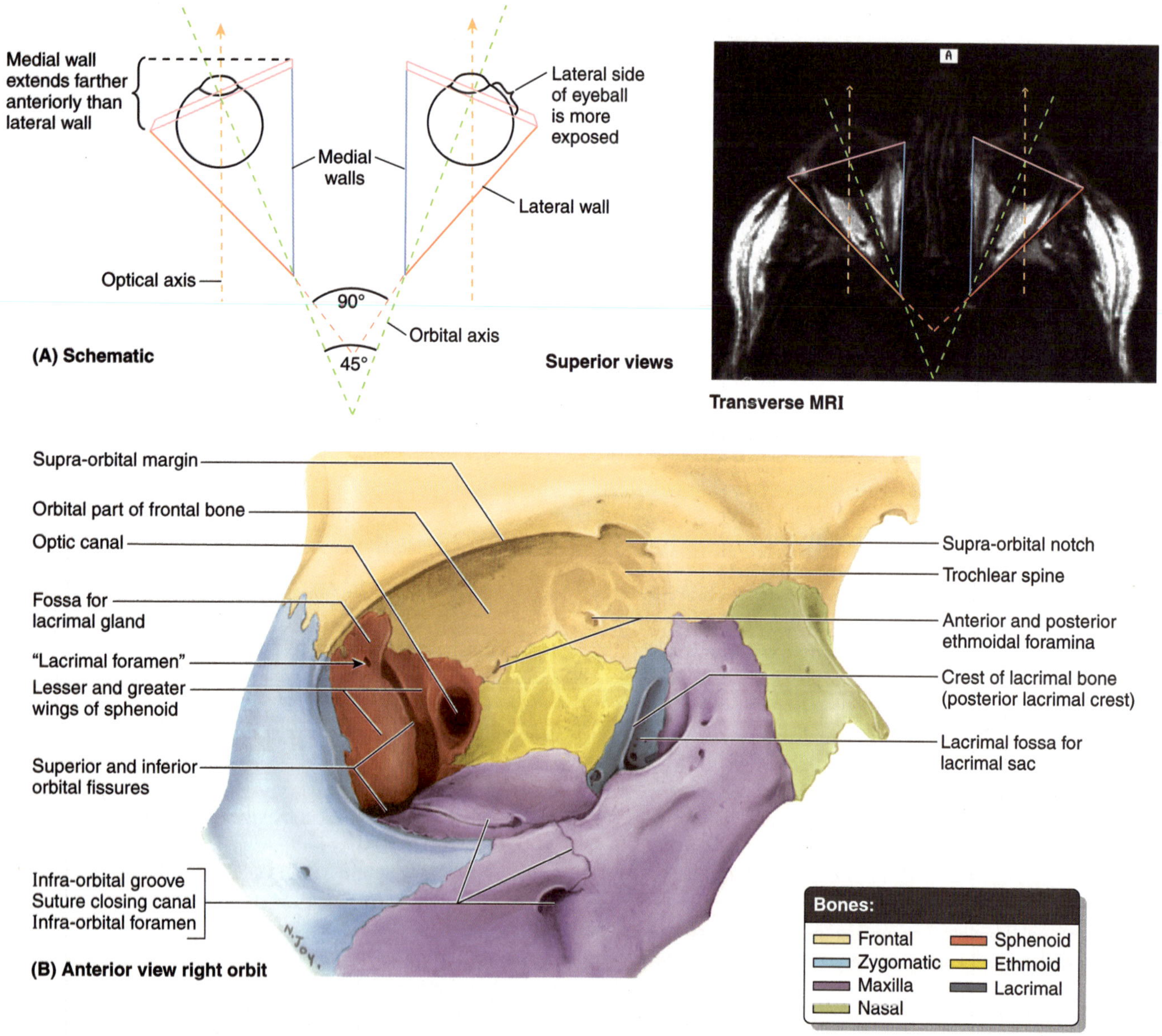

FIGURE 8.44. Orbits and placement of eyeballs within them. A. Note the orbits' disposition relative to each other and to the optical axes (line of gaze). The orbits are separated by ethmoidal cells and the upper nasal cavity and septum. **B.** The bony walls of the orbit are shown. This anterolateral view allows a view of the orbit and apex, which lie in the sagittal plane and are not well seen in an anterior view.

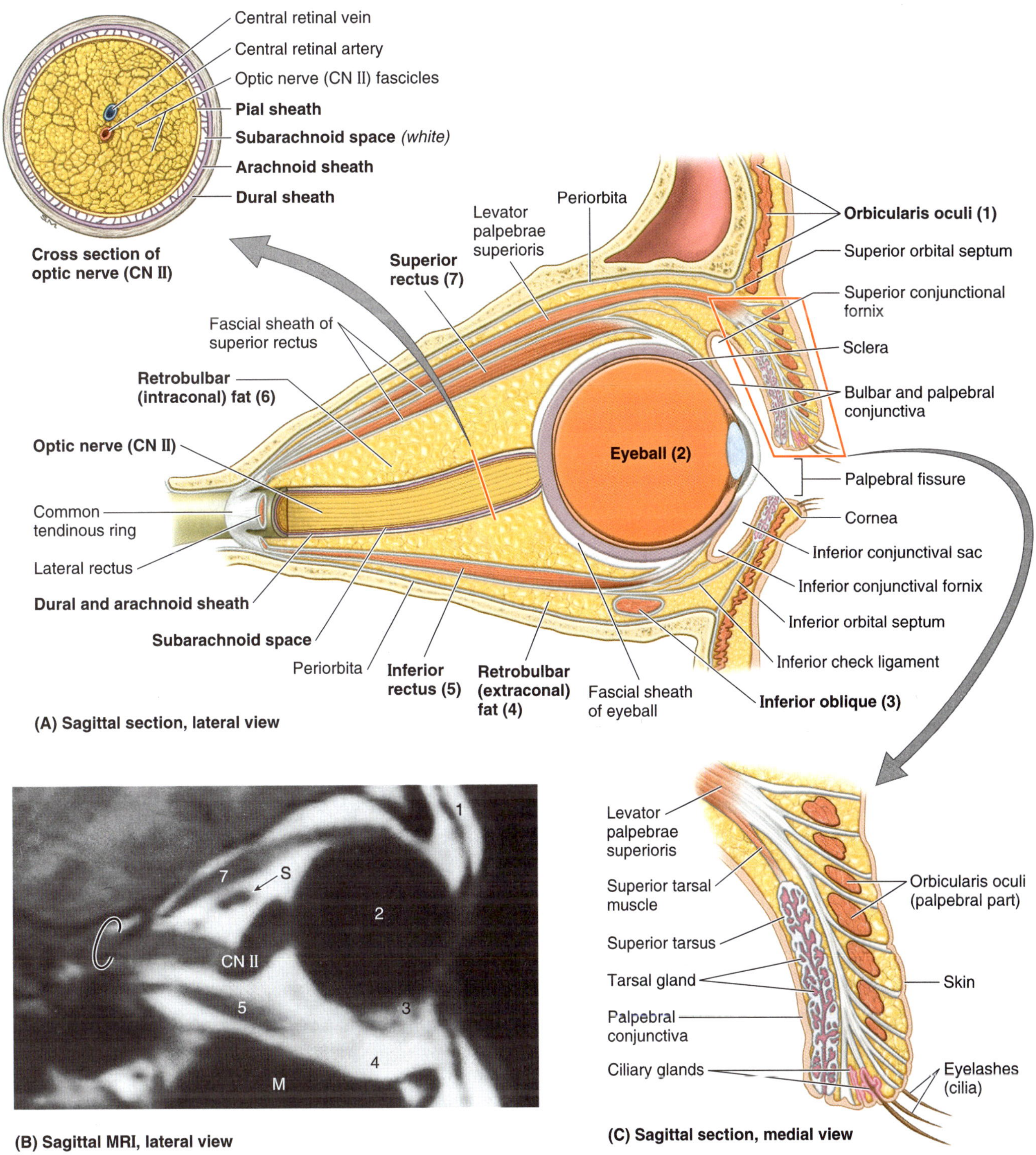

FIGURE 8.45. Orbit, eyeball, and eyelids. A. Sagittal section of orbit demonstrating the contents of the orbit. **Inset**, cross-section of optic nerve (CN II). The subarachnoid space around the optic nerve is continuous with the space between the arachnoid and the pia covering the brain. The numbers refer to structures labeled in part B. **B.** MRI study providing a sagittal section similar to **A**. *M*, maxillary sinus; *S*, superior ophthalmic vein; *arc*, optic canal. **C.** Detail of the superior eyelid. The tarsus forms the skeleton of the eyelid and contains tarsal glands. (Part **B** courtesy of Dr. W. Kucharczyk, Professor and Neuroradiologist Senior Scientist, Department of Medical Imaging, University Health Network, Toronto, Ontario, Canada.)

- *extra-ocular muscles*, which position the eyeballs and raise the superior eyelids.
- *nerves and vessels* in transit to the eyeballs and muscles.
- *orbital fascia* surrounding the eyeballs and muscles.
- *mucous membrane (conjunctiva)* lining the eyelids and anterior aspect of the eyeballs, and most of the *lacrimal apparatus*, which lubricates it.

All space within the orbits not occupied by these structures is filled with orbital fat; thus, it forms a matrix in which the structures of the orbit are embedded.

The quadrangular pyramidal **orbit** has a base, four walls, and an apex (Fig. 8.44B):

- The **base of the orbit** is outlined by the **orbital margin**, which surrounds the **orbital opening**. The bone forming the orbital margin is reinforced to afford protection to the orbital contents and provides attachment for the *orbital septum*, a fibrous membrane that extends into the eyelids.
- The **superior wall** (roof) is approximately horizontal and is formed mainly by the *orbital part of the frontal bone*, which separates the orbital cavity from the anterior cranial fossa. Near the apex of the orbit, the superior wall is formed by the *lesser wing of the sphenoid*. Anterolaterally, a shallow depression in the orbital part of the frontal bone, called the **fossa for lacrimal gland** (lacrimal fossa), accommodates the lacrimal gland.
- The **medial walls** of the contralateral orbits are essentially parallel and are formed primarily by the **orbital plate of ethmoid bone**, along with contributions from the *frontal process of the maxilla*, *lacrimal*, and *sphenoid bones*. Anteriorly, the medial wall is indented by the **lacrimal groove** and **fossa for lacrimal sac**; the *trochlea* (pulley) for the tendon of one of the extra-ocular muscles is located superiorly. Much of the bone forming the medial wall is paper thin. The ethmoid bone is highly pneumatized with ethmoidal cells (air sinuses), often visible through the bone of a dried cranium.
- The **inferior wall** (orbital floor) is formed mainly by the *maxilla* and partly by the zygomatic and palatine bones. The thin inferior wall is shared by the orbit and maxillary sinus. It slants inferiorly from the apex to the inferior orbital margin. The inferior wall is demarcated from the lateral wall of the orbit by the inferior orbital fissure, a gap between the orbital surfaces of the maxilla and the sphenoid.
- The **lateral wall** is formed by the **frontal process of the zygomatic bone** and the *greater wing of the sphenoid*. This is the strongest and thickest of the four walls, which is important because it is most exposed and vulnerable to direct trauma. Its posterior part separates the orbit from the temporal and middle cranial fossae. The lateral walls of the contralateral orbits are nearly perpendicular to each other.
- The **apex of the orbit** is at the **optic canal** in the *lesser wing of the sphenoid* just medial to the *superior orbital fissure*.

The widest part of the orbit corresponds to the equator of the eyeball (Fig. 8.45A), an imaginary line encircling the eyeball equidistant from its anterior and posterior poles. The bones forming the orbit are lined with **periorbita**, the periosteum of the orbit. The periorbita is continuous

- at the optic canal and superior orbital fissure with the periosteal layer of the dura mater.
- over the orbital margins and through the inferior orbital fissure with the periosteum covering the external surface of the cranium (pericranium).
- with the orbital septa at the orbital margins.
- with the fascial sheaths of the extra-ocular muscles.
- with the orbital fascia that forms the *fascial sheath of the eyeball*.

Eyelids and Lacrimal Apparatus

The eyelids and lacrimal fluid, secreted by the lacrimal glands, protect the cornea and eyeballs from injury and irritation (e.g., from dust and small particles).

EYELIDS

The **eyelids** are moveable folds that cover the eyeball anteriorly when closed, thereby protecting it from injury and excessive light. They also keep the cornea moist by spreading the lacrimal fluid. The eyelids are covered externally by thin skin and internally by transparent mucous membrane, the **palpebral conjunctiva** (Fig. 8.45A, C). The palpebral conjunctiva is reflected onto the eyeball, where it is continuous with the bulbar conjunctiva. The **bulbar conjunctiva** is thin, transparent and loosely attached to the anterior surface (sclera or "white") of the eyeball where it contains small, visible blood vessels. It is adherent to the periphery of the cornea (Fig. 8.46B). The lines of reflection of the palpebral conjunctiva onto the eyeball form continuous recesses or "pockets," the **superior** and **inferior conjunctival fornices** (singular = fornix; Figs. 8.45A and 8.46).

For microanatomy of eyelids, refer *diFiore's Atlas of Histology with Functional Correlations*, 1st South Asian Edition, Chapter 22, Organs of Special Senses: Visual Auditory Systems, p. 627. AN43.3

The **conjunctival sac** is the space bound by the palpebral and bulbar conjunctivae. It is a closed space when the eyelids are closed, but opens via an anterior aperture, the *palpebral fissure* (L. *rima palpebrae*, the gap between the eyelids), when the eye is open (eyelids are parted) (Fig. 8.45A). The conjunctival sac is a specialized form of mucosal "bursa" that enables the eyelids to move freely over the surface of the eyeball as they open and close.

The superior (upper) and inferior (lower) eyelids are strengthened by dense bands of connective tissue, the **superior** and **inferior tarsi** (singular = tarsus), which form the "skeleton" of the eyelids (Figs. 8.45C and 8.47A). Fibers of the palpebral portion of the *orbicularis oculi* (the sphincter of the palpebral fissure) are in the connective tissue superficial to the tarsi and deep to the skin of the eyelids (Fig. 8.45C). Embedded in the tarsi are **tarsal glands** that produce a lipid secretion that lubricates the edges of the eyelids and prevents them from sticking together when they close. The lipid secretion also forms a barrier that lacrimal fluid does not

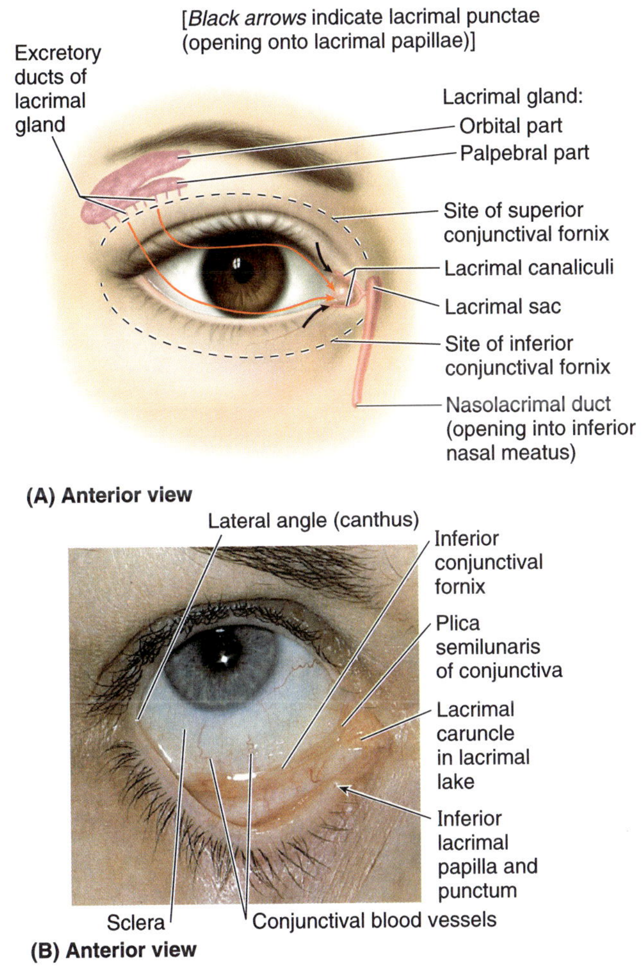

FIGURE 8.46. Lacrimal apparatus and anterior eyeball. A. The components of the lacrimal apparatus, by which tears flow from the superolateral aspect of the conjunctival sac (*dashed lines*) to the nasal cavity, are demonstrated. **B.** The surface features of the eye are shown. The fibrous outer coat of the eyeball includes the tough white sclera and the central transparent cornea, through which the pigmented iris with its aperture, the pupil, can be seen. The inferior eyelid has been everted to show the reflection of conjunctiva from the anterior surface of the eyeball to the inner surface of the eyelid. The semilunar fold is a vertical fold of conjunctiva near the medial angle, at the lacrimal caruncle.

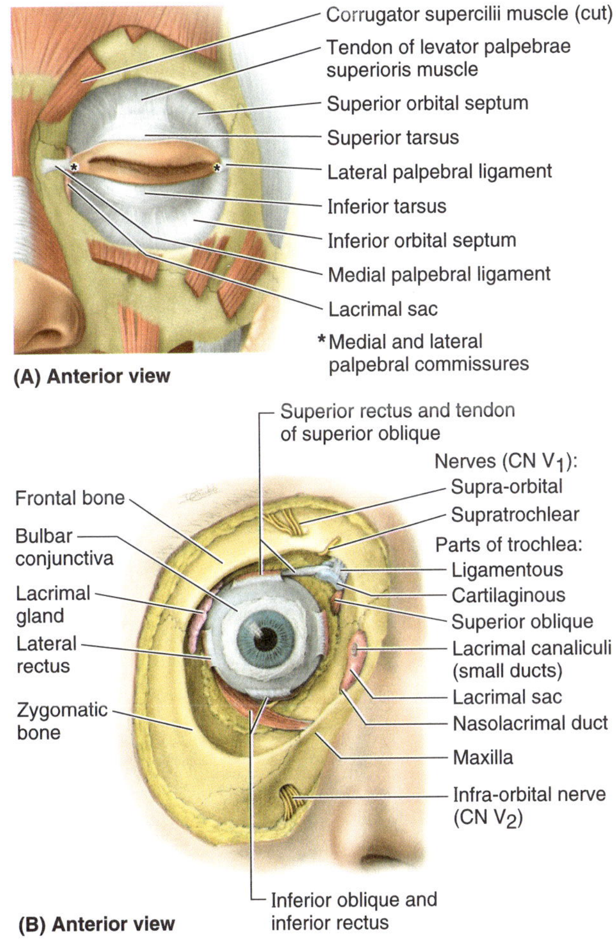

FIGURE 8.47. Skeleton of eyelids, and anterior approach to orbit. A. The superior and inferior tarsi and their attachments are shown. Their ciliary margins are free; however, they are attached peripherally to the orbital septum (palpebral fascia in the eyelid). **B.** In this dissection of the orbit, the eyelids, orbital septum, levator palpebrae superioris, and some fat have been removed. Part of the lacrimal gland is seen between the bony orbital wall laterally and the eyeball and lateral rectus muscle medially. Structures receiving lacrimal drainage from the conjunctival sac are seen medially.

cross when produced in normal amounts. When production is excessive, it spills over the barrier onto the cheeks as tears.

The **eyelashes** (L. *cilia*) are in the margins of the eyelids. The large sebaceous glands associated with the eyelashes are **ciliary glands**. The junctions of the superior and inferior eyelids make up the **medial** and **lateral palpebral commissures**, defining the **medial** and **lateral angles of the eye** (G. *kanthos*, corner of eye), or *canthi* (singular = canthus; Figs. 8.46B and 8.47A).

Between the nose and the medial angle of the eye is the **medial palpebral ligament**, which connects the tarsi to the medial margin of the orbit (Fig. 8.47A). The orbicularis oculi originates from and inserts onto this ligament. A similar **lateral palpebral ligament** attaches the tarsi to the lateral margin of the orbit, but it does not provide for direct muscle attachment.

The **orbital septum** is a fibrous membrane that spans from the tarsi to the margins of the orbit, where it becomes continuous with the periosteum (Figs. 8.45A and 8.47A). It keeps the orbital fat contained and, owing to its continuity with the periorbita, can limit the spread of infection to and from the orbit. The septum constitutes in large part the posterior fascia of the orbicularis oculi muscle.

8

LACRIMAL APPARATUS

The lacrimal apparatus (Figs. 8.46A and 8.47B) consists of the following: AN31.

- **Lacrimal gland**: secretes **lacrimal fluid**, a watery physiological saline containing the bacteriocidal enzyme lysozyme. The fluid moistens and lubricates the surfaces of the conjunctiva and cornea and provides some nutrients and dissolved oxygen to the cornea. When produced in excess, the overflowing fluid becomes tears.
- **Excretory ducts of lacrimal gland**: convey lacrimal fluid from the lacrimal glands to the conjunctival sac (Fig. 8.46A).

- **Lacrimal canaliculi** (L. small canals): commence at a **lacrimal punctum** (opening) on the **lacrimal papilla** near the medial angle of the eye and drain lacrimal fluid from the **lacrimal lake** (L. *lacus lacrimalis*; a triangular space at the medial angle of the eye where the tears collect) to the **lacrimal sac** (dilated superior part of the nasolacrimal duct) (Figs. 8.46A and 8.47B).
- **Nasolacrimal duct**: conveys the lacrimal fluid to the *inferior nasal meatus* (a cavity below the inferior nasal concha, the lowest of three downward-curving ridges on the lateral wall of the nasal cavity).

The *lacrimal gland*, almond shaped and approximately 2 cm long, lies in the *fossa for the lacrimal gland* in the superolateral part of each orbit (Figs. 8.44B, 8.46A, and 8.47B). The gland is divided into a superior **orbital** and **inferior palpebral parts** by the lateral expansion of the tendon of the *levator palpebrae superioris* (Fig. 8.46A). **Accessory lacrimal glands** may also be present, sometimes in the middle part of the eyelid, or along the superior or inferior fornices of the conjunctival sac. They are more numerous in the superior eyelid than in the inferior eyelid.

Production of lacrimal fluid is stimulated by parasympathetic impulses from CN VII. It is secreted through 8–12 *excretory ducts*, which open into the lateral part of the *superior conjunctival fornix* of the conjunctival sac. The fluid flows inferiorly within the sac under the influence of gravity. When the cornea becomes dry, the eye blinks. The eyelids come together in a lateral to medial sequence pushing a film of fluid medially over the cornea, somewhat like windshield wipers. In this way, lacrimal fluid, containing foreign material such as dust, is pushed toward the medial angle of the eye, accumulating in the lacrimal lake. Capillary action drains fluid into the lacrimal canaliculi through the lacrimal puncta. Action of the orbicular oculi muscle, attached in part to the lacrimal sac, assists in pulling fluid into the sac (Figs. 8.46A, B and 8.47B; Fernandez-Valencia et al., 1990).

From this sac, the fluid drains to the inferior nasal meatus of the nasal cavity through the nasolacrimal duct. It then flows posteriorly across the floor of the nasal cavity to the nasopharynx and is eventually swallowed. In addition to cleansing particles and irritants from the conjunctival sac, lacrimal fluid provides the cornea with nutrients and oxygen.

The **nerve supply of the lacrimal gland** is both sympathetic and parasympathetic (Fig. 8.48). The *presynaptic parasympathetic secretomotor fibers* are conveyed from the facial nerve by the *greater petrosal nerve* and then by the *nerve of the pterygoid canal* to the *pterygopalatine ganglion*, where they synapse with the cell body of the postsynaptic fiber. Vasoconstrictive, postsynaptic sympathetic fibers, brought from the *superior cervical ganglion* by the *internal carotid plexus* and deep petrosal nerve, join the parasympathetic fibers to form the nerve of the pterygoid canal and traverse the pterygopalatine ganglion. The terminal communicating branch of the zygomatic nerve (from CN V_2) brings both types of fibers to the lacrimal branch of the ophthalmic nerve, the merger of branches occurring immediately before or just after entering the gland (see Chapter 10, Summary of Cranial Nerves).

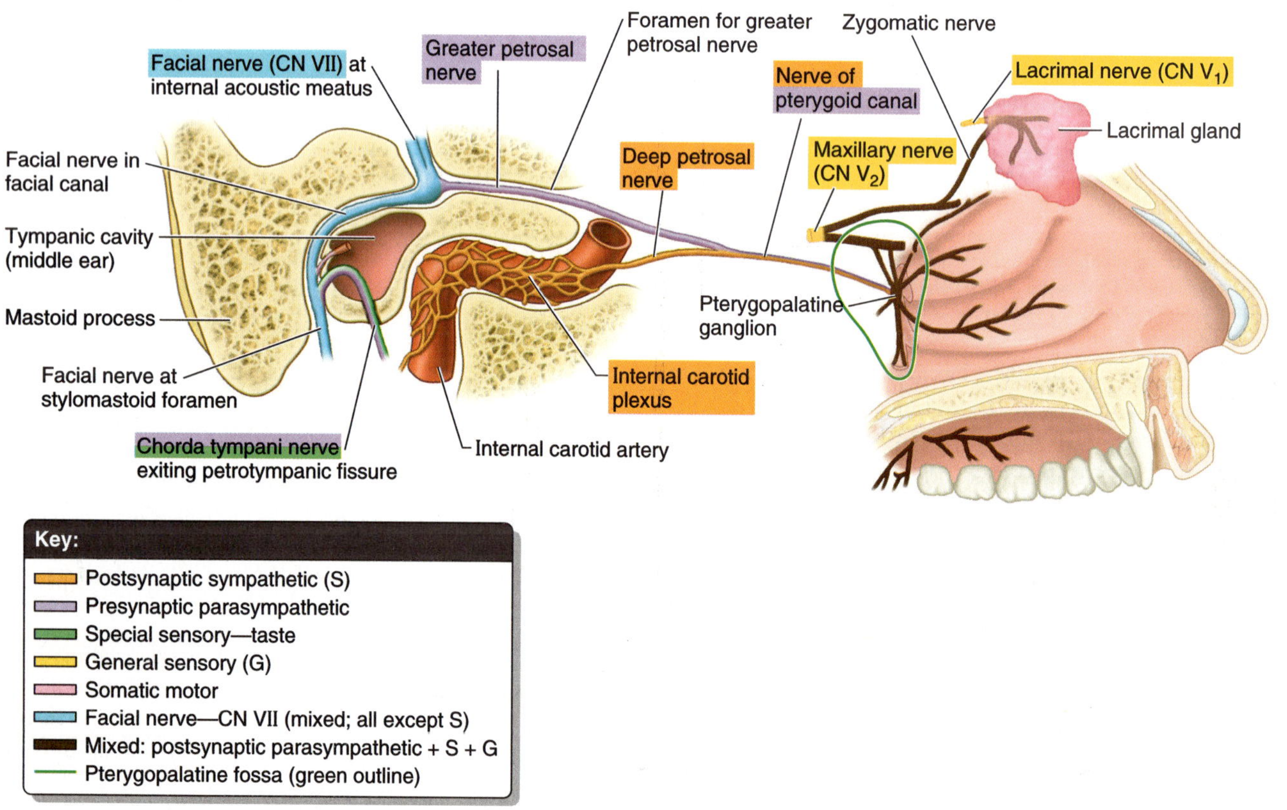

FIGURE 8.48. Innervation of lacrimal gland. The facial nerve (CN VII), greater petrosal nerve, and nerve of pterygoid canal deliver presynaptic parasympathetic fibers to the pterygopalatine ganglion. The synapse between presynaptic and postsynaptic fibers occurs here. The maxillary, infra-orbital, zygomatic, and lacrimal nerves convey the postsynaptic fibers to the gland.

AN41.1

Eyeball

The eyeball contains the optical apparatus of the visual system (Fig. 8.45A). It occupies most of the anterior portion of the orbit, suspended by six extrinsic muscles that control its movement, and a fascial *suspensory apparatus*. It measures approximately 25 mm in diameter. All anatomical structures within the eyeball have a circular or spherical arrangement. The *eyeball proper* has three layers; however, there is an additional connective tissue layer that surrounds the eyeball, supporting it within the orbit. The connective tissue layer is composed posteriorly of the **fascial sheath of the eyeball** (bulbar fascia or Tenon capsule), which forms the actual socket for the eyeball, and anteriorly of bulbar conjunctiva. The fascial sheath is the most substantial portion of the suspensory apparatus. A very loose connective tissue layer, the **episcleral space** (a potential space) lies between the fascial sheath and the outer layer of the eyeball, facilitating movements of the eyeball within the fascial sheath.

The *three layers of the eyeball* are as follows (Fig. 8.49):

1. *Fibrous layer* (outer coat or tunic), consisting of the *sclera* and *cornea*.
2. *Vascular layer* (middle coat), consisting of the *choroid*, *ciliary body*, and *iris*.
3. *Inner layer* (inner coat), consisting of the *retina*, which has both *optic* and *nonvisual parts*.

FIBROUS LAYER OF EYEBALL

The **fibrous layer of the eyeball** is the external fibrous skeleton of the eyeball, providing shape and resistance. The sclera is the tough opaque part of the fibrous layer of the eyeball, covering the posterior five sixths of the eyeball (Figs. 8.49A and 8.50). It provides attachment for both the extrinsic (extraocular) and intrinsic muscles of the eye. The anterior part of the sclera is visible through the transparent bulbar conjunctiva as "the white of the eye" (Fig. 8.46B). The **cornea** is the transparent part of the fibrous layer covering the anterior one sixth of the eyeball (Figs. 8.49A and 8.50). The convexity of the cornea is greater than that of the sclera, and so it appears to protrude from the eyeball when viewed laterally.

The two parts of the fibrous layer differ primarily in terms of the regularity of arrangement of the collagen fibers of which they are composed and the degree of hydration of each. While the sclera is relatively avascular, the cornea is completely avascular, receiving its nourishment from capillary beds around its periphery and fluids on its external and internal surfaces (*lacrimal fluid* and *aqueous humor*, respectively). Lacrimal fluid also provides oxygen absorbed from the air.

The cornea is highly sensitive to touch; its innervation is provided by the ophthalmic nerve (CN V_1). Even very small foreign bodies (e.g., dust particles) elicit blinking, flow of tears, and sometimes severe pain. Its nourishment is derived from the capillary beds at its periphery, the *aqueous humor*, and *lacrimal fluid*. The lacrimal fluid also provides oxygen absorbed from air. Drying of the corneal surface may cause development of an ulcer (open sore).

The **corneal limbus** is the angle formed by the intersecting curvatures of sclera and cornea at the **corneoscleral junction**. The junction is a 1-mm-wide, gray, translucent circle that includes numerous capillary loops involved in nourishing the avascular cornea.

For microanatomy of cornea, refer *diFiore's Atlas of Histology with Functional Correlations*, 1st South Asian Edition, Chapter 22, Organs of Special Senses: Visual Auditory Systems, pp. 629–630. AN4

For microanatomy of sclerocorneal junction, refer *diFiore's Atlas of Histology with Functional Correlations*, 1st South Asian Edition, Chapter 22, Organs of Special Senses: Visual Auditory Systems, pp. 629–630. AN4

VASCULAR LAYER OF EYEBALL

The middle **vascular layer of the eyeball** (also called the uvea or uveal tract) consists of the choroid, ciliary body, and iris (Fig. 8.49B). The **choroid** is a dark reddish brown layer

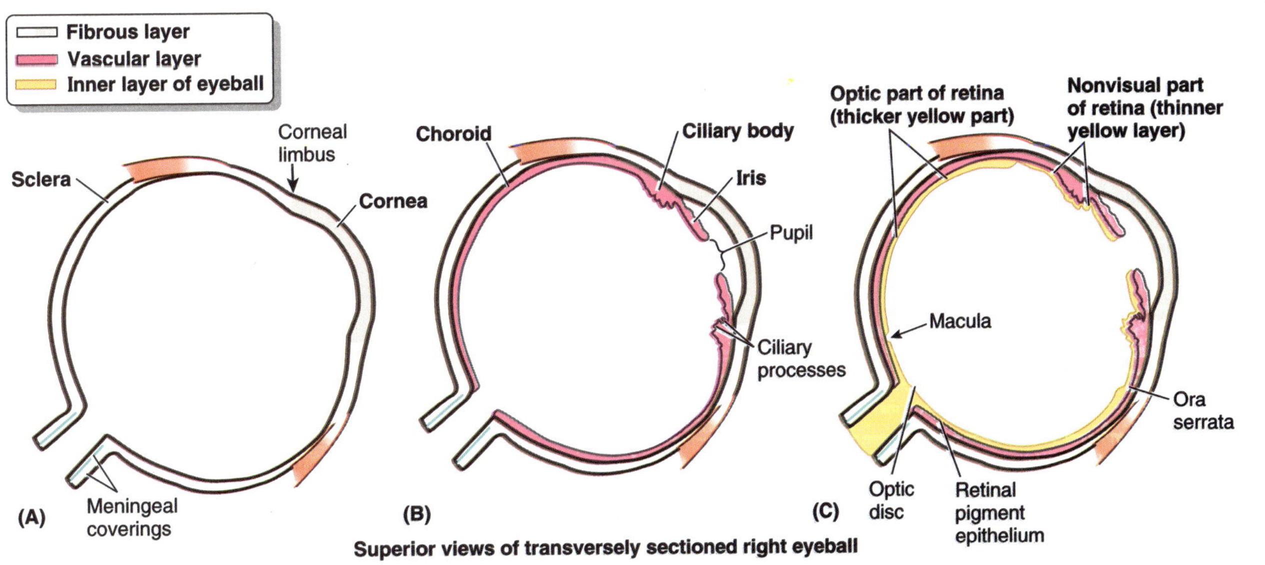

FIGURE 8.49. Layers of eyeball. The three layers are added sequentially. **A.** Outer fibrous layer. **B.** Middle vascular layer. **C.** Inner layer (retina).

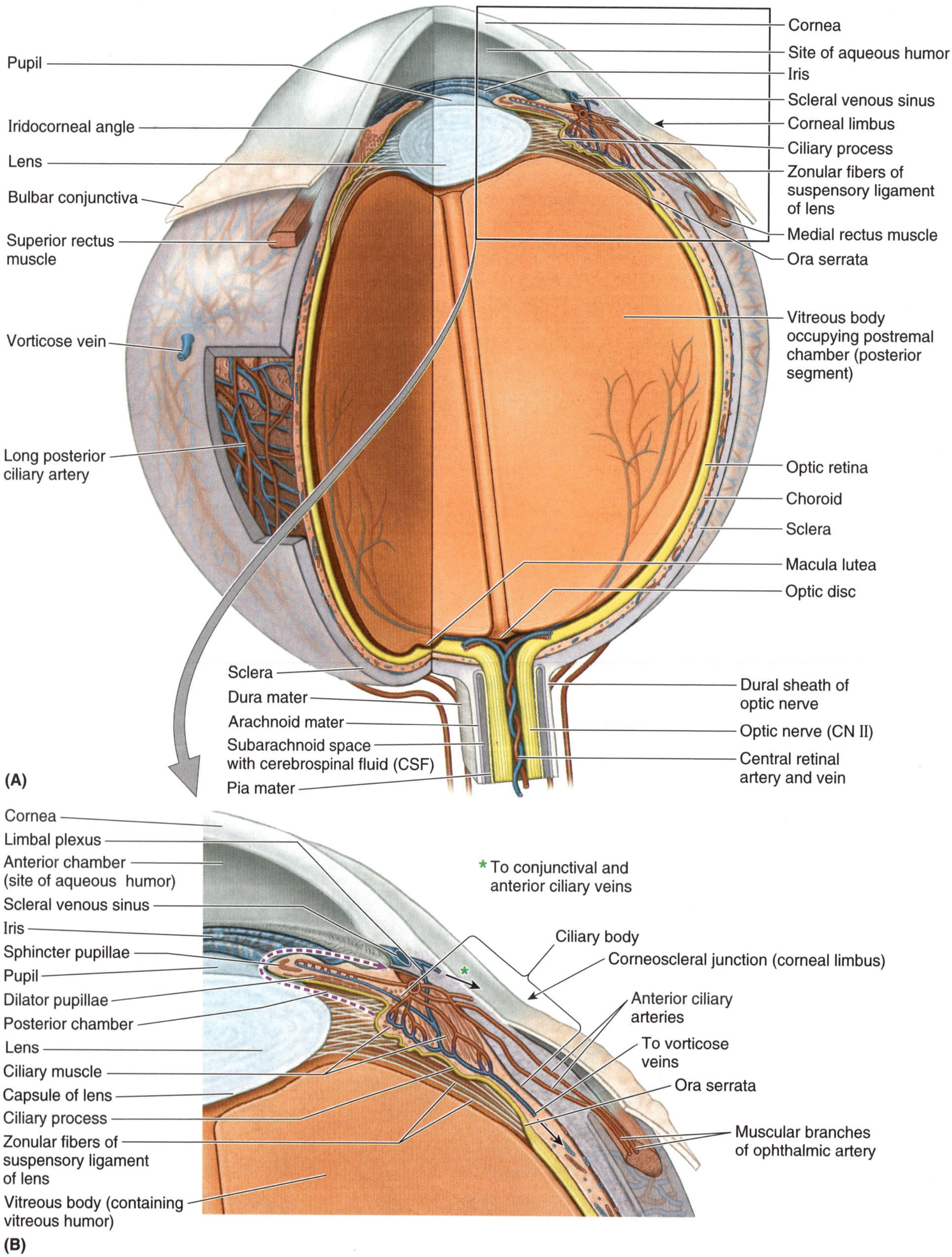

FIGURE 8.50. Eyeball with quarter section removed. A. The inner aspect of the optic part of the retina is supplied by the central retinal artery, whereas the outer, light-sensitive aspect is nourished by the capillary lamina of the choroid (Fig. 8.64). The central retinal artery courses through the optic nerve and divides at the optic disc into superior and inferior branches. The branches of the central retinal artery are end arteries that do not anastomose with each other or any other vessel. **B.** The structural details of the ciliary region are shown. The ciliary body is both muscular and vascular, as is the iris. The latter includes two muscles: the sphincter pupillae and dilator pupillae muscles. Venous blood from this region and the aqueous humor in the anterior chamber drain into the scleral venous sinus.

between the sclera and retina. It forms the largest part of the vascular layer of the eyeball and lines most of the sclera (Fig. 8.50A). Within this pigmented and dense vascular bed, larger vessels are located externally (near the sclera). The finest vessels (the **capillary lamina of the choroid**, or *choriocapillaris*, an extensive capillary bed) are innermost, adjacent to the avascular light-sensitive layer of the retina, which it supplies with oxygen and nutrients. The choroid is engorged with blood in life (it has the highest perfusion rate per gram of tissue of all vascular beds of the body). Consequently, this layer is responsible for the "red eye" reflection that occurs in flash photography. The choroid attaches firmly to the pigment layer of the retina, but can easily be stripped from the sclera. The choroid is continuous anteriorly with the ciliary body.

AN41.3 The **ciliary body** is a ring-like thickening of the vascular layer posterior to the corneoscleral junction that is muscular as well as vascular (Figs. 8.49B and 8.50). It connects the choroid with the circumference of the iris. The ciliary body provides attachment for the lens. The contraction and relaxation of the circularly arranged smooth muscle of the ciliary body controls the thickness, and therefore the focus, of the lens. Folds on the internal surface of the ciliary body, the **ciliary processes**, secrete *aqueous humor*. A clear watery fluid, aqueous humor fills the **anterior segment of the eyeball**, the interior of the eyeball anterior to the lens, suspensory ligament, and ciliary body (Fig. 8.50B).

The **iris**, which literally lies on the anterior surface of the lens, is a thin contractile diaphragm with a central aperture, the **pupil**, for transmitting light (Figs. 8.49B, 8.50, and 8.51A). When a person is awake, the size of the pupil varies continually to regulate the amount of light entering the eye (Fig. 8.51B). Two involuntary muscles control the size of the pupil: the parasympathetically stimulated, circularly arranged **sphincter pupillae** decreases its diameter (constrict or contracts the pupil, *pupillary miosis*), and the sympathetically stimulated, radially arranged **dilator pupillae** increases its diameter (dilates the pupil). The nature of the pupillary responses is paradoxical: sympathetic responses usually occur immediately, yet it may take up to 20 minutes for the pupil to dilate in response to low lighting, as in a darkened theater. Parasympathetic responses are typically slower than sympa-

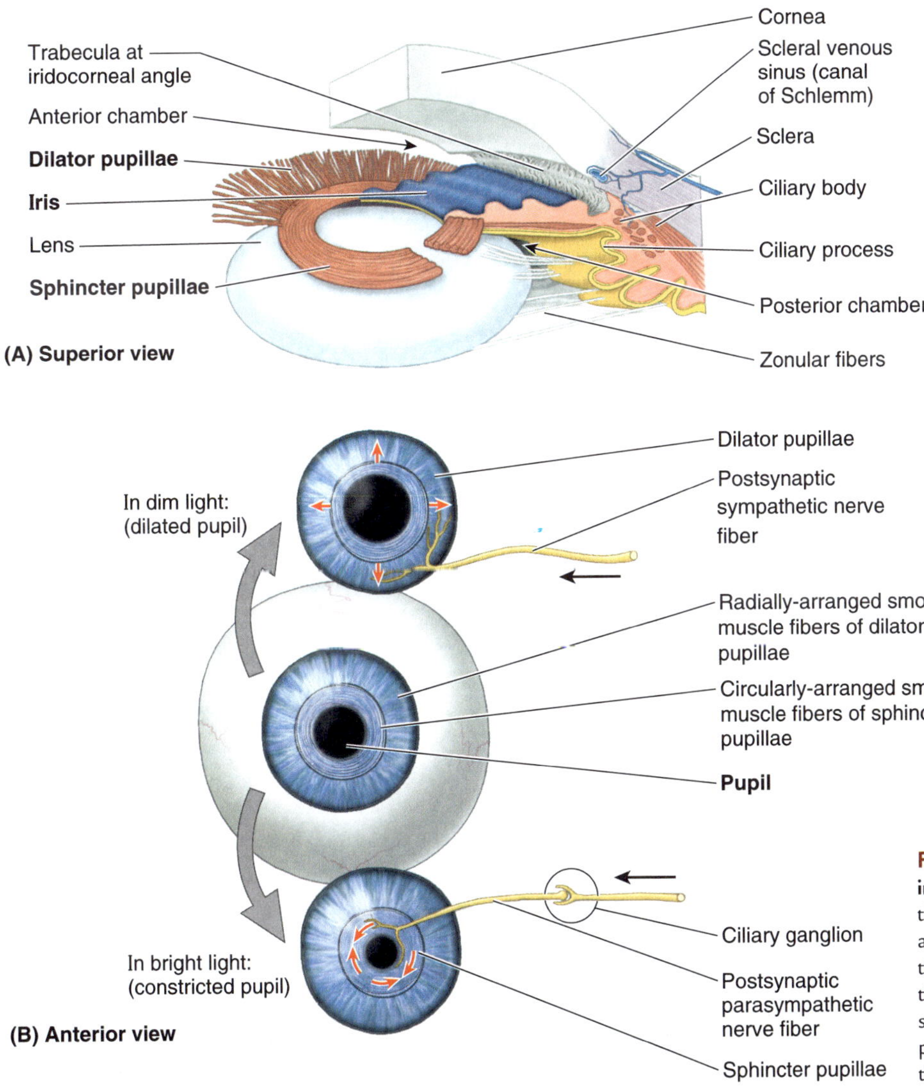

FIGURE 8.51. Structure and function of the iris. A. Iris dissected in situ. The iris separates the anterior and posterior chambers of the anterior segment of the eyeball as it bounds the pupil. **B.** Dilation and constriction of the pupil. In dim light, sympathetic fibers stimulate dilation of the pupil. In bright light, parasympathetic fibers stimulate constricting the pupil.

thetic responses, yet parasympathetically stimulated papillary constriction is normally instantaneous. Abnormal sustained pupillary dilation (*mydriasis*) may occur in certain diseases or as a result of trauma or the use of certain drugs.

INNER LAYER OF EYEBALL

The inner layer of the eyeball is the **retina** (Figs. 8.49C and 8.50). It is the sensory neural layer of the eyeball. Grossly, the retina consists of two functional parts with distinct locations: an optic part and a nonvisual retina. The **optic part of the retina** is sensitive to visual light rays and has two layers: a neural layer and pigmented layer. The **neural layer** is light receptive. The **pigmented layer** consists of a single layer of cells that reinforces the light-absorbing property of the choroid in reducing the scattering of light in the eyeball. The **nonvisual retina** is an anterior continuation of the pigmented layer and a layer of supporting cells. The nonvisual retina extends over the ciliary body (**ciliary part of the retina**) and the posterior surface of the iris (**iridial part of the retina**), to the pupillary margin.

Clinically, the internal aspect of the posterior part of the eyeball, where light entering the eyeball is focused, is referred to as the **fundus of the eyeball** (ocular fundus). The retina of the fundus includes a distinctive circular area called the **optic disc** (optic papilla), where the sensory fibers and vessels conveyed by the optic nerve (CN II) enter the eyeball (Figs. 8.49C, 8.50A, and 8.52A, B). Because it contains no photoreceptors, the optic disc is insensitive to light. Consequently, this part of the retina is commonly called the *blind spot*.

Just lateral to the optic disc is the **macula of the retina** or macula lutea (L. yellow spot). The yellow color of the macula

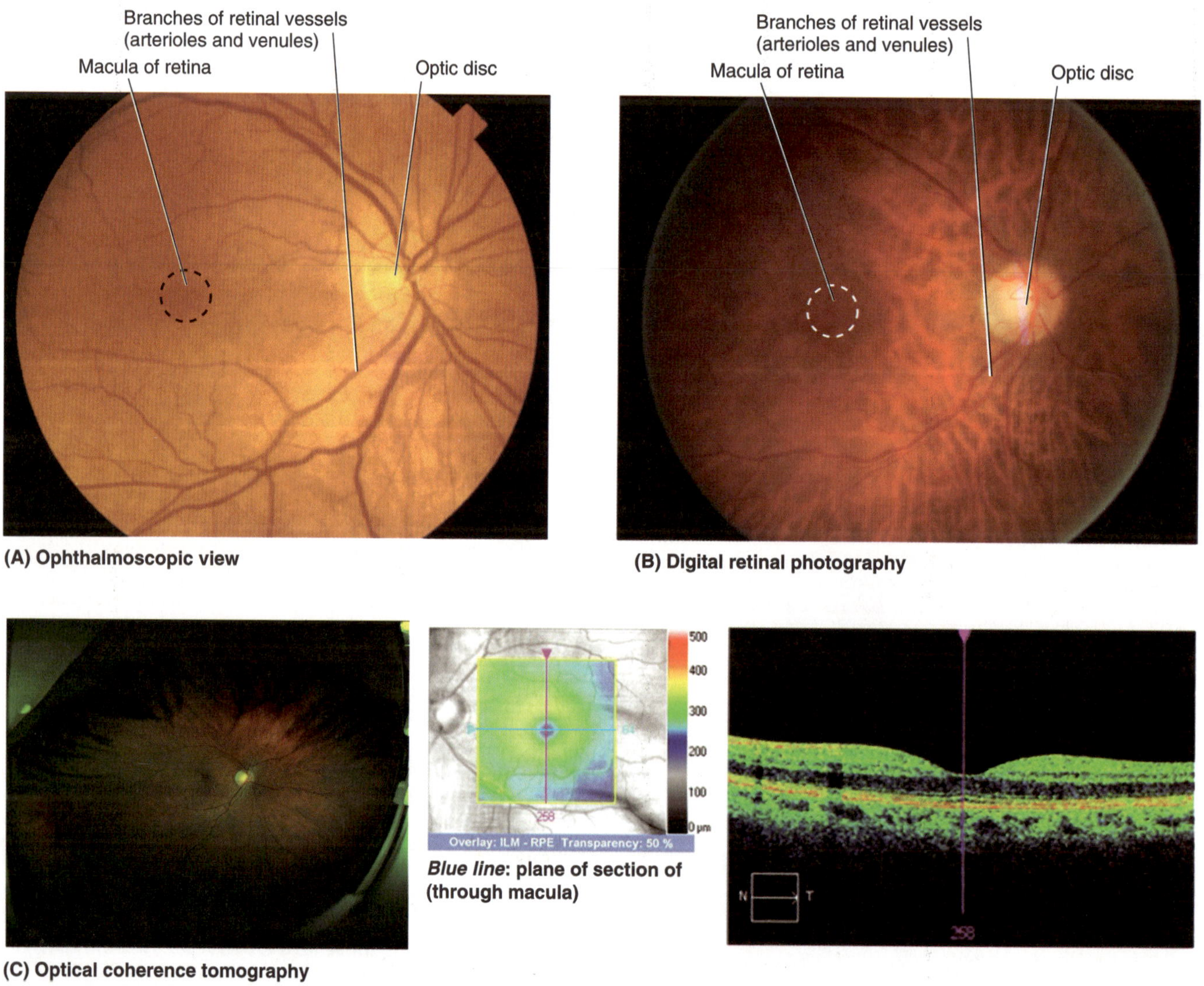

FIGURE 8.52. Fundus of right eyeball. A and B. Retinal venules (wider) and retinal arterioles (narrower) radiate from the center of the oval optic disc. The dark area lateral to the disc is the macula. Branches of retinal vessels extend toward this area, but do not reach its center, the fovea centralis, shown in part C. **C.** Optical coherence tomography measures macular thickness, especially important within the avascular foveola of the fovea centralis—the area of most acute vision. The technique produces the right sectional image of the macula.

is apparent only when the retina is examined with red-free light. The macula is a small oval area of the retina with special photoreceptor cones that is specialized for acuity of vision. It is not normally observed with an *ophthalmoscope* (a device for viewing the interior of the eyeball through the pupil). At the center of the macula, a depression, the **fovea centralis** (L., central pit), is the area of most acute vision (Fig. 8.52C). The fovea is approximately 1.5 mm in diameter; its center, the **foveola**, does not have the capillary network visible elsewhere deep to the retina.

The optic part of the retina terminates anteriorly along the **ora serrata** (L. serrated edge), the irregular posterior border of the ciliary body (Figs. 8.49C and 8.50A). Except for the cones and rods of the neural layer, the retina is supplied by the *central retinal artery*, a branch of the ophthalmic artery. The cones and rods of the outer neural layer receive nutrients from the *capillary lamina of the choroid*, or choriocapillaris (discussed in "Vasculature of Orbit," see p. 963). It has the finest vessels of the inner surface of the choroid, against which the retina is pressed. A corresponding system of retinal veins unites to form the *central retinal vein*.

AN43.2 For microanatomy of retina, refer *diFiore's Atlas of Histology with Functional Correlations*, 1st South Asian Edition, Chapter 22, Organs of Special Senses: Visual Auditory Systems, pp. 631–637.

REFRACTIVE MEDIA AND COMPARTMENTS OF EYEBALL

On their way to the retina, light waves pass through the refractive media of the eyeball: cornea, aqueous humor, lens, and vitreous humor (Fig. 8.50A). The *cornea* is the primary refractory medium of the eyeball, that is, it bends light to the greatest degree, focusing an inverted image on the light-sensitive retina of the *fundus of the eyeball*.

The **aqueous humor** ("aqueous") occupies the *anterior segment of the eyeball* (Figs. 8.50B and 8.51A). The anterior segment is subdivided by the iris and pupil. The **anterior chamber of the eye** is the space between the cornea anteriorly and the iris/pupil posteriorly. The **posterior chamber of the eye** is between the iris/pupil anteriorly and the lens and ciliary body posteriorly. Aqueous humor is produced in the posterior chamber by the *ciliary processes* of the ciliary body. This clear watery solution provides nutrients for the avascular cornea and lens. After passing through the pupil into the anterior chamber, the aqueous humor drains through a trabecular meshwork at the **iridocorneal angle** into the **scleral venous sinus** (L. *sinus venosus sclerae*, canal of Schlemm) (Fig. 8.51A). The humor is removed by the **limbal plexus**, a network of scleral veins close to the limbus, which drain in turn into both tributaries of the *vorticose* and *anterior ciliary veins* (Fig. 8.50B). Intra-ocular pressure (IOP) is a balance between production and outflow of aqueous humor.

The **lens** is posterior to the iris and anterior to the vitreous humor of the *vitreous body* (Figs. 8.50 and 8.51A). It is a transparent, biconvex structure enclosed in a capsule. The highly elastic **capsule of the lens** is anchored by **zonular fibers** (collectively constituting the **suspensory ligament of the lens**) to the encircling ciliary processes. Although most refraction is produced by the cornea, the convexity of the lens, particularly its anterior surface, constantly varies to fine-tune the focus of near or distant objects on the retina (Fig. 8.53). The isolated unattached lens assumes a nearly spherical shape. In other words, in the absence of external attachment and stretching, it becomes nearly round. The **ciliary muscle** of the ciliary body changes the shape of the lens. In the absence of nerve stimulation, the diameter of the relaxed muscular ring is larger. The lens suspended within the ring is under tension as its periphery is stretched, causing it to be thinner (less convex). The less convex lens brings more distant objects into focus (far vision). Parasympathetic stimulation via the oculomotor nerve (CN III) causes sphincter-like contraction of the ciliary muscle. The ring becomes smaller, and tension on the lens is reduced. The relaxed lens thickens (becomes more convex), bringing near objects into focus (near vision). The active process of changing the shape of the lens for near vision is called **accommodation**. The thickness of the lens increases with aging so that the ability to accommodate typically becomes restricted after age 40.

The **vitreous humor** is a watery fluid enclosed in the meshes of the **vitreous body**, a transparent jelly-like substance in the posterior four fifths of the eyeball posterior to the lens (**posterior segment of the eyeball**, also called the *postremal* or *vitreous chamber*) (Fig. 8.50A). In addition to transmitting light, the vitreous humor holds the retina in place and supports the lens.

Extra-Ocular Muscles of Orbit

AN31

The **extra-ocular muscles of the orbit** are the *levator palpebrae superioris*, four *recti* (*superior*, *inferior*, *medial*, and *lateral*), and two *obliques* (*superior* and *inferior*). These seven muscles work together to elevate the superior eyelids and move the eyeballs on three axes (Fig. 8.54). They are illustrated in Figures 8.54 to 8.59 and the attachments, nerve supply, and main actions of the orbital muscles, beginning from the primary position, are outlined in Table 8.8. Additional details are provided in the following sections.

LEVATOR PALPEBRAE SUPERIORIS

The **levator palpebrae superioris** broadens into a wide bilaminar aponeurosis as it approaches its distal attachments. The superficial lamina attaches to the skin of the superior eyelid, and the deep lamina to the superior tarsus (Fig. 8.54B). This muscle is opposed most of the time by gravity and is the antagonist of the superior half of the orbicularis oculi, the sphincter of the palpebral fissure. The deep lamina of the distal (palpebral) part of the muscle includes smooth muscle fibers, the **superior tarsal muscle**, that produce additional widening of the palpebral fissure, especially during a sympathetic response (e.g., fright). However, they seem to func-

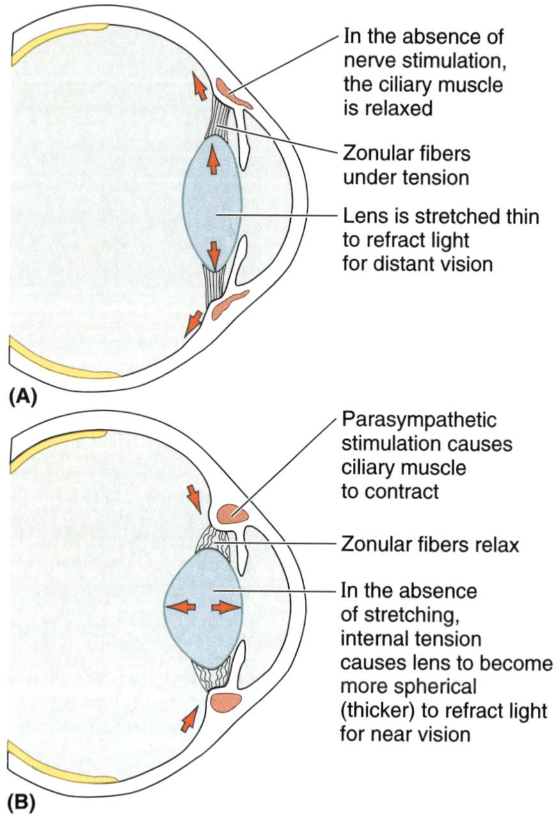

FIGURE 8.53. Changing lens shape (accommodation). A. Distant vision. **B.** Near vision.

tion continuously (in the absence of a sympathetic response) because an interruption of the sympathetic supply produces a constant *ptosis*—drooping of the upper eyelid.

MOVEMENTS OF EYEBALL

Movements of the eyeball occur as rotations around three *axes—vertical*, *transverse*, and *anteroposterior* (Fig. 8.54A)—and are described according to the direction of movement of the pupil from the primary position or of the superior pole of the eyeball from the neutral position. Rotation of the eyeball around the vertical axis moves the pupil medially (toward the midline, **adduction**) or laterally (away from the midline, **abduction**). Rotation around the transverse axis moves the pupil superiorly (**elevation**) or inferiorly (**depression**). Movements around the anteroposterior (AP) axis (corresponding to the axis of gaze in the primary position) move the superior pole of the eyeball medially (**medial rotation**, or intorsion) or laterally (**lateral rotation**, or extorsion). These rotational movements accommodate changes in the tilt of the head. Absence of these movements resulting from nerve lesions contributes to double vision. Movements may occur around the three axes simultaneously, requiring three terms to describe the direction of movement from the primarily position (e.g., the pupil is elevated, adducted, and medially rotated).

RECTI AND OBLIQUE MUSCLES

The four **recti muscles** (L. *rectos*, straight) run anteriorly to the eyeball, arising from a fibrous cuff, the **common tendinous ring**, that surrounds the optic canal and from part of the superior orbital fissure at the apex of the orbit (Figs. 8.54B, C, 8.55A, 8.55B). Structures that enter the orbit through the optic canal and the adjacent part of the fissure lie initially within the cone of recti (Figs. 8.54B, C and 8.55B). The four recti muscles are named for their individual positions relative to the eyeball. Because they mainly run anteriorly to attach to the superior, inferior, medial, and lateral aspects of the eyeball anterior to its equator, the primary actions of the four recti in producing elevation, depression, adduction, and abduction are relatively intuitive.

Several factors make the actions of the obliques and the secondary actions of the superior and inferior recti more challenging to understand. The *apex of the orbit* is medially placed relative to the orbit, so that the *axis of the orbit* does not coincide with the *optical axis* (Figs. 8.44A, 8.54C, 8.56). Therefore, *when the eye is in the primary position*, the **superior rectus (SR)** and **inferior rectus (IR)** muscles also approach the eyeball from its medial side, their line of pull passing medial to the vertical axis. This gives both muscles a secondary action of *adduction*. The SR and IR also extend

(*continued on p.* 959)

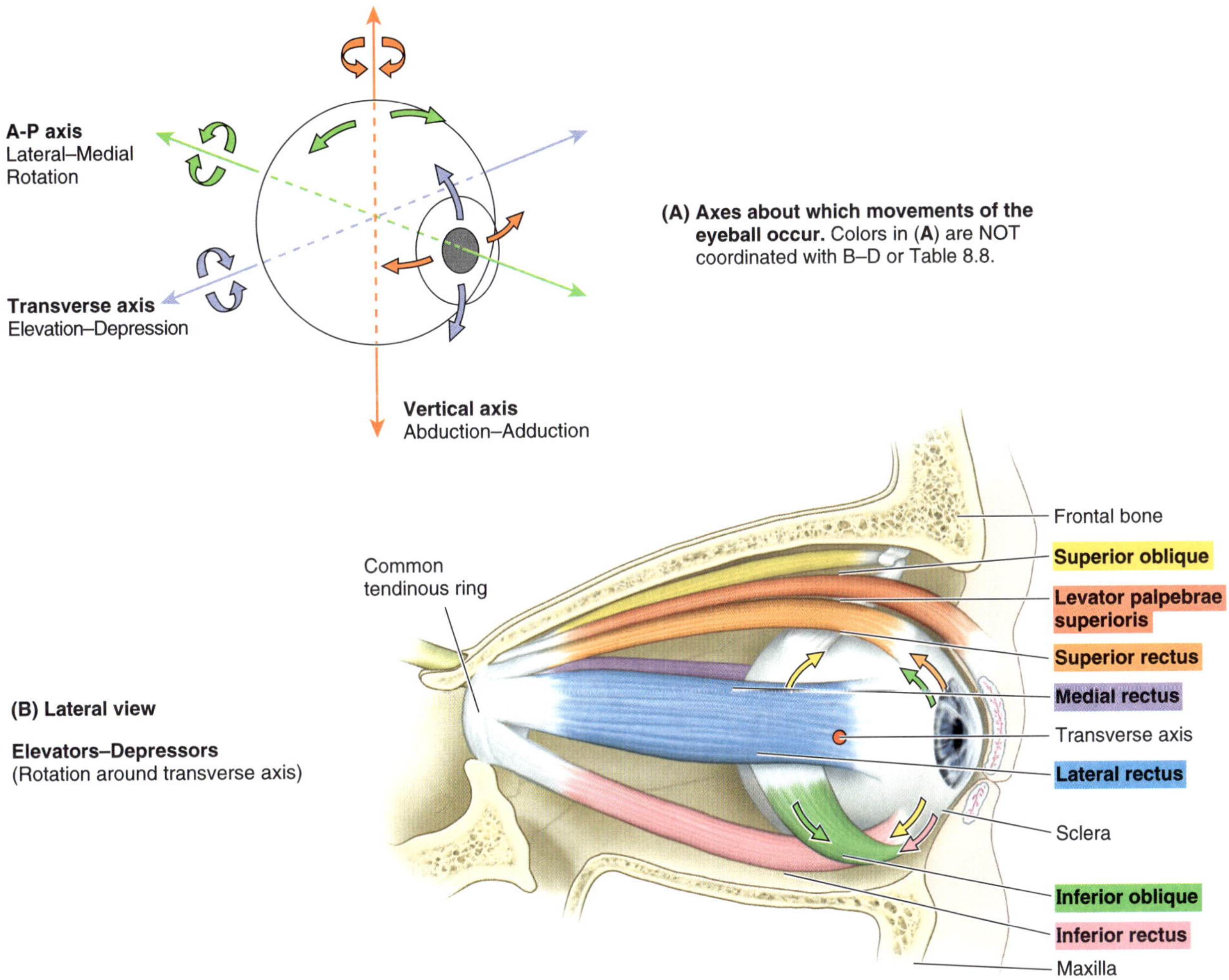

FIGURE 8.54. Extra-ocular muscles and their movements. A. Axes around which movements of the eyeball occur. **B.** Position of muscles in right orbit. *Arrows*, movements of the eyeball around the transverse axis.

TABLE 8.8. EXTRA-OCULAR MUSCLES OF ORBIT

Muscle	Origin	Insertion	Innervation	Main Action[a]
Levator palpebrae superioris	Lesser wing of sphenoid bone, superior and anterior to optic canal	Superior tarsus and skin of superior eyelid	Oculomotor nerve (CN III); deep layer (superior tarsal muscle) is supplied by sympathetic fibers.	Elevates superior eyelid
Superior oblique (SO)	Body of sphenoid bone	Its tendon passes through a fibrous ring or trochlea, changes its direction, and inserts into sclera deep to superior rectus muscle.	Trochlear nerve (CN IV)	Abducts, depresses, and medially rotates eyeball
Inferior oblique (IO)	Anterior part of floor of orbit	Sclera deep to lateral rectus muscle	Oculomotor nerve (CN III)	Abducts, elevates, and laterally rotates eyeball
Superior rectus (SR)	Common tendinous ring	Sclera just posterior to corneoscleral junction		Elevates, adducts, and rotates eyeball medially
Inferior rectus (IR)				Depresses, adducts, and rotates eyeball laterally
Medial rectus (MR)				Adducts eyeball
Lateral rectus (LR)			Abducent nerve (CN VI)	Abducts eyeball

[a]The actions described are for muscles acting alone, starting from the primary position (gaze directed anteriorly). In fact, muscles rarely act independently and almost always work together in synergistic and antagonistic groups. Clinical testing requires maneuvers to isolate muscle actions. Only the actions of the medial and lateral rectus are tested, starting from the primary position (Fig. 8.57E).

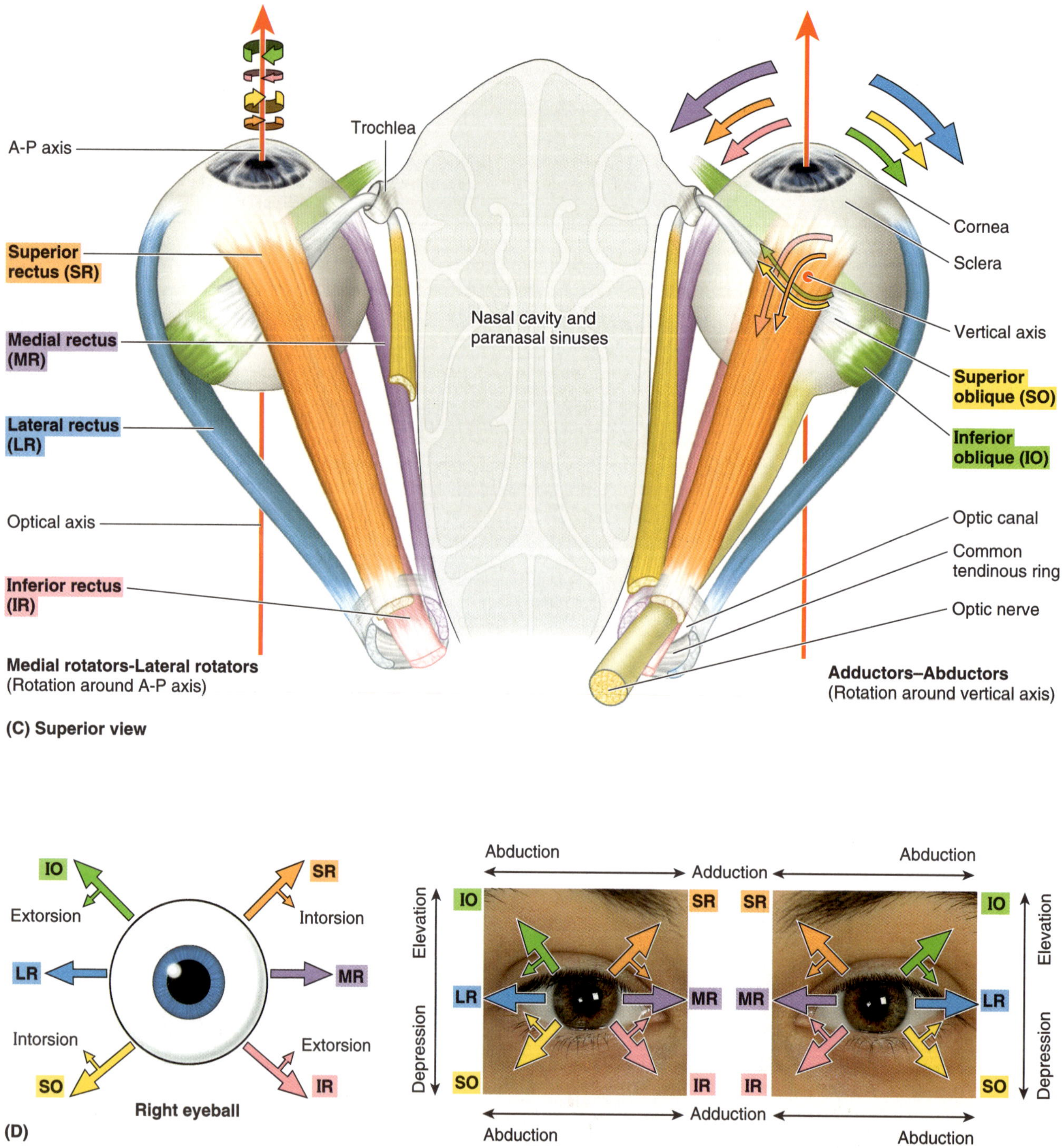

FIGURE 8.54. **(Continued) C.** Position of muscles in right and left orbits. *Arrows at left*, movements of the eyeball around the AP axis; *arrows at right*, movements of the eyeball around the vertical axis. To understand the actions produced by muscles starting from the primary position, it is necessary to observe the placement and line of pull of the muscle relative to the axes about which the movements occur. **D.** Unilateral and bilateral demonstration of extra-ocular muscle actions, starting from the primary position. For movements in any of the six cardinal directions (*large arrows*) the indicated muscle is the prime mover. Movements in directions between *large arrows* require synergistic actions by the adjacent muscles. For example, direct elevation requires the synergistic actions of IO and SR; direct depression requires synergistic action of SO and IR. *Small arrows*, muscles producing rotational movements around the AP axis. Coordinated action of the contralateral yoke muscles is required to direct the gaze. For example, in directing the gaze to the right, the right LR and left MR are yoke muscles.

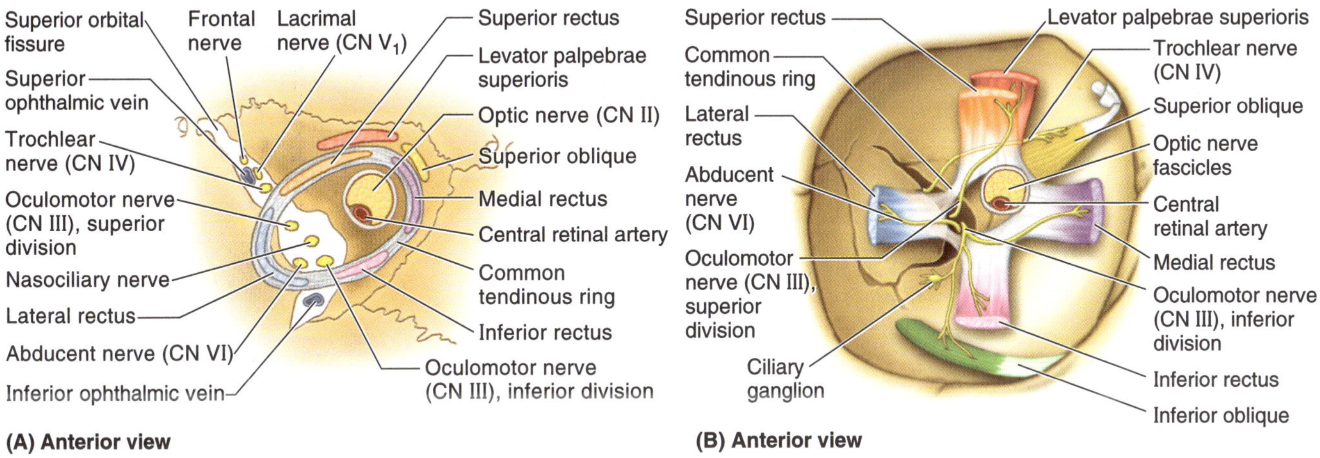

FIGURE 8.55. Relationship at apex of orbit. A. Common tendinous ring. The ring is formed by the origin of the four recti muscles and encircles the optic sheath of CN II, the superior and inferior divisions of CN III, the nasociliary nerve (CN V_1), and CN VI. The nerves supplying the extra-ocular muscles enter the orbit through the superior orbital fissure: oculomotor (CN III), trochlear (CN IV), and abducent (CN VI). **B.** Muscles and motor nerves. The fat and fascia have also been removed.

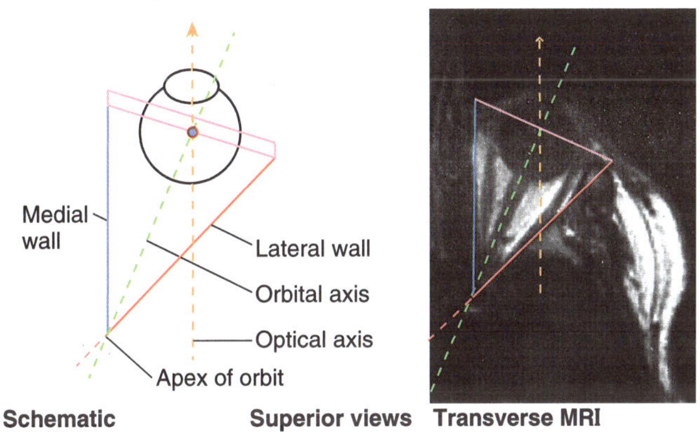

FIGURE 8.56. Orbital versus optical axis. Because the apex is located medial as well as posterior to the eyeball, the two axes do not coincide, resulting in secondary movements produced by the superior and inferior recti and oblique muscles.

laterally, passing superior and inferior to the AP axis, respectively, giving the SR a secondary action of *medial rotation*, and the IR a secondary action of *lateral rotation*.

If the gaze is first directed laterally (abducted by the **lateral rectus [LR]**) so that the line of gaze coincides with the plane of the IR and SR, *the SR produces elevation only* (and is solely responsible for the movement) (Fig. 8.57A), and *the IR produces depression only* (and is likewise solely responsible) (Fig. 8.57B). During a physical examination, the physician directs the patient to follow his or her finger laterally (testing the LR and abducent nerve [CN VI]), then superiorly and inferiorly to isolate and test the function of the SR and IR and the integrity of the oculomotor nerve (CN III), which supplies both (Fig. 8.57E).

The **inferior oblique (IO)** is the only muscle to originate from the anterior part of the orbit (immediately lateral to the lacrimal fossa) (Fig. 8.47B). The **superior oblique (SO)** originates from the apex region like the rectus muscles (but super medial to the common tendinous ring) (Fig. 8.55A). However, its tendon traverses the *trochlea* just inside the super medial orbital rim, redirecting its line of pull (Figs. 8.54B, C and 8.55B). Therefore, the inserting tendons of the oblique muscles lie in the same oblique vertical plane. When the inserting tendons are viewed anteriorly (Fig. 8.47B) or superiorly (Fig. 8.54C) with the eyeball in the primary position, it can be seen that the tendons of the oblique muscles pass mainly laterally to insert on the lateral half of the eyeball, posterior to its equator. Because they pass inferior and superior to the AP axis as they pass laterally, the IO is the primary lateral rotator, and the SO is the primary medial rotator of the eye. However, in the primary position, the obliques also pass posteriorly across the transverse axis (Fig. 8.54B) and posterior to the vertical axis (Fig. 8.54C), giving the SO a secondary function as a depressor, the IO a secondary function as an elevator, and both muscles a secondary function as abductors (Fig. 8.54B, C).

If the gaze is first directed medially (adducted by the **medial rectus [MR]**) so that the line of gaze coincides with plane of the inserting tendons of the SO and IO, *the SO produces depression only* (and is solely responsible for the movement) (Fig. 8.57C), and *the IO produces elevation only* (and is

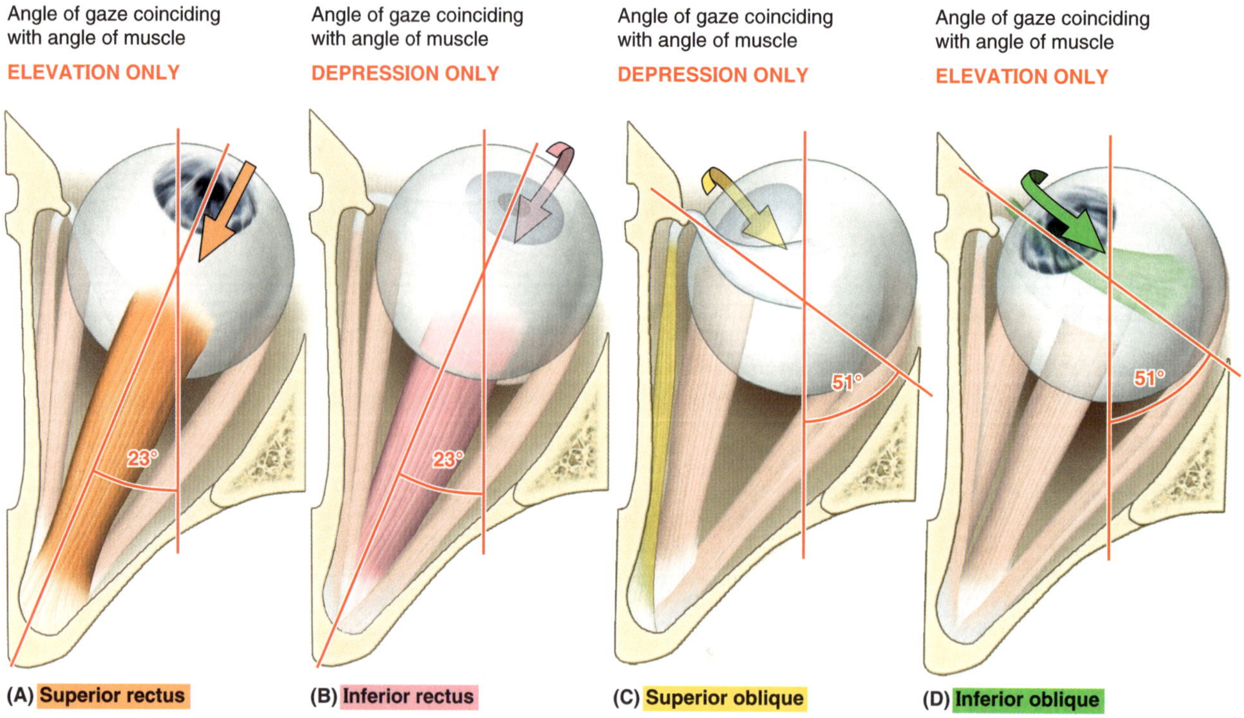

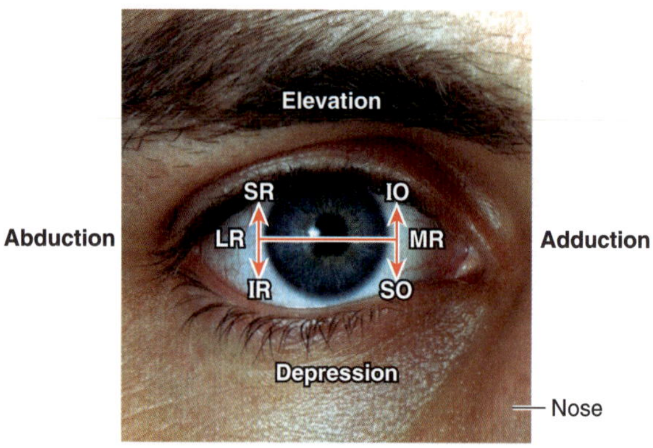

(E) Actions of muscles of orbit as tested clinically (right eye)

FIGURE 8.57. Clinical testing of extra-ocular muscles. A, B. When the eye is initially abducted by LR, only the rectus muscles can produce elevation and depression. **C, D.** When the eye is initially adducted by MR, only the oblique muscles can produce elevation and depression. **E.** Following movements of the examiner's finger, the pupil is moved in an extended H-pattern to isolate and test individual extra-ocular muscles and the integrity of their nerves.

likewise solely responsible) (Fig. 8.57D). During a physical examination, the physician directs the patient to follow his or her finger medially (testing the MR and oculomotor nerve) and then inferiorly and superiorly to isolate and test the functions of the SO and IO and the integrity of the trochlear nerve (CN IV), which supplies the SO, and of the inferior division of CN III, which supplies the IO (Fig. 8.57E). In practice

- the main action of the superior oblique is depression of the pupil in the adducted position (e.g., directing the gaze down the page when the gaze of both eyes is directed medially [*converged*] for reading).
- the main action of the inferior oblique is elevation of the pupil in the adducted position (e.g., directing the gaze up the page during **convergence** for reading).

Although the actions produced by the extra-ocular muscles have been considered individually, all motions require the action of several muscles in the same eye, assisting each other as synergists or opposing each other as antagonists. Muscles that are synergistic for one action may be antagonistic for another. For example, no single muscle can act to elevate the pupil directly from the primary position (Fig. 8.54D). The two elevators (SR and IO) act as synergists to do so. However, these muscles are antagonistic as rotators and so neutralize each other so that no rotation occurs as they work together to elevate the pupil. Similarly, no single muscle can act to depress the pupil directly from the primary position. The two depressors, the SO and IR, both produce depression when acting alone and also produce opposing actions in terms of adduction–abduction and medial–lateral rotation. However, when the SO and IR act simultaneously, their synergistic

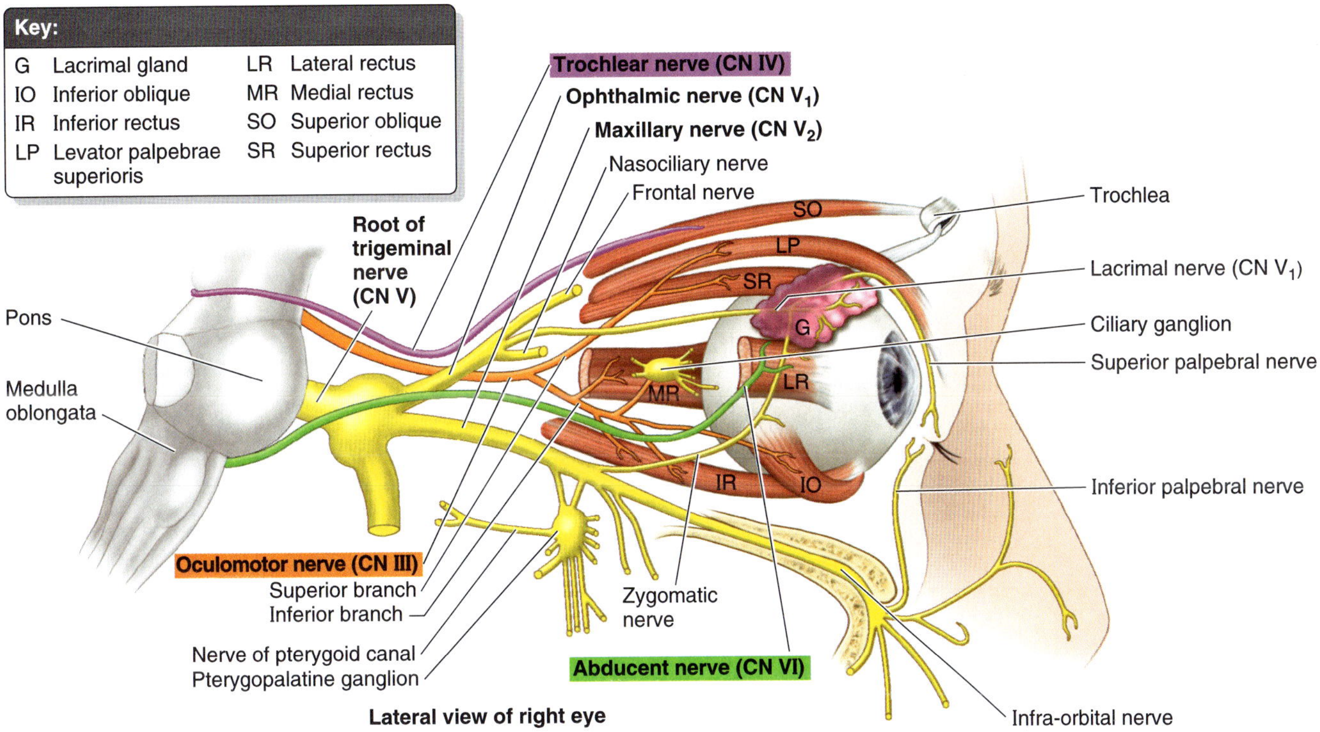

FIGURE 8.58. Nerves of orbit. Three cranial nerves (CN III, IV, and VI) supply the seven voluntary extra-ocular muscles. CN IV supplies the superior oblique, CN VI supplies the lateral rectus, and CN III supplies the remaining five muscles. The CN III also brings presynaptic parasympathetic fibers to the ciliary ganglion. The trigeminal nerve (CN V) supplies sensory fibers to the orbit, orbital region, and eyeball.

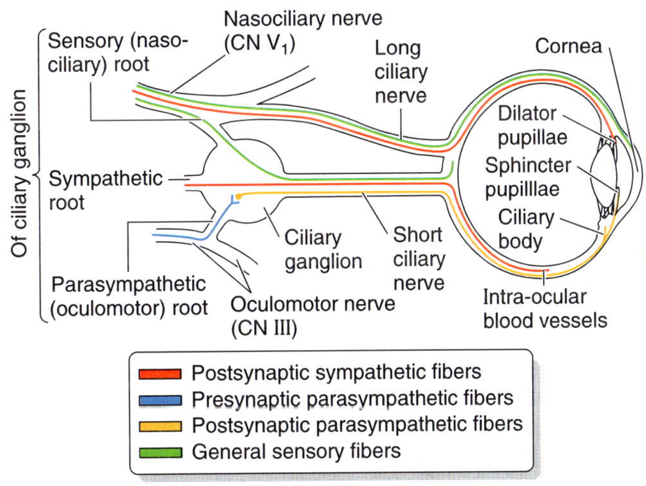

FIGURE 8.59. Distribution of nerve fibers to ciliary ganglion and eyeball. The ciliary ganglion receives three types of nerve fibers from three separate sources. All parasympathetic innervation but only some of the sensory and sympathetic innervation to the eyeball traverses the ganglion. Sympathetic and sensory fibers in the long ciliary nerve bypass the ganglion.

actions depress the pupil because their antagonistic actions neutralize each other; therefore, pure depression results.

To direct the gaze, coordination of both eyes must be accomplished by the paired action of contralateral **yoke muscles** (functionally paired contralateral extra-ocular muscles). For example, in directing the gaze to the right, the right lateral rectus and left medial rectus act as yoke muscles (Fig. 8.60).

SUPPORTING APPARATUS OF EYEBALL

The *fascial sheath of the eyeball* envelops the eyeball, extending posteriorly from the conjunctival fornices to the optic nerve, forming the actual socket for the eyeball (Figs. 8.45A; 8.61C). The cup-like fascial sheath is pierced by the tendons of the extra-ocular muscles and is reflected onto each of them as a tubular *muscle sheath*. The muscle sheaths of the levator and superior rectus muscles are fused.

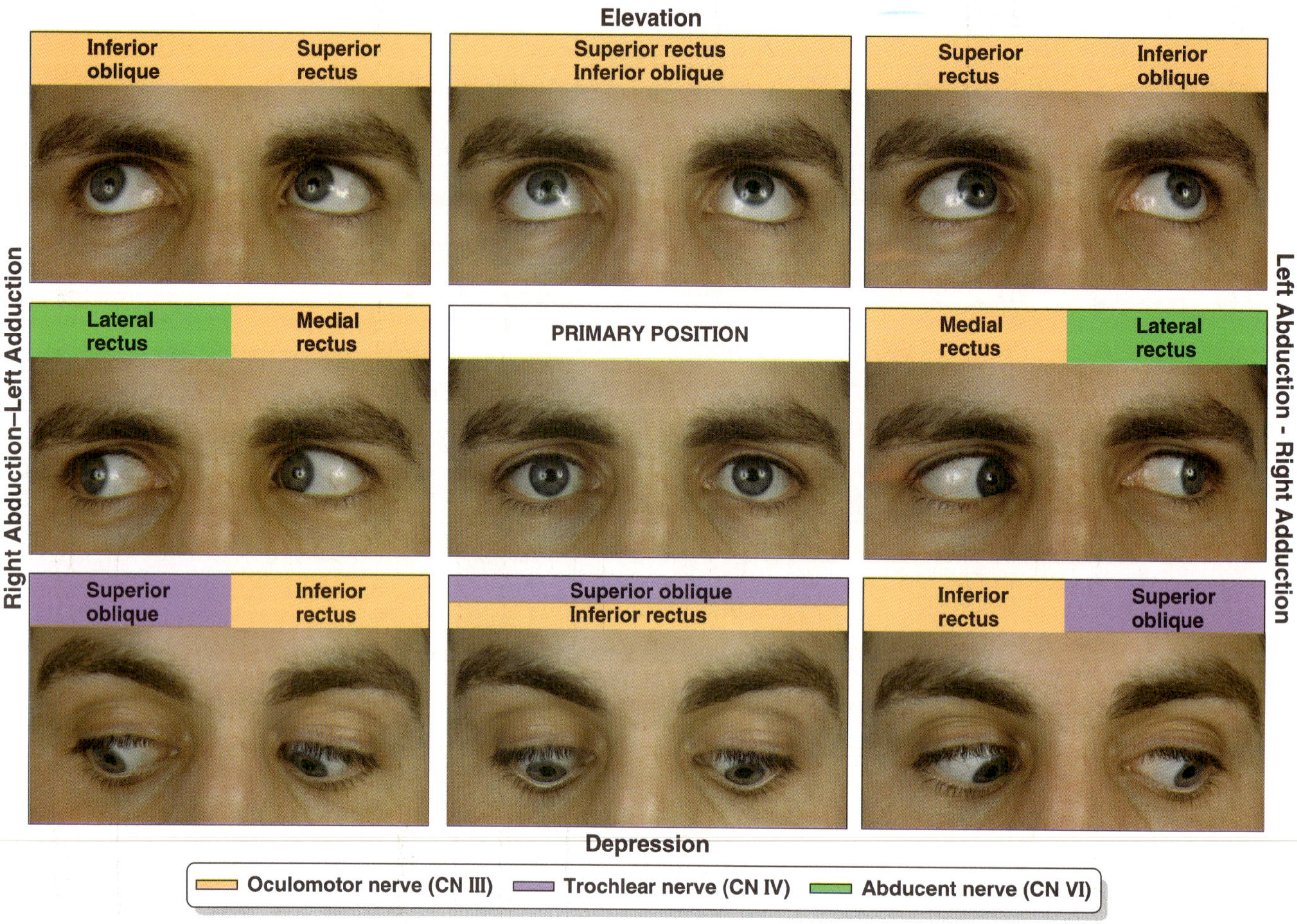

N43.5 **FIGURE 8.60. Binocular movements and muscles producing them.** All movements start from the primary position.

Therefore, when the gaze is directed superiorly, the superior eyelid is further elevated out of the line of vision. Triangular expansions from the sheaths of the medial and lateral rectus muscles, called the **medial** and **lateral check ligaments**, are attached to the lacrimal and zygomatic bones, respectively (Fig. 8.61C). These ligaments limit abduction and adduction. A blending of the check ligaments with the fascia of the inferior rectus and inferior oblique muscles forms a hammock-like sling, the **suspensory ligament of the eyeball**. A similar **inferior check ligament** from the fascial sheath of the inferior rectus retracts the inferior eyelid when the gaze is directed downward (Fig. 8.45A). Collectively, the check ligaments act with the oblique muscles and the retrobulbar fat to resist the posterior pull on the eyeball produced by the rectus muscles. In diseases or starvation that reduce the **retrobulbar fat**, the eyeball is retracted into the orbit (*enophthalmos*).

Nerves of Orbit

N31.2 The large optic nerves convey purely sensory nerves that transmit impulses generated by optical stimuli (Figs. 8.45A and 8.50A). They are cranial nerves (CN II) by convention, but develop as paired anterior extensions of the forebrain, and therefore are central nervous system (CNS) fiber tracts formed of second-order neurons. The optic nerves begin at the **lamina cribrosa of the sclera**, where the unmyelinated nerve fibers pierce the sclera and become myelinated, posterior to the *optic disc*. They exit the orbits via the optic canals. Throughout their course in the orbit, the optic nerves are surrounded by extensions of the *cranial meninges* and *subarachnoid space*, the latter occupied by a thin layer of *CSF* (Figs. 8.61C; 8.45A, *inset*). The intra-orbital extensions of the cranial dura and arachnoid constitute the **optic nerve sheath**, which becomes continuous anteriorly with the fascial sheath of the eyeball and the sclera. A layer of pia mater covers the surface of the optic nerve within the sheath.

In addition to the optic nerve (CN II), the nerves of the orbit include those that enter through the *superior orbital fissure* and supply the ocular muscles: **oculomotor** (CN III), **trochlear** (CN IV), and **abducent** (CN VI) nerves (Figs. 8.55 and 8.58). A memory device for the innervation of the extra-ocular muscles moving the eyeball is similar to a chemical formula: $LR_6SO_4AO_3$ (lateral rectus, CN **VI**; superior oblique, CN **IV**; all others, CN **III**). The trochlear and abducent nerves pass directly to the single muscle supplied

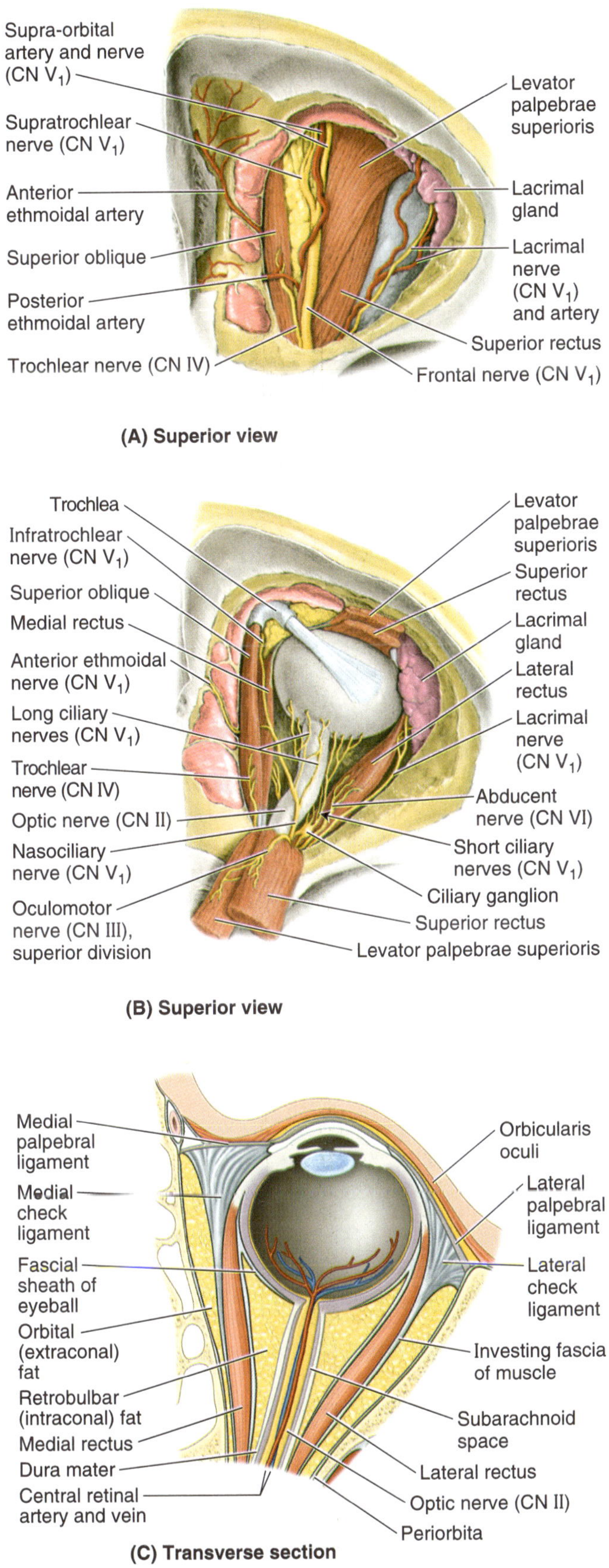

FIGURE 8.61. Dissection of right orbit. A. Super cial dissection of orbit. **B.** Deep dissection of orbit. **C.** Demonstration of fascial sheath of eyeball and check ligaments.

by each nerve. The oculomotor nerve divides into a superior and an inferior division. The superior division supplies the superior rectus and levator palpebrae superioris. The inferior division supplies the medial and inferior rectus and inferior oblique and carries presynaptic parasympathetic fibers to the ciliary ganglion (Fig. 8.59). The movements are stimulated by the oculomotor, trochlear, and abducent nerves, starting from the primary position in the right and left orbits, and produce binocular vision, demonstrated in Figure 8.60.

The three terminal branches of the *ophthalmic nerve*, CN V_1 (the frontal, nasociliary, and lacrimal nerves—Figs. 8.58, 8.61A), pass through the superior orbital fissure and supply structures related to the anterior orbit (e.g., lacrimal gland and eyelids), face, and scalp (Fig. 8.62). The cutaneous branches of CN V_1 (lacrimal, frontal, and infratrochlear nerves) are described in "Cutaneous Nerves of Face and Scalp" and in Table 8.5.

The **ciliary ganglion** is a small group of postsynaptic parasympathetic nerve cell bodies associated with CN V_1. It is located between the optic nerve and the lateral rectus toward the posterior limit of the orbit (Figs. 8.58, 8.61B). The ciliary ganglion receives nerve fibers from three sources (Fig. 8.59):

1. Sensory fibers from CN V_1 via the **sensory** or **nasociliary root of the ciliary ganglion**.
2. Presynaptic parasympathetic fibers from CN III via the **parasympathetic** or **oculomotor root of the ciliary ganglion**.
3. Postsynaptic sympathetic fibers from the *internal carotid plexus* via the **sympathetic root of the ciliary ganglion**.

The **short ciliary nerves** arise from the ciliary ganglion and are considered to be branches of CN V_1 (Figs. 8.59, 8.61B, and 8.62). They carry parasympathetic and sympathetic fibers to the ciliary body and iris. The short ciliary nerves consist of postsynaptic parasympathetic fibers originating in the ciliary ganglion, afferent fibers from the nasociliary nerve that pass through the ganglion, and postsynaptic sympathetic fibers that also pass through it. **Long ciliary nerves**, branches of the nasociliary nerve (CN V_1) that pass to the eyeball, bypassing the ciliary ganglion, convey postsynaptic sympathetic fibers to the dilator pupillae and afferent fibers from the iris and cornea.

The *posterior* and *anterior ethmoidal nerves*, branches of the nasociliary nerve arising in the orbit, exit via openings in the medial wall of the orbit to supply the mucous membrane of the sphenoidal and ethmoidal sinuses and the nasal cavities, as well as the dura of the anterior cranial fossa.

Vasculature of Orbit

ARTERIES OF ORBIT

The blood supply of the orbit is mainly from the **ophthalmic artery**, a branch of the internal carotid artery (Fig. 8.63;

(*continued on p.* 965)

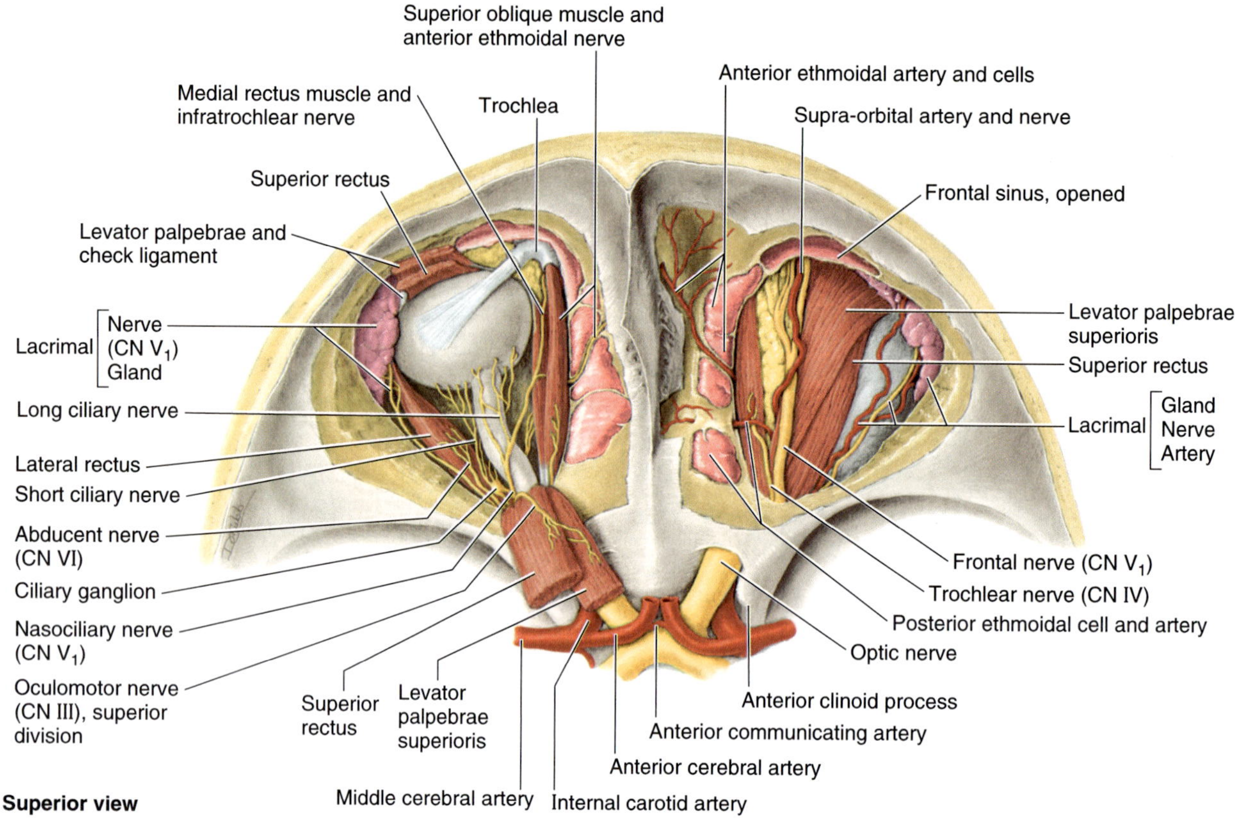

FIGURE 8.62. Dissection of orbit. In this superior approach, the orbital part of the frontal bone has been removed. On the right side, three nerves applied to the roof of the orbit (trochlear, frontal, and lacrimal) are evident. On the left side, the levator palpebrae superioris and superior rectus have been cut and reflected and the orbital fat removed to demonstrate the nerves that traverse the intraconal fat.

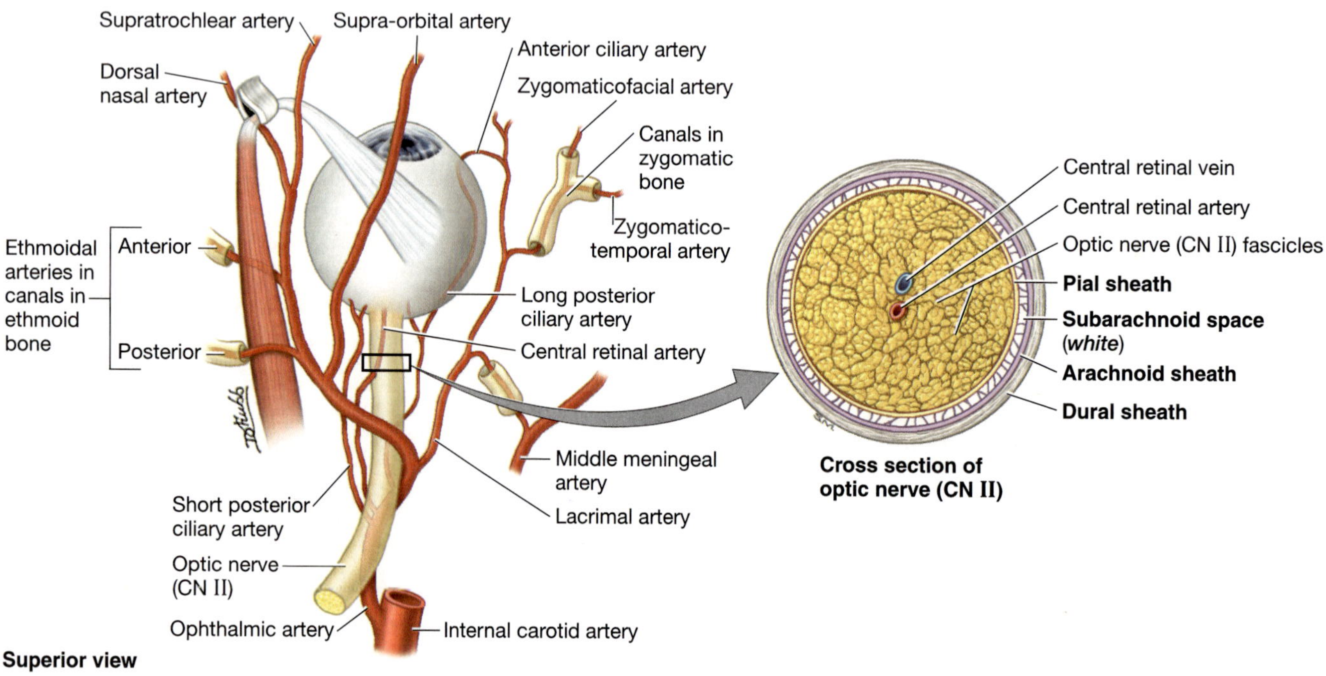

FIGURE 8.63. Arteries of orbit and arteries and veins of eyeball. Branches of ophthalmic artery. *Inset,* cross-section of optic nerve (CN II).

TABLE 8.9. **ARTERIES OF ORBIT**

Artery	Origin	Course and Distribution
Ophthalmic	Internal carotid artery	Traverses optic foramen to reach orbital cavity
Central retinal artery	Ophthalmic artery	Pierces dural sheath of optic nerve and runs to eyeball; branches from center of optic disc; supplies optic retina (except cones and rods)
Supra-orbital		Passes superiorly and posteriorly from supra-orbital foramen to supply forehead and scalp
Supratrochlear		Passes from supra-orbital margin to forehead and scalp
Lacrimal		Passes along superior border of lateral rectus muscle to supply lacrimal gland, conjunctiva, and eyelids
Dorsal nasal		Courses along dorsal aspect of nose and supplies its surface
Short posterior ciliaries		Pierce sclera at periphery of optic nerve to supply choroid, which in turn supplies cones and rods of optic retina
Long posterior ciliaries		Pierce sclera to supply ciliary body and iris
Posterior ethmoidal		Passes through posterior ethmoidal foramen to posterior ethmoidal cells
Anterior ethmoidal		Passes through anterior ethmoidal foramen to anterior cranial fossa; supplies anterior and middle ethmoidal cells, frontal sinus, nasal cavity, and skin on dorsum of nose
Anterior ciliary	Muscular (rectus) branches of ophthalmic and infra-orbital arteries	Pierce sclera at attachments of rectus muscles and form networks in iris and ciliary body
Infra-orbital	Third part of maxillary artery	Passes along infra-orbital groove and foramen to face

Table 8.9); the **infra-orbital artery**, from the external carotid artery, also contributes blood to structures related to the orbital floor. The **central retinal artery**, a branch of the ophthalmic artery arising inferior to the optic nerve, pierces the sheath of the optic nerve and runs within the nerve to the eyeball, emerging at the optic disc (Fig. 8.45A, *inset*). Its branches spread over the internal surface of the retina (Figs. 8.52 and 8.64). The terminal branches are *end arteries (arterioles)*, which provide the only blood supply to the internal aspect of the retina.

The external aspect of the retina is also supplied by the *capillary lamina of the choroid (choriocapillaris)*. Of the eight or so *posterior ciliary arteries* (also branches of the ophthalmic artery), six **short posterior ciliary arteries** directly supply the choroid, which nourishes the outer nonvascular layer of the retina. Two **long posterior ciliary arteries**, one on each side of the eyeball, pass between the sclera and the choroid to anastomose with the **anterior ciliary arteries** (continuations of the **muscular branches of the ophthalmic artery** to the rectus muscles) to supply the ciliary plexus.

VEINS OF ORBIT

Venous drainage of the orbit is through the **superior** and **inferior ophthalmic veins**, which pass through the superior orbital fissure and enter the cavernous sinus (Fig. 8.65). The **central retinal vein** (Fig. 8.63 *inset*; Fig. 8.64) usually enters the cavernous sinus directly, but it may join one of the ophthalmic veins. The vortex, or **vorticose veins**, from the vascular layer of the eyeball drain into the inferior ophthalmic vein. The **scleral venous sinus** is a vascular structure encircling the anterior chamber of the eyeball through which the aqueous humor is returned to the blood circulation.

Surface Anatomy of Eye and Lacrimal Apparatus

For a description of the surface anatomy of the eyelids, see "Surface Anatomy of Face." The anterior part of the sclera (the "white" of the eye) is covered by the transparent *bulbar conjunctiva*, which contains minute but apparent conjunctival blood vessels (Fig. 8.66B). When irritated, the vessels may enlarge noticeably, and the bulbar conjunctiva may take on a distinctly pink appearance when inflamed ("red" eyes). The normal tough, opaque sclera often appears slightly blue in infants and children and commonly has a yellow hue in many older people.

The anterior transparent part of the eye is the *cornea*, which is continuous with the sclera at its margins. In a lateral view (Fig. 8.66A), most of the visible part of the eyeball protrudes slightly through the *palpebral fissure*. It is apparent that the cornea has a greater curvature (convexity) than that of the rest of the eyeball (the part covered by sclera); thus, a shallow angle occurs at the *corneoscleral junction*, the *corneal limbus* (Fig. 8.66B). The prominence of the cornea also makes movements of the eyeball apparent when the eyelids are closed.

The dark circular opening through which light enters the eyeball, the *pupil*, is surrounded by the *iris* (plural = irides), a circular pigmented diaphragm. The relative size of the pupil and iris varies with the brightness of the entering light; however, the size of the contralateral pupils and irides should be uniform.

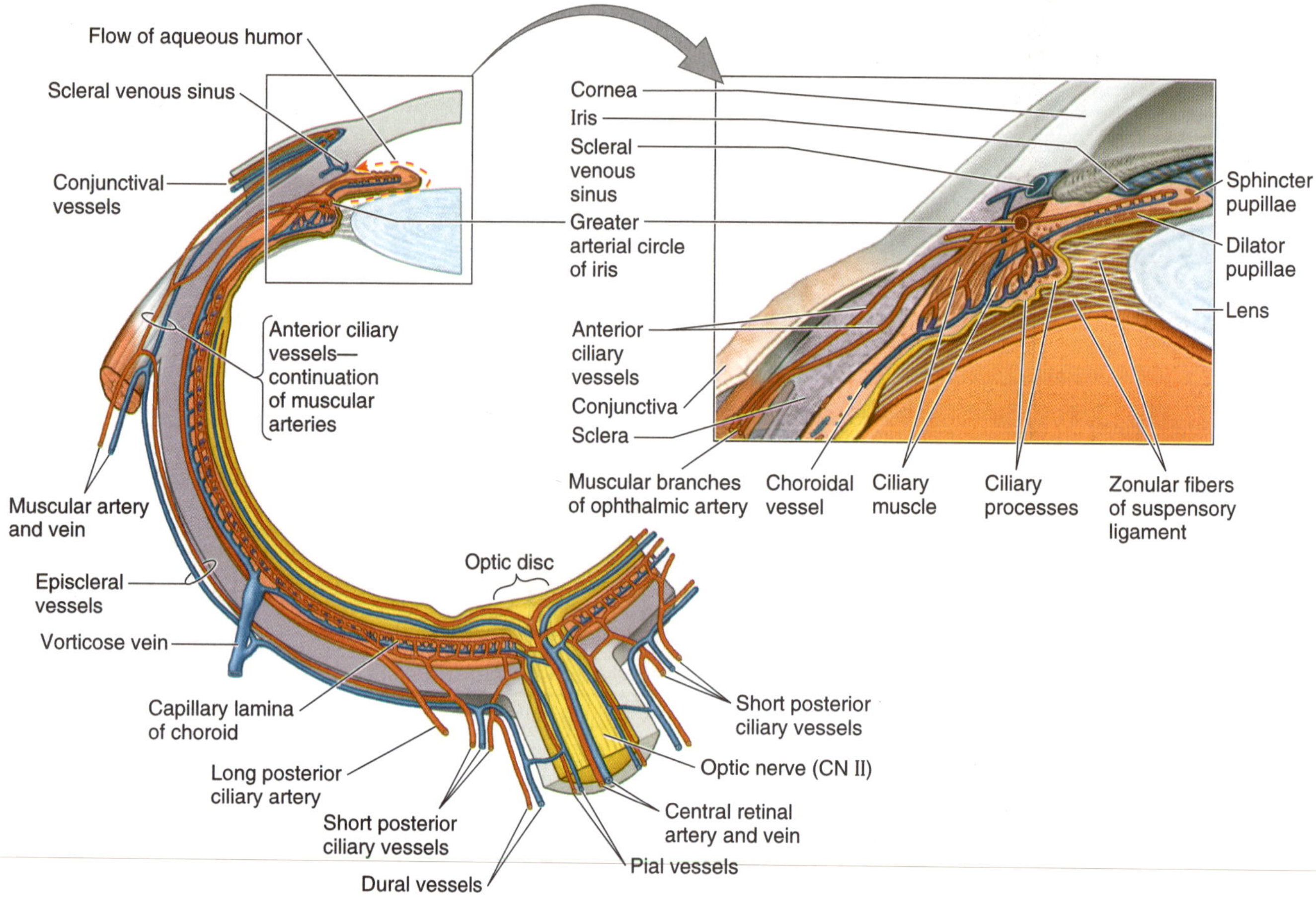

FIGURE 8.64. Partial horizontal section of right eyeball. The artery supplying the inner part of the retina (central retinal artery) and the choroid, which in turn nourishes the outer nonvascular layer of the retina, are shown. The choroid is arranged so that the supplying vessels and larger choroidal vessels are externally placed, and the smallest vessels (the capillary lamina) are most internal, adjacent to the nonvascular layer of the retina. The vorticose vein (one of four to five) drains venous blood from the choroid into the posterior ciliary and ophthalmic veins. The scleral venous sinus returns the aqueous humor, secreted into the anterior chamber by the ciliary processes, to the venous circulation.

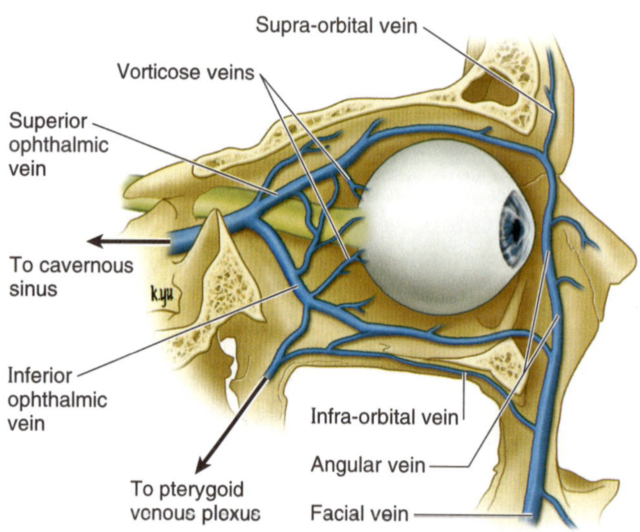

FIGURE 8.65. Ophthalmic veins. The superior ophthalmic vein empties into the cavernous sinus, and the inferior ophthalmic vein empties into the pterygoid venous plexus. They communicate with the facial and supra-orbital veins anteriorly and each other posteriorly. The superior ophthalmic vein accompanies the ophthalmic artery and its branches.

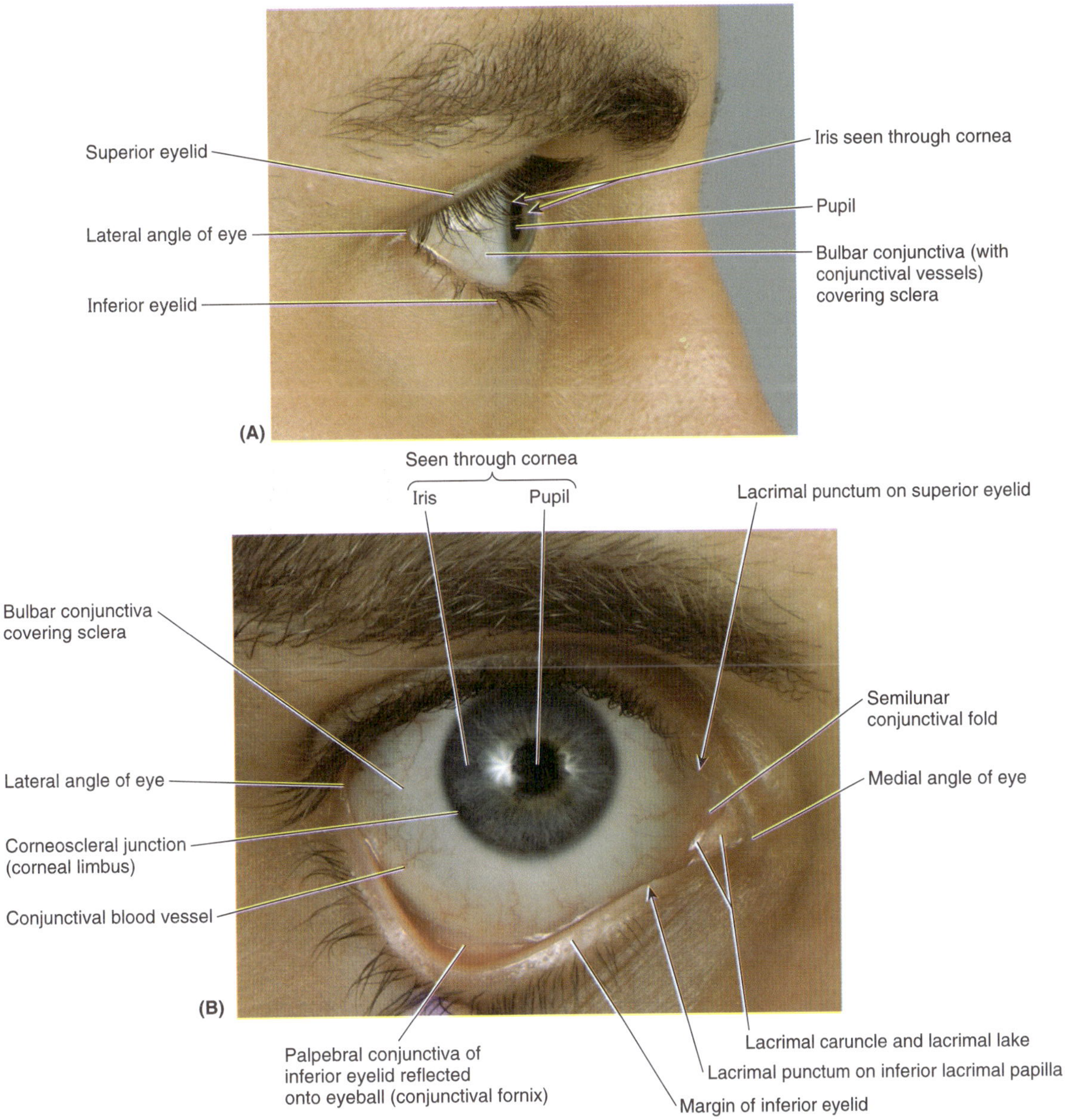

FIGURE 8.66. Surface anatomy of the eye (A) and lacrimal apparatus (B).

Normally, when the eyes are open and the gaze is directed anteriorly, the superior part of the cornea and iris are covered by the edge of the *superior eyelid*, and the inferior part of the cornea and iris are fully exposed above the *inferior eyelid*, usually exposing a narrow rim of sclera. Even slight variations in the position of the eyeballs are noticeable, causing a change in facial expression to a surprised look when the superior eyelid is elevated (as occurs in *exophthalmos*, or protrusion of the eyeballs, caused by hyperthyroidism) or a sleepy appearance (as occurs when the superior eyelid droops, *ptosis*, owing to an absence of sympathetic innervation in Horner syndrome).

The *bulbar conjunctiva* is reflected from the sclera onto the deep surface of the eyelid. The *palpebral conjunctiva* is normally red and vascular. With experience, examination of the palpebral conjunctiva can provide some assessment of hemoglobin levels. It is commonly examined in cases of suspected *anemia*, a blood condition commonly manifested by pallor (paleness) of the mucous membranes. When the superior eyelid is everted ("flipped" so that the palpebral conjunctiva is superficial), the size and extent of the enclosed *superior tarsus* can be appreciated, and commonly, the *tarsal glands* can be distinguished through the palpebral conjunctiva as slightly yellow vertical stripes. Under close examination, the openings of these glands (approximately 20 per eyelid) can be seen on the margins of the eyelids, posterior to the two to three rows of emerging cilia or *eyelashes*. As the bulbar conjunctiva is continuous with the anterior epithelium of the cornea and the palpebral conjunctiva, it forms the *conjunctival sac*. The palpebral fissure is the "mouth," or anterior aperture, of the conjunctival sac.

In the *medial angle of the eye*, a reddish shallow reservoir of tears, the *lacrimal lake*, can be observed. Within the lake is the *lacrimal caruncle*, a small mound of moist modified skin. Lateral to the caruncle is a *semilunar conjunctival fold*, which slightly overlaps the eyeball. When the edges of the eyelids are everted, a small pit, the *lacrimal punctum*, is visible at its medial end on the summit of a small elevation, the *lacrimal papilla*.

For development and developmental basis of congenital AN43.4
anomalies of eye, refer *Langman's Medical Embryology*, South Asian Edition, Chapter 20, Eye, p. 370.

CLINICAL BOX

ORBITAL REGION, ORBIT, AND EYEBALL

Fractures of Orbit

The orbital margin is strong to protect the orbital content. However, when the blows are powerful enough and the impact is directly on the bony rim, the resulting fractures usually occur at the three sutures between the bones forming the orbital margin. Because of the thinness of the medial and inferior walls of the orbit, a blow to the eye may fracture the orbital walls while the margin remains intact (Fig. B8.24). Indirect traumatic injury that displaces the orbital walls is called a *blowout fracture of the orbit*. Fractures of the medial wall may involve the ethmoidal and sphenoidal sinuses, whereas fractures of the inferior wall (orbital floor) may involve the maxillary sinus.

Although the superior wall is stronger than the medial and inferior walls, it is thin enough to be translucent and may be readily penetrated. Thus, a sharp object may pass through it and enter the frontal lobe of the brain.[2]

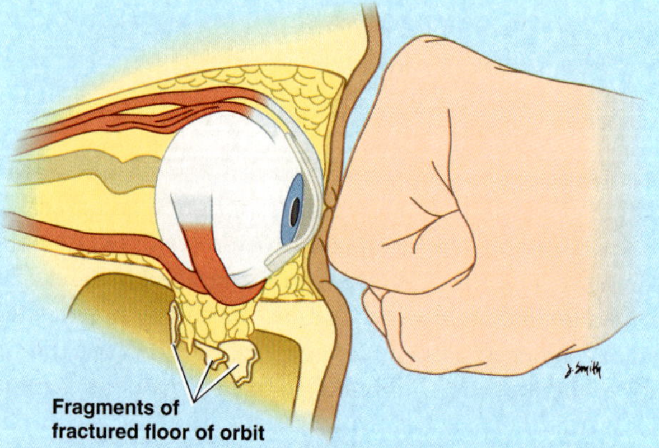

FIGURE B8.24. Blowout fracture of orbit.

[2]This is the anatomical basis of the historical psychosurgery procedure, transorbital prefrontal lobotomy—an interesting but most unfortunate episode in the history of medicine preceding the development of tranquilizing drugs. See https://www.britannica.com/topic/transorbital-lobotomy.

Orbital fractures often result in intra-orbital bleeding, which exerts pressure on the eyeball, causing *exophthalmos* (protrusion of the eyeball). Any trauma to the eye may affect adjacent structures, for example, bleeding into the maxillary sinus, displacement of maxillary teeth, and fracture of nasal bones resulting in hemorrhage, airway obstruction, and infection that could spread to the cavernous sinus through the ophthalmic vein.

Orbital Tumors

Because of the closeness of the optic nerve to the sphenoidal and posterior ethmoidal sinuses, a malignant tumor in these sinuses may erode the thin bony walls of the orbit and compress the optic nerve and orbital contents. Tumors in the orbit produce *exophthalmos* (protrusion of the eyeball). The easiest entrance to the orbital cavity for a tumor in the middle cranial fossa is through the superior orbital fissure. Tumors in the temporal or infratemporal fossa gain access to this cavity through the inferior orbital fissure. Although the lateral wall of the orbit is nearly as long as the medial wall, because it extends laterally and anteriorly, it does not reach as far anteriorly as the medial wall does, which occupies essentially a sagittal plane (Fig. 8.44A). Nearly 2.5 cm of the eyeball is exposed when the pupil is turned medially as far as possible. Therefore, the lateral side of the orbit affords a good approach for operations on the eyeball.

Injury to Nerves Supplying Eyelids

Because it supplies the levator palpebrae superioris, a lesion of the oculomotor nerve causes paralysis of the muscle, and the superior eyelid droops (*ptosis*). Damage to the facial nerve involves paralysis of the orbicularis oculi, preventing the eyelids from closing fully. Normal rapid protective blinking of the eye is also lost.

The loss of tonus of the muscle in the inferior eyelid causes the lid to fall away (evert) from the surface of the eyeball, leading to drying of the cornea. This leaves the eyeball unprotected from dust and small particles. Thus, irritation of the unprotected eyeball results in excessive but inefficient lacrimation (tear formation). *Excessive lacrimal fluid* also forms when the lacrimal drainage apparatus is obstructed, thereby preventing the fluid from reaching the inferior part of the eyeball. People often dab their eyes constantly to wipe the tears, resulting in further irritation.

Inflammation of Palpebral Glands

Any of the glands in the eyelid may become inflamed and swollen from infection or obstruction of their ducts. If the ducts of the ciliary glands are obstructed, a painful red suppurative (pus-producing) swelling, a sty (*hordeolum*), develops on the eyelid. *Cysts of the sebaceous glands* of the eyelid, called *chalazia*, may also form. Obstruction of a tarsal gland produces inflammation, a *tarsal chalazion*, that protrudes toward the eyeball and rubs against it as the eyelids blink.

Hyperemia of Conjunctiva

The conjunctiva is colorless, except when its vessels are dilated and congested ("bloodshot eyes"). Hyperemia of the conjunctiva is caused by local irritation (e.g., from dust, chlorine, or smoke). An inflamed conjunctiva, *conjunctivitis* ("pinkeye"), is a common contagious infection of the eye.

Subconjunctival Hemorrhages

Subconjunctival hemorrhages are common and are manifested by bright or dark red patches deep to and within the bulbar conjunctiva. The hemorrhages may result from injury or inflammation. A blow to the eye, excessively hard blowing of the nose, and paroxysms of coughing or violent sneezing can cause hemorrhages resulting from rupture of small subconjunctival capillaries.

Development of Retina

The retina and optic nerve develop from the **optic cup**, a cup-like outgrowth of the embryonic forebrain, the **optic vesicle** (Fig. B8.25A). As it evaginates from the forebrain (Fig. B8.25B), the optic vesicle carries the developing meninges with it. Hence, the optic nerve is invested with cranial meninges and an extension of the subarachnoid space (Fig. B8.25C). The central retinal artery and vein cross the subarachnoid space and run within the distal part of the optic nerve. The pigment cell layer of the retina develops from the outer layer of the optic cup, and the neural layer develops from the inner layer of the cup (Moore et al., 2016).

Retinal Detachment

The layers of the developing retina are separated in the embryo by an *intraretinal space* (Fig. B8.25B). During the early fetal period, the layers fuse, obliterating this space. Although the pigment cell layer becomes firmly fixed to the choroid, its attachment to the neural layer is not firm. Consequently, detachment of the retina may follow a blow to the eye (Fig. B8.26). A detached retina usually results from seepage of fluid between the neural and pigment cell layers of the retina, perhaps days or even weeks after trauma to the eye. Persons with a retinal detachment may complain of flashes of light or specks floating in front of the eye.

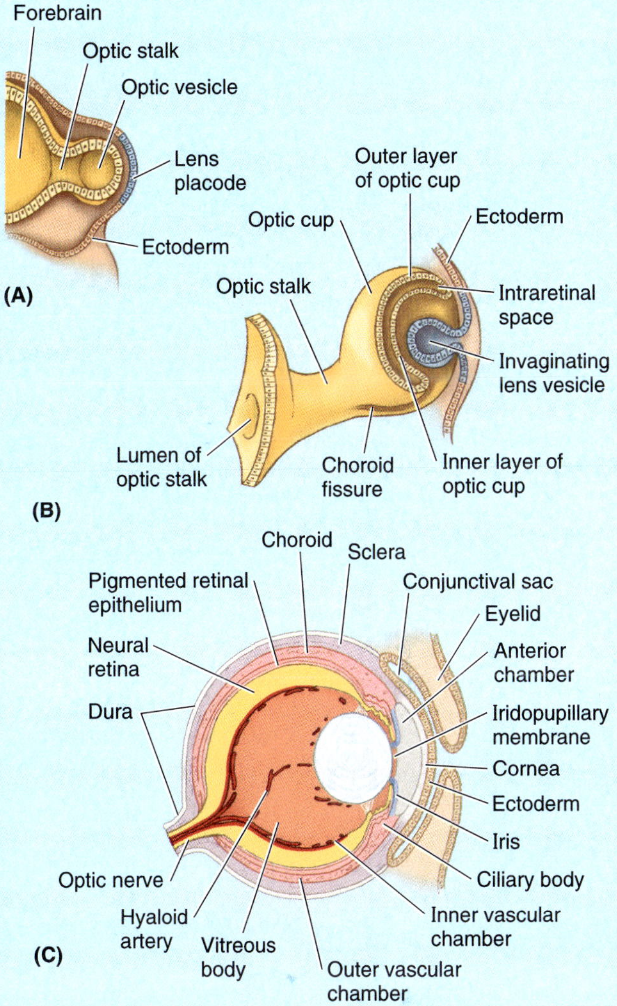

FIGURE B8.25. Development of retina.

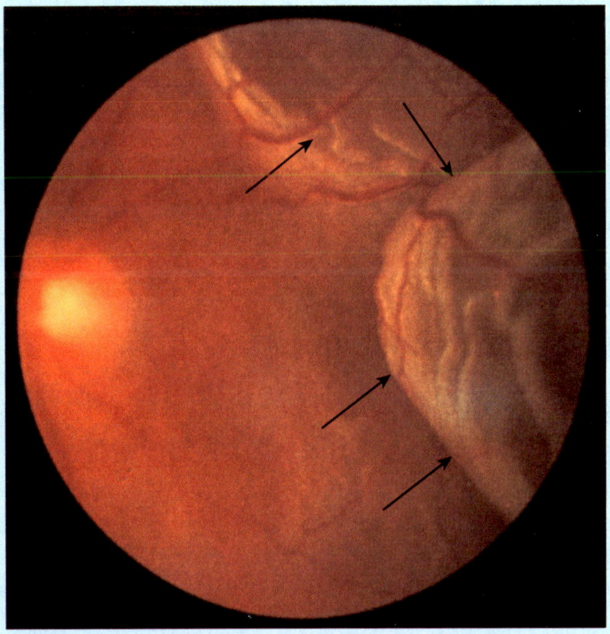

Ophthalmoscopic view (*arrows*, wrinkles in detached retina)

FIGURE B8.26. Retinal detachment.

Pupillary Light Reflex

The *pupillary light reflex* is tested using a penlight during a neurological examination. This reflex, involving CN II (afferent limb) and CN III (efferent limb), is the rapid constriction of the pupil in response to light. When light enters one eye, both pupils constrict because each retina sends fibers into the optic tracts of both sides. The sphincter pupillae muscle is innervated by parasympathetic fibers. Consequently, interruption of these fibers causes dilation of the pupil because of the unopposed action of the sympathetically innervated dilator pupillae muscle. The first sign of *compression of the oculomotor nerve* is ipsilateral slowness of the pupillary response to light.

Uveitis

Uveitis, inflammation of the vascular layer of the eyeball (uvea), may progress to severe visual impairment and blindness if the inflammation is not treated by a specialist in ophthalmology.

Ophthalmoscopy

Physicians use an *ophthalmoscope* (funduscope) to view the fundus of the eyeball (Fig. 8.52). The retinal arteries and veins radiate over the fundus from the optic disc. The pale, oval disc appears on the medial side with the retinal vessels radiating from its center. Pulsation of the retinal arteries is usually visible. Centrally, at the posterior pole of the eyeball, the macula appears darker than the reddish hue of surrounding areas of the retina because the black melanin pigment in the choroid and pigment cell layer is not screened by capillary blood.

Papilledema

An increase in CSF pressure slows venous return from the retina, causing *edema of the retina* (fluid accumulation). The edema is viewed during ophthalmoscopy as swelling of the optic disc, a condition called *papilledema*. Normally, the disc is flat and does not form a papilla. Papilledema results from increased intracranial pressure and increased CSF pressure in the extension of the subarachnoid space around the optic nerve (Fig. 8.50A).

Presbyopia and Cataracts

N41.2 As people age, their lenses become harder and more flattened. These changes gradually reduce the focusing power of the lenses, a condition known as *presbyopia* (G. presbyos, old). Some people also experience a loss of transparency (cloudiness) of the lens from areas of opaqueness (*cataracts*). *Cataract extraction* combined with an *intra-ocular lens implant* has become a common operation. An extracapsular cataract extraction involves removing the lens but leaving the capsule of the lens intact to receive a synthetic intra-ocular lens (Fig. B8.27A, B). Intracapsular lens extraction involves removing the lens and lens capsule and implanting a synthetic intra-ocular lens in the anterior chamber (Fig. B8.27C).

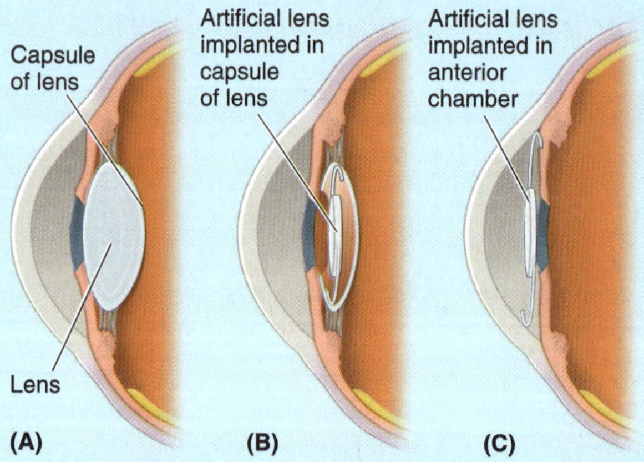

FIGURE B8.27. Synthetic lens implant.

Coloboma of Iris

The absence of a section of the iris (Fig. B8.28) may result from a birth defect, in which the choroid (retinal) fissure fails to close properly (Fig. B8.25B),

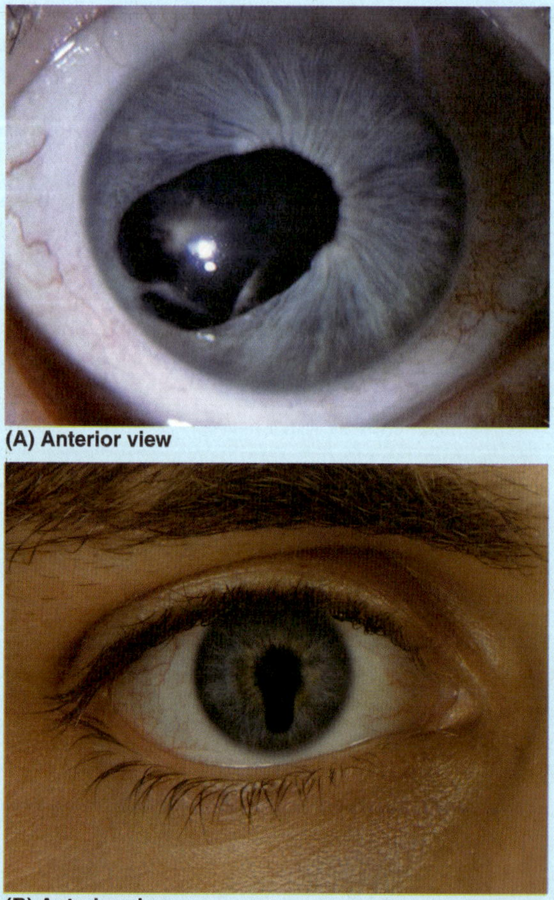

(A) Anterior view

(B) Anterior view

FIGURE B8.28. Coloboma of iris.

from penetrating or nonpenetrating injuries to the eyeball, or a surgical iridectomy. When the iris is injured in such a manner, the iridial fissure does not heal.

Glaucoma

AN41.2

Outflow of aqueous humor through the scleral venous sinus into the blood circulation must occur at the same rate at which the aqueous is produced. If the outflow decreases significantly because the outflow pathway is blocked (Fig. B8.29), pressure builds up in the anterior and posterior chambers of the eye, a condition called *glaucoma*. Blindness can result from compression of the inner layer of the eyeball (retina) and the retinal arteries if aqueous humor production is not reduced to maintain normal intra-ocular pressure.

Hemorrhage into Anterior Chamber

Hemorrhage within the anterior chamber of the eyeball (*hyphema*) usually results from blunt trauma to the eyeball, (e.g., from a squash or racquet ball or a hockey stick) (Fig. B8.30). Initially, the anterior chamber is tinged red; however, blood soon accumulates in this chamber. The initial hemorrhage usually stops in a few days and recovery is usually good.

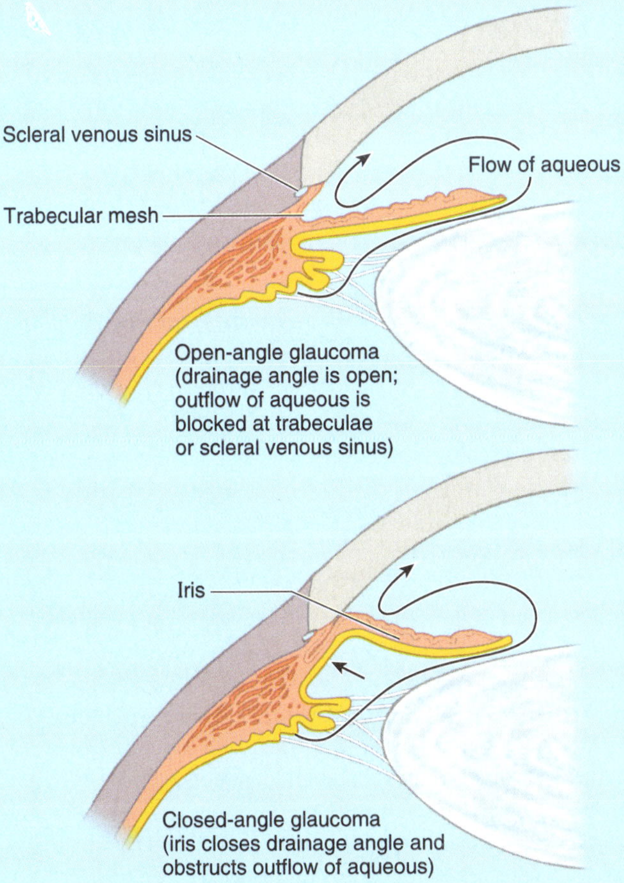

FIGURE B8.29. Open- vs. closed-angle glaucoma.

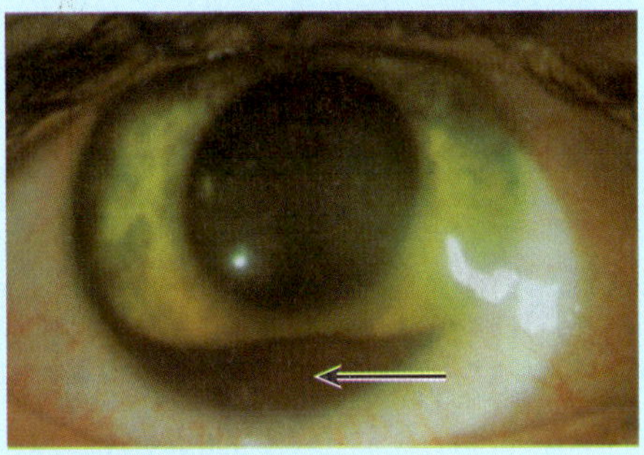

Anterior view

FIGURE B8.30. Hyphema (*arrow*).

Artificial Eye

The fascial sheath of the eyeball forms a socket for an artificial eye when the eyeball is removed (*enucleated*). After this operation, the eye muscles cannot retract too far because their fascial sheaths remain attached to the fascial sheath of the eyeball. Therefore, some coordinated movement of a properly fitted artificial eyeball is possible. Because the suspensory ligament supports the eyeball (see Figs. 8.61C and 8.64), it is preserved when surgical removal of the bony floor of the orbit is performed (e.g., during the removal of a tumor).

Corneal Reflex

During a neurological examination, the examiner touches the cornea with a wisp of cotton (Fig. B8.14). A normal (positive) response is a blink. Absence of a blink suggests a lesion of CN V_1; a lesion of CN VII (the motor nerve to the orbicularis oculi) may also impair this reflex. The examiner must be certain to touch the cornea (not just the sclera) to evoke the reflex. The presence of a contact lens may hamper or abolish the ability to evoke this reflex.

Corneal Abrasions and Lacerations

Foreign objects such as sand or metal filings (particles) produce *corneal abrasions* that cause sudden, stabbing pain in the eyeball and tears. Opening and closing the eyelids is also painful. *Corneal lacerations* are caused by sharp objects, such as a tree branch, fingernails, or the corner of a page of a book.

Corneal Ulcers and Transplants

Damage to the sensory innervation of the cornea from CN V_1 leaves the cornea vulnerable to injury by foreign particles. People with corneal lesions (scarred or opaque corneas) may receive *corneal transplants* from donors or implants of nonreactive plastic material.

Horner Syndrome

Horner syndrome results from interruption of a cervical sympathetic trunk and is manifest by the absence of sympathetically stimulated AN31.3

functions on the ipsilateral side of the head. The syndrome includes the following signs: constriction of the pupil (miosis), drooping of the superior eyelid (ptosis), redness and increased temperature of the skin (vasodilation), and absence of sweating (anhydrosis). Constriction of the pupil occurs because the parasympathetically stimulated sphincter of the pupil is unopposed. The ptosis is a consequence of paralysis of the smooth muscle fibers interdigitated with the aponeurosis of the levator palpebrae superioris that collectively constitute the superior tarsal muscle, supplied by sympathetic fibers.

Paralysis of Extra-Ocular Muscles/ Palsies of Orbital Nerves

One or more extra-ocular muscles may be paralyzed by disease in the brainstem or by a head injury, resulting in *diplopia* (double vision). Paralysis of a muscle is apparent by the limitation of movement of the eyeball in the field of action of the muscle and by the production of two images when one attempts to use the muscle.

OCULOMOTOR NERVE PALSY

AN31.5 Complete *oculomotor nerve palsy* affects most of the ocular muscles, the levator palpebrae superioris, and the sphincter pupillae. The superior eyelid droops and cannot be raised voluntarily because of the unopposed activity of the orbicularis oculi (supplied by the facial nerve) (Fig. B8.31A). The pupil is also fully dilated and nonreactive because of the unopposed dilator pupillae. The pupil is fully abducted and depressed ("down and out") because of the unopposed activity of the lateral rectus and superior oblique, respectively. Also refer *Snell's Clinical Neuroanatomy*, South Asian Edition, Chapter 11, Cranial Nerve Nuclei, p. 358.

ABDUCENT NERVE PALSY

When the abducent nerve (CN VI) supplying only the lateral rectus is paralyzed, the individual cannot abduct the pupil on the affected side (abducent nerve palsy or paralysis). The pupil is fully adducted by the unopposed pull of the medial rectus (Fig. B8.31B).

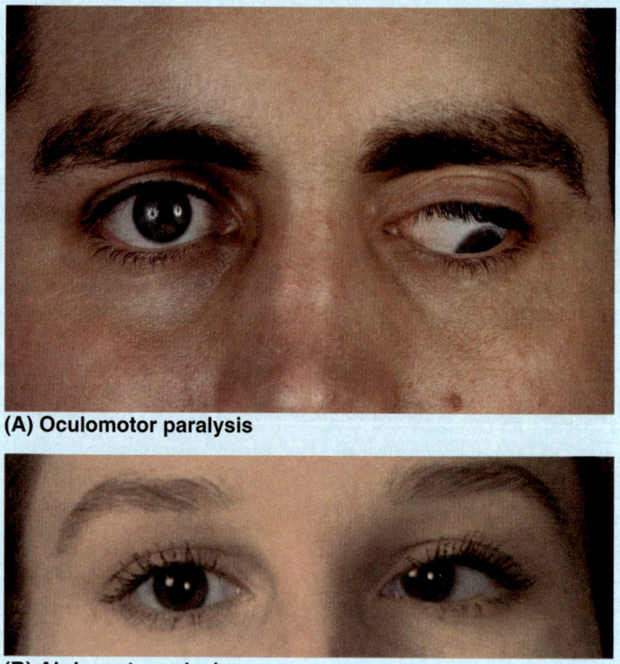

(A) Oculomotor paralysis

(B) Abducent paralysis

FIGURE B8.31. Orbital nerve palsies.

Blockage of Central Retinal Artery

Because terminal branches of the central retinal artery AN41.2 are end arteries, obstruction of them by an embolus results in instant and total blindness. Blockage of the artery is usually unilateral and occurs in older people.

Blockage of Central Retinal Vein

Because the central retinal vein enters the cavernous sinus, *thrombophlebitis* of this sinus may result in the passage of a thrombus to the central retinal vein and produce blockage of the small retinal veins. Occlusion of a branch of the central retinal vein usually results in slow, painless loss of vision.

The Bottom Line: Orbits, Eyeball, and Accessory Visual Structures

Orbits: The orbits are pyramidal cavities, with bases directed anteriorly and apices posteriorly, that house the eyeballs and accessory visual structures. • The medial walls of the contralateral orbits are parallel, and the lateral walls are perpendicular to each other. • The margins and lateral walls of the orbits, being most vulnerable to direct trauma, are strong. • The superior wall (roof) and inferior wall (floor) are shared with the anterior cranial fossa and the maxillary sinus, respectively, and much of the paper-thin medial wall is common to the ethmoidal cells. • The medial wall and floor are thus vulnerable to the spread of disease processes from the paranasal sinuses and to blowout fractures when blunt force is applied to the orbital contents, suddenly increasing intra-orbital pressure. • The optic canal and superior orbital fissure at the apex of the orbit are the primary paths by which structures enter and exit the orbits.

Accessory visual structures: The eyelids and lacrimal apparatus are protective devices for the eyeball. • The

continued on next page

The Bottom Line (continued)

conjunctival sac is a special form of mucosal bursa, which enables the eyelids to move over the surface of the eyeball as they open and close, spreading the moistening and lubricating film of lacrimal fluid within the sac. • The fluid is secreted into the lateral superior fornix of the sac and is spread by gravity and blinking across the anterior eyeball, cleansing and providing the cornea with nutrients and oxygen as it is pushed toward the medial angle of the eye. • The fluid and contained irritants accumulate in the lacrimal lake. • They are drained from here by capillary action through superior and inferior lacrimal puncta into lacrimal canaliculi that pass to the lacrimal sac. • The sac drains via the nasolacrimal duct into the nasal cavity, where the fluid flows posteriorly and is eventually swallowed. • Although the conjunctival sac opens anteriorly via the palpebral fissure, the watery lacrimal fluid will not cross the lipid barrier secreted by the tarsal glands onto the margins of the fissure, unless it is produced in excess, as when crying.

Eyeball: The eyeball contains the optical apparatus of the visual system. • It has a trilaminar construction, with (1) a supporting outer fibrous layer, consisting of the opaque sclera and transparent anterior cornea; (2) a middle vascular layer, consisting of the choroid (largely concerned with providing nourishment to the cones and rods of the retina), the ciliary body (producer of the aqueous humor and adjuster of the lens), and the iris (protector of the retina); and (3) an inner layer, consisting of optic and nonvisual parts of the retina. • The cornea is the major refractive component of the eyeball, with focusing adjustments made by the lens. • Parasympathetic stimulation of the ciliary body reduces tension on the lens, allowing it to thicken for near vision. • Relaxation of the ciliary body in the absence of stimulation stretches the lens, making it thinner for far vision. • Parasympathetic stimulation also constricts the sphincter of the iris, which closes the pupil in response to bright light. • Sympathetic stimulation of the dilator of the iris opens the pupil to admit more light. • The anterior segment of the eyeball is filled with aqueous humor, produced by the ciliary processes in the posterior chamber. • The aqueous humor passes through the pupil into the anterior chamber and is absorbed into the venous circulation at the scleral venous sinus. • The posterior segment or vitreous chamber is filled with vitreous humor, which maintains the shape of the eye, transmits light, and holds the retina in place against the choroid.

Extra-ocular muscles: There are seven extra-ocular muscles: four recti, two obliques, and a levator of the superior eyelid. • Six muscles originate from the apex of the orbit, and the four rectus muscles arise from a common tendinous ring. • Only the inferior oblique arises anteriorly in the orbit. The levator palpebrae superioris elevates the superior eyelid. • Associated smooth muscle (superior tarsal muscle) widens the palpebral fissure even more during sympathetic responses; ptosis results from the absence of sympathetic innervation to the head (Horner syndrome). • When the eyes are adducted (converged) as for close reading, the superior and inferior obliques produce depression and elevation, respectively, directing the gaze down or up the page. • Coordination of the contralateral extra-ocular muscles as yoke muscles is necessary to direct the gaze in a particular direction.

Nerves of orbit: All muscles of the orbit are supplied by CN III, except for the superior oblique and lateral rectus, which are supplied by CN IV and VI, respectively. • Memory device: $LR_6SO_4AO_3$.

Vasculature of orbit: Extra-ocular circulation is provided mainly by the ophthalmic (internal carotid) and infra-orbital (external carotid) arteries, the latter supplying structures near the orbital floor. • Superior and inferior ophthalmic veins drain anteriorly to the facial vein, posteriorly to the cavernous sinus, and inferiorly to the pterygoid venous plexus. • Intra-ocular circulation is exclusively from the ophthalmic artery, with the central retinal artery supplying all of the retina except the layer of cones and rods, which is nourished by the capillary lamina of the choroid. • The ciliary–iridial structures receive blood from anterior ciliary arteries (from the rectus muscle branches of the ophthalmic artery) and two long posterior ciliary arteries. • Multiple short posterior ciliary arteries supply the choroid. • Superior and inferior vorticose veins drain the eyeballs to the respective ophthalmic veins.

PAROTID AND TEMPORAL REGIONS, INFRATEMPORAL FOSSA, AND TEMPOROMANDIBULAR JOINT

Parotid Region

The **parotid region** is the posterolateral part of the facial region (Fig. 8.23A), bounded by the

- zygomatic arch superiorly.
- external ear and anterior border of the sternocleidomastoid posteriorly.
- ramus of the mandible medially.
- anterior border of the masseter muscle anteriorly.
- angle and inferior border of the mandible inferiorly.

The parotid region includes the parotid gland and duct, the parotid plexus of the facial nerve (CN VII), the retromandibular vein, the external carotid artery, and the masseter muscle.

PAROTID GLAND

The **parotid gland** is the largest of three paired salivary glands. AN28.9 From a functional viewpoint, it would seem logical to discuss all three glands simultaneously in association with the anatomy of the mouth. However, from an anatomical viewpoint, particularly in dissection courses, the parotid gland is usually examined with or immediately subsequent to the dissection of the face for complete exposure of the facial nerve. Although the parotid plexus of the facial nerve (CN VII) is embedded within the parotid gland, the branches extending from the gland to innervate the muscles of facial expression are encountered during the dissection of the face, and were discussed and illustrated previously in this chapter. Dissection of the parotid region must be completed before dissection of the infratemporal region and muscles of mastication or the carotid triangle of the neck. The *submandibular gland* is encountered primarily during dissection of the submandibular triangle of the neck, and the *sublingual glands* when dissecting the floor of the mouth.

The parotid gland is enclosed within a tough, unyielding, fascial capsule, the **parotid sheath** (capsule), derived from the *investing layer of deep cervical fascia* (Figs. 8.67, 9.4 and 9.16). The parotid gland has an irregular shape because the area occupied by the gland, the **parotid bed**, is anteroinferior to the external acoustic meatus, where it is wedged between the ramus of the mandible and the mastoid process (Figs. 8.23A, C and 8.67). Fatty tissue between the lobes of the gland confers the flexibility the gland must have to accommodate the motion of the mandible. The apex of the parotid gland is posterior to the angle of the mandible, and its base is related to the zygomatic arch. The subcutaneous lateral surface of the parotid gland is almost flat.

The **parotid duct** passes horizontally from the anterior edge of the gland (Fig. 8.67). At the anterior border of the masseter, the duct turns medially, pierces the buccinator, and enters the oral cavity through a small orifice opposite the 2nd maxillary molar tooth. Embedded within the substance of the parotid gland, from superficial to deep, are the *parotid plexus of the facial nerve* (CN VII) and its branches (Figs. 8.23A, C and 8.67), the *retromandibular vein*, and the *external carotid artery*. On the parotid sheath and within the gland are *parotid lymph nodes*.

INNERVATION OF PAROTID GLAND AND RELATED STRUCTURES

Although the parotid plexus of CN VII is embedded within it, CN VII does not provide innervation to the gland. The *auriculotemporal nerve*, a branch of CN V_3, is closely related to the parotid gland and passes superior to it with the superficial temporal vessels. The auriculotemporal nerve and the **great auricular nerve**, a branch of the cervical plexus composed AN28.9

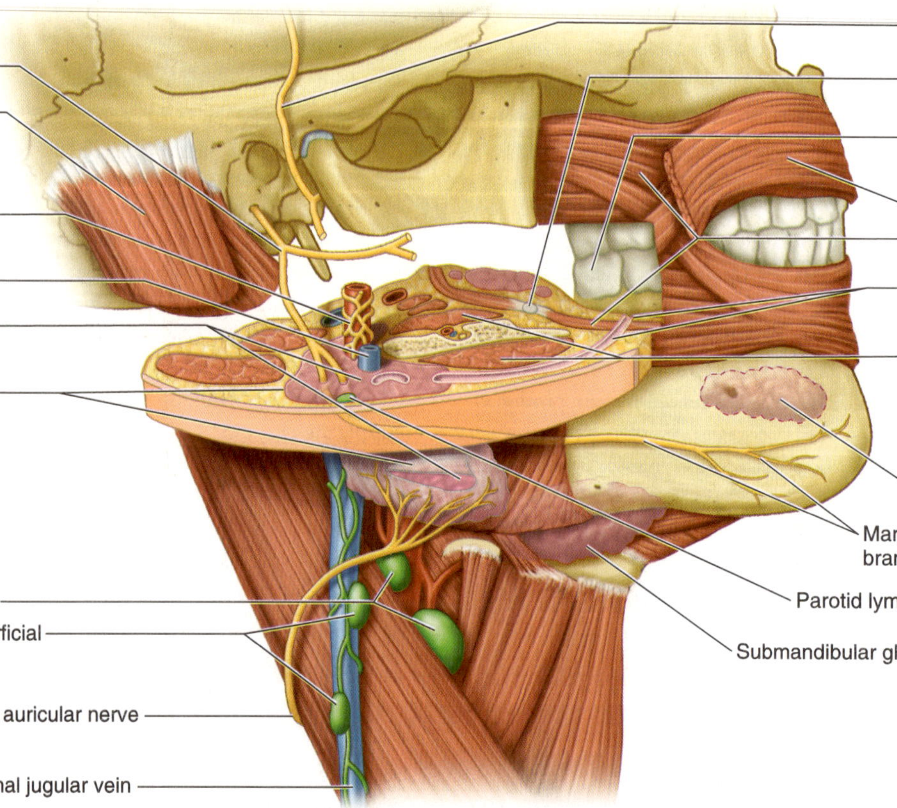

FIGURE 8.67. Relationships of parotid gland. A transverse slice through the bed of the parotid gland demonstrates the relationship of the gland to the surrounding structures. The gland passes deeply between the ramus of the mandible, flanked by the muscles of mastication anteriorly and the mastoid process and sternocleidomastoid muscle posteriorly. The dimensions of the parotid bed change with movements of the mandible. The external carotid artery and peri-arterial plexus, retromandibular vein, and parotid plexus of the facial nerve (CN VII) are embedded within the gland itself. The parotid duct turns medially at the anterior border of the masseter muscle and pierces the buccinator muscle.

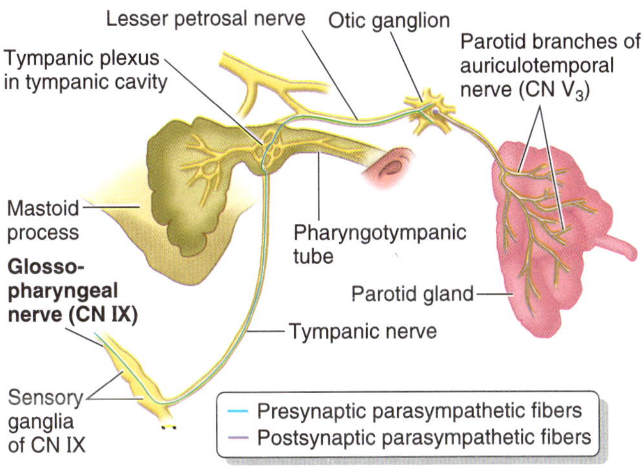

FIGURE 8.68. Innervation of parotid gland.

of fibers from C2 and C3 spinal nerves, innervates the parotid sheath (Fig. 8.67) as well as the overlying skin.

The parasympathetic component of the **glossopharyngeal nerve** (CN IX) supplies presynpatic secretory fibers to the **otic ganglion** (Fig. 8.68). The postsynaptic parasympathetic fibers are conveyed from the ganglion to the parotid gland by the auriculotemporal nerve. Stimulation of the parasympathetic fibers produces a thin, watery saliva. Sympathetic fibers are derived from the cervical ganglia through the **external carotid nerve plexus** on the external carotid artery (Fig. 8.67). The vasomotor activity of these fibers may reduce secretion from the gland. Sensory nerve fibers pass to the gland through the great auricular and auriculotempo-
AN43.2 ral nerves. For microanatomy of serous salivary glands, refer *diFiore's Atlas of Histology with Functional Correlations*, 1st South Asian Edition, Chapter 13, Digestive System Part I: Oral Cavity and Major Salivary Glands, pp. 334–335.

Temporal Region

AN33.1 The **temporal region** of the head includes the lateral area of the scalp and the deeper soft tissues overlying the temporal fossa of the cranium, superior to the zygomatic arch (Figs. 8.14 and 8.69A, *inset*). The **temporal fossa**, occupied primarily by the upper portion of the *temporalis muscle*, is bounded (Figs. 8.1A and 8.69A) as follows:

- Posteriorly and superiorly by the temporal lines.
- Anteriorly by the frontal and zygomatic bones.
- Laterally by the zygomatic arch.
- Inferiorly by the infratemporal crest (Fig. 8.69B).

The *floor of the temporal fossa* is formed by parts of the four bones that form the *pterion*: frontal, parietal, temporal, and greater wing of the sphenoid. The fan-shaped *temporalis muscle* arises from the bony floor and overlying **temporal fascia** (Fig. 8.70), which forms the *roof of the temporal fossa*. This tough fascia covers the temporalis, attaching superiorly to the *superior temporal line*. Inferiorly, the fascia splits into two layers, which attach to the lateral and medial surfaces of the zygomatic arch. The temporal fascia also tethers the zygomatic arch superiorly. The powerful masseter muscle is attached to the inferior border of the arch. When it contracts, exerting a strong downward pull on the zygomatic arch, the temporal fascia provides resistance.

Infratemporal Fossa

The **infratemporal fossa** is an irregularly shaped space AN33.2 deep and inferior to the zygomatic arch, deep to the ramus of the mandible, and posterior to the maxilla (Fig. 8.69A, B). It communicates with the temporal fossa through the interval between (deep to) the zygomatic arch and (superficial to) the cranial bones.

The *boundaries of the infratemporal fossa* are as follows (Fig. 8.69):

- Laterally: the ramus of the mandible.
- Medially: the lateral pterygoid plate.
- Anteriorly: the posterior aspect of the maxilla.
- Posteriorly: the tympanic plate and the mastoid and styloid processes of the temporal bone.
- Superiorly: the inferior (infratemporal) surface of the greater wing of the sphenoid.
- Inferiorly: where the medial pterygoid muscle attaches to the mandible near its angle (see Fig. 8.74D).

The *infratemporal fossa contains* the (Figs. 8.70 to 8.72)

- inferior part of the temporalis muscle.
- lateral and medial pterygoid muscles.
- maxillary artery.
- pterygoid venous plexus.
- mandibular, inferior alveolar, lingual, buccal, and chorda tympani nerves.
- otic ganglion (see Fig. 8.77).

The parotid and temporal regions and the infratemporal fossa collectively include the *temporomandibular joint* and the *muscles of mastication* that produce its movements.

TEMPOROMANDIBULAR JOINT AN33.3

The **temporomandibular joint (TMJ)** is a modified hinge type of synovial joint, permitting gliding (translation) and a small degree of rotation (pivoting) in addition to flexion (elevation) and extension (depression) movements typical for hinge joints. The bony articular surfaces involved are the *mandibular fossa* and *articular tubercle of the temporal bone* superiorly and the *head of the mandible* inferiorly (Figs. 8.9B and 8.71A–D). The loose *fibrous layer of the joint capsule* attaches to the margins of the articular cartilage on the temporal bone and around the neck of the mandible (Figs. 8.71E and 8.72A, C). The two bony articular surfaces are completely separated by intervening fibrocartilage, the articular disc of the TMJ, attached at its periphery to the internal aspect of the fibrous capsule. This creates separate **superior** and **inferior articular cavities**, or compartments, lined by separate **superior** and **inferior synovial membranes** (Figs. 8.71A, B and 8.72B, C).

(*continued on p.* 979)

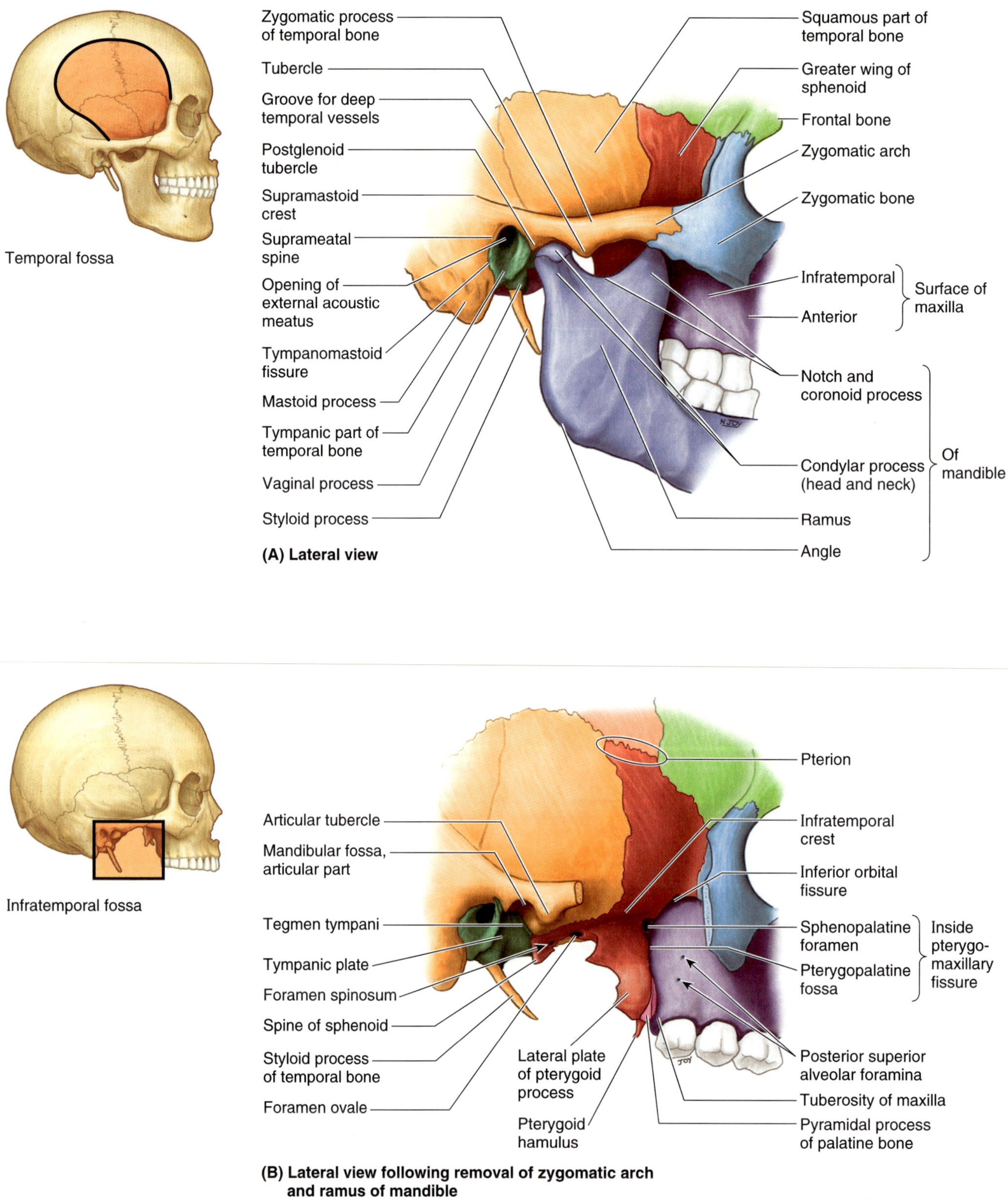

FIGURE 8.69. Bony boundaries of temporal and infratemporal fossae. A. The lateral wall of the infratemporal fossa is formed by the ramus of the mandible. The space is deep to the zygomatic arch and is traversed by the temporal muscle and the deep temporal nerves and vessels. Through this interval, the temporal fossa communicates inferiorly with the infratemporal fossa. **B.** The roof and three walls of the infratemporal fossa are shown. The fossa is an irregularly shaped space posterior to the maxilla (anterior wall). The roof of the fossa is formed by the infratemporal surface of the greater wing of the sphenoid. The medial wall is formed by the lateral pterygoid plate. The posterior wall is formed by the tympanic plate, styloid process, and mastoid process of the temporal bone. The infratemporal fossa communicates with the pterygopalatine fossa through the pterygomaxillary fissure.

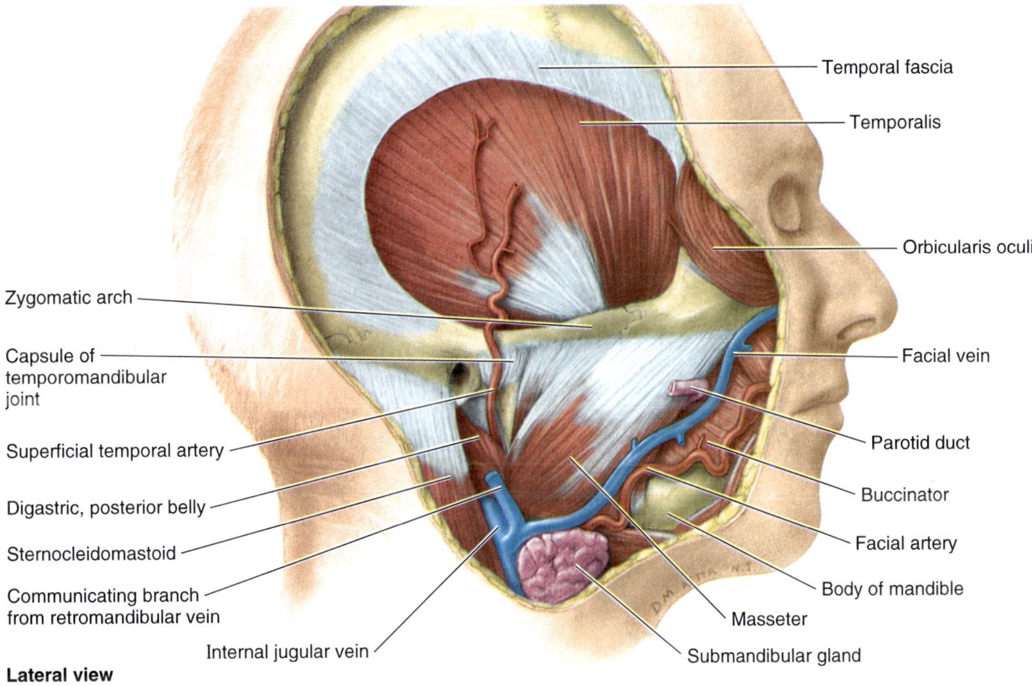

FIGURE 8.70. Dissections of temporal and infratemporal regions. In this superficial dissection of the great muscles on the side of the cranium, the parotid gland and most of the temporal fascia have been removed. The temporal and masseter muscles are both supplied by the trigeminal nerve (CN V) and both close the jaw. The facial artery passes deep to the submandibular gland, whereas the facial vein passes superficial to it.

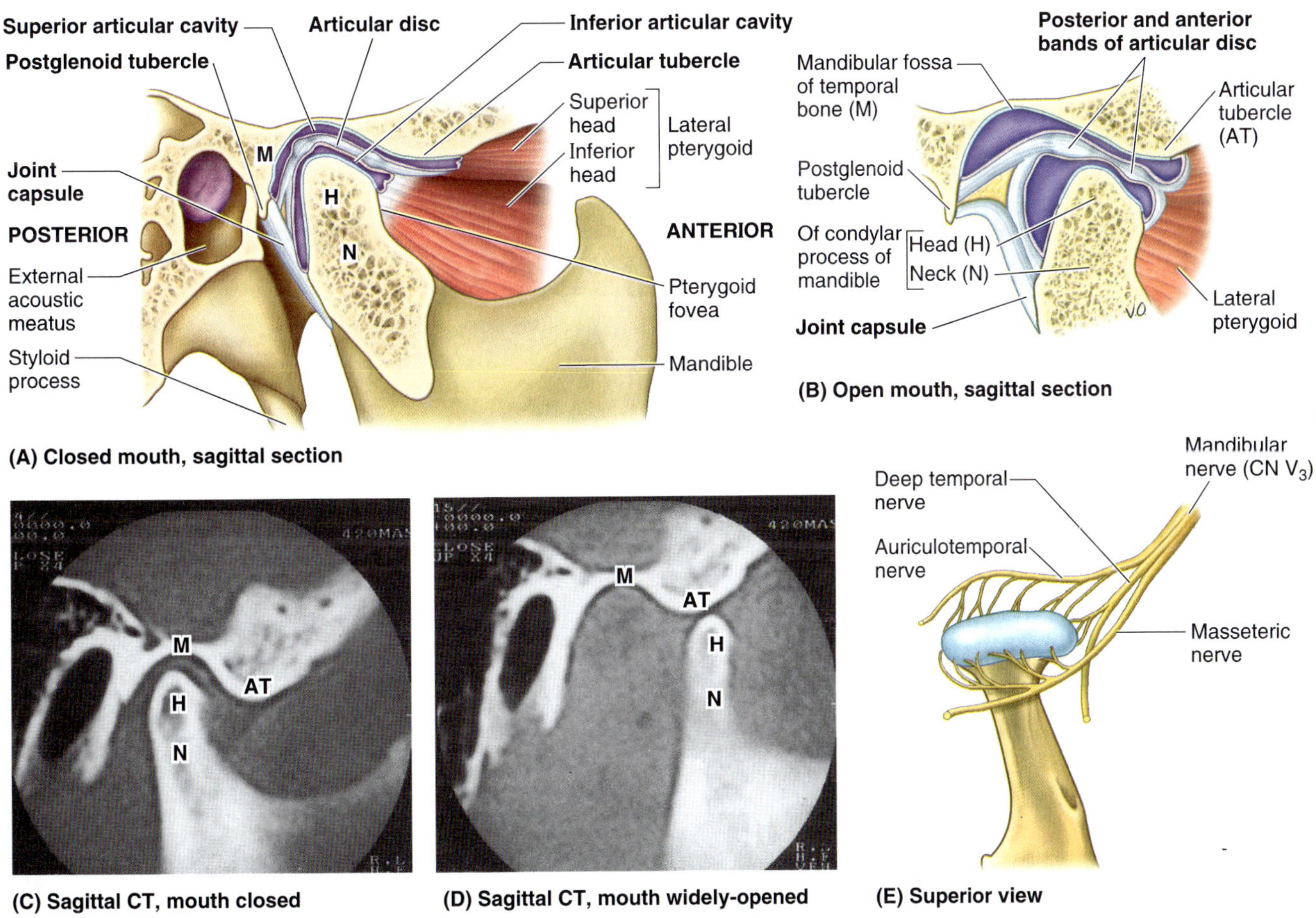

FIGURE 8.71. Temporomandibular joint (TMJ). A–D. Anatomical and CT images of the TMJ in the closed- and open-mouth positions. **E.** Innervation of TMJ.

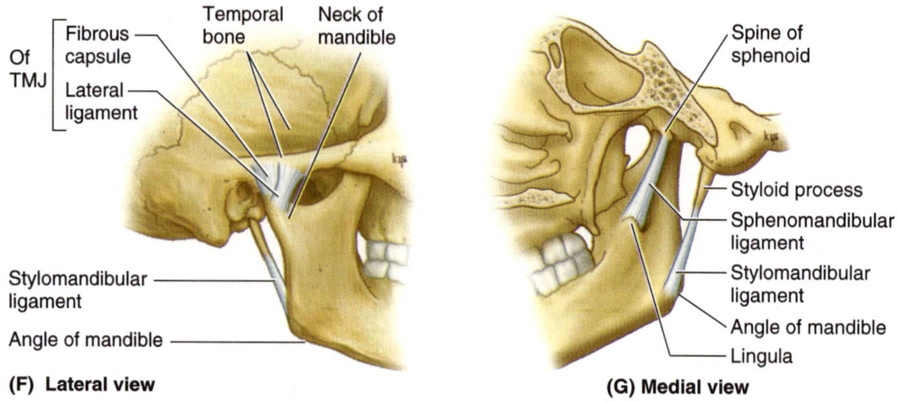

FIGURE 8.71. (Continued) F, G. The TMJ and the extrinsic stylomandibular and sphenomandibular ligaments are shown. The sphenomandibular ligament passively bears the weight of the lower jaw and is the "swinging hinge" of the mandible, permitting protrusion and retrusion as well as elevation and depression.

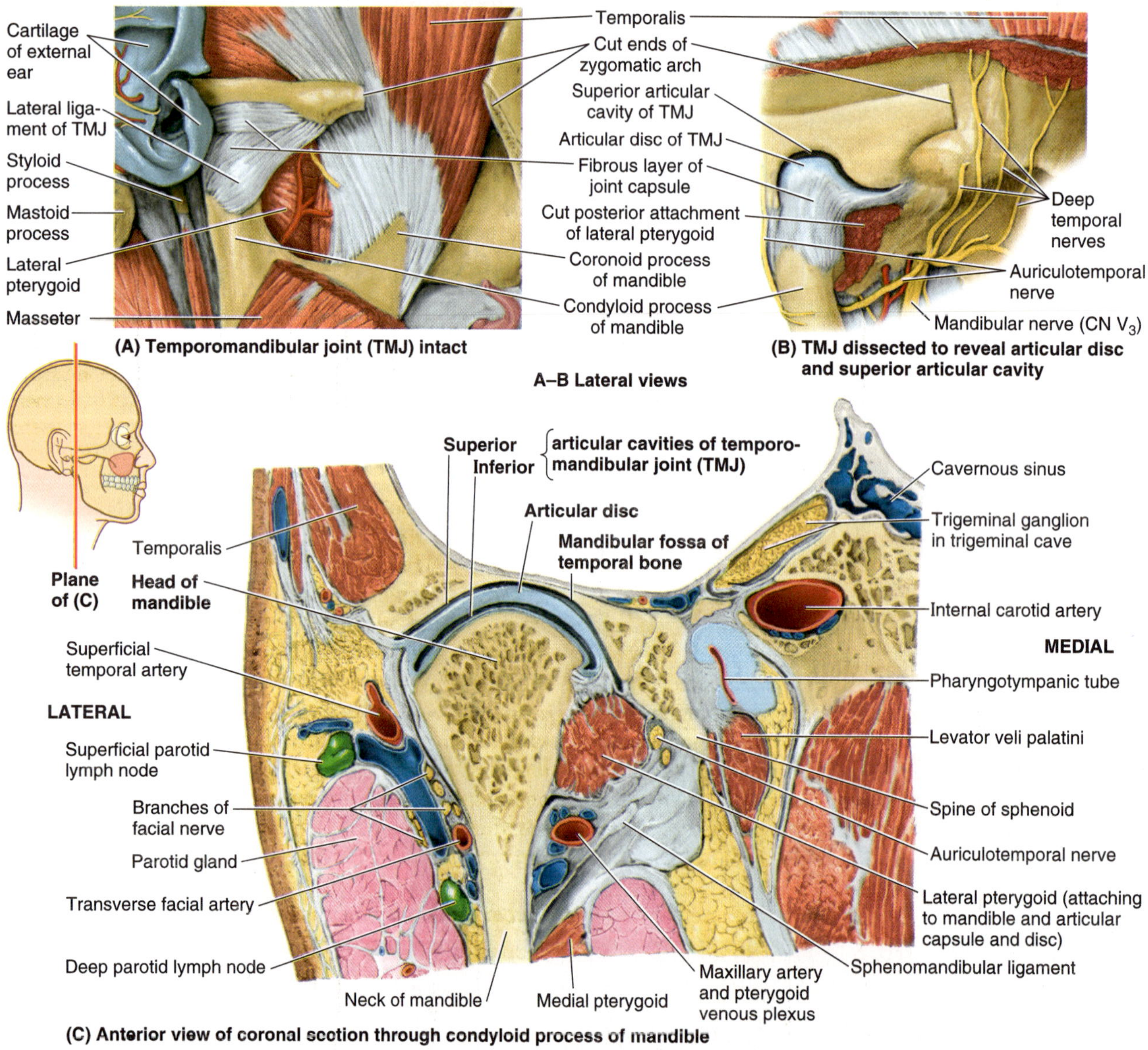

FIGURE 8.72. Dissections and coronal sections of TMJ. A. The fibrous layer of the joint capsule is thickened to form the lateral ligament of the TMJ, which with the postglenoid tubercle prevents excessive posterior displacement of the head of the mandible. **B.** The upper portion of the fibrous capsule has been removed, demonstrating the superior compartment of the TMJ between the mandibular fossa and the articular disc. The auriculotemporal nerve provides articular branches to the joint. **C.** Coronal section of the right TMJ demonstrating the articular disc dividing the joint cavity into superior and inferior compartments.

The gliding movements of protrusion and retrusion (translation) occur between the temporal bone and the articular disc (superior cavity) (Fig. 8.73). The hinge movements of depression and elevation and the rotational or pivoting movements occur in the inferior compartment. A thickened part of the joint capsule forms the intrinsic **lateral ligament of the TMJ** (Figs. 8.71E and 8.72A), which strengthens the joint laterally and, with the **postglenoid tubercle** (Fig. 8.71A), acts to prevent posterior dislocation of the joint.

Two extrinsic ligaments and the lateral ligament connect the mandible to the cranium. The **stylomandibular ligament**, which is actually a thickening of the fibrous capsule of the parotid gland, runs from the styloid process to the angle of the mandible (Fig. 8.71E, F). It does not contribute significantly to the strength of the joint. The **sphenomandibular ligament** runs from the spine of the sphenoid to the lingula of the mandible (Figs. 8.71F and 8.72C). It is the primary passive support of the mandible, although the tonus of the muscles of mastication usually bears the mandible's weight. However, the sphenomandibular ligaments serve as a "swinging hinge" for the mandible, serving both as a fulcrum and as a check ligament for the movements of the mandible at the TMJs.

The movements of the mandible at the TMJs are shown in Figure 8.73, and the muscles (or forces) producing the movements are summarized in Table 8.10. When the mouth is closed and at rest, the heads of the mandible are held in the retracted position in the mandibular fossae, and the chin is elevated by the tonus of the retractors and elevators of the mandible (Figs. 8.71A, C, 8.72B, C, and 8.73A). When sleeping in the supine or sitting position (head upright), as one enters a state of deep sleep, the tonic contraction relaxes and gravity causes depression of the mandible (the mouth falls open).

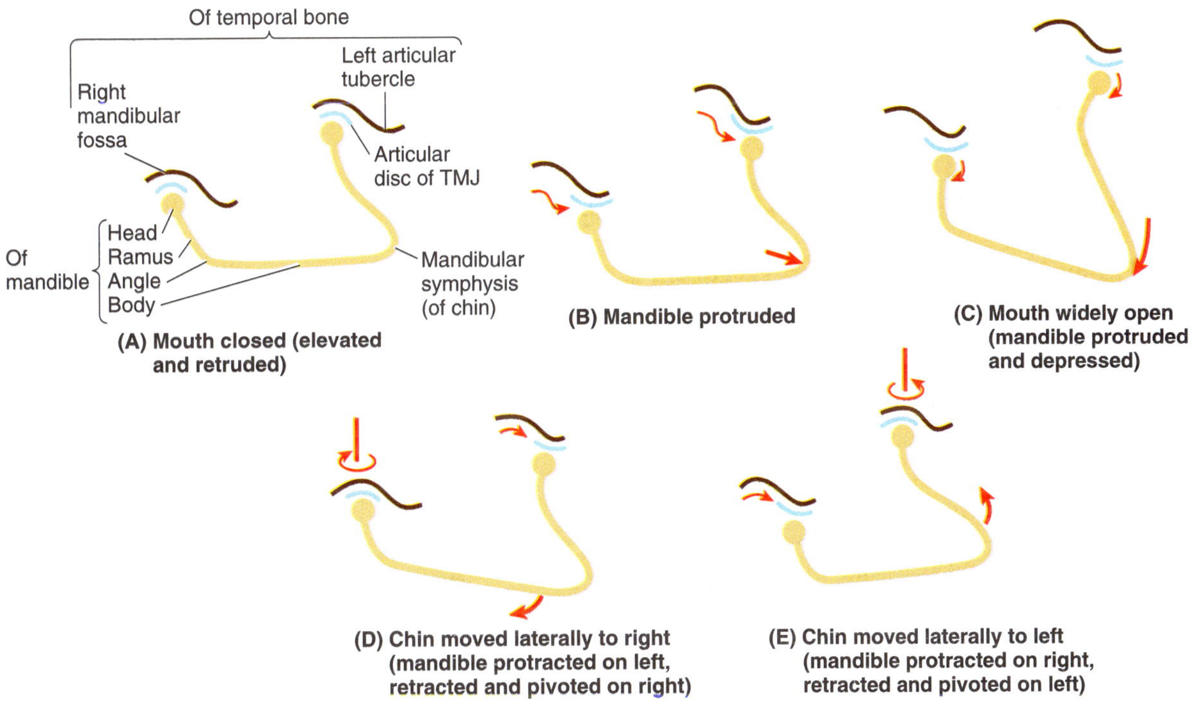

FIGURE 8.73. Movements of mandible consequent to movement at TMJs.

TABLE 8.10. MOVEMENTS OF TEMPOROMANDIBULAR JOINT

Movements of Mandible	Muscle(s)
Elevation (close mouth)	Temporalis, masseter, and medial pterygoid
Depression (open mouth)	Lateral pterygoid, suprahyoid, and infrahyoid muscles[a]
Protrusion (protrude chin)	Lateral pterygoid, masseter, and medial pterygoid[b]
Retrusion (retrude chin)	Temporalis (posterior oblique and near horizontal fibers) and masseter
Lateral movements (grinding and chewing)	Temporalis of same side, pterygoids of opposite side, and masseter

[a]The prime mover is normally gravity; these muscles are mainly active against resistance.
[b]The lateral pterygoid is the prime mover here, with minor secondary roles played by the masseter and medial pterygoid.

To enable more than a small amount of depression of the mandible—that is, to open the mouth wider than just to separate the upper and lower teeth—the head of the mandible and articular disc must move anteriorly on the articular surface until the head lies inferior to the articular tubercle (a movement referred to as "translation" by dentists) (Fig. 8.73B). If this occurs without depression, the chin protrudes. Most often, the mandible is depressed (the mouth is opened) as the head of the mandible and articular disc glide toward the articular tubercle, with full depression possible only when the heads and discs are fully protracted (Figs. 8.71B, D and 8.73C). If protraction of head and disc occurs unilaterally, the contralateral head rotates (pivots) on the inferior surface of the articular disc in the retracted position, permitting simple side-to-side chewing or grinding movements over a small range (Fig. 8.73D, E). During protrusion and retrusion of the mandible, the head and articular disc slide anteriorly and posteriorly on the articular surface of the temporal bone, with both sides moving together (Fig. 8.73A, B).

MUSCLES OF MASTICATION

N33.2 TMJ movements are produced chiefly by the **muscles of mastication**. These four muscles (**temporal**, **masseter**, and **medial** and **lateral pterygoid muscles**) develop from the mesoderm of the embryonic first pharyngeal arch. Consequently, they are all innervated by the nerve of that arch, the *(motor root of the) mandibular nerve* (CN V_3). The muscles of mastication are shown in isolation in Figure 8.74 and in situ in Figures 8.70 and 8.76; their attachments, details concerning their innervation, and their main actions are described in Table 8.11. In addition to the movements listed, studies indicate that the superior head of the lateral pterygoid muscle is active during the retraction movement produced by the posterior fibers of the temporalis. Traction is applied to the articular disc so that it is not pushed posteriorly ahead of the retracting mandible.

Generally, depression of the mandible is produced by gravity. The *suprahyoid* and *infrahyoid muscles* are strap-like muscles on each side of the neck (Fig. 8.74E; Table 8.11). They are primarily used to raise and depress the hyoid bone and larynx, respectively—for example, during swallowing (see Chapter 9, Neck). Indirectly, they can also help depress the mandible, especially when opening the mouth suddenly, against resistance, or when inverted (e.g., standing on one's head). The platysma can be similarly used.

NEUROVASCULATURE OF INFRATEMPORAL FOSSA

The **maxillary artery** is the larger of the two terminal branches of the external carotid artery. It arises posterior to the neck of the mandible and is divided into three parts based on its relation to the lateral pterygoid muscle. The three parts of the maxillary artery and their branches are illustrated in isolation in Figure 8.75, and their courses and distributions are listed in Table 8.12. Relationships of the maxillary artery and many of its branches are shown in Figure 8.76.

The **pterygoid venous plexus** is located partly between AN33.4
the temporalis and pterygoid muscles (Fig. 8.25). It is the venous equivalent of most of the maxillary artery, that is, most of the veins that accompany the branches of the maxillary artery drain into this plexus. The plexus anastomoses anteriorly with the facial vein via the deep facial vein and superiorly with the cavernous sinus via emissary veins. The extensive nature and volume of the pterygoid venous plexus is difficult to appreciate in the cadaver, in which it is usually drained of blood.

The **mandibular nerve** arises from the trigeminal ganglion in the middle cranial fossa. It immediately receives the motor root of the trigeminal nerve and descends through the foramen ovale into the infratemporal fossa (Fig. 8.77). The branches of CN V_3 are the auriculotemporal, inferior alveolar, lingual, and buccal nerves. Branches of CN V_3 also supply the four muscles of mastication but not the buccinator, which is supplied by the facial nerve.

The **auriculotemporal nerve** encircles the middle meningeal artery and divides into numerous branches, the largest of which passes posteriorly, medial to the neck of the mandible, and supplies sensory fibers to the auricle and temporal region. The auriculotemporal nerve also sends articular (sensory) fibers to the TMJ (Fig. 8.71E). It conveys postsynaptic parasympathetic secretomotor fibers from the *otic ganglion* to the parotid gland.

The **inferior alveolar nerve** enters the mandibular foramen and passes through the mandibular canal, forming the *inferior dental plexus*, which sends branches to all mandibular teeth on its side. Another branch of the dental plexus, the *mental nerve*, passes through the mental foramen and supplies the skin and mucous membrane of the lower lip, the skin of the chin, and the vestibular gingiva of the mandibular incisor teeth.

The **lingual nerve** lies anterior to the inferior alveolar nerve (Fig. 8.76). It is sensory to the anterior two thirds of the tongue, the floor of the mouth, and the lingual gingivae. It enters the mouth between the medial pterygoid muscle and the ramus of the mandible and passes anteriorly under cover of the oral mucosa, medial and inferior to the 3rd molar tooth. The **chorda tympani nerve**, a branch of CN VII carrying taste fibers from the anterior two thirds of the tongue, joins the lingual nerve in the infratemporal fossa (Fig. 8.76B). The chorda tympani also carries secretomotor fibers for the submandibular and sublingual salivary glands.

The **otic ganglion** (parasympathetic) is located in the infratemporal fossa, just inferior to the foramen ovale, medial to CN V_3 and posterior to the medial pterygoid muscle (Fig. 8.77). Presynaptic parasympathetic fibers, derived mainly from the glossopharyngeal nerve, synapse in the otic ganglion (Fig. 8.68). Postsynaptic parasympathetic fibers, which are secretory to the parotid gland, pass from the otic ganglion to this gland through the auriculotemporal nerve.

(continued on p. 987)

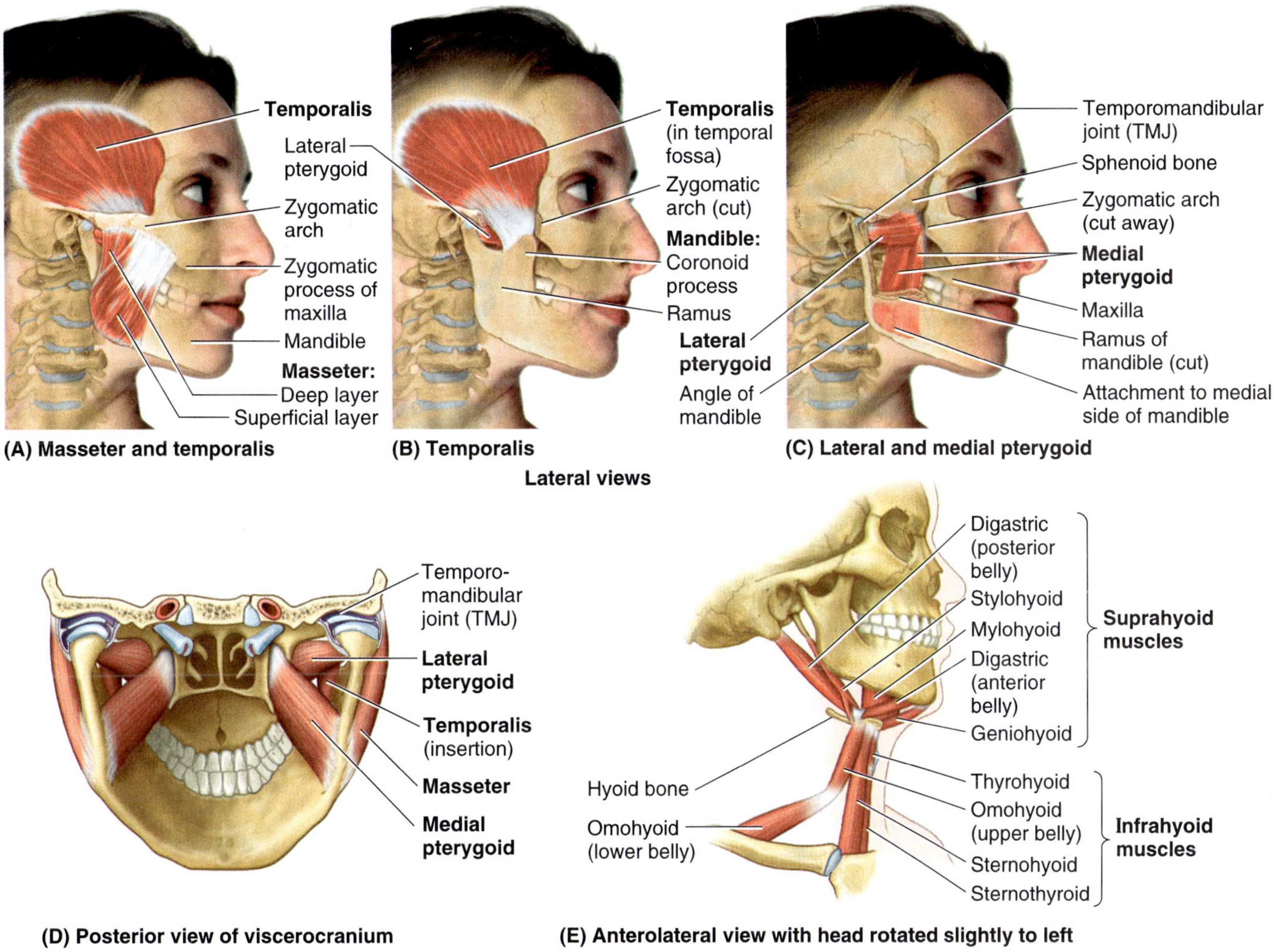

FIGURE 8.74. Muscles acting on mandible/temporomandibular joint.

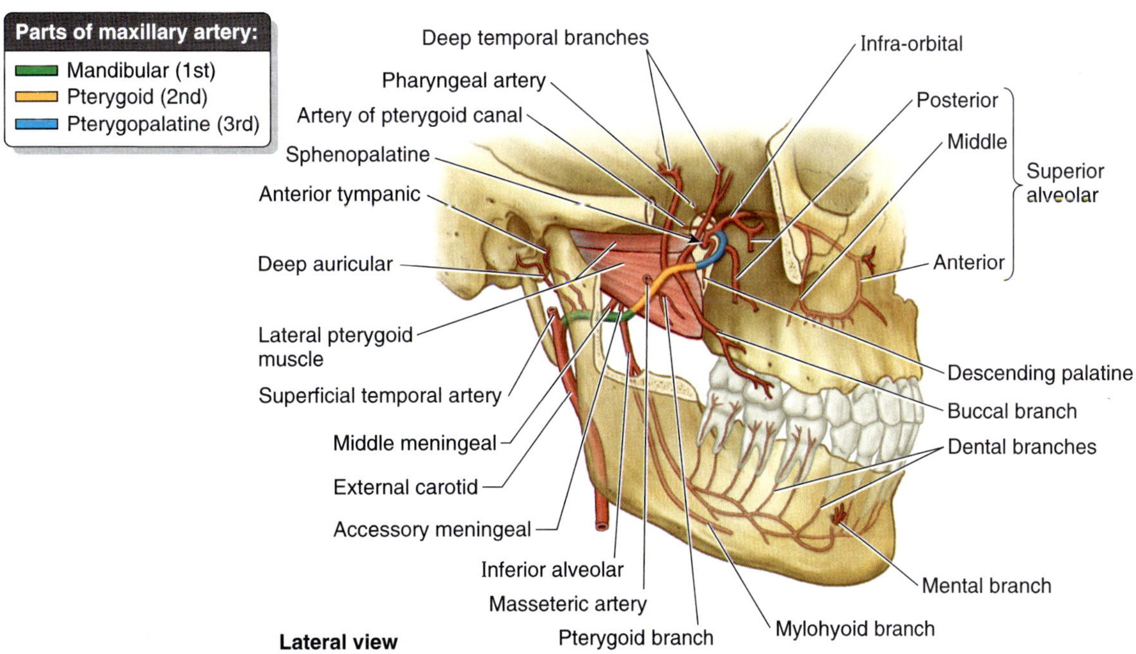

FIGURE 8.75. Parts and branches of maxillary artery.

TABLE 8.11. MUSCLES ACTING ON MANDIBLE/TEMPOROMANDIBULAR JOINT

Muscle(s)	Proximal Attachment	Distal Attachment	Innervation		Action on Mandible
Muscles of mastication					
Temporalis	Triangular muscle with broad attachment to floor of temporal fossa and deep surface of temporal fascia	Narrow attachment to tip and medial surface of coronoid process and anterior border of ramus of mandible	Anterior trunk of mandibular nerve ($CN\ V_3$)	Via deep temporal branches	Elevates mandible, closing jaws; posterior, more horizontal fibers are 1° retractors of mandible.
Masseter	Quadrate muscle attaching to inferior border and medial surface of maxillary process of zygomatic bone and the zygomatic arch	Angle and lateral surface of ramus of mandible		Via masseteric nerve	Elevates mandible, closing jaws; superficial fibers make limited contribution to protrusion of mandible.
Lateral pterygoid	Triangular two-headed muscle from (1) infratemporal surface and crest of greater wing of sphenoid and (2) lateral surface of lateral pterygoid plate	Superior head attaches primarily to joint capsule and articular disc of TMJ; inferior head attaches primarily to pterygoid fovea on anteromedial aspect of neck of condyloid process of mandible.		Via lateral pterygoid nerve	Acting bilaterally, protracts mandible and depresses chin; acting unilaterally, swings jaw toward contralateral side; alternate unilateral contraction produces larger lateral chewing movements.
Medial pterygoid	Quadrangular two-headed muscle from (1) medial surface of lateral pterygoid plate and pyramidal process of palatine bone and (2) tuberosity of maxilla	Medial surface of ramus of mandible, inferior to mandibular foramen; in essence, a "mirror image" of ipsilateral masseter, two muscles flanking ramus		Via medial pterygoid nerve	Acts synergistically with masseter to elevate mandible; contributes to protrusion; alternate unilateral activity produces smaller grinding movements.
Suprahyoid muscles					
Digastric	Base of cranium	Hyoid bone	Facial and mandibular nerves		Depresses mandible against resistance when infrahyoid muscles fix or depress hyoid bone
Stylohyoid	Styloid process		Facial nerve (CN VII)		
Mylohyoid	Medial body of mandible		Mandibular nerve ($CN\ V_3$)		
Geniohyoid	Anterior body of mandible		Nerve to geniohyoid (C1–C2)		
Infrahyoid muscles					
Omohyoid	Scapula	Hyoid bone	Ansa cervicalis from cervical plexus (C1–C3)		Fixes or depresses hyoid bone
Sternohyoid	Manubrium of sternum				
Sternothyroid		Thyroid cartilage			
Thyrohyoid	Thyroid cartilage	Hyoid bone	C1 (via hypoglossal n.–CN XII)		
Muscle of facial expression					
Platysma	Subcutaneous tissue of infraclavicular and supraclavicular regions	Base of mandible, skin of cheek and lower lip, angle of mouth (modiolus), and orbicularis oris	Cervical branch of facial nerve (CN VII)		Depresses mandible against resistance

TABLE 8.12. PARTS AND BRANCHES OF MAXILLARY ARTERY

Part	Course	Branches	Distribution
First (mandibular)	Proximal (posterior) to lateral pterygoid muscle; runs horizontally, deep (medial) to neck of condylar process of mandible and lateral to stylomandibular ligament	Deep auricular artery	Supplies external acoustic meatus, external tympanic membrane, and temporomandibular joint
		Anterior tympanic artery	Supplies internal aspect of tympanic membrane
		Middle meningeal artery	Enters cranial cavity via foramen spinosum to supply periosteum, bone, red bone marrow, dura mater of lateral wall and calvaria of neurocranium, trigeminal ganglion, facial nerve and geniculate ganglion, tympanic cavity, and tensor tympani muscle
		Accessory meningeal artery	Enters cranial cavity via foramen ovale; its distribution is mainly extracranial to muscles of infratemporal fossa, sphenoid bone, mandibular nerve, and otic ganglion.
		Inferior alveolar artery	Descends to enter mandibular canal of mandible via mandibular foramen; supplies mandible, mandibular teeth, chin, mylohyoid muscle
Second (pterygoid)	Adjacent (superficial or deep) to lateral pterygoid muscle; ascends obliquely anterosuperiorly, medial to temporalis muscle	Masseteric artery	Traverses mandibular notch, supplying temporomandibular joint and masseter muscle
		Deep temporal arteries	Anterior and posterior arteries ascend between temporalis muscle and bone of temporal fossa, supplying mainly muscle.
		Pterygoid branches	Irregular in number and origin; supply pterygoid muscle
		Buccal artery	Runs antero-inferiorly with buccal nerve to supply buccal fat-pad, buccinator, and buccal oral mucosa
Third (pterygoid–palatine)	Distal (anteromedial) to lateral pterygoid muscle; passes between heads of lateral pterygoid and through pterygomaxillary fissure into pterygopalatine fossa	Posterior superior alveolar artery	Descends on maxilla's infratemporal surface with branches traversing alveolar canals to supply maxillary molar and premolar teeth, adjacent gingiva, and mucous membrane of maxillary sinus
		Infra-orbital artery	Traverses inferior orbital fissure, infra-orbital groove, canal, and foramen; supplies inferior oblique and rectus muscles, lacrimal sac, maxillary canines and incisors teeth, mucous membrane of maxillary sinus, and skin of infra-orbital region of face
		Artery of pterygoid canal	Passes posteriorly through pterygoid canal; supplies mucosa of upper pharynx, pharyngotympanic tube, and tympanic cavity
		Pharyngeal branch	Passes through palatovaginal canal to supply mucosa of nasal roof, nasopharynx, sphenoidal air sinus, and pharyngotympanic tube
		Descending palatine artery	Descends through palatine canal, dividing into greater and lesser palatine arteries to mucosa and glands of hard and soft palate
		Sphenopalatine artery	Terminal branch of maxillary artery, traverses sphenopalatine foramen to supply walls and septum of nasal cavity; frontal, ethmoidal, sphenoid, and maxillary sinuses; and anteriormost palate

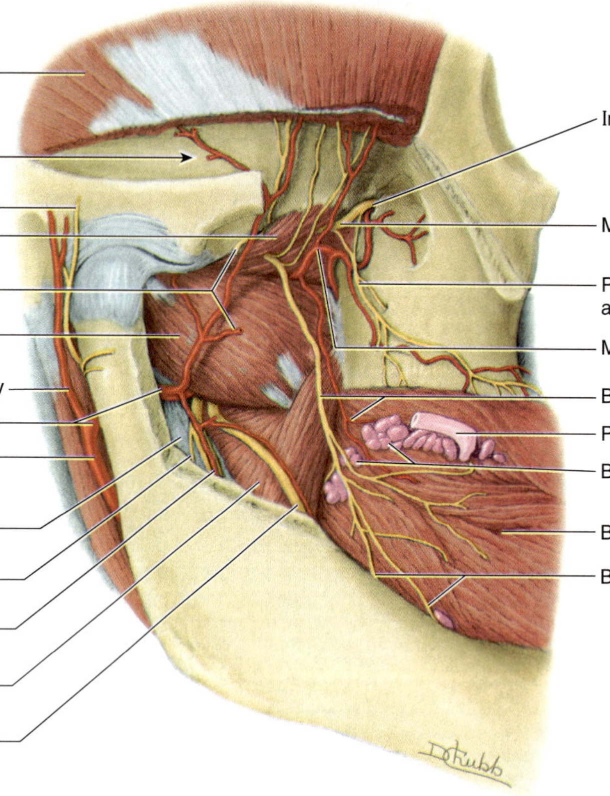

(A) Lateral view

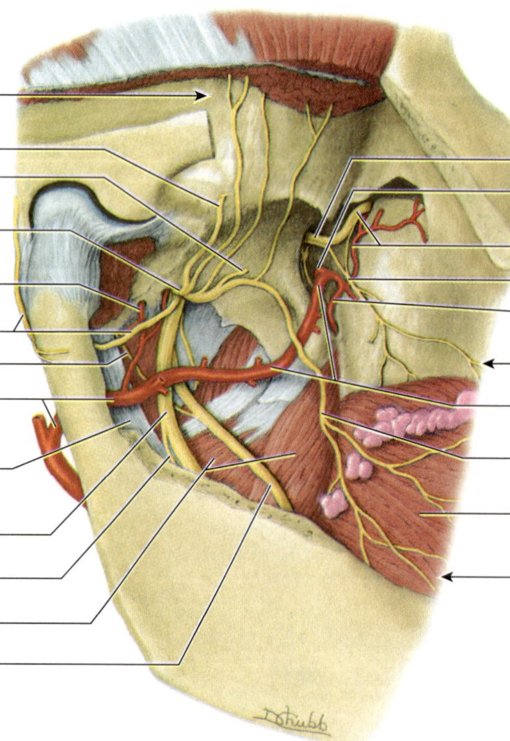

(B) Lateral view

FIGURE 8.76. Dissections of infratemporal region. A. In this superficial dissection, most of the zygomatic arch and attached masseter, the coronoid process and adjacent parts of the ramus of the mandible, and the inferior half of the temporal muscle have been removed. The first part of the maxillary artery, the larger of the two end branches of the external carotid, run anteriorly, deep to the neck of the mandible, and then pass deeply between the lateral and the medial pterygoid muscles. **B.** In this deep dissection, more of the ramus of the mandible, the lateral pterygoid muscle, and most branches of the maxillary artery have been removed. Branches of the mandibular nerve (CN V_3), including the auriculotemporal nerve, and the second part of the maxillary artery pass between the sphenomandibular ligament and the neck of the mandible.

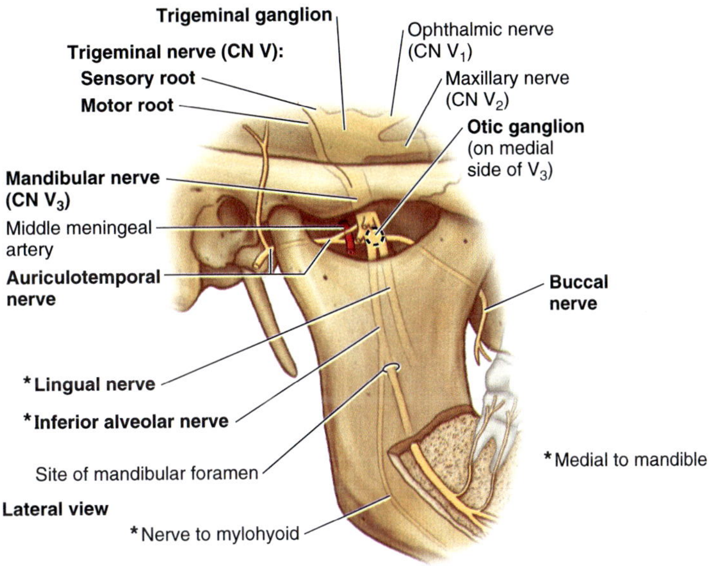

FIGURE 8.77. Nerves of infratemporal fossa.

CLINICAL BOX

AN28.9 PAROTID AND TEMPORAL REGIONS, INFRATEMPORAL FOSSA, AND TEMPOROMANDIBULAR JOINT

Parotidectomy

Most tumors of the parotid glands are benign. However, most (80% of) salivary gland cancers begin in the parotid glands. Surgical excision of the parotid gland (*parotidectomy*) is often performed as part of the treatment. Because the parotid plexus of CN VII is embedded in the parotid gland, the plexus and its branches are in jeopardy during surgery (see Fig. 8.23A, C). An important step in parotidectomy is the identification, dissection, isolation, and preservation of the facial nerve. A superficial portion of the gland (often erroneously referred to as a "lobe") is removed, after which the parotid plexus, which occupies a distinct plane within the gland, can be retracted to enable dissection of the deep portion of the gland. The parotid gland makes a substantial contribution to the posterolateral contour of the face, the extent of its contribution being especially evident after it has been surgically removed. See the clinical box "Paralysis of Facial Muscles" for a discussion of the functional consequences of injury
AN28.10 to the facial nerve. For the anatomical basis of Frey's syndrome, refer *Snell's Clinical Anatomy by Regions*, South Asian Edition, Chapter 11, Head and Neck, p. 728.

Infection of Parotid Gland

The parotid gland may become infected by infectious agents that pass through the bloodstream, as occurs in *mumps*, an acute communicable viral disease that primarily effects the parotid glands. Infection of the gland causes inflammation (*parotiditis*) and swelling of the gland, visible as marked distension of the cheek. Severe pain occurs because the parotid sheath resists swelling. Often, the pain is worse during chewing because the enlarged gland is wrapped around the posterior border of the ramus of the mandible and is compressed against the mastoid process of the temporal bone when the mouth is opened. The mumps virus may also cause *inflammation of the parotid duct*, producing *redness of the parotid papilla*, the small projection at the opening of the duct into the superior oral vestibule (Fig. 8.67). Because the pain produced by mumps may be confused with a toothache, redness of the papilla is often an early sign that the disease involves the parotid gland and not a tooth.

Parotid gland disease often causes pain in the auricle and external acoustic meatus of the external ear, the temporal region, and TMJ because the auriculotemporal and great auricular nerves, from which the parotid gland and sheath receive sensory fibers, also supply sensory fibers to the skin over the temporal fossa and auricle.

Abscess in Parotid Gland

A bacterial infection localized in the parotid gland usually produces an abscess (pus formation). The infection could result from extremely poor dental hygiene, or the infection could spread to the gland through the parotid ducts. Physicians and dentists must determine whether a swelling of the cheek results from infection of the parotid gland or from an abscess of dental origin.

Sialography of Parotid Duct

A radiopaque fluid can be injected into the duct system of the parotid gland through a cannula inserted through the orifice of the parotid duct in the mucous membrane of the cheek. This technique (*sialography*) is followed by radiography of the gland. *Parotid sialograms* (G. *sialon*, saliva + G. *grapho*, to write) demonstrate parts of the parotid duct system that may be displaced or dilated by disease.

Blockage of Parotid Duct

The parotid duct may be blocked by a calcified deposit, called a *sialolith* or *calculus* (L. pebble). The resulting pain in the parotid gland is made worse by eating. Sucking a lemon slice is painful because of the buildup of saliva in the proximal part of the blocked parotid duct.

Accessory Parotid Gland

Sometimes, an additional *accessory parotid gland* lies on the masseter muscle between the parotid duct and the zygomatic arch. Several ducts open from this accessory gland into the parotid duct.

Mandibular Nerve Block

To produce a mandibular nerve block, an anesthetic agent is injected near the mandibular nerve where it enters the infratemporal fossa (Fig. 8.69B). In the extra-oral approach, the needle passes through the mandibular notch of the ramus of the mandible into the infratemporal fossa. The injection usually anesthetizes the auriculotemporal, inferior alveolar, lingual, and buccal branches of CN V_3.

Inferior Alveolar Nerve Block

An inferior alveolar nerve block anesthetizes the inferior alveolar nerve, a branch of CN V_3. The site of the anesthetic injection is around the *mandibular foramen*, the opening into the mandibular canal on the medial aspect of the ramus of the mandible (Fig. 8.77). This canal gives passage to the inferior alveolar nerve, artery, and vein. When this nerve block is successful, all mandibular teeth are anesthetized to the median plane. The skin and mucous membrane of the lower lip, the labial alveolar mucosa and gingivae, and the skin of the chin are also anesthetized because they are supplied by the mental nerve, a branch of the inferior alveolar nerve (Fig. 8.81A). There are possible problems associated with an inferior alveolar nerve block, such as injection of the anesthetic into the parotid gland or the medial pterygoid muscle. This would affect ability to open the mouth (*pterygoid trismus*).

Dislocation of Temporomandibular Joint (TMJ)

N33.5 Sometimes during yawning or taking a large bite, excessive contraction of the lateral pterygoids may cause the heads of the mandible to dislocate anteriorly (pass anterior to the articular tubercles) (Fig. B8.32). In this position, the mandible remains depressed and the person is unable to close his or her mouth. Most common, a sideways blow to the chin by a clenched hand (fist) when the mouth is open dislocates the TMJ on the side that received the blow. Dislocation of the TMJ may also accompany fractures of the mandible. Posterior dislocation is uncommon, being resisted by the presence of the postglenoid tubercle and the strong intrinsic lateral ligament. Usually in falls on or direct blows to the chin, the neck of the mandible fractures before dislocation occurs. Because of the close relationship of the facial and auriculotemporal nerves to the TMJ, care must be taken during surgical procedures to preserve both the branches of the facial nerve overlying it and the articular branches of the auriculotemporal nerve that enter the posterior part of the joint. Injury to articular branches of the auriculotemporal nerve supplying the TMJ, associated with traumatic dislocation and rupture of the articular capsule and lateral ligament, leads to laxity and instability of the TMJ.

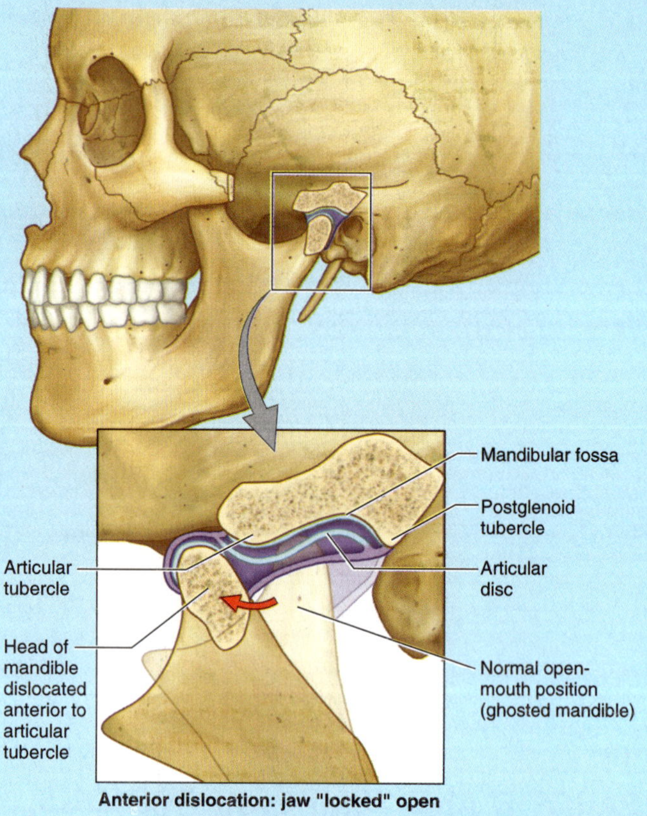

FIGURE B8.32. Dislocation of TMJ.

Arthritis of TMJ

The TMJ may become inflamed from degenerative arthritis, for example. Abnormal function of the TMJ may result in structural problems such as dental occlusion and joint clicking (*crepitus*). The clicking is thought to result from delayed anterior disc movements during mandibular depression and elevation.

The Bottom Line: Parotid and Temporal Regions, Infratemporal Fossa, and Temporomandibular Joint

Parotid region: The largest of the salivary glands, the parotid gland makes a substantial contribution to the contour of the face. • Occupying a complex space anterior to the auricle of the ear, the gland straddles most of the posterior aspect of the ramus of the mandible. • Fatty tissue in the gland gives it flexibility to accommodate the motions of the mandible. • The parotid duct passes anteriorly across the masseter, parallel and about a finger's breadth inferior to the zygomatic arch, and then turns medially to enter the superior oral vestibule opposite the 2nd maxillary molar. • Parotid fascia, continuous with the investing layer of deep cervical fascia, invests the gland as the parotid sheath. • The sheath is innervated by the great auricular nerve, but the gland receives parasympathetic secretomotor innervation from the glossopharyngeal nerve via a complex route involving the otic ganglion. • Medial and anterior to the parotid gland, one of the muscles of mastication—the masseter—lies lateral to the ramus of the mandible, receiving its innervation via masseteric branches of the mandibular nerve and maxillary artery that traverse the mandibular notch.

Temporal and infratemporal fossa: The temporal fossa and its inferior continuation deep to the zygomatic arch and ramus of the mandible, the infratemporal fossa, are largely occupied by derivatives of the embryonic first pharyngeal arch: three of the four muscles of mastication (temporalis muscle and two pterygoid muscles) and the nerve that conveys motor fibers to them, the mandibular nerve (CN V_3).

TMJ and muscles of mastication: The TMJ is a hinge joint, modified by the presence of an articular disc that intervenes between the mandibular head and the articular surfaces of the temporal bone. • Gliding movements between the mandibular fossa and articular eminence occur in the upper compartment and are produced by the lateral pterygoid (protraction) and posterior fibers of the temporalis (retraction). • The mandible must be protracted for full opening of the mouth. • Hinge and pivoting movements occur in the lower compartment and are produced by gravity (depression) and three of the four muscles of mastication (elevation): masseter, medial pterygoid, and anterior portion of the temporalis.

Neurovasculature of infratemporal fossa: Also contained in the infratemporal fossa is the second part of the maxillary artery and its venous equivalent, the pterygoid venous plexus. • Adjacent cranial compartments communicate with the fossae, and neurovascular structures pass to and from the fossae via bony passages, including the (1) foramen ovale, through which the mandibular nerve enters from the middle cranial fossa; (2) foramen spinosum, through which the middle meningeal artery enters and the meningeal branch of CN V_3 returns to the middle cranial fossa; (3) pterygomaxillary fissure, through which the maxillary artery passes into the pterygopalatine fossa for further distribution; (4) inferior orbital fissure, through which the inferior ophthalmic veins drain to the pterygoid venous plexus; and (5) mandibular foramen, through which the inferior alveolar nerve passes to mandibular canal for distribution to the mandible and teeth.

ORAL REGION

The **oral region** includes the oral cavity, teeth, gingivae, tongue, palate, and the region of the palatine tonsils. The oral cavity is where food is ingested and prepared for digestion in the stomach and small intestine. Food is chewed by the teeth, and saliva from the salivary glands facilitates the formation of a manageable *food bolus* (L. lump). *Deglutition* (swallowing) is voluntarily initiated in the oral cavity. The voluntary phase of the process pushes the bolus from the oral cavity into the pharynx, the expanded part of the alimentary (digestive) system, where the involuntary (automatic) phase of swallowing occurs.

Oral Cavity

The **oral cavity** (mouth) consists of two parts: the *oral vestibule* and the *oral cavity proper* (Fig. 8.78). It is in the oral cavity that food and drinks are tasted and where mastication (chewing) and lingual manipulation of food occur. The **oral vestibule** is the slit-like space between the teeth and gingivae (gums) and the lips and cheeks. The vestibule communicates with the exterior through the **oral fissure** (opening). The size of the fissure is controlled by the peri-oral muscles, such as the orbicularis oris (the sphincter of the oral fissure), buccinator, risorius, and depressors and elevators of the lips (dilators of the fissure).

The **oral cavity proper** is the space between the upper and the lower **dental arches** or arcades (maxillary and mandibular alveolar arches and the teeth they bear). The oral cavity is limited laterally and anteriorly by the dental arches. The *roof of the oral cavity* is formed by the palate. Posteriorly, the oral cavity communicates with the oropharynx (oral part of the pharynx). When the mouth is closed and at rest, the oral cavity is fully occupied by the tongue.

Lips, Cheeks, and Gingivae

LIPS AND CHEEKS

The **lips** are mobile, musculofibrous folds surrounding the mouth, extending from the *nasolabial sulci* and *nares* laterally, and superiorly to the *mentolabial sulcus* inferiorly (Fig. 8.79).

8

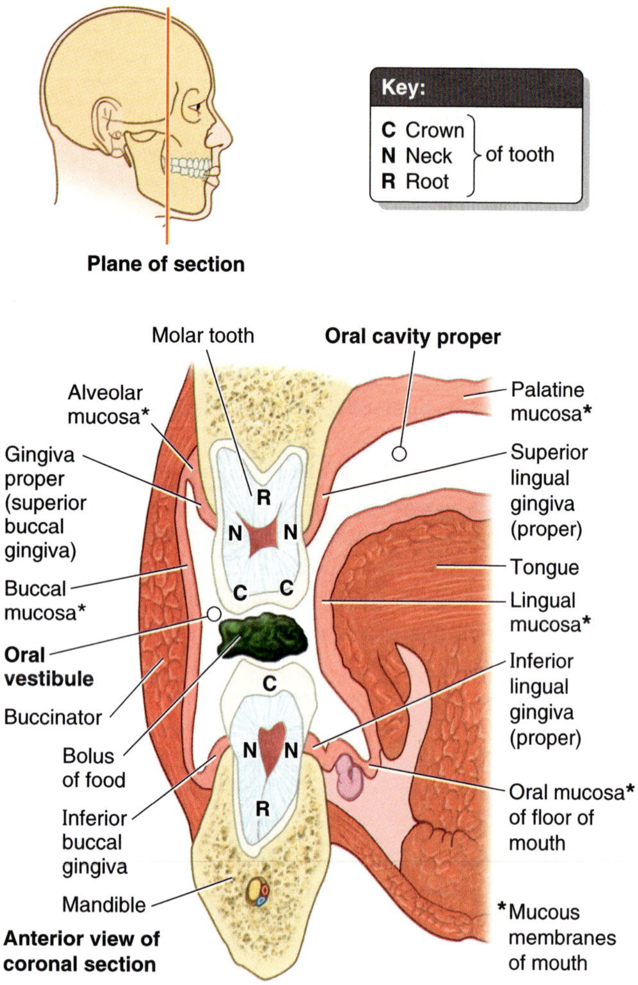

FIGURE 8.78. Coronal section of mouth region. The orientation drawing shows the plane of the section. During chewing, the tongue (centrally), buccinator (laterally), and orbicularis oris (anteriorly) work together to retain the bolus of food between the occlusive surfaces of the molar teeth.

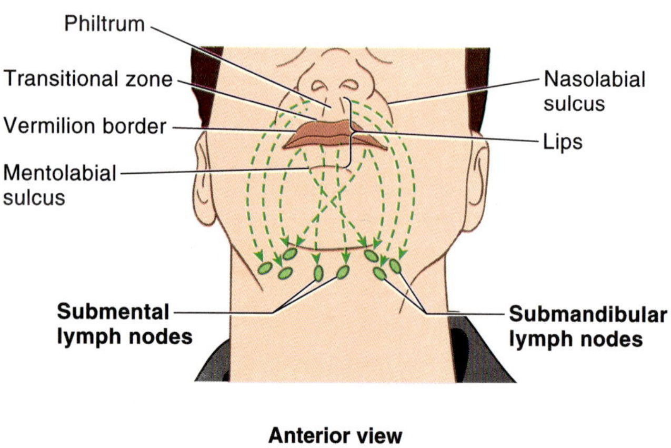

FIGURE 8.79. Lymphatic drainage of lips. Lymph from the upper lip and lateral parts of the lower lip drains to the submandibular nodes. Lymph from the middle part of the lower lip drains to the submental nodes.

They contain the orbicularis oris and superior and inferior labial muscles, vessels, and nerves (Fig. 8.16). The lips are covered externally by skin and internally by mucous membrane. The lips function as the valves of the *oral fissure*, containing the sphincter (orbicularis oris) that controls entry and exit from the mouth and upper alimentary and respiratory tracts. The lips are used for grasping food, sucking liquids, keeping food out of the oral vestibule, forming speech, and osculation (kissing).

The *transitional zone of the lips* (commonly considered by itself to be the lip), ranging from brown to red, continues into the oral cavity where it is continuous with the mucous membrane of the mouth (labial mucosa). This membrane covers the intra-oral, vestibular part of the lips (Fig. 8.80). The **labial frenula** (frena) are free-edged folds of mucous membrane in the midline, extending from the vestibular gingiva to the mucosa of the upper and lower lips. The frenula (frenum) extending to the upper lip is larger. Other smaller frenula sometimes appear laterally in the premolar vestibular regions.

The **superior** and **inferior labial arteries**, branches of the facial arteries, anastomose with each other in the lips to form an arterial ring (Fig. 8.24; Table 8.5). The pulse of these arteries may be palpated by grasping the upper or lower lip lightly between the first two digits. The upper lip is supplied by superior labial branches of the *facial* and *infra-orbital arteries*. The lower lip is supplied by inferior labial branches of the *facial* and *mental arteries*.

The upper lip is supplied by the superior labial branches of the *infra-orbital nerves* (of CN V_2), and the lower lip is supplied by the inferior labial branches of the mental nerves (of CN V_3). Lymph from the upper lip and lateral parts of the lower lip passes primarily to the *submandibular lymph nodes* (Fig. 8.79), whereas lymph from the medial part of the lower lip passes initially to the *submental lymph nodes*.

The **cheeks** (L. *buccae*) have essentially the same structure as the lips with which they are continuous. The cheeks form the movable walls of the oral cavity. Anatomically, the external aspect of the cheeks constitutes the *buccal region*, bounded anteriorly by the *oral* and *mental regions* (lips and chin), superiorly by the *zygomatic region*, posteriorly by the *parotid region*, and inferiorly by the inferior border of the *mandible* (Fig. 8.14). The *prominence of the cheek* occurs at the junction of the zygomatic and buccal regions. The zygomatic bone underlying the prominence and the zygomatic arch, which continues posteriorly, are commonly referred to as the "cheek bone" (Fig. 8.3). Lay persons consider the zygomatic and parotid regions also to be part of the cheek.

The principal muscles of the cheeks are the buccinators (Fig. 8.78). Numerous small **buccal glands** lie between the mucous membrane and the buccinators (Fig. 8.76A). Superficial to the buccinators are encapsulated collections of fat. These *buccal fat-pads* are proportionately much larger in infants, presumably to reinforce the cheeks and keep them from collapsing during sucking. The cheeks are supplied by buccal branches of the maxillary artery and innervated by buccal branches of the mandibular nerve.

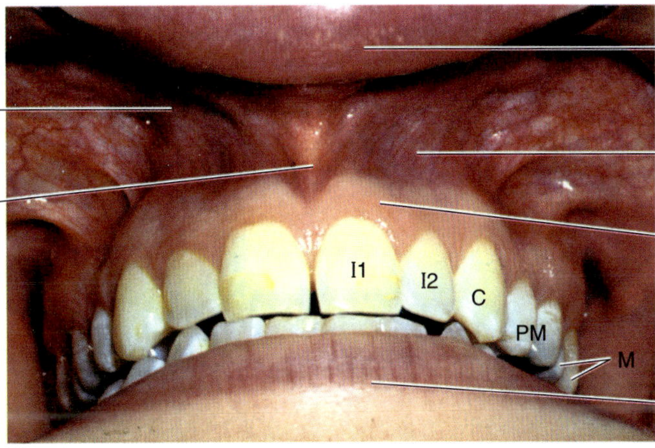

(A)

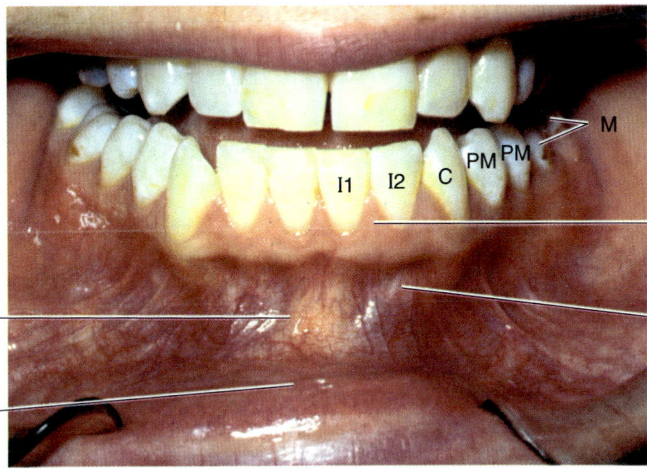

(B)

FIGURE 8.80. Oral vestibule and gingivae. A. The vestibule and gingivae of the maxilla are shown. **B.** The vestibule and gingivae of the mandible are shown. As the alveolar mucosa approaches the necks of the teeth, it changes in texture and color to become the gingiva proper. (Courtesy of Dr. B. Liebgott, Professor, Division of Anatomy, Department of Surgery, University of Toronto, Toronto, Ontario, Canada.)

GINGIVAE

The **gingivae** (gums) are composed of fibrous tissue covered with mucous membrane. The **gingiva proper** (attached gingiva) is firmly attached to the alveolar part of the mandible and alveolar process of the maxilla and the necks of the teeth (Figs. 8.78 and 8.80). The gingiva proper adjacent to the tongue is the superior and inferior lingual gingivae, and that adjacent to the lips and cheeks is the **maxillary** and **mandibular labial** or **buccal gingiva**, respectively. The gingiva proper is normally pink, stippled, and keratinized. The **alveolar mucosa** (unattached gingiva) is normally shiny red and nonkeratinizing. The nerves and vessels supplying the gingiva, underlying alveolar bone, and *periodontium* (which surrounds the root[s] of a tooth, anchoring it to the tooth socket), are presented in Figure 8.81A, C.

Teeth

The *chief functions of teeth* are as follows:

- Incise (cut), reduce, and mix food material with saliva during mastication (chewing).
- Help sustain themselves in the tooth sockets by assisting the development and protection of the tissues that support them.
- Participate in articulation (distinct connected speech).

The teeth are set in the *tooth sockets* and are used in mastication and in assisting in articulation. A tooth is identified and described as **deciduous** (primary) or **permanent** (secondary), the type of tooth, and its proximity to the midline or front of the mouth (e.g., medial and lateral incisors; the 1st molar is anterior to the 2nd).

Children have 20 deciduous teeth; adults normally have 32 permanent teeth (Fig. 8.82A, C). The usual ages of the eruption ("cutting") of these teeth are demonstrated in Figure 8.83 and listed in Tables 8.13A and 8.13B. Before eruption, the developing teeth reside in the alveolar arches as **tooth buds** (Fig. 8.82B).

The types of teeth are identified by their characteristics: **incisors**, thin cutting edges; **canines**, single prominent cones; **premolars** (bicuspids), two cusps; and **molars**, three or more cusps (Fig. 8.82A, C). The **vestibular surface** (labial or buccal) of each tooth is directed outwardly, and the

(*continued on p.* 991)

8

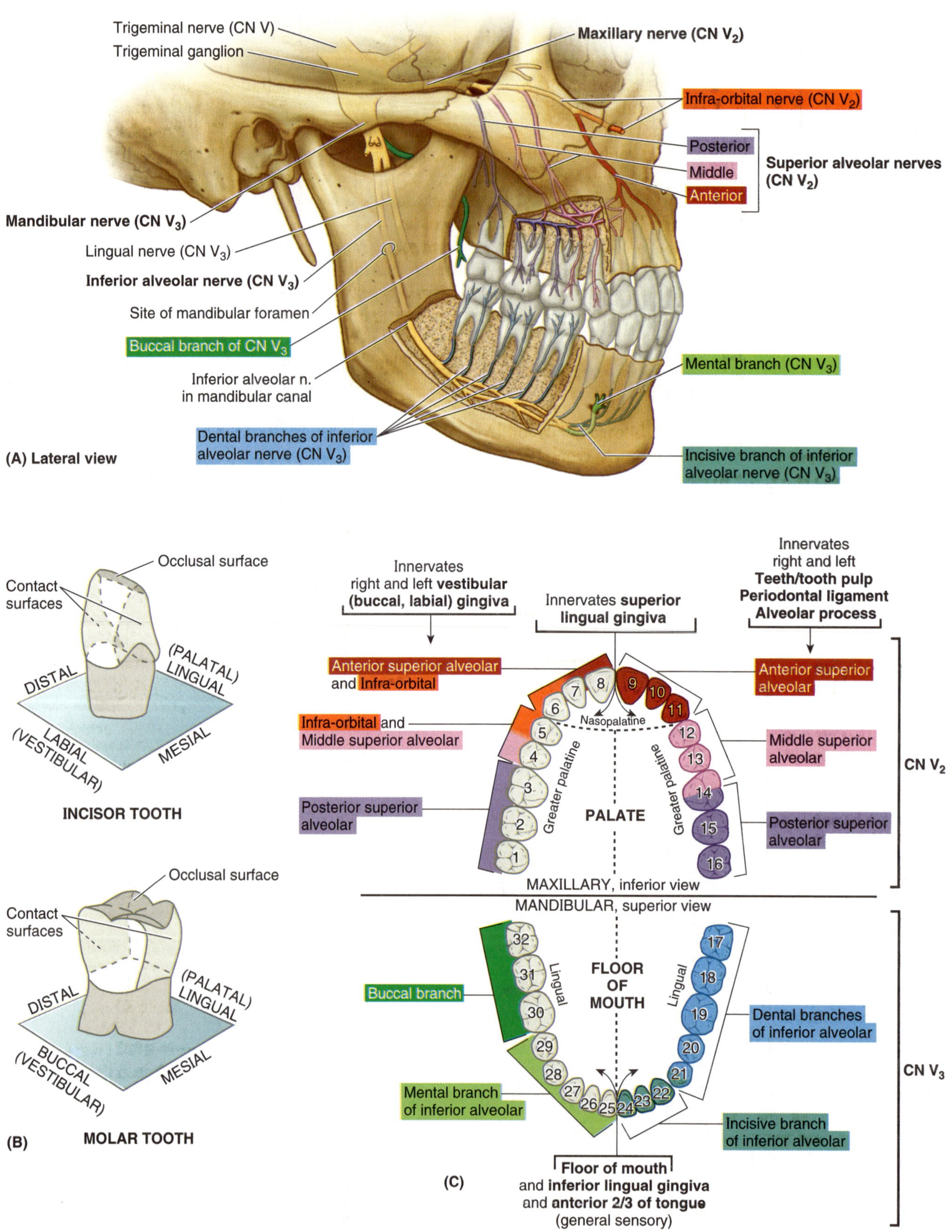

FIGURE 8.81. Innervation of teeth and gingiva. A. Superior and inferior alveolar nerves. **B.** Surfaces of an incisor and molar tooth. **C.** Innervation of the mouth and teeth.

lingual surface is directed inwardly (Fig. 8.81B). As used in clinical (dental) practice, the **mesial surface** of a tooth is directed toward the median plane of the facial part of the cranium. The **distal surface** is directed away from this plane. Both mesial and distal surfaces are *contact surfaces*, that is, surfaces that contact adjacent teeth. The masticatory surface is the **occlusal surface**.

PARTS AND STRUCTURE OF TEETH

A tooth has a crown, neck, and root (Fig. 8.84). The **crown** projects from the gingiva. The **neck** is between the crown and root. The **root** is fixed in the tooth socket by the *periodontium* (connective tissue surrounding the roots). The number of roots varies. Most of the tooth is composed of **dentine** (L. *dentinium*), which is covered by **enamel** over the crown and cement (L. *cementum*) over the root. The **pulp cavity** contains connective tissue, blood vessels, and nerves. The **root canal** (pulp canal) transmits the nerves and vessels to and from the pulp cavity through the **apical foramen**.

The **dental alveoli** (tooth sockets; Figs. 8.83B and 8.84B) are in the *alveolar processes* of the maxillae and the *alveolar part* of the mandible (Fig. 8.82A); they are the skeletal features that display the greatest change during a lifetime (Fig. 8.83B). Adjacent alveoli are separated by **interalveolear septa**. Within the alveolus, the roots of teeth with more than one root are separated by **interradicular septa** (Figs. 8.83B and 8.84B). The bone of the socket has a thin cortex separated

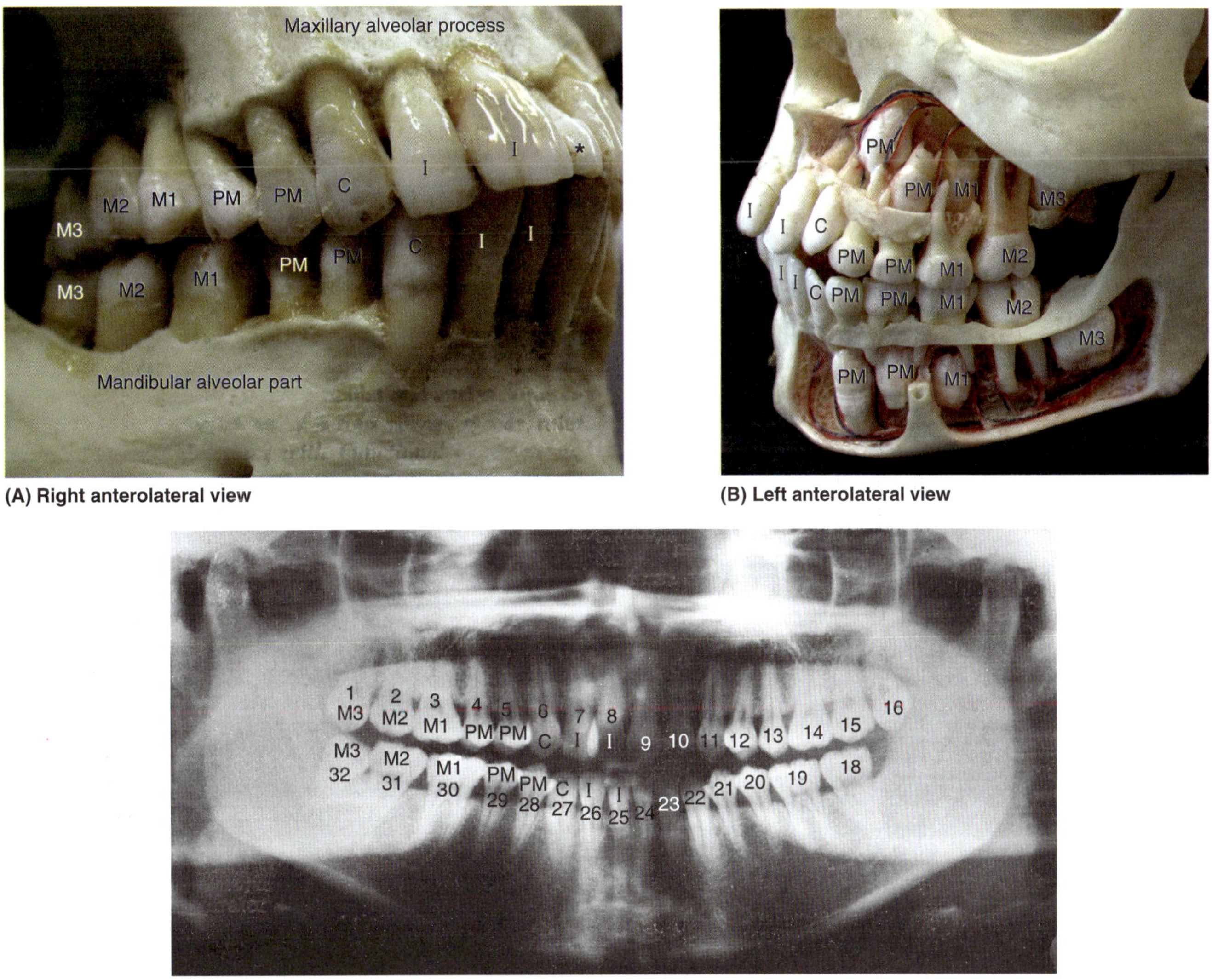

(A) Right anterolateral view

(B) Left anterolateral view

(C) Panoramic view

FIGURE 8.82. Secondary dentition. A. The teeth are shown in occlusion. There is a supernumerary midline tooth (mesiodens) in this specimen (*). **B.** Maxillary and mandibular jaws of a child acquiring secondary dentition are shown. The alveolar process of the maxilla and alveolar part of the mandible are carved to reveal the roots of the teeth and tooth buds. **C.** A pantomographic radiograph of an adult mandible and maxilla is shown. The left lower 3rd molar is not present. *I*, incisor; *C*, canine; *PM*, premolar; *M1*, *M2*, and *M3*, 1st, 2nd, and 3rd molars. (Part **C** courtesy of M. J. Pharoah, Associate Professor of Dental Radiology, Faculty of Dentistry, University of Toronto, Toronto, Ontario, Canada.)

TABLE 8.13A. DECIDUOUS TEETH

Deciduous Teeth	Central Incisor	Lateral Incisor	Canine	1st Molar	2nd Molar
Eruption (months)[a]	6–8	8–10	16–20	12–16	20–24
Shedding (years)	6–7	7–8	10–12	9–11	10–12

[a]In some normal infants, the first teeth (medial incisors) may not erupt until 12–13 months of age.

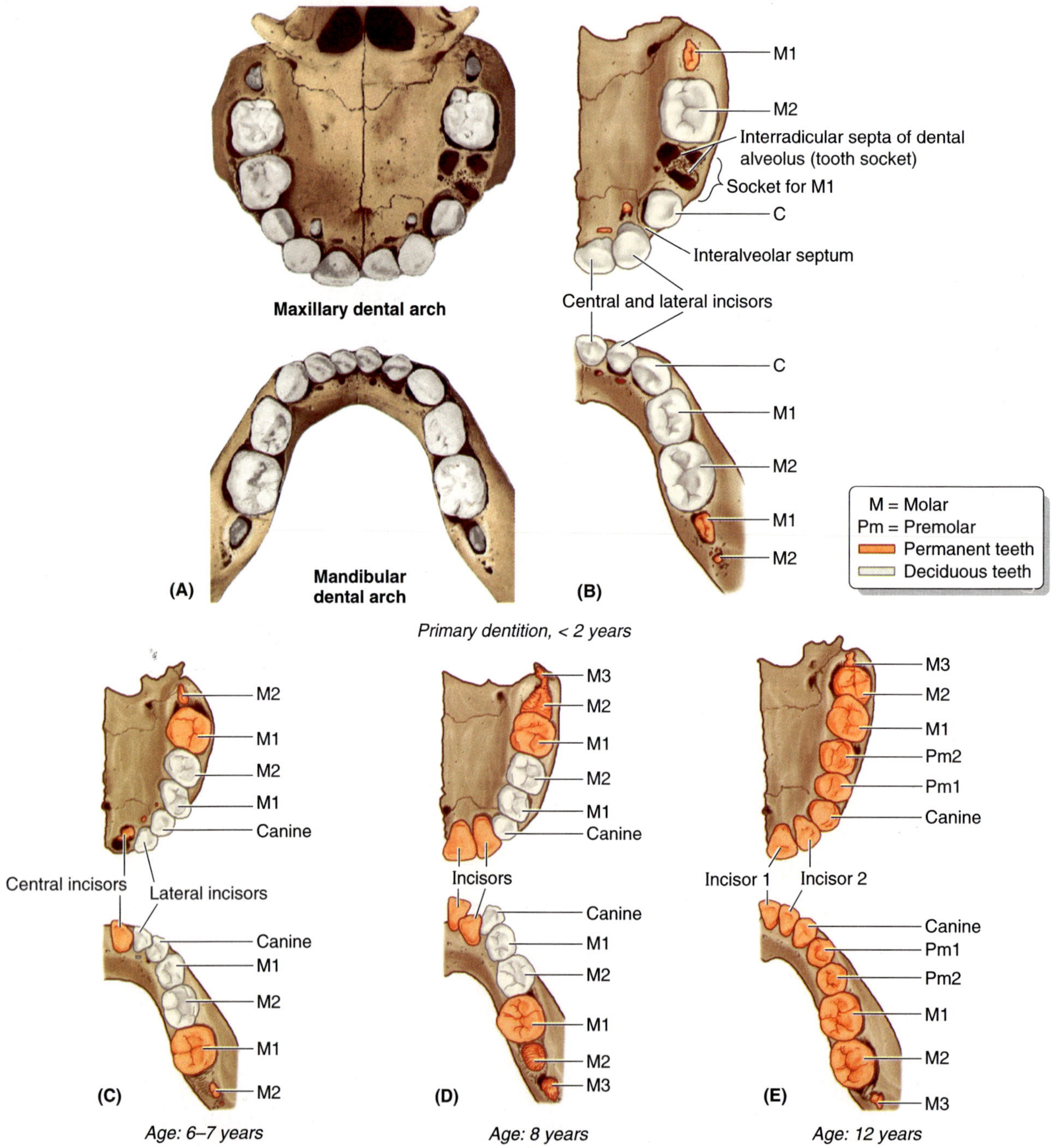

FIGURE 8.83. Primary dentition (deciduous teeth) and eruption of permanent teeth.

TABLE 8.13B. PERMANENT TEETH

Permanent Teeth	Central Incisor	Lateral Incisor	Canine	1st Premolar	2nd Premolar	1st Molar	2nd Molar	3rd Molar
Eruption (years)	7–8	8–9	10–12	10–11	11–12	6–7	12	13–25

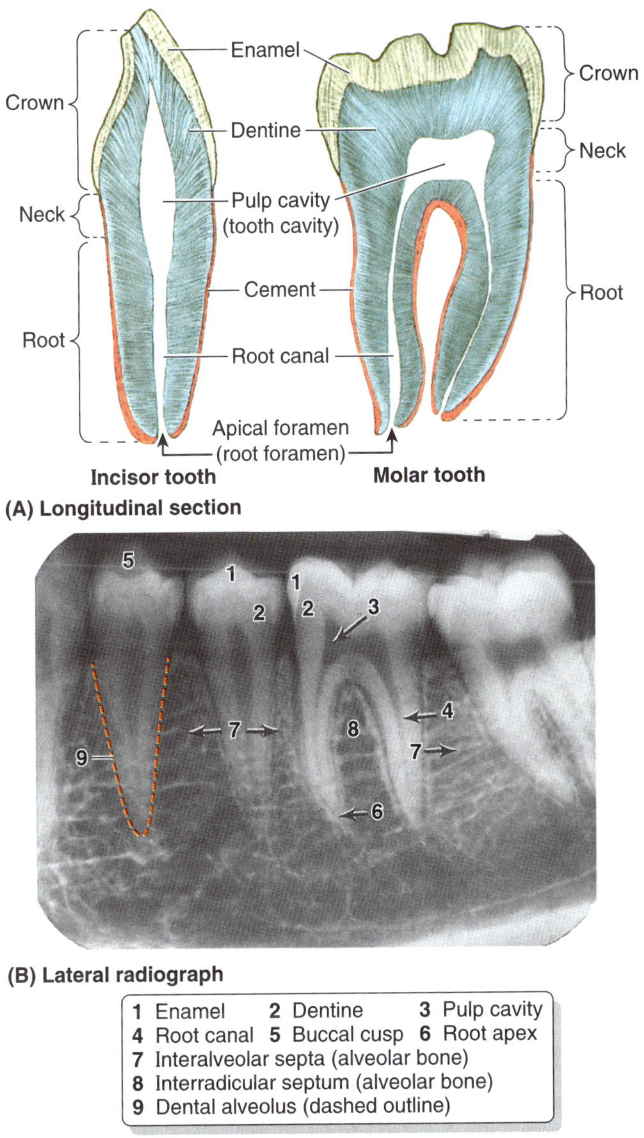

FIGURE 8.84. Sections of teeth. A. An incisor and a molar tooth are shown. In living people, the pulp cavity is a hollow space within the crown and neck of the tooth containing connective tissue, blood vessels, and nerves. The cavity narrows down to the root canal in a single-rooted tooth or to one canal per root of a multirooted tooth. The vessels and nerves enter or leave through the apical foramen. **B.** Bite-wing radiograph of maxillary premolar and molar teeth demonstrating features shown and described in part **A**.

from the adjacent labial and lingual cortices by a variable amount of trabeculated bone. The labial wall of the socket is particularly thin over the incisor teeth. The reverse is true for the molars, where the lingual wall is thinner. Therefore, the labial surface commonly is broken to extract incisors and the lingual surface is broken to extract molars.

The roots of the teeth are connected to the bone of the alveolus by a springy suspension forming a special type of fibrous joint called a **dento-alveolar syndesmosis** or **gomphosis**. The **periodontium** (periodontal membrane) is composed of collagenous fibers that extend between the cement of the root and the periosteum of the alveolus. It is abundantly supplied with tactile, pressoreceptive nerve endings, lymph capillaries, and glomerular blood vessels that act as hydraulic cushioning to curb axial masticatory pressure. *Pressoreceptive nerve endings* are capable of receiving changes in pressure as stimuli.

VASCULATURE OF TEETH

The **superior** and **inferior alveolar arteries**, branches of the maxillary artery, supply the maxillary and mandibular teeth, respectively (Figs. 8.75 and 8.76A; Table 8.12). The **alveolar veins** have the same names and distribution accompany the arteries. **Lymphatic vessels** from the teeth and gingivae pass mainly to the *submandibular lymph nodes* (Fig. 8.79).

INNERVATION OF TEETH

The *nerves supplying the teeth* are illustrated in Figure 8.81A. The named branches of the *superior* (CN V_2) and *inferior* (CN V_3) *alveolar nerves* give rise to **dental plexuses** that supply the maxillary and mandibular teeth.

Palate

The **palate** forms the arched roof of the mouth and the floor of the nasal cavities (Fig. 8.85). It separates the oral cavity from the nasal cavities and the nasopharynx, the part of the pharynx superior to the soft palate. The superior (nasal) surface of the palate is covered with respiratory mucosa, and the inferior (oral) surface is covered with oral mucosa, densely packed with glands. The palate consists of two regions: the hard palate anteriorly and the soft palate posteriorly.

HARD PALATE

The **hard palate** is vaulted (concave). This space is mostly filled by the tongue when it is at rest. The anterior two thirds of the palate have a bony skeleton formed by the palatine processes of the maxillae and the horizontal plates of the palatine bones (Fig. 8.86A). The **incisive fossa** is a depression in the midline of the bony palate posterior to the central incisor teeth into which the incisive canals open. The nasopalatine nerves pass from the nose through a variable number of incisive canals and foramina that open into the incisive fossa (Fig. 8.89B).

Medial to the 3rd molar tooth, the *greater palatine foramen* pierces the lateral border of the bony palate (Fig. 8.86A). The *greater palatine vessels and nerve* emerge from this foramen and run anteriorly on the palate. The *lesser palatine foramina* posterior to the greater palatine foramen pierce the pyramidal process of the palatine bone. These foramina transmit the *lesser palatine nerves and vessels* to the soft palate and adjacent structures (Fig. 8.89).

SOFT PALATE

The **soft palate** is the movable posterior third of the palate and is suspended from the posterior border of the hard palate

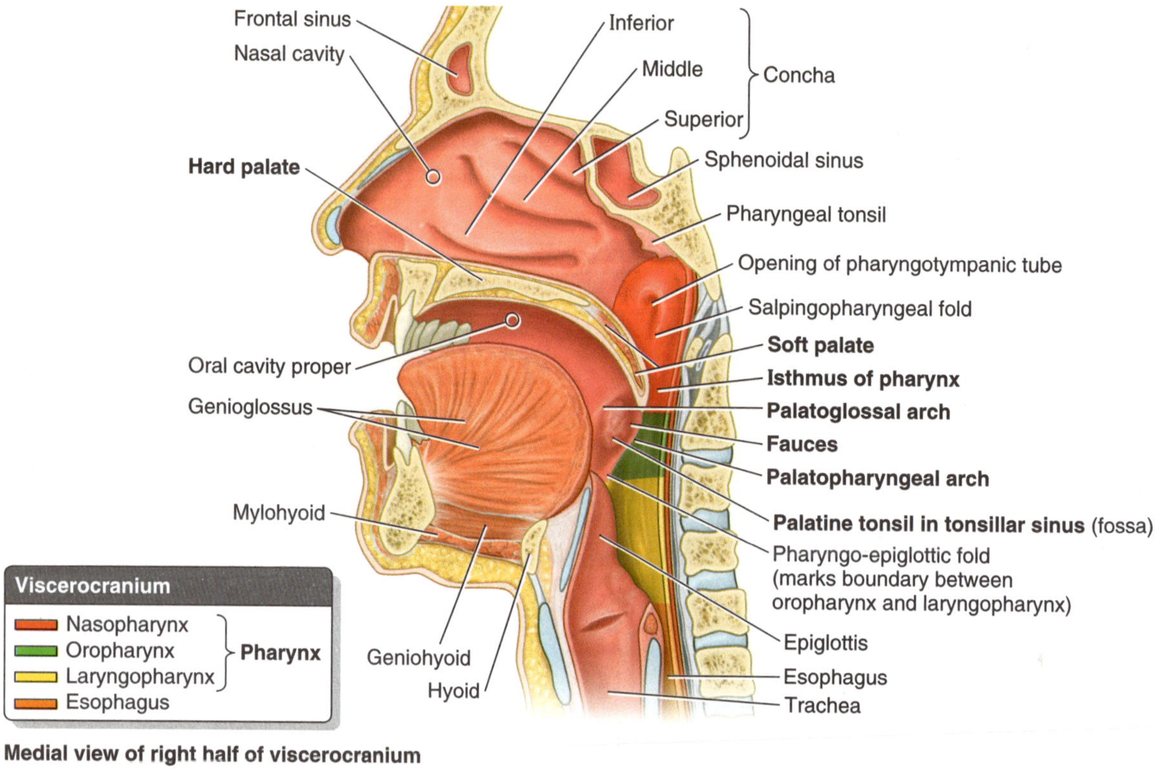

FIGURE 8.85. Median section of head and neck. The airway and food passageways cross in the pharynx. The soft palate acts as a valve, elevating to seal the pharyngeal isthmus connecting the nasal cavity and nasopharynx with the oral cavity and oropharynx.

(Figs. 8.85 and 8.86B). The soft palate has no bony skeleton; however, its anterior *aponeurotic part* is strengthened by the **palatine aponeurosis**, which attaches to the posterior edge of the hard palate. The aponeurosis is thick anteriorly and thin posteriorly, where it blends with a posterior *muscular part of the soft palate*. Postero-inferiorly, the soft palate has a curved free margin from which hangs a conical process, the **uvula**.

When swallowing, the soft palate is initially tensed to allow the tongue to press against it, squeezing the bolus (masticated mass) of food to the back of the mouth. The soft palate is then elevated posteriorly and superiorly against the wall of the pharynx, thereby preventing passage of food into the nasal cavity.

Laterally, the soft palate is continuous with the wall of the pharynx and is joined to the tongue and pharynx by the **palatoglossal** and **palatopharyngeal arches**, respectively (Fig. 8.85). A few taste buds are located in the epithelium covering the oral surface of the soft palate, the posterior wall of the oropharynx, and the epiglottis.

The **fauces** (L. throat) is the space between the oral cavity and the pharynx. The fauces is bounded superiorly by the soft palate, inferiorly by the root of the tongue, and laterally by the **pillars of the fauces**, the *palatoglossal* and *palatopharyngeal arches*. The **isthmus of the fauces** is the short, constricted space that establishes the connection between the oral cavity proper and oropharynx. The isthmus is bounded anteriorly by the palatoglossal folds and posteriorly by the palatopharyngeal folds. The **palatine tonsils**, often referred to as "the tonsils," are masses of lymphoid tissue, one on each side of the oropharynx. Each tonsil is in a **tonsillar sinus (fossa)**, bounded by the palatoglossal and palatopharyngeal arches and the tongue.

SUPERFICIAL FEATURES OF PALATE

The mucosa of the hard palate is tightly bound to the underlying bone (Fig. 8.87A). Consequently, submucous injections here are extremely painful. The *superior lingual gingiva*, the part of the gingiva covering the lingual surface of the teeth and the alveolar process, is continuous with the mucosa of the palate. Therefore, injection of an anesthetic agent into the gingiva of a tooth anesthetizes the adjacent palatal mucosa.

Deep to the mucosa of the palate are mucus-secreting **palatine glands** (Fig. 8.87B). The openings of the ducts of these glands give the palatine mucosa a pitted (orange-peel) appearance. In the midline, posterior to the maxillary incisor teeth, is the **incisive papilla**. This elevation of the mucosa lies directly anterior to the underlying *incisive fossa* (Fig. 8.86A).

Radiating laterally from the incisive papilla are several parallel **transverse palatine folds** or rugae (Fig. 8.87A, B). These folds assist with manipulation of food during mastication. Passing posteriorly in the midline of the palate from the incisive papilla is a narrow whitish streak, the **palatine**

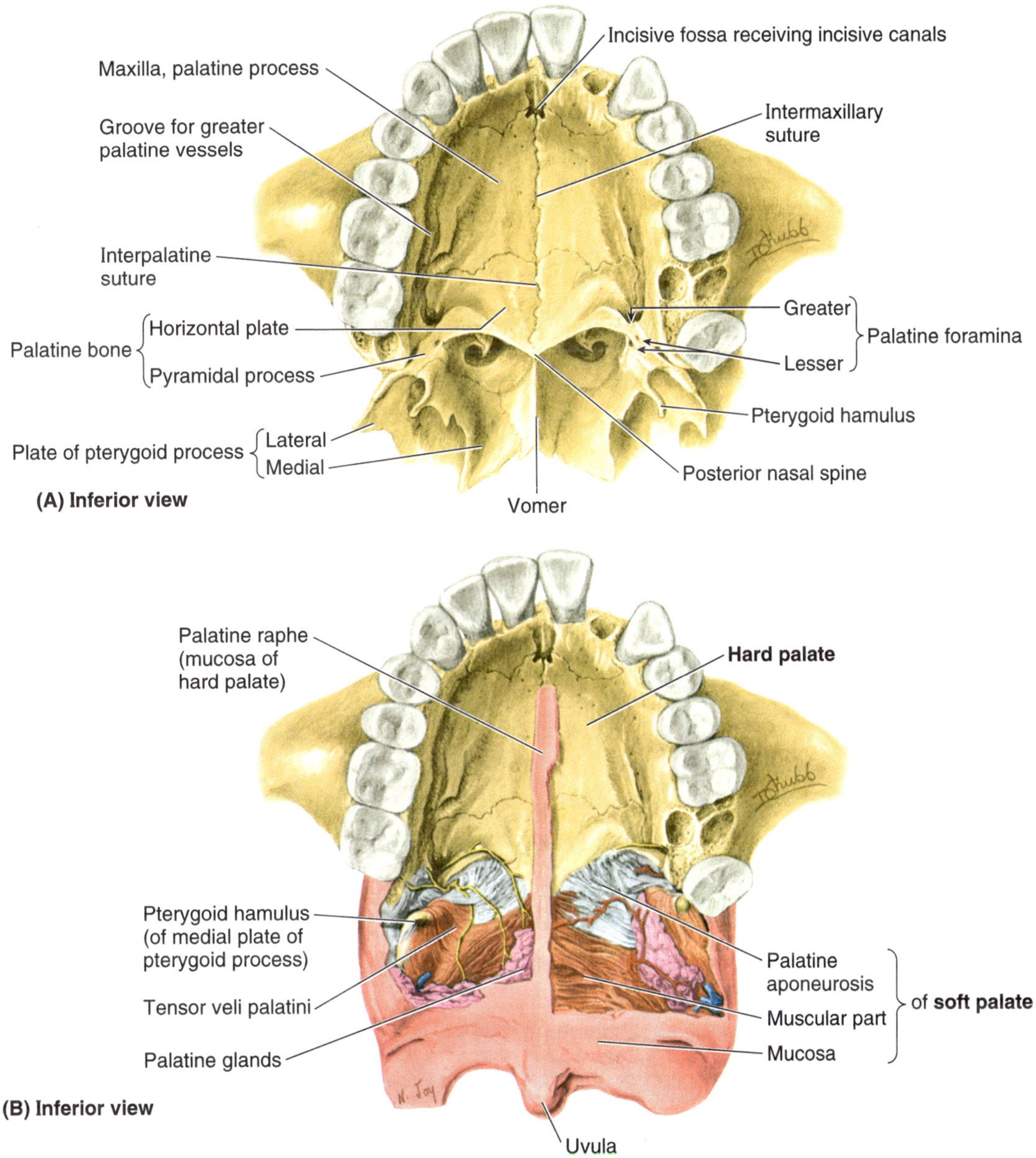

FIGURE 8.86. Palate. The bones and structures of the hard palate and soft palate are shown. The palate has bony **(A)**, aponeurotic, and muscular parts **(B)**. The mucosa has been removed on each side of the palatine raphe in part **B**. The palatine aponeurosis is formed by the merging of the flattened tendons of the right and left tensor veli palatini muscles. Before they become flattened, each tendon uses the pterygoid hamulus as a trochlea or pulley, redirecting its line of pull approximately 90°.

raphe. It may present as a ridge anteriorly and a groove posteriorly. The palatine raphe marks the site of fusion of the embryonic palatal processes (palatal shelves) (Moore et al., 2016). You can feel the transverse palatine folds and the palatine raphe with your tongue.

MUSCLES OF SOFT PALATE

The soft palate may be elevated so that it is in contact with the posterior wall of the pharynx. This closes the *isthmus of the pharynx*, requiring that one breathes through the mouth. The soft palate may also be drawn inferiorly so that it is in contact with the posterior part of the tongue. This closes the *isthmus of the fauces*, so that expired air passes through the nose (even when the mouth is open) and prevents substances in the oral cavity from passing to the pharynx. Tensing the soft palate pulls it tight at an intermediate level so that the tongue may push against it, compressing masticated food and propelling it into the pharynx for swallowing.

The five muscles of the soft palate arise from the base of the cranium and descend to the palate. The muscles of the soft palate are illustrated in Figure 8.88 and their attachments, nerve supply, and actions are described in Table 8.14. Note that the direction of pull of the belly of the *tensor veli palatini* is redirected approximately 90° because its tendon uses the pterygoid hamulus as a pulley or trochlea, allow-

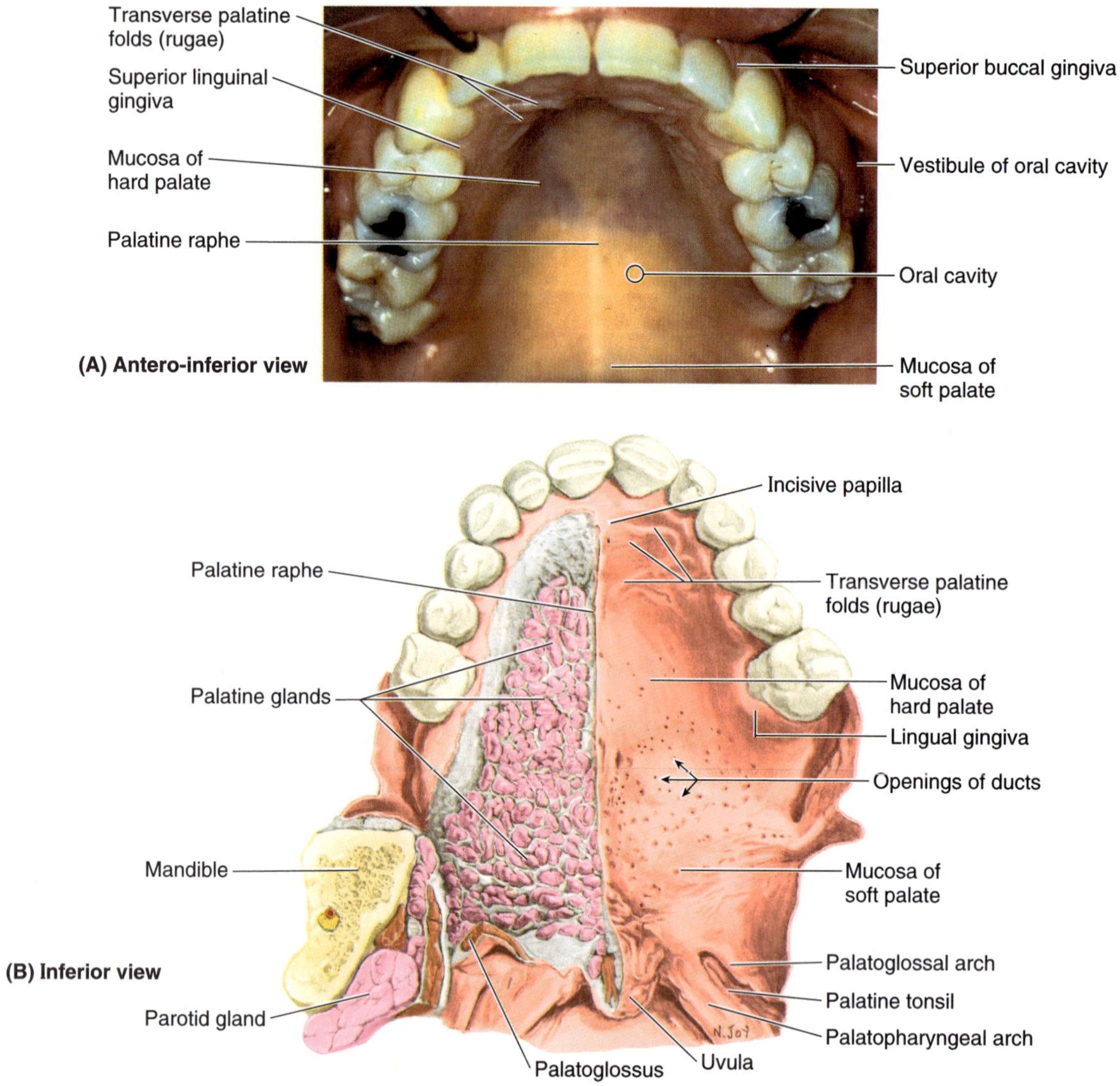

FIGURE 8.87. Maxillary teeth and palate. A. The maxillary teeth and the mucosa covering the hard palate in a living person are shown. **B.** The mucous membrane and glands of the palate are demonstrated. The orifices of the ducts of the palatine glands give the mucous membrane an orange-skin appearance. The palatine glands form a thick layer in the soft palate and a thin one in the hard palate; they are absent in the region of the incisive fossa and the anterior part of the palatine raphe. (Part **A** Courtesy of Dr. B. Liebgott, Professor, Division of Anatomy, Department of Surgery, University of Toronto, Toronto, Ontario, Canada.)

ing it to pull horizontally on the aponeurosis (Figs. 8.86B and 8.88).

VASCULATURE AND INNERVATION OF PALATE

The palate has a rich blood supply, chiefly from the **greater palatine artery** on each side, a branch of the descending palatine artery (Fig. 8.89). The greater palatine artery passes through the greater palatine foramen and runs anteromedially. The **lesser palatine artery**, a smaller branch of the descending palatine artery, enters the palate through the lesser palatine foramen and anastomoses with the **ascending palatine artery**, a branch of the facial artery (Fig. 8.89B). The **veins of the palate** are tributaries of the *pterygoid venous plexus*.

The *sensory nerves of the palate* are branches of the maxillary nerve (CNV_2), which branch from the *pterygopalatine ganglion* (Fig. 8.89A). The **greater palatine nerve** supplies the gingivae, mucous membrane, and glands of most of the hard palate. The **nasopalatine nerve** supplies the mucous membrane of the anterior part of the hard palate (Fig. 8.89B). The **lesser palatine nerves** supply the soft palate. The palatine nerves accompany the arteries through the greater and lesser palatine foramina, respectively. Except for the tensor veli palatini supplied by CN V_3, all muscles of the soft palate are supplied through the *pharyngeal plexus of nerves* (see Chapter 9, Neck).

For development and developmental basis of congenital anomalies of palate, refer *Langman's Medical Embryology*, South Asian Edition Chapter 17, Head and Neck, pp. 310, 313. AN43.4

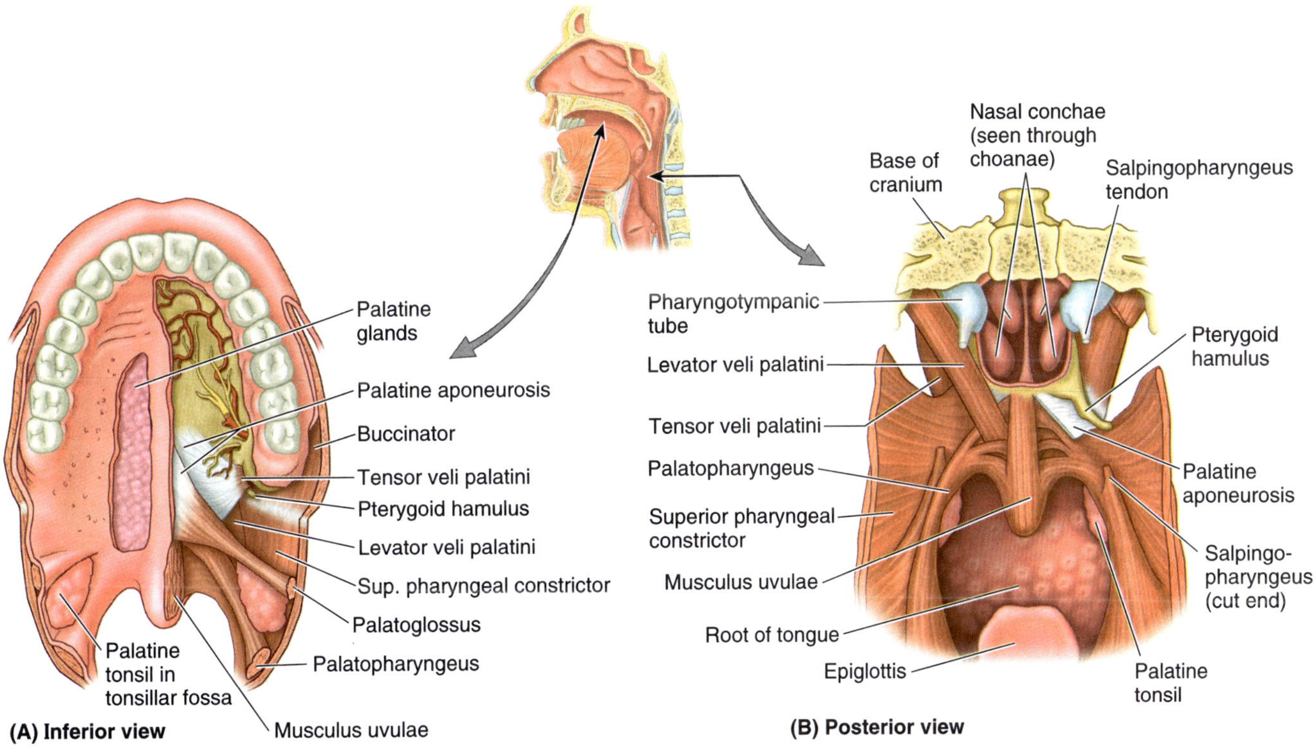

FIGURE 8.88. Muscles of soft palate.

TABLE 8.14. MUSCLES OF SOFT PALATE

Muscle	Superior Attachment	Inferior Attachment	Innervation	Main Action
Tensor veli palatini	Scaphoid fossa of medial pterygoid plate, spine of sphenoid bone, and cartilage of pharyngotympanic tube	Palatine aponeurosis	Medial pterygoid nerve (a branch of mandibular nerve, CN V_3) via otic ganglion	Tenses soft palate and opens mouth of pharyngotympanic tube during swallowing and yawning
Levator veli palatini	Cartilage of pharyngotympanic tube and petrous part of temporal bone		Pharyngeal branch of vagus nerve (CN X) via pharyngeal plexus	Elevates soft palate during swallowing and yawning
Palatoglossus	Palatine aponeurosis	Side of tongue		Elevates posterior part of tongue and draws soft palate onto tongue
Palatopharyngeus	Hard palate and palatine aponeurosis	Lateral wall of pharynx		Tenses soft palate and pulls walls of pharynx superiorly, anteriorly, and medially during swallowing
Musculus uvulae	Posterior nasal spine and palatine aponeurosis	Mucosa of uvula		Shortens uvula and pulls it superiorly

Tongue

AN39.1 The **tongue** (L. *lingua*; G. *glossa*) is a mobile muscular organ covered with mucous membrane. It can assume a variety of shapes and positions. It is partly in the oral cavity and partly in the oropharynx. The tongue's main functions are articulation (forming words during speaking) and squeezing food into the oropharynx as part of deglutition (swallowing). The tongue is also involved with mastication (chewing), taste, and oral cleansing.

PARTS AND SURFACES OF TONGUE

The tongue has a root, body, and apex (Fig. 8.90A). The **root of the tongue** is the attached posterior portion, extending between the mandible, hyoid, and the nearly vertical posterior surface of the tongue. The **body of the tongue** is the anterior, approximately two thirds of the tongue between root and apex. The **apex** (tip) of the tongue is the anterior end of the body, which rests against the incisor teeth. The body and apex of the tongue are extremely mobile.

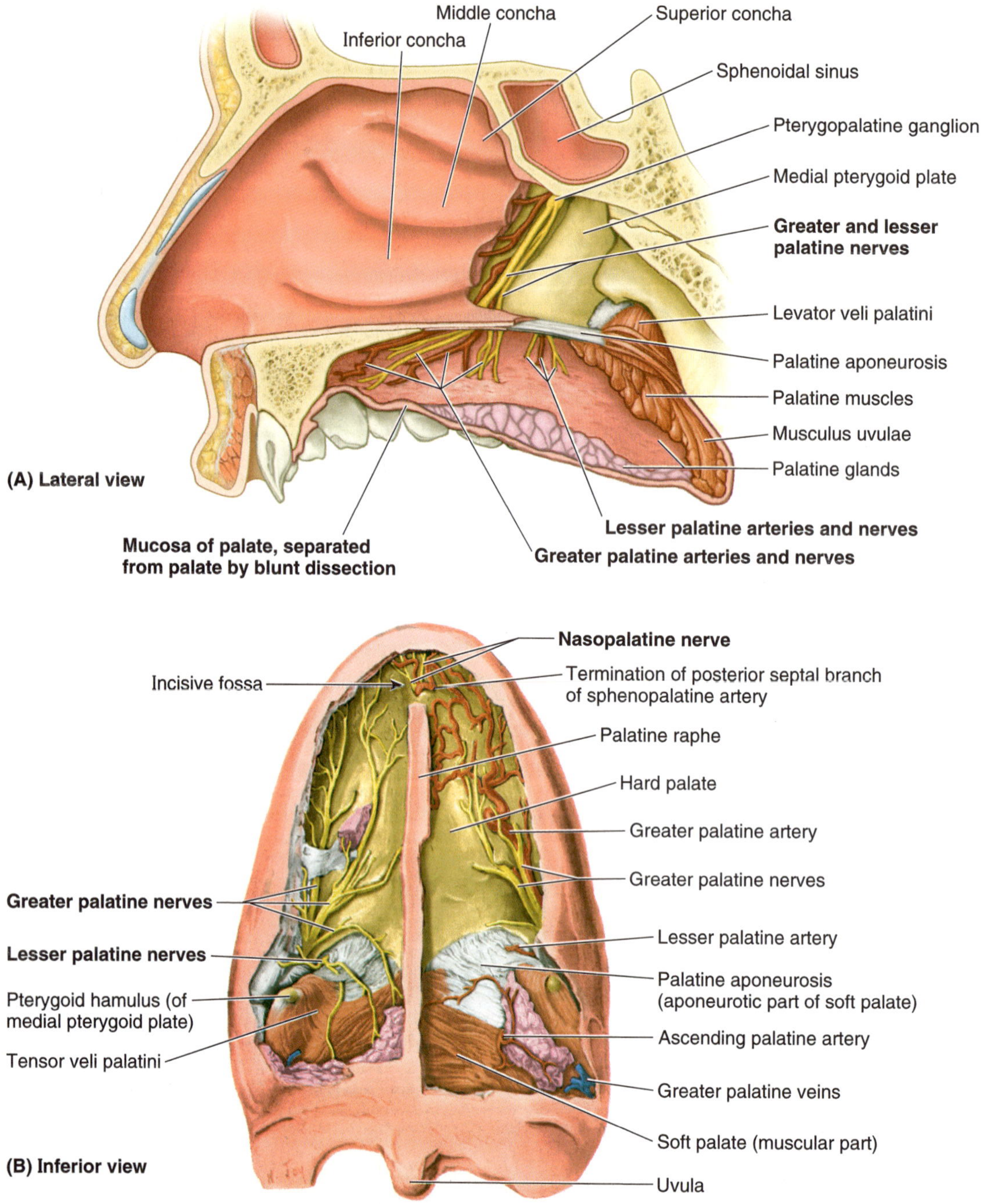

FIGURE 8.89. Nerves and vessels of palate. A. In this dissection of the posterior part of the lateral wall of the nasal cavity and the palate, the mucous membrane of the palate, containing a layer of mucous glands, has been separated from the hard and soft regions of the palate by blunt dissection. The posterior ends of the middle and inferior nasal conchae are cut through; these and the mucoperiosteum are pulled off the side wall of the nose as far as the posterior border of the medial pterygoid plate. The perpendicular plate of the palatine bone is broken through to expose the palatine nerves and arteries descending from the pterygopalatine fossa in the palatine canal. **B.** The nerves and vessels of an edentulous palate are shown. The mucosa has been removed on each side of the palatine raphe, demonstrating a branch of the greater palatine nerve on each side and the artery on the lateral side. There are four palatine arteries, two on the hard palate (greater palatine and the terminal branch of posterior nasal septal/sphenopalatine artery) and two on the soft palate (lesser palatine and ascending palatine).

The tongue features two surfaces. The more extensive, superior and posterior surface is the *dorsum of the tongue* ("top" of the tongue). The *inferior surface of the tongue* (commonly referred to as its "underside") usually rests against the floor of the mouth. The margin of the tongue separating the two surfaces is related on each side to the lingual gingivae and lateral teeth (see Fig. 8.92C). The **dorsum of the tongue** is characterized by a V-shaped groove, the **terminal sulcus of the tongue**, the angle of which points posteriorly to the *foramen cecum* (Fig. 8.90B). This small pit, frequently absent, is the nonfunctional remnant of the proximal part of the embryonic thyroglossal duct from which the thyroid gland developed. The terminal sulcus divides the dorsum of the tongue transversely into a presulcal **anterior**

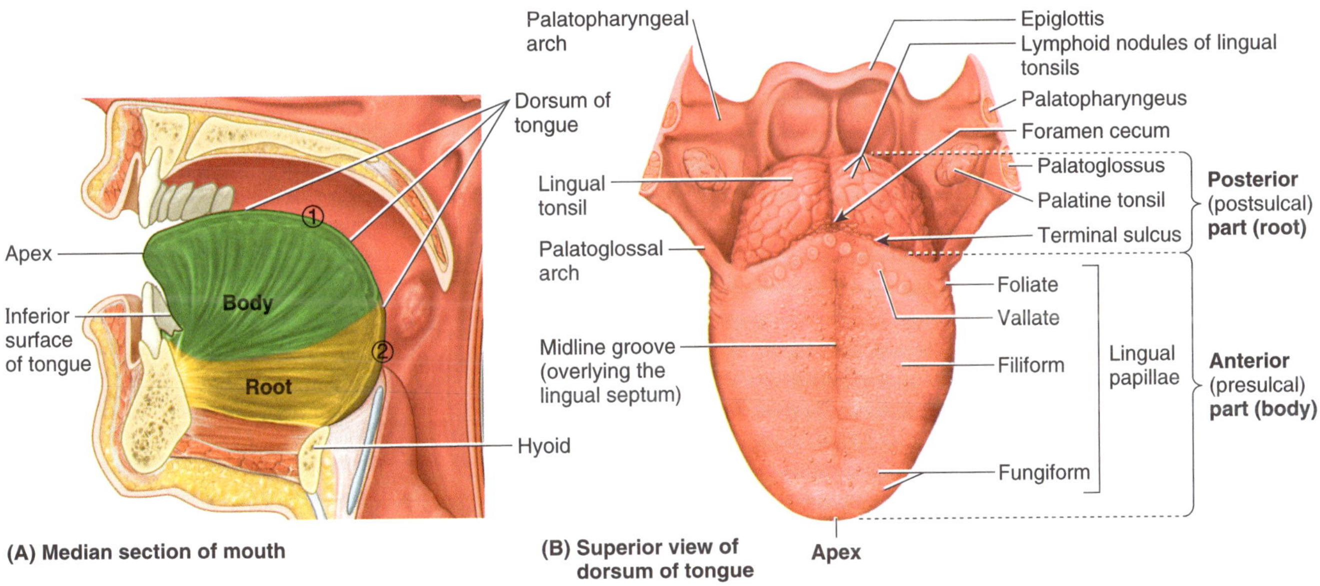

FIGURE 8.90. Parts and features of tongue. A. The anterior free part constituting the majority of the mass of the tongue is the body of the tongue. The superior surface of the body in the oral cavity (1) is the dorsum. The posterior attached portion with an oropharyngeal surface (2) is the root of the tongue. **B.** The anterior (two thirds) and posterior (third) parts of the dorsum of the tongue are separated by the terminal sulcus (groove) and foramen cecum. *Brackets*, indicate parts of the dorsum of the tongue and do not embrace specific labels.

part in the oral cavity proper and a postsulcal **posterior part** in the oropharynx.

A midline groove divides the anterior part of the tongue into right and left parts. The *mucosa of the anterior part* of the tongue is relatively thin and closely attached to the underlying muscle. It has a rough texture because of numerous small **lingual papillae**:

- **Vallate papillae**: large and flat topped, lie directly anterior to the terminal sulcus and are arranged in a V-shaped row. They are surrounded by deep circular trenches, the walls of which are studded with *taste buds*. The ducts of the serous glands of the tongue open into the trenches.
- **Foliate papillae**: small lateral folds of the lingual mucosa. They are poorly developed in humans.
- **Filiform papillae**: long and numerous, contain afferent nerve endings that are sensitive to touch. These scaly, conical projections are pinkish gray and are arranged in V-shaped rows that are parallel to the terminal sulcus, except at the apex, where they tend to be arranged transversely.
- **Fungiform papillae**: mushroom-shaped pink or red spots scattered among the filiform papillae, but most numerous at the apex and margins of the tongue.

The vallate, foliate, and most of the fungiform papillae contain taste receptors in the taste buds.

The *mucosa of the posterior part* of the tongue is thick and freely movable. It has no lingual papillae, but the underlying **lymphoid nodules** give this part of the tongue an irregular, cobblestone appearance. The lymphoid nodules are known collectively as the **lingual tonsil**. The pharyngeal part of the tongue constitutes the anterior wall of the oropharynx. It can be inspected only with a mirror or downward pressure on the tongue with a tongue depressor.

The **inferior surface of the tongue** is covered with a thin, transparent mucous membrane (Fig. 8.91). This surface is connected to the floor of the mouth by a midline fold called the **frenulum of the tongue**. The frenulum allows the anterior part of the tongue to move freely. On each side of the frenulum, a deep lingual vein is visible through the thin mucous membrane. A **sublingual caruncle** (papilla) is present on each side of the base of the frenulum of the tongue that includes the *opening of the submandibular duct* from the submandibular salivary gland.

MUSCLES OF TONGUE

AN39.

The tongue is essentially a mass of muscles that is mostly covered by mucosa (mucous membrane—Fig. 8.92; Table 8.15). As with the orbital muscles, it is traditional to provide descriptions of the actions of tongue muscles (1) ascribing a single action to a specific muscle or (2) implying that a particular movement is the consequence of a single muscle acting. This approach facilitates learning but greatly oversimplifies the actions of the tongue. The muscles of the tongue do not act in isolation, and some muscles perform multiple actions. Parts of a single muscle are capable of acting independently, producing different, even antagonistic actions. In general, *extrinsic muscles alter the position of the tongue*, and *intrinsic muscles alter its shape*. The four intrinsic and four extrinsic muscles in each half of the tongue are separated by a median fibrous **lingual septum** (Fig. 8.92C), which merges posteriorly with the lingual aponeurosis (a tough sheet of connective tissue, the lamina propria, deep to the dorsal mucous membrane of the tongue, into which lingual muscles insert—Fig. 8.92B).

Extrinsic Muscles of Tongue. The **extrinsic muscles of the tongue** (genioglossus, hyoglossus, styloglossus, and palatoglossus) originate outside the tongue and attach to it. They

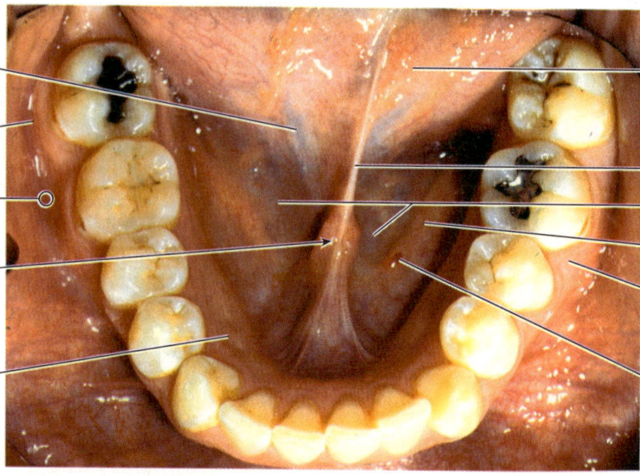

FIGURE 8.91. Floor of mouth and oral vestibule. The tongue is elevated and retracted superiorly. (Courtesy of Dr. B. Liebgott, Professor, Division of Anatomy, Department of Surgery, University of Toronto, Toronto, Ontario, Canada.)

mainly move the tongue but they can alter its shape as well. They are illustrated in Figure 8.92, and their shape, position, attachments, and main actions are described in Table 8.15.

Intrinsic Muscles of Tongue. The superior and inferior longitudinal, transverse, and vertical muscles are confined to the tongue. They have their attachments entirely within the tongue and are not attached to bone. They are illustrated in Figure 8.92, and their shape, position, attachments, and main actions are described in Table 8.15. The **superior** and **inferior longitudinal muscles** act together to make the tongue short and thick and to retract the protruded tongue. The **transverse** and **vertical muscles** act simultaneously to make the tongue long and narrow, which may push the tongue against the incisor teeth or protrude the tongue from the open mouth (especially when acting with the posterior inferior part of the genioglossus).

INNERVATION OF TONGUE

AN39.1 All muscles of the tongue, except the *palatoglossus*, receive motor innervation from CN XII, the **hypoglossal nerve** (Fig. 8.93). Palatoglossus is a palatine muscle supplied by the *pharyngeal plexus* (see Fig. 8.46A). For general sensation (touch and temperature), the mucosa of the anterior two thirds of the tongue is supplied by the *lingual nerve*, a branch of CN V_3 (Figs. 8.93, 8.97, and 8.98). For special sensation (taste), this part of the tongue, except for the vallate papillae, is supplied the *chorda tympani nerve*, a branch of CN VII. The chorda tympani joins the lingual nerve in the infratemporal fossa and runs anteriorly in its sheath. The mucosa of the posterior third of the tongue and the vallate papillae are supplied by the lingual branch of the *glossopharyngeal nerve* (CN IX) for both general and special sensation (Fig. 8.93). Twigs of the **internal laryngeal nerve**, a branch of the vagus nerve (CN X), supply mostly general but some special sensation to a small area of the tongue just anterior to the epiglottis. These mostly sensory nerves also carry **parasympathetic secretomotor fibers** to serous glands in the tongue.

Traditionally, *four basic taste sensations are described: sweet, salty, sour,* and *bitter*. A fifth basic taste (*umami*-stimulated by monosodium glutamate) has more recently been identified. Certain areas of the tongue have been described as being most sensitive to the different tastes, but evidence indicates all areas are capable of detecting all tastes. Other "tastes" expressed by gourmets are influenced by olfactory sensation (smell and aroma).

VASCULATURE OF TONGUE

The *arteries of the tongue* are derived from the **lingual artery**, AN39.1 which arises from the *external carotid artery* (Fig. 8.94). On entering the tongue, the lingual artery passes deep to the hyoglossus muscle. The **dorsal lingual arteries** supply the root of the tongue; the **deep lingual arteries** supply the body of the tongue. The deep lingual arteries communicate with each other near the apex of the tongue. The dorsal lingual arteries are prevented from communicating by the *lingual septum* (Fig. 8.92C).

The *veins of the tongue* are the **dorsal lingual veins**, which accompany the lingual artery. The **deep lingual veins**, which begin at the apex of the tongue, run posteriorly beside the lingual frenulum to join the **sublingual vein** (Fig. 8.95). The sublingual veins in elderly people are often varicose (enlarged and tortuous). Some or all of the veins may drain into the IJV, or they may do so indirectly, joining first to form a **lingual vein** that accompanies the initial part of the lingual artery.

The **lymphatic drainage of the tongue** is exceptional. Most of the lymphatic drainage converges toward and follows the venous drainage; however, lymph from the tip of the tongue, frenulum, and central lower lip runs an independent course (Fig. 8.96). *Lymph from different areas of the tongue drains via four routes*:

1. Lymph from the *root of the tongue* drains bilaterally into the **superior deep cervical lymph nodes**.
2. Lymph from the *medial part of the body* drains bilaterally and directly to the **inferior deep cervical lymph nodes**.
3. Lymph from the right and left *lateral parts of body* drains to the submandibular **lymph nodes on the ipsilateral side**.
4. The *apex and frenulum* drain to the **submental lymph nodes**, the medial portion draining bilaterally.

(*continued on p.* 1002)

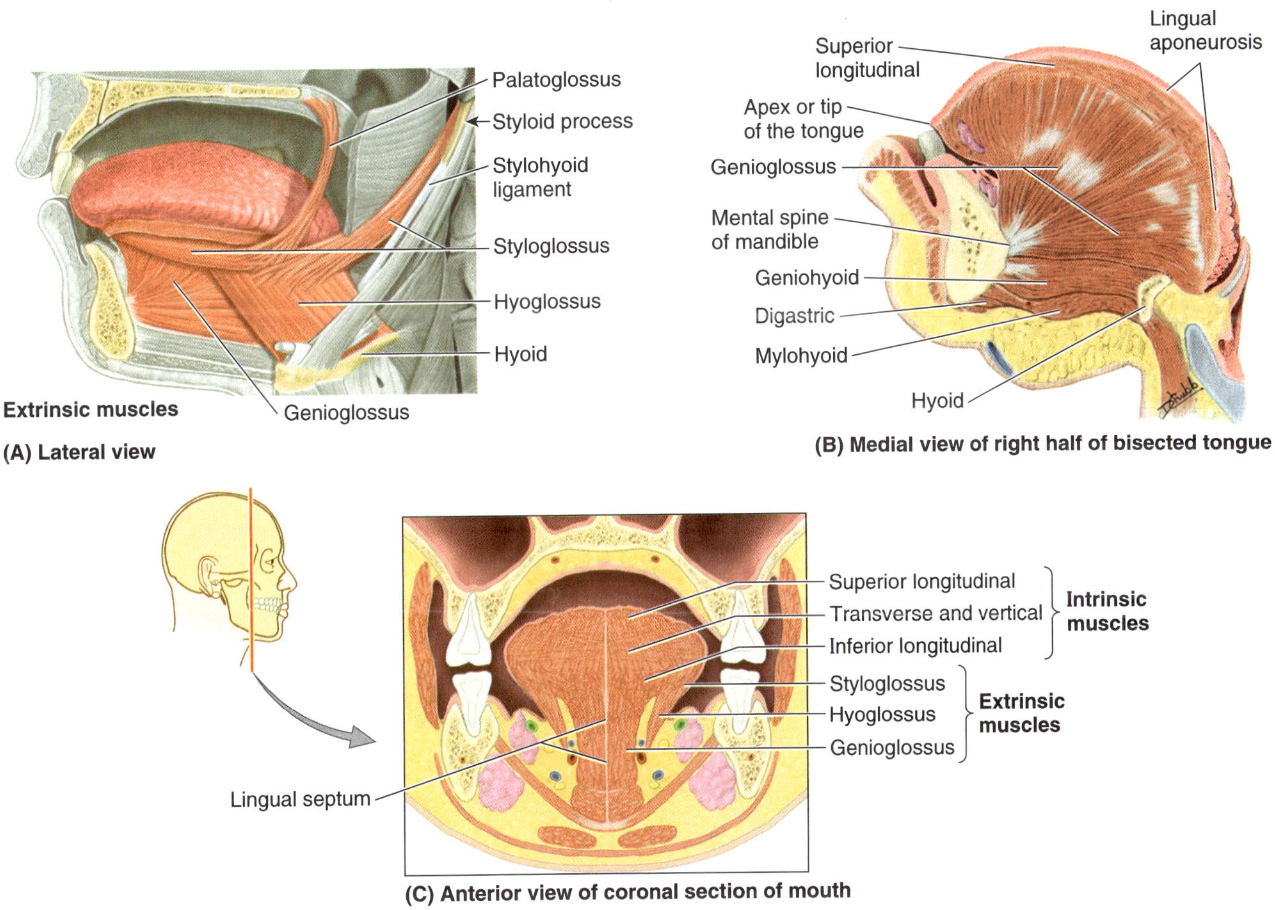

FIGURE 8.92. Muscles of tongue.

TABLE 8.15. MUSCLES OF TONGUE

Muscle	Shape and Position	Proximal Attachment	Distal Attachment	Main Action(s)
Extrinsic muscles of tongue[a]				
Genioglossus	Fan-shaped muscle; constitutes bulk of tongue	Via a short tendon from superior part of mental spine of mandible	Entire dorsum of tongue; inferiormost and posteriormost fibers attach to body of hyoid bone.	Bilateral activity depresses tongue, especially central part, creating a longitudinal furrow; posterior part pulls tongue anteriorly for protrusion; most anterior part retracts apex of protruded tongue; unilateral contraction deviates tongue to contralateral side.
Hyoglossus	Thin, quadrilateral muscle	Body and greater horn of hyoid bone	Inferior aspects of lateral part of tongue	Depresses tongue, especially pulling its sides inferiorly; helps shorten (retrude) tongue
Styloglossus	Small, short triangular muscle	Anterior border of distal styloid process; stylohyoid ligament	Sides of tongue posteriorly, interdigitating with hyoglossus	Retrudes tongue and curls (elevates) its sides, working with genioglossus to form a central trough during swallowing
Palatoglossus[b]	Narrow crescent-shaped palatine muscle; forms posterior column of isthmus of fauces	Palatine aponeurosis of soft palate	Enters posterolateral tongue transversely, blending with intrinsic transverse muscles	Capable of elevating posterior tongue or depressing soft palate; most commonly acts to constrict isthmus of fauces.

TABLE 8.15. MUSCLES OF TONGUE (Continued)

Muscle	Shape and Position	Proximal Attachment	Distal Attachment	Main Action(s)
Intrinsic muscles of tongue[a]				
Superior longitudinal	Thin layer deep to mucous membrane of dorsum	Submucosal fibrous layer and median fibrous septum	Margins of tongue and mucous membrane	Curls tongue longitudinally upward, elevating apex and sides of tongue; shortens (retrudes) tongue
Inferior longitudinal	Narrow band close to inferior surface	Root of tongue and body of hyoid bone	Apex of tongue	Curls tongue longitudinally downward, depressing apex; shortens (retrudes) tongue
Transverse	Deep to superior longitudinal muscle	Median fibrous septum	Fibrous tissue at lateral lingual margins	Narrows and elongates (protrudes) tongue[c]
Vertical	Fibers intersect transverse muscle	Submucosal fibrous layer of dorsum of tongue	Inferior surface of borders of tongue	Flattens and broadens tongue[c]

[a]Except for palatoglossus, the muscles of the tongue are innervated by the hypoglossal nerve (CN XII).
[b]A palatine muscle, the palatoglossus is innervated by the vagus nerve (CN X).
[c]Act simultaneously to protrude tongue.

All lymph from the tongue ultimately drains to the deep cervical nodes and passes via the jugular venous trunks into the venous system at the right and left venous angles.

N43.2 For microanatomy of tongue, refer *diFiore's Atlas of Histology with Functional Correlations*, 1st South Asian Edition, Chapter 13, Digestive System Part I: Oral Cavity and Major Salivary Glands, p. 322.

N43.4 For development and developmental basis of congenital anomalies of tongue, refer *Langman's Medical Embryology*, South Asian Edition, Chapter 17, Head and Neck, p. 306.

Salivary Glands

The **salivary glands** are the parotid, submandibular, and sublingual glands (Fig. 8.97). The clear, tasteless, odorless viscid fluid, **saliva**, secreted by these glands and the mucous glands of the oral cavity

- keeps the mucous membrane of the mouth moist.
- lubricates the food during mastication.
- begins the digestion of starches.
- serves as an intrinsic "mouthwash."
- plays significant roles in the prevention of tooth decay and in the ability to taste.

In addition to the main salivary glands, small **accessory salivary glands** are scattered over the palate, lips, cheeks, tonsils, and tongue. The *parotid glands*, the largest of the

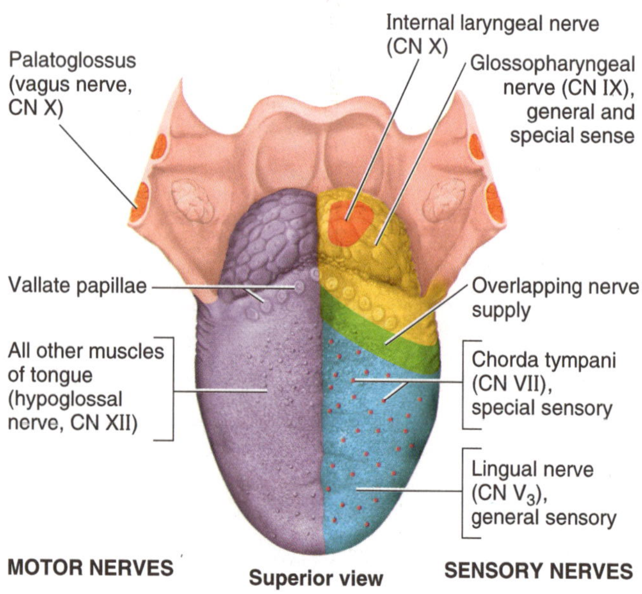

FIGURE 8.93. **Nerve supply to parts of tongue.**

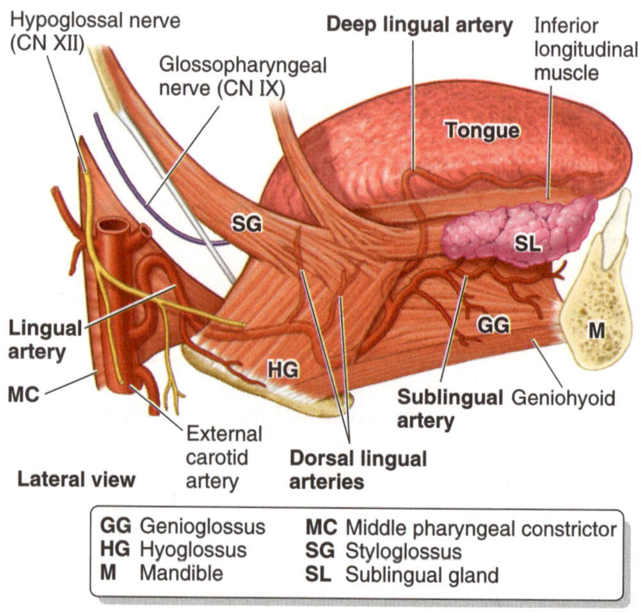

FIGURE 8.94. **Blood supply of tongue.** The main artery to the tongue is the lingual artery, a branch of the external carotid artery. The dorsal lingual arteries provide the blood supply to the root of the tongue and a branch to the palatine tonsil. The deep lingual arteries supply the body of the tongue. The sublingual arteries provide the blood supply to the floor of the mouth, including the sublingual glands.

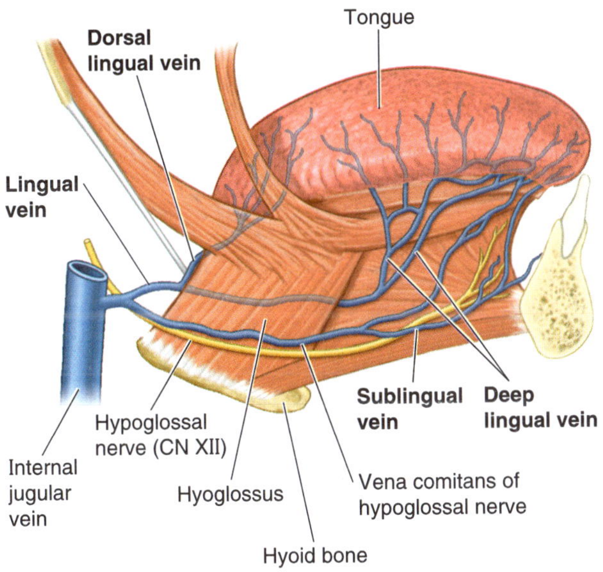

FIGURE 8.95. **Venous drainage of tongue.**

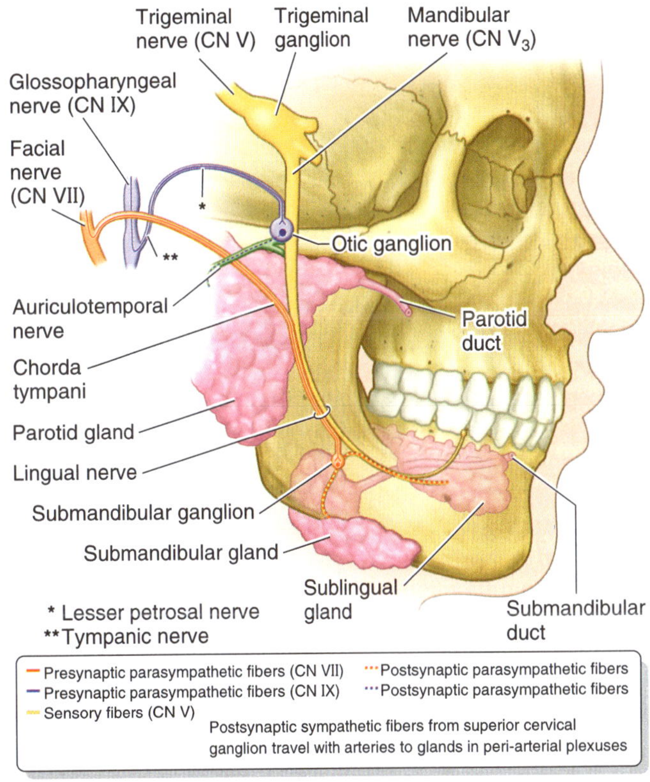

FIGURE 8.97. **Innervation of salivary glands.**

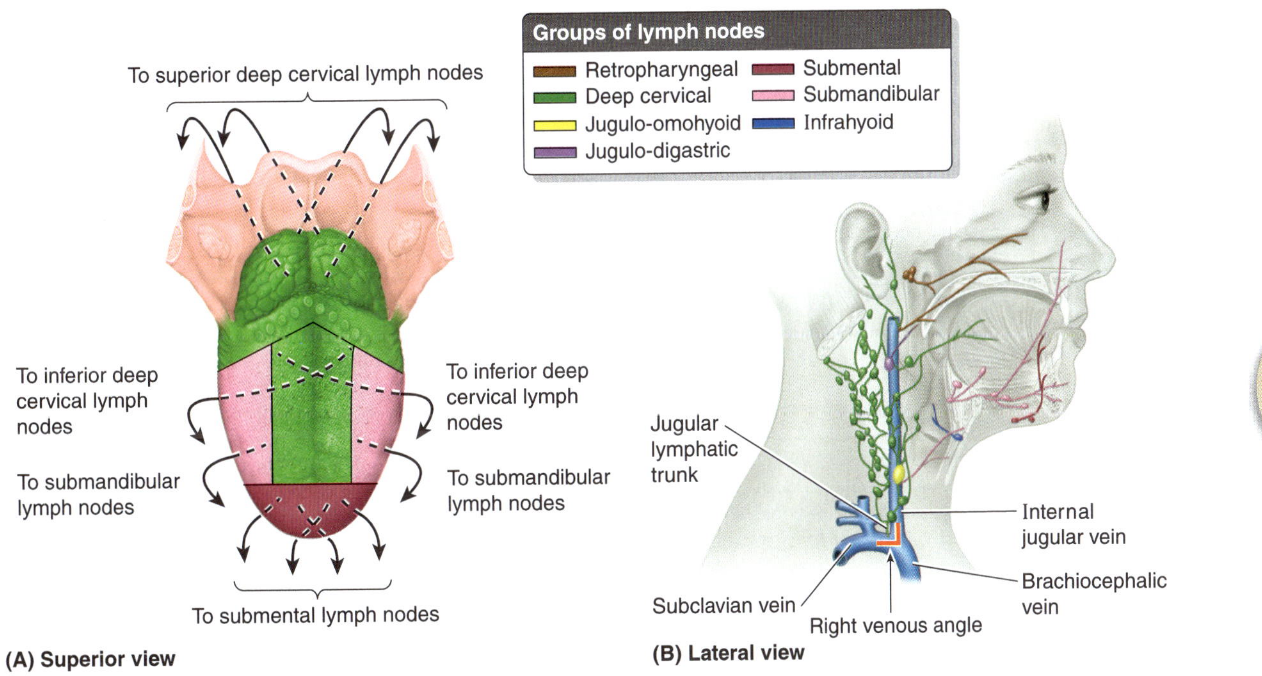

FIGURE 8.96. **Lymphatic drainage of tongue.** **A.** The dorsum of the tongue is shown. **B.** Lymph drains to the submental, submandibular, and superior and inferior deep cervical lymph nodes, including the jugulodigastric and jugulo-omohyoid nodes. Extensive communications occur across the midline of the tongue.

three paired salivary glands, were discussed earlier in this chapter. The parotid glands are located lateral and posterior to the rami of the mandible and masseter muscles, within unyielding fibrous sheaths. The parotid glands drain anteriorly via single ducts that enter the oral vestibule opposite the second maxillary molar teeth (see Fig. 8.67).

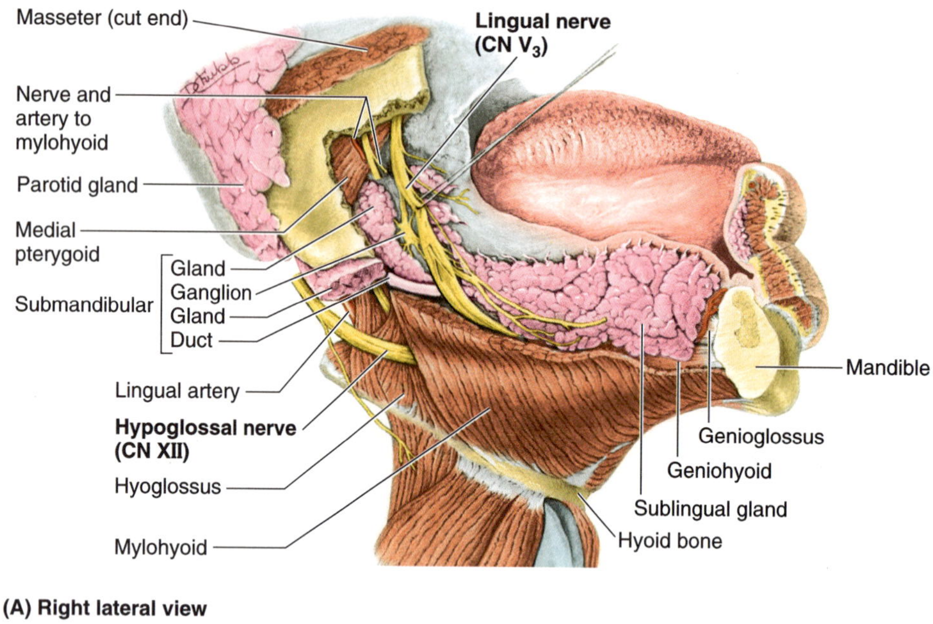

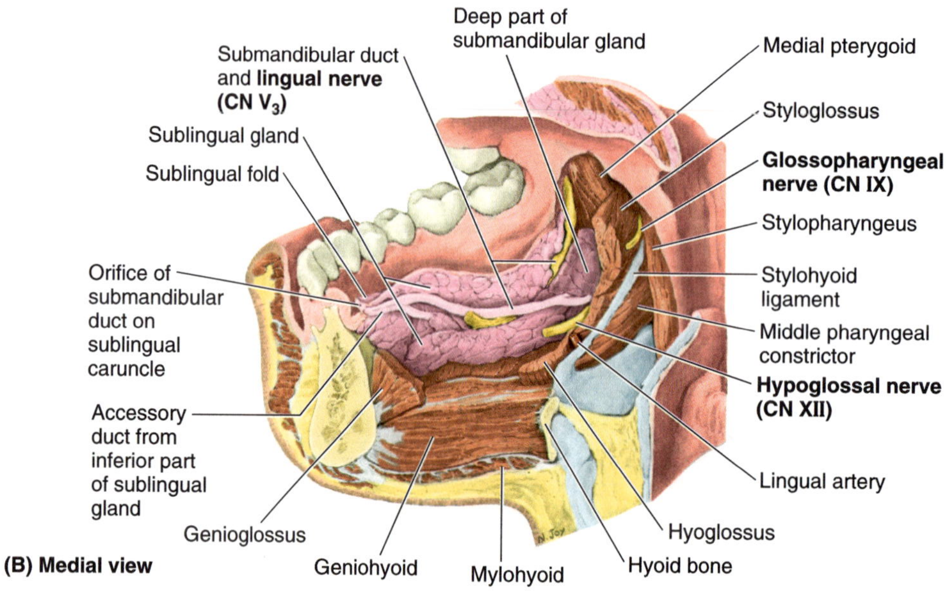

FIGURE 8.98. Parotid, submandibular, and sublingual salivary glands. A. The body and parts of the ramus of the mandible have been removed. The parotid gland contacts the deep part of the submandibular gland posteriorly. Fine ducts passing from the superior border of the sublingual gland open on the sublingual fold. **B.** The right sublingual and submandibular glands and the floor of the mouth are shown. The tongue has been excised. The orifice of the duct of the submandibular gland is visible at the anterior end of the sublingual fold. The submandibular duct adheres to the medial side of the sublingual gland. Here it is receiving, as it sometimes does, a large accessory duct from the inferior part of the sublingual gland. The sublingual caruncluae are bilateral papillae flanking the frenulum of the tongue, each bearing the opening of the ipsilateral submandibular duct.

SUBMANDIBULAR GLANDS

AN34.1 The **submandibular glands** lie along the body of the mandible, partly superior and partly inferior to the posterior half of the mandible, and partly superficial and partly deep to the mylohyoid muscle (Fig. 8.98). The **submandibular duct**, approximately 5 cm long, arises from the portion of the gland that lies between the mylohyoid and hyoglossus muscles. Passing from lateral to medial, the *lingual nerve* loops under the duct that runs anteriorly, opening by one to three orifices on a small sublingual papilla beside the base of the frenulum of the tongue (Fig. 8.98B). The orifices of the submandibular ducts are visible, and saliva can often be seen trickling from them (or spraying from them during yawning). The **arterial supply of the submandibular glands** is from the **submental arteries** (Fig. 8.94). The **veins** accompany the arteries. The **lymphatic vessels** of the glands end in the *deep cervical lymph nodes*, particularly the *jugulo-omohyoid node* (Fig. 8.96B).

N43.2 For microanatomy of mixed salivary gland, refer *diFiore's Atlas of Histology with Functional Correlations*, 1st South Asian Edition, Chapter 13, Digestive System Part I: Oral Cavity and Major Salivary Glands, pp. 336–337.

The submandibular glands are supplied by presynaptic parasympathetic secretomotor fibers conveyed from the facial nerve to the lingual nerve by the chorda tympani nerve, which synapse with postsynaptic neurons in the submandibular ganglion (Fig. 8.97). The latter fibers accompany arteries to reach the gland, along with vasoconstrictive postsynaptic sympathetic fibers from the superior cervical ganglion.

Submandibular ganglion is related to the lingual nerve AN34.1 but functionally to the chorda tympani nerve. It lies deep to the submandibular salivary gland on the surface of the hyoglossus muscle and is attached to the lingual nerve by small nerves (Fig. 8.99).

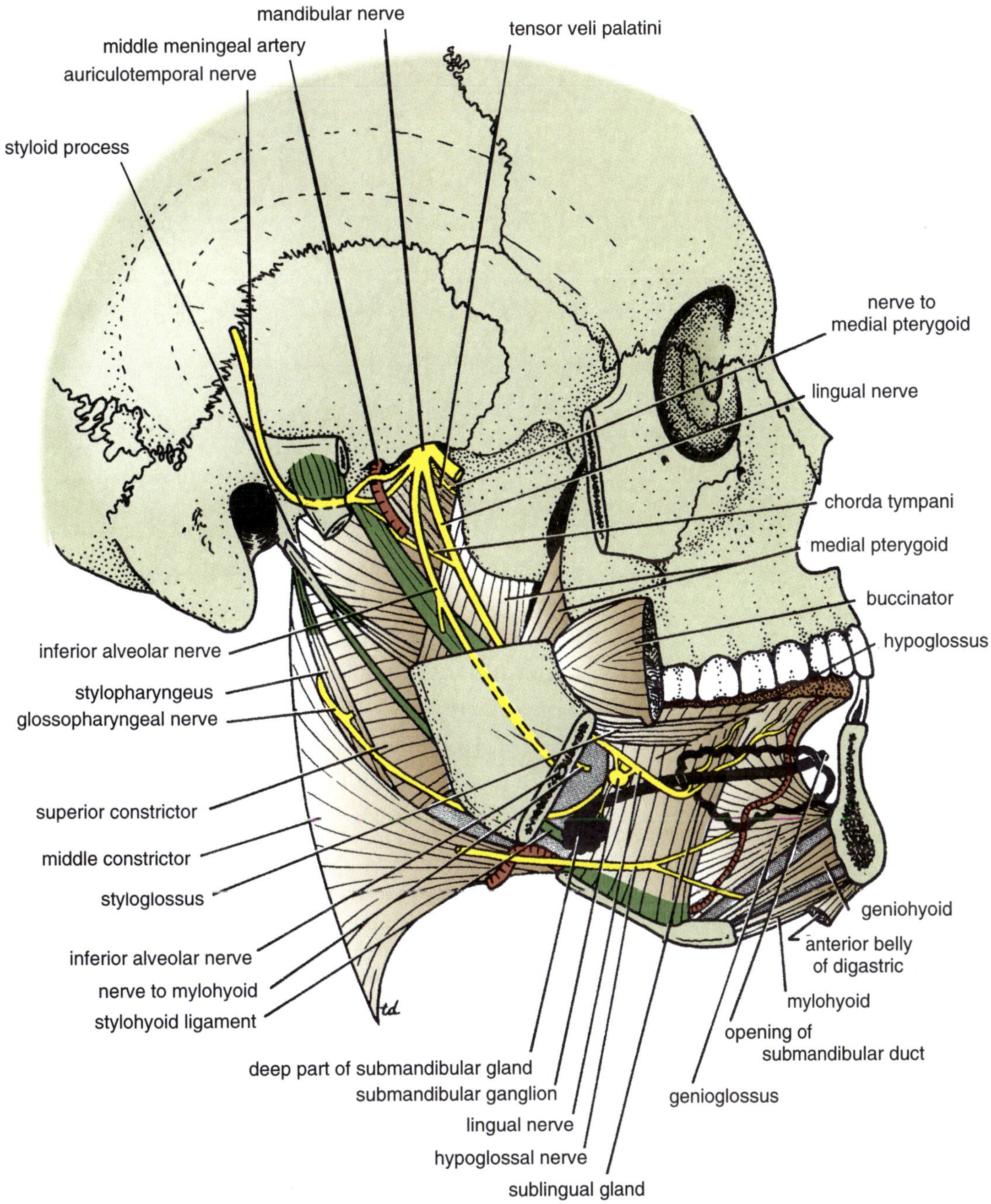

FIGURE 8.99. Infratemporal and submandibular regions. Parts of the zygomatic arch, the ramus, and the body of the mandible have been removed. Mylohyoid and lateral pterygoid muscles have also been removed to display deeper structures. The outline of the sublingual gland is shown as a solid black wavy line.

8

SUBLINGUAL GLANDS

The **sublingual glands** are the smallest and most deeply situated of the salivary glands (Fig. 8.98). Each almond-shaped gland lies in the floor of the mouth between the mandible and the genioglossus muscle. The glands from each side unite to form a horseshoe-shaped mass around the connective tissue core of the frenulum of the tongue. Numerous small **sublingual ducts** open into the floor of the mouth along the sublingual folds. The **arterial supply of the sublingual glands** is from the *sublingual* and *submental arteries*, branches of the lingual and facial arteries, respectively (Fig. 8.94). The **nerves of the glands** accompany those of the submandibular gland. Presynaptic parasympathetic secretomotor fibers are conveyed by the facial, chorda tympani, and lingual nerves to synapse in the submandibular ganglion (Fig. 8.97).

For microanatomy of mucus salivary gland, refer *diFiore's Atlas of Histology with Functional Correlations*, 1st South Asian Edition, Chapter 13, Digestive System Part I: Oral Cavity and Major Salivary Glands, pp. 337–338. AN43

CLINICAL BOX

ORAL REGION

Cleft Lip

Cleft lip (*harelip*, a misnomer) is a birth defect (usually of the upper lip) that occurs in 1 of 1,000 births; 60–80% of affected infants are males. The clefts vary from a small notch in the transitional zone of the lip and vermilion border to a notch that extends through the lip into the nose (Fig. B8.33). In severe cases, the cleft extends deeper and is continuous with a cleft in the palate. Cleft lip may be unilateral or bilateral (Moore et al., 2016).

Cyanosis of Lips

The lips, like fingers, have an abundant, relatively superficial arterial blood flow. Because of this, they can lose a disproportionate amount of body heat when exposed to a cold environment. Both lips are provided with sympathetically innervated arteriovenous anastomoses, capable of redirecting a considerable portion of the blood back to the body core, reducing heat loss while producing cyanosis of the lips and fingers. *Cyanosis*, a dark bluish or purplish coloration of the lips and mucous membranes, results from deficient oxygenation of capillary blood and is a sign of many pathologic conditions. The common blue discoloration of the lips owing to cold exposure does not indicate pathology. Instead, it results from the decreased blood flow in the capillary beds supplied by the superior and inferior labial arteries and the increased extraction of oxygen. Simple warming restores the normal coloring of the lips.

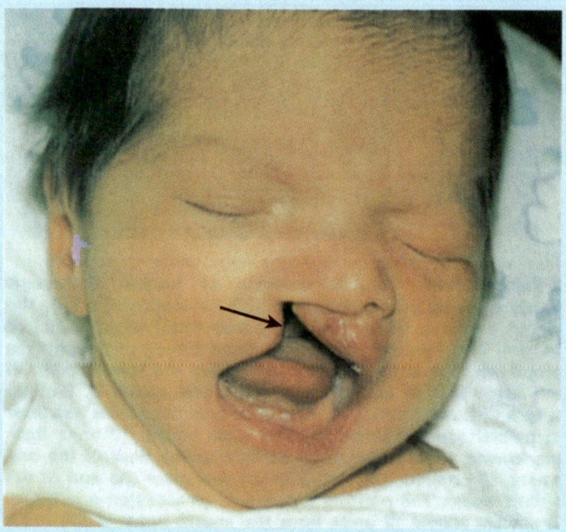

FIGURE B8.33. Unilateral cleft lip (*arrow*).

Large Labial Frenulum

An excessively large superior labial frenulum in children may cause a space between the central incisor teeth. Resection of the frenulum and the underlying connective tissue (*frenulectomy*) between the incisors allows approximation of the teeth, which may require an orthodontic appliance ("brace"). A large lower labial frenulum in adults may pull on the labial gingiva and contribute to *gingival recession*, which results in an abnormal exposure of the roots of the teeth.

Gingivitis

Improper oral hygiene results in food and bacterial deposits in tooth and gingival crevices that may cause inflammation of the gingivae (*gingivitis*). The gingivae swell and redden as a result. If untreated, the disease spreads to other supporting structures, including alveolar bone, producing *periodontitis* (inflammation and destruction of bone and periodontium). *Dento-alveolar abscesses* (collections of pus resulting from death of inflamed tissues) may drain to the oral cavity and lips.

Dental Caries, Pulpitis, and Tooth Abscesses

Acid, enzymes, or both produced by oral bacteria may break down (decay) the hard tissues of a tooth. This results in the formation of *dental caries* (*cavities*) (Fig. B8.34A–C). Neglected dental caries eventually invade and inflame tissues in the pulp cavity (Fig. B8.34B, C). Invasion of the pulp by a deep carious lesion results in infection and irritation of the tissues (*pulpitis*). Because the pulp cavity is a rigid space, the swollen tissues cause considerable pain (*toothache*). If untreated, the small vessels in the root canal may die from the pressure of the swollen tissue, and the infected material may pass through the apical canal and foramen into the periodontal tissues (Fig. B8.34C). An infective process develops and spreads through the root canal to the alveolar bone, producing an *abscess* (*peri-apical disease*). If untreated, loss of the tooth may occur with an abscess remaining (Fig. B8.34D). Treatment involves removal of the decayed tissue and restoration of the anatomy of the tooth with prosthetic dental material (commonly referred to as a "filling") (Fig. B8.34E).

Pus from an abscess of a maxillary molar tooth may extend into the nasal cavity or the maxillary sinus. The roots of the maxillary molar teeth are closely related to the floor of this sinus. As a consequence, infection of the pulp cavity may also cause sinusitis, or sinusitis may stimulate nerves entering the teeth and simulate a toothache. The roots of mandibular teeth are closely related to the mandibular canal (Fig. B8.34E), and abscess formation may compress the nerve causing pain that may be referred to (perceived as coming from) more anterior teeth.

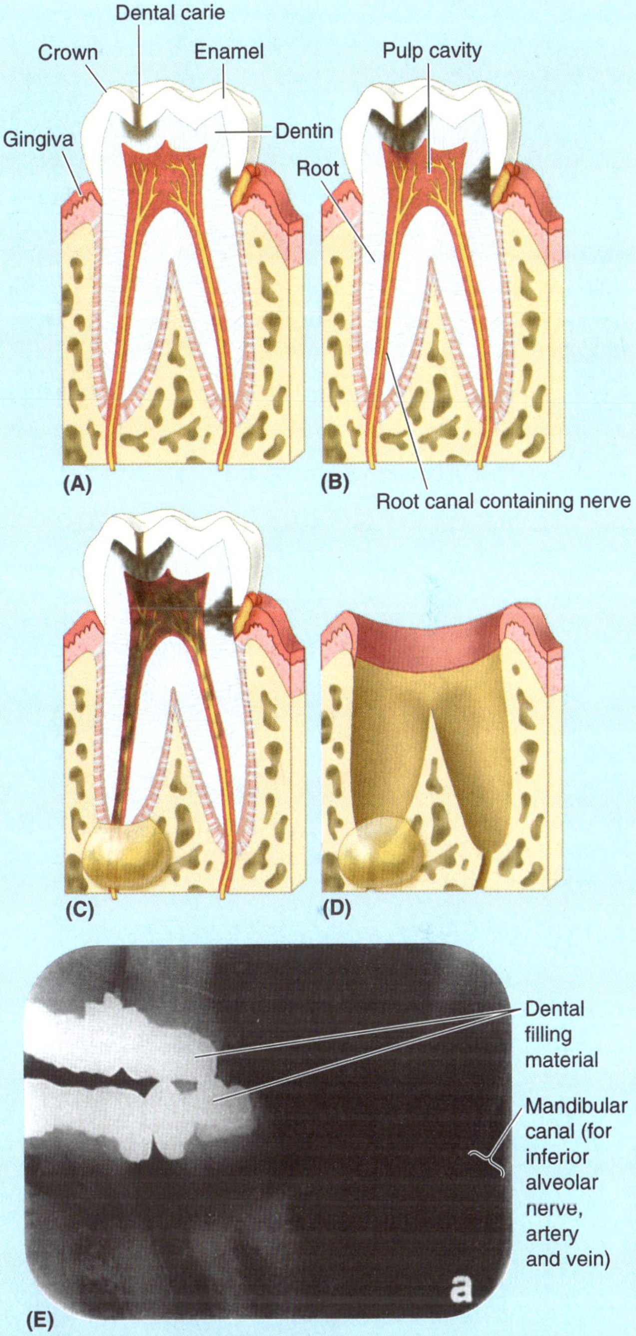

FIGURE B8.34. Dental caries and peri-apical disease.

Supernumerary Teeth (Hyperdontia)

Supernumerary teeth are teeth present in addition to the normal complement (number) of teeth. They may be single, multiple, unilateral or bilateral, erupted or unerupted, and in one or both maxillary and mandibular alveolar arches (Fig. B8.35). They may occur in both deciduous and permanent dentitions, but more commonly occur in the latter. The presence of a single supernumerary (accessory) tooth is usually seen in the anterior maxilla. The most common supernumerary tooth is a *mesiodens*, which is a malformed, peg-like tooth that occurs between the maxillary central incisor teeth (Fig. B8.35A). A *supernumerary tooth* occurs in addition to the normal number but resembles the size, shape, or placement of normal teeth. An *accessory tooth* does not resemble the form or disposition of a normal tooth (Fig. B8.35B).

Multiple supernumerary teeth are rare in individuals with no other associated diseases or syndromes, such as cleft lip or cleft palate or cranial dysplasia (malformation). The supernumerary teeth can cause problems for the eruption and alignment of normal dentition and are usually surgically extracted.

Extraction of Teeth

Sometimes, it is not practical to restore a tooth because of extreme tooth destruction. The only alternative is tooth extraction. A tooth may lose its blood supply as a result of trauma. The blow to the tooth disrupts the blood vessels entering and leaving the apical foramen. It is not always possible to save the tooth. Supernumerary teeth are also extracted.

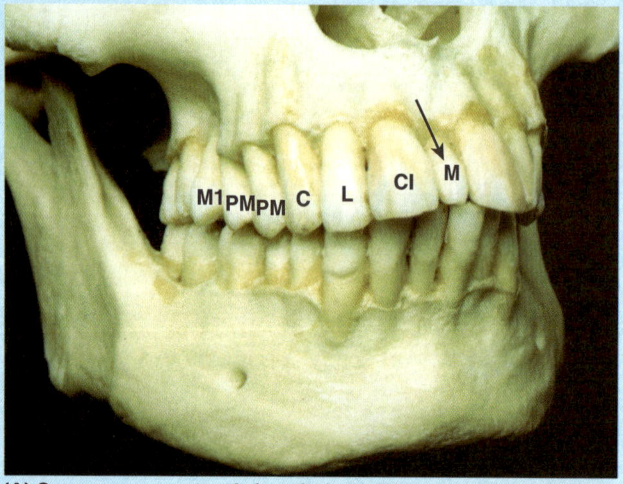

(A) Supernumerary tooth (mesiodens–M)

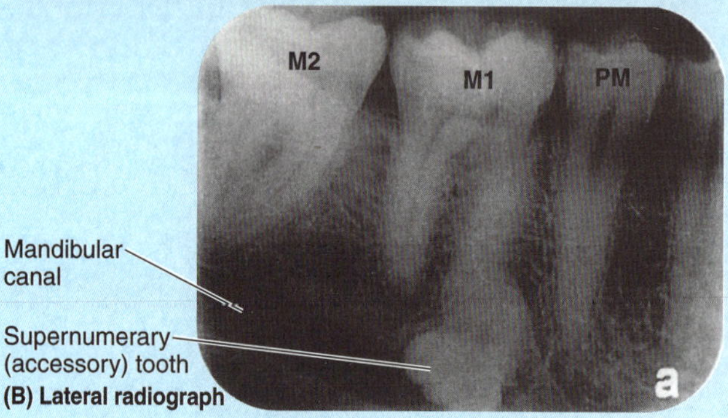

(B) Lateral radiograph

FIGURE B8.35. Supernumerary teeth. *C*, canine; *CI*, central incisor; *LI*, lateral incisor; *M*, mesiodens; *M1*, 1st molar; *M2*, 2nd molar; *PM*, premolar; *arrow*, supernumerary tooth.

The *lingual nerve* is closely related to the medial aspect of the 3rd molar teeth; therefore, caution is taken to avoid injuring this nerve during their extraction. Damage to this nerve results in altered sensation to the ipsilateral side of the tongue.

Unerupted 3rd molars are common dental problems. These teeth are the last to erupt, usually when people are in their late teens or early 20s. Often, there is not enough room for these molars to erupt, and they become lodged (impacted) under or against the 2nd molar teeth (Fig. B8.36, *insets*). If impacted 3rd molars become painful, they are usually removed. When doing so, the surgeon takes care not to injure the alveolar nerves (Figs. 8.81A and B8.34E).

Dental Implants

Following extraction of a tooth, or fracture of a tooth at its neck, a prosthetic crown may be placed on an abutment (metal peg) inserted into a metal socket surgically implanted into the alveolar bone (Fig. B8.37). A procedure to augment the alveolar bone with calf or cadaveric bone may be required before the socket can be implanted. A waiting period of several months may be necessary to allow bone growth around the implanted socket before the abutment and prosthetic crown are mounted.

Nasopalatine Block

The nasopalatine nerves can be anesthetized by injecting anesthetic into the incisive fossa in the hard palate. The needle is inserted immediately

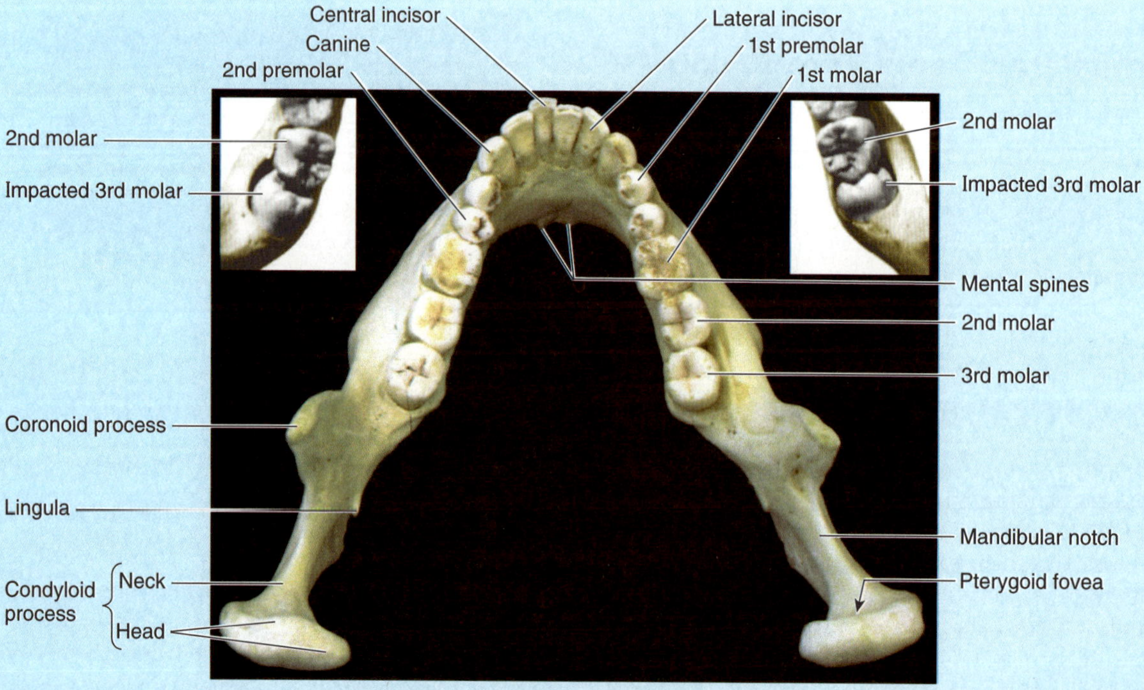

FIGURE B8.36. Normal adult mandible with full dentition. Insets, impacted 3rd molars.

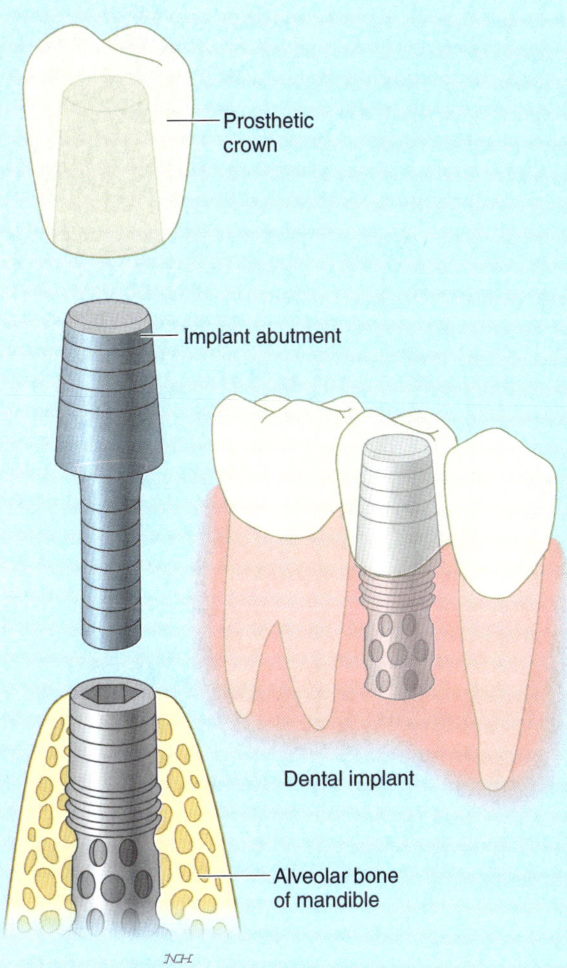

FIGURE B8.37. Dental implants.

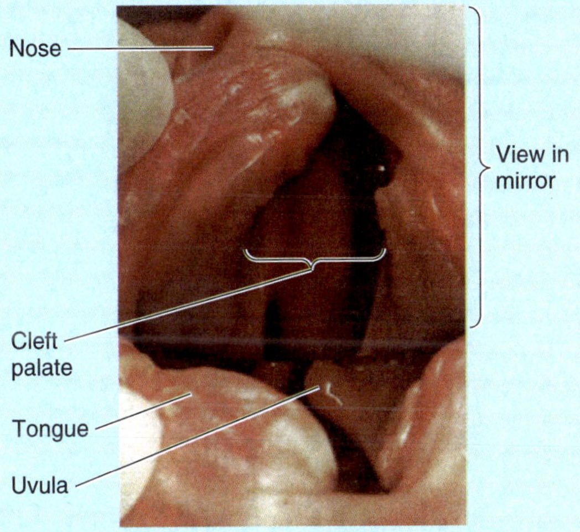

FIGURE B8.38. Bilateral cleft palate.

posterior to the incisive papilla. Both nerves are anesthetized by the same injection where they emerge through the incisive fossa (Fig. 8.89B). The affected tissues are the palatal mucosa, the lingual gingivae and alveolar bone of the six anterior maxillary teeth, and the hard palate.

Greater Palatine Block

The greater palatine nerve can be anesthetized by injecting anesthetic into the greater palatine foramen. The nerve emerges between the 2nd and the 3rd molar teeth. This nerve block anesthetizes all the palatal mucosa and lingual gingivae posterior to the maxillary canine teeth and the underlying bone of the palate. Branches of the greater palatine arteries should be avoided. The anesthetic should be injected slowly to prevent stripping of the mucosa from the hard palate.

AN43.4 Cleft Palate

Cleft palate, with or without cleft lip, occurs in approximately 1 of 2,500 births and is more common in females than in males. The cleft may involve only the uvula, giving it a fishtail appearance, or it may extend through the soft and hard regions of the palate (Fig. B8.38). In severe cases associated with cleft lip, the cleft palate extends through the alveolar processes of the maxillae and the lips on both sides. The embryological basis of cleft palate is failure of mesenchymal masses in the lateral palatine processes to meet and fuse with each other, with the nasal septum, and/or with the posterior margin of the median palatine process (Moore et al., 2016).

Gag Reflex

It is possible to touch the anterior part of the tongue without feeling discomfort. However, when the posterior part is touched, the individual gags. CN IX and CN X are responsible for the muscular contraction of each side of the pharynx. Glossopharyngeal branches provide the afferent limb of the gag reflex.

Paralysis of Genioglossus

When the genioglossus muscle is paralyzed, the tongue has a tendency to fall posteriorly, obstructing the airway and presenting the risk of suffocation. Total relaxation of the genioglossus muscles occurs during general anesthesia. Thus, an airway is inserted in an anesthetized person to prevent the tongue from relapsing.

Injury to Hypoglossal Nerve

AN39.

Trauma, such as a fractured mandible, may injure the hypoglossal nerve (CN XII), resulting in paralysis and eventual atrophy of one side of the tongue. The tongue deviates to the paralyzed side during protrusion because of the action of the unaffected genioglossus muscle on the other side.

Sublingual Absorption of Drugs

For quick absorption of a drug, for example, when nitroglycerin is used as a vasodilator in persons with *angina pectoris* (chest pain due to cardiac ischemia), the pill or spray is put under the tongue where it dissolves and enters the deep lingual veins in <1 minute (Figs. 8.91 and B8.39).

Lingual Carcinoma

A *lingual carcinoma* in the posterior part of the tongue metastasizes to the superior deep cervical lymph nodes on both sides. However, a tumor in the anterior part usually does not metastasize to the inferior deep cervical lymph nodes until late in the disease. Because the nodes are closely related to the IJV, metastases from the tongue may be distributed through the submental and submandibular regions and along the IJVs in the neck (Fig. 8.96).

Lingual Frenectomy

A frenulum (frenum) of the tongue extending farther anteriorly toward the apex (tongue-tie) interferes with tongue movements and may affect speech. In unusual cases, a *frenectomy* (cutting the frenulum) in infants may be necessary to free the tongue for normal movements and speech.

Excision of Submandibular Gland and Removal of a Calculus

Excision of a submandibular gland because of a calculus (stone) in the submandibular duct or a tumor in the gland is not uncommon. Skin incision is made at least 2.5 cm inferior to the angle of the mandible to avoid injury to the marginal mandibular branch of the facial nerve (see Fig. 8.67). Caution must also be taken not to injure the lingual nerve when incising the duct. The submandibular duct passes directly over the nerve inferior to the neck of the 3rd molar tooth (Fig. 8.98). AN34.2

Sialography of Submandibular Ducts

The submandibular salivary glands may be examined radiographically after injection of a contrast medium into their ducts (Fig. B8.40). This special type of radiograph (*sialogram*) demonstrates the salivary ducts and some secretory units. Because of the small size of the ducts of the sublingual glands and their multiplicity, one cannot usually inject contrast medium into the ducts.

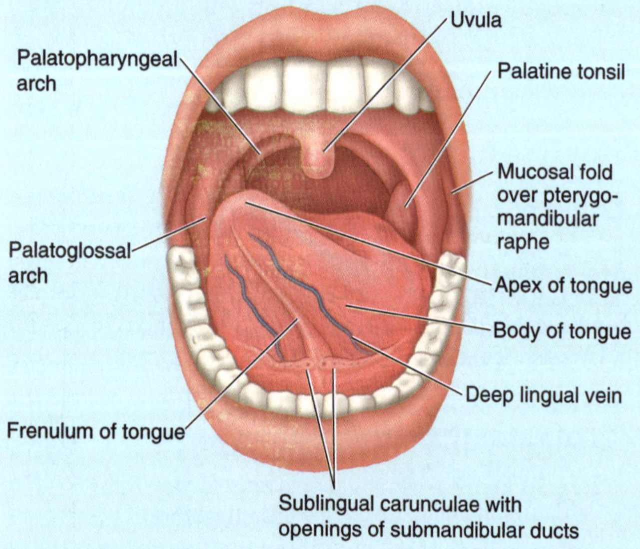

FIGURE B8.39. Floor of mouth and inferior surface of tongue.

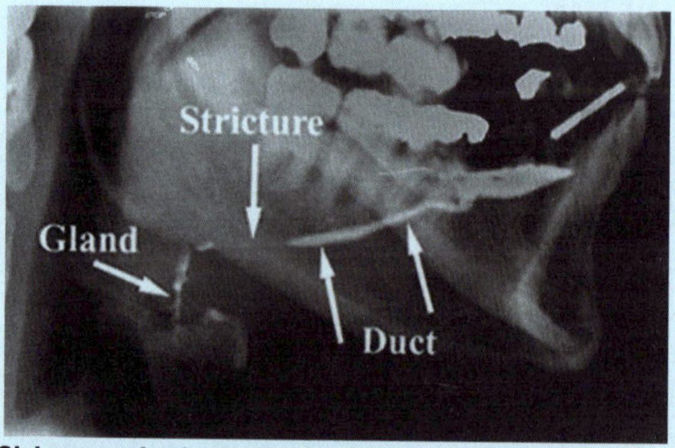

Sialogram of submandibular duct and gland. Lateral view.

FIGURE B8.40. Sialogram of submandibular duct and gland.

The Bottom Line: Oral Region

Oral cavity: The oral cavity (mouth) is the primary portal of the alimentary system, and a secondary portal for the respiratory system, especially important for speech in the latter case. • The oral cavity extends from the oral fissure to the oropharyngeal isthmus. • The oral cavity is divided by the upper and lower jaws and their dental arches into a superficial oral vestibule (between the lips and cheeks and the gingival and teeth) and a deeper oral cavity proper (internal to the jaws and dental arcades). • The oral cavity (and specifically the oral vestibule) is bounded by the lips and cheeks, which

continued on next page

The Bottom Line (continued)

are flexible dynamic musculofibrous folds containing muscles, neurovasculature, and mucosal glands, covered superficially with skin and deeply with oral mucosa. • The cheeks also include buccal fat-pads.

Teeth: The strong alveolar parts of the maxilla and mandible contain, in sequence, two sets of teeth (20 deciduous and 32 permanent teeth). • The crowns of the teeth project from the gingiva, and the roots are anchored in tooth sockets by periodontium. • The maxilla, its teeth, gingivae, and adjacent vestibule are supplied by branches of the maxillary nerve (CN V_2), the alveolar arteries, and accompanying veins. • The same features of the mandible are supplied by the mandibular nerve (CN V_3) and inferior alveolar vessels.

Palate: The roof of the oral cavity proper is formed by the hard (anterior two thirds) and soft (posterior one third) palates, the latter being a controlled flap that allows or limits communication with the nasal cavity. • The mucosa of the hard palate includes abundant palatine glands. • Branches of the maxillary (greater and lesser palatine arteries) and facial (ascending palatine artery) arteries supply the palate; its venous blood drains to the pterygoid plexus. The palate receives sensory innervation from the maxillary nerve (CN V_2); the muscles of the soft palate receive motor innervation from the pharyngeal plexus (CN X) plus a branch from the mandibular nerve (CN V_3) for the tensor veli palatini.

Tongue: The tongue is a mass of striated muscle, innervated by CN XII, and covered with a specialized mucosa textured with lingual papillae. • It occupies most of the oral cavity when the mouth is closed. • Its extrinsic muscles primarily control its placement, whereas its intrinsic muscles primarily control its shape, for manipulation of food during chewing, swallowing, and speech. • It is highly sensitive, with four cranial nerves contributing sensory fibers to it. • The terminal sulcus divides it into an anterior two thirds, receiving general sensation from the lingual nerve (CN V_3) and taste fibers from CN VII, and a posterior third receiving all sensory innervation from CN IX. • Adjacent to the epiglottis, CN X provides general and special sensory innervation.

Salivary glands: Salivary glands secrete saliva to initiate digestion by facilitating chewing and swallowing. • The parotid gland, the largest, receives parasympathetic innervation from CN IX via the otic ganglion. • The submandibular and sublingual glands receive parasympathetic innervation from CN VII by way of the chorda tympani nerve, lingual nerve, and submandibular ganglion. Their ducts open into the oral cavity under the tongue.

PTERYGOPALATINE FOSSA

The **pterygopalatine fossa** is a small pyramidal space inferior to the apex of the orbit and medial to the infratemporal fossa (Fig. 8.100). It lies between the *pterygoid process of the sphenoid* posteriorly and the rounded posterior aspect of the maxilla anteriorly. The fragile *perpendicular plate of the palatine bone* forms its medial wall. The incomplete roof of the pterygopalatine fossa is formed by the medial continuation of the *infratemporal surface of the greater wing of the sphenoid*. The floor of the pterygopalatine fossa is formed by the *pyramidal process of the palatine bone*. Its superior larger end opens anterosuperiorly into the *inferior orbital fissure*. Its inferior end narrows, continuing as the *greater and lesser palatine canals*. The pterygopalatine fossa communicates through many passageways, distributing and receiving nerves and vessels to and from most of the major compartments of the viscerocranium (Fig. 8.101A).

The **contents of the pterygopalatine fossa** (Fig. 8.101B, C) are as follows:

- Terminal (pterygopalatine or third) part of the maxillary artery, and the initial parts of its branches, and accompanying veins (tributaries of the pterygoid venous plexus).
- Maxillary nerve (CN V_2), with which the pterygopalatine ganglion is associated. Branches arising from the ganglion within the fossa are considered to be branches of the maxillary nerve.
- Neurovascular sheaths of the vessels and nerves and a fatty matrix occupy all remaining space.

Pterygopalatine Part of Maxillary Artery

The *maxillary artery*, a terminal branch of the external carotid artery, passes anteriorly through the infratemporal fossa, as described previously. The **pterygopalatine part of the maxillary artery**, its third part (i.e., the part located anterior to the lateral pterygoid), passes medially through the *pterygomaxillary fissure* and enters the pterygopalatine fossa (Figs. 8.101B and 8.102A). The artery lies anterior to the pterygopalatine ganglion and gives rise to branches that accompany all nerves entering and exiting the fossa, sharing the same names with many (Table 8.12).

Maxillary Nerve

The **maxillary nerve** runs anteriorly through the *foramen rotundum*, which enters posterior wall of the fossa (Figs. 8.101C, 8.102B, and 8.103C). Within the pterygopalatine fossa, the maxillary nerve gives off the *zygomatic nerve*, which in turn divides into zygomaticofacial and zygomaticotemporal nerves (Figs. 8.102B and 8.103A). These nerves emerge from the zygomatic bone through cranial foramina of the same name and supply general sensation to the lateral region of the cheek and temple. The **zygomaticotemporal nerve** also gives rise to a communicating branch, which conveys postsynaptic parasympathetic secretomotor fibers to the lacrimal gland by way of the heretofore purely sensory lacrimal nerve from CN V_1 (Fig. 8.103A, B).

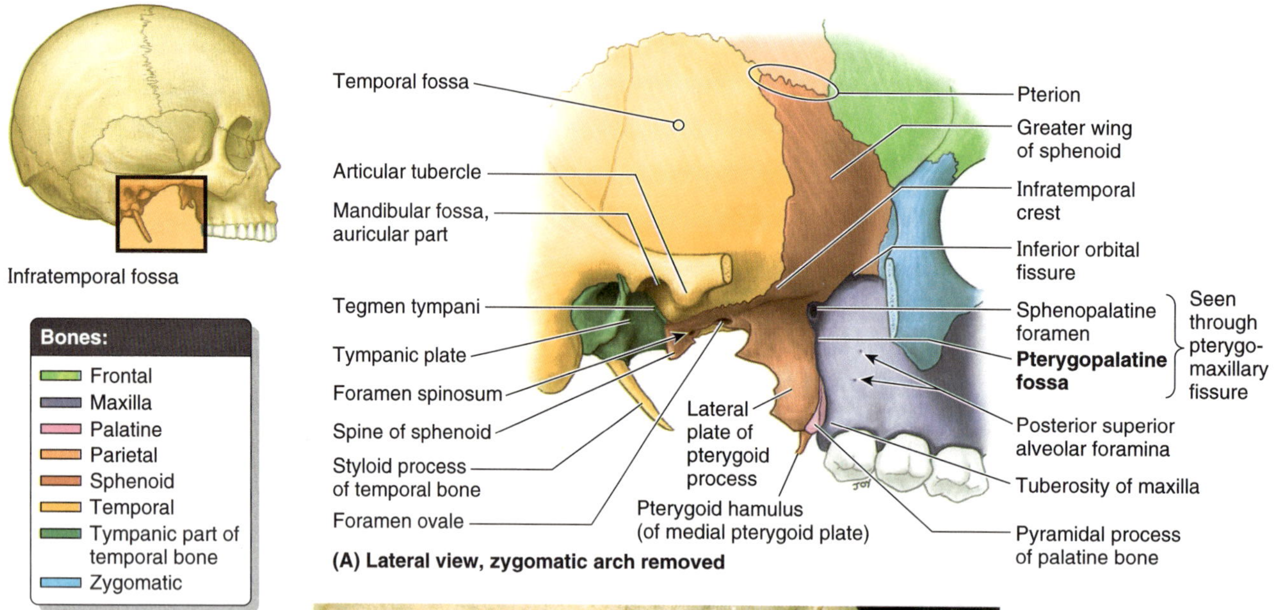

(A) Lateral view, zygomatic arch removed

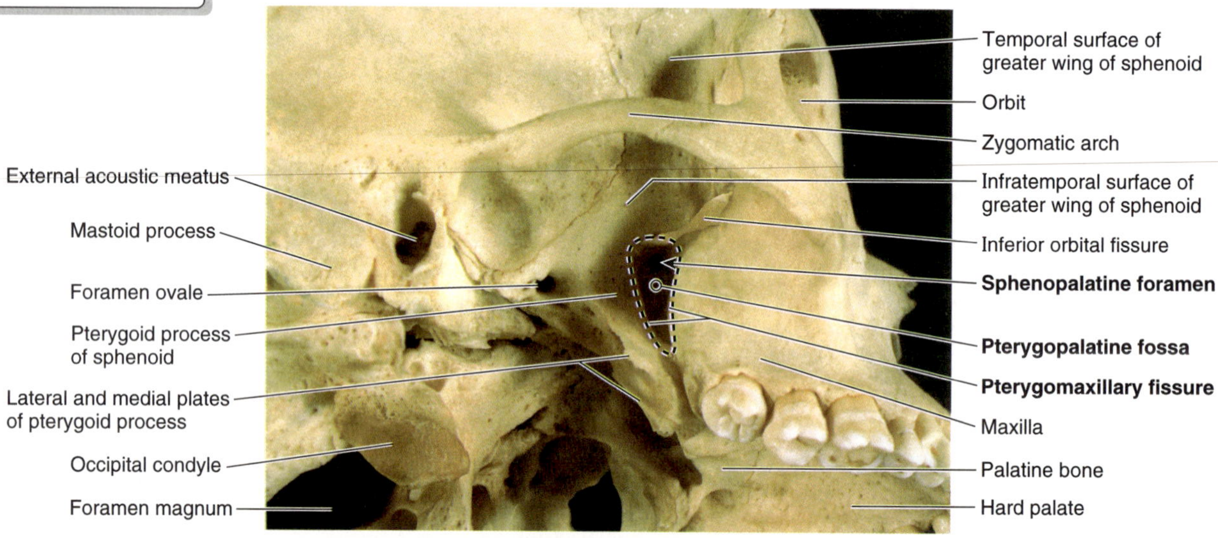

(B) Inferolateral and slightly posterior view, looking into infratemporal and pterygopalatine fossae

FIGURE 8.100. Temporal, infratemporal, and pterygopalatine fossae. The pterygopalatine fossa is seen medial to the infratemporal fossa through the pterygomaxillary fissure, between the pterygoid process and the maxilla. The sphenopalatine foramen is an opening into the nasal cavity at the top of the palatine bone.

While in the pterygopalatine fossa, the maxillary nerve also gives off the two *ganglionic branches to the pterygopalatine ganglion* (sensory roots of the pterygopalatine ganglion) that suspend the parasympathetic **pterygopalatine ganglion** in the superior part of the pterygopalatine fossa (Figs. 8.101C and 8.103A). The pterygopalatine nerves convey general sensory fibers of the maxillary nerve, which pass through the pterygopalatine ganglion without synapsing to supply the nose, palate, and pharynx (Fig. 8.103C). The maxillary nerve leaves the pterygopalatine fossa through the inferior orbital fissure, after which it is known as the *infra-orbital nerve* (Figs. 8.101C and 8.102B).

The **parasympathetic fibers to the pterygopalatine ganglion** come from the facial nerve by way of its first branch, the *greater petrosal nerve* (Figs. 8.101C and 8.103A, B). This nerve joins the *deep petrosal nerve* as it passes through the foramen lacerum to form the **nerve of the pterygoid canal**, which passes anteriorly through this canal to the pterygopalatine fossa. The parasympathetic fibers of the greater petrosal nerve synapse in the pterygopalatine ganglion. The **deep petrosal nerve** is a sympathetic nerve arising from the *internal carotid peri-arterial plexus* as the artery exits the carotid canal (Figs. 8.101C and 8.103A, C). It conveys postsynaptic fibers from nerve cell bodies in the *superior cervical sympathetic ganglion* to the pterygopalatine ganglion by joining the *nerve of the pterygoid canal*. The fibers do not synapse in the ganglion but pass directly through it into the branches (of CN V_2) arising from it (Fig. 8.103C). The postsynaptic sympathetic fibers pass to the palatine glands, and the mucosal glands of the nasal cavity and superior pharynx.

(*continued on p.* 1015)

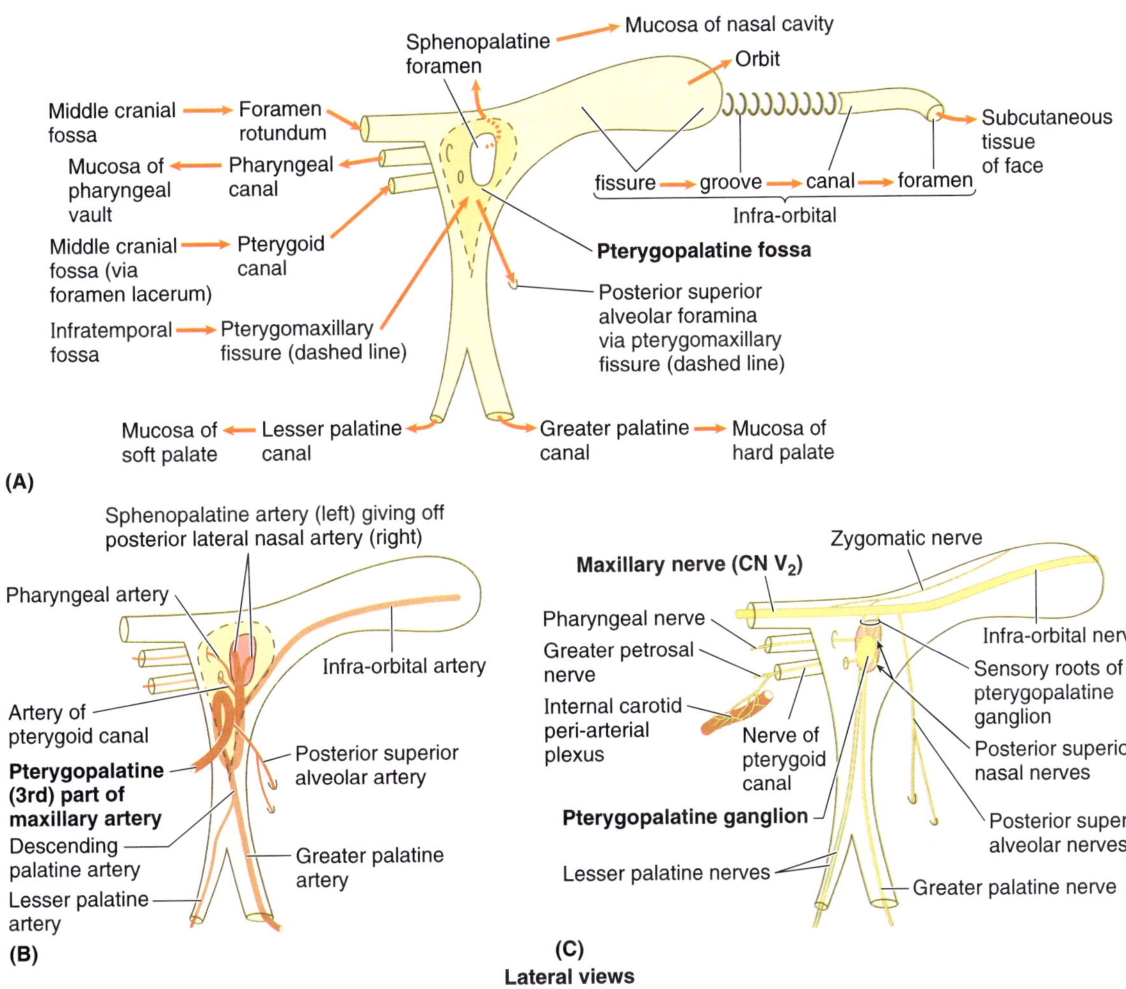

FIGURE 8.101. Pterygopalatine fossa—communications and contents. A. Communications of the pterygopalatine fossa and the passageways by which structures enter and exit fossae are shown. **B.** The distribution of branches of the pterygopalatine part of the maxillary artery is demonstrated. **C.** Branches of the maxillary nerve and pterygopalatine ganglion enter and exit the fossa.

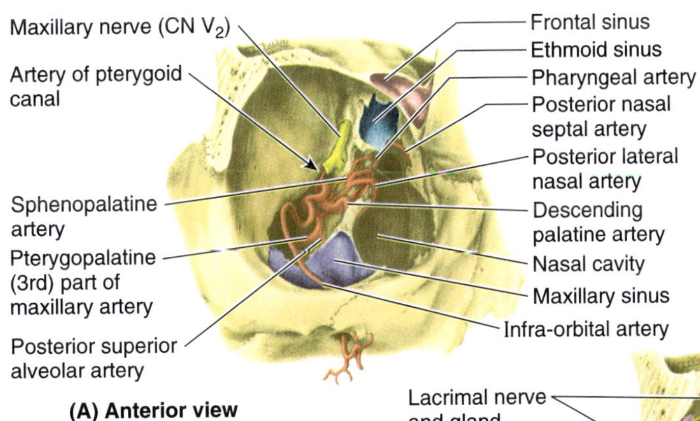

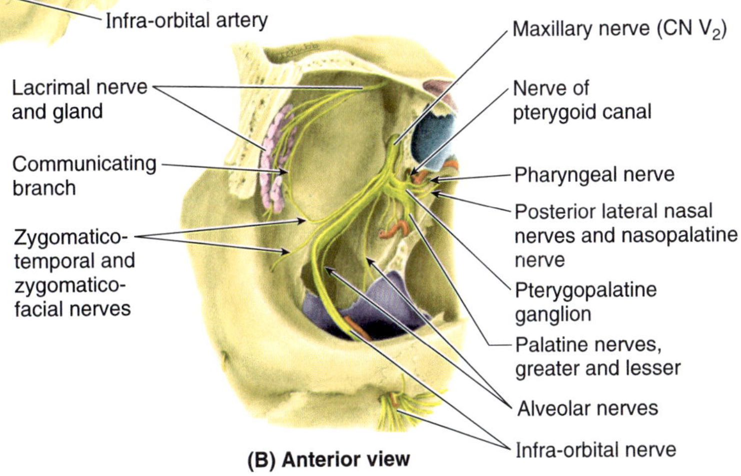

FIGURE 8.102. Orbital approach to contents of pterygopalatine fossa. A. The pterygopalatine (third) part of the maxillary artery lies anterior to the lateral pterygoid muscle (Table 8.12). The branches of the third part arise just before and within the pterygopalatine fossa. **B.** The maxillary nerve (CN V_2) traverses the posterior wall of the pterygopalatine fossa via the foramen rotundum, sending two nerves (roots) to the pterygopalatine ganglion within the fossa. The branches arising from the ganglion are considered to be branches of CN V_2.

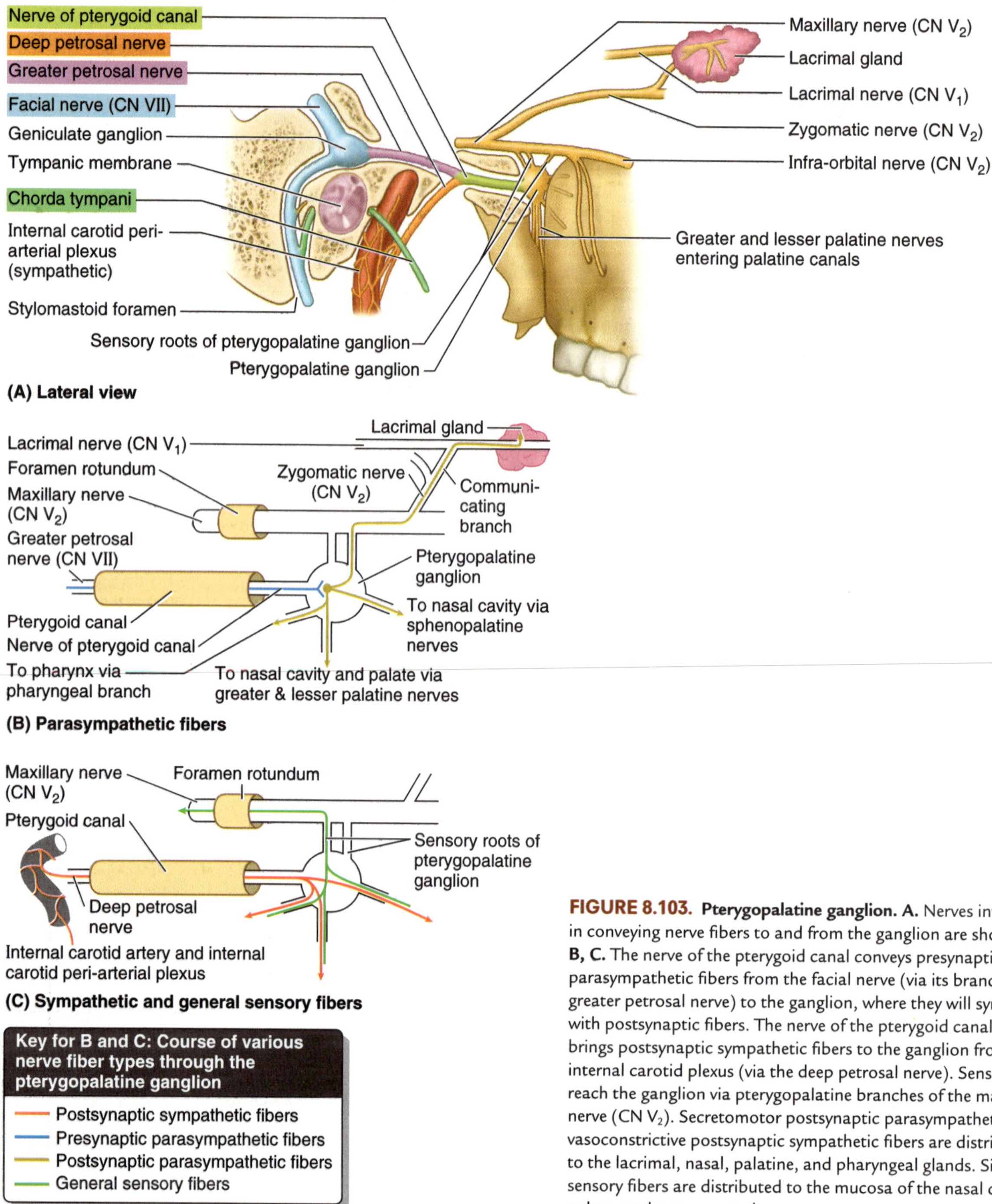

FIGURE 8.103. Pterygopalatine ganglion. A. Nerves involved in conveying nerve fibers to and from the ganglion are shown. **B, C.** The nerve of the pterygoid canal conveys presynaptic parasympathetic fibers from the facial nerve (via its branch, the greater petrosal nerve) to the ganglion, where they will synapse with postsynaptic fibers. The nerve of the pterygoid canal also brings postsynaptic sympathetic fibers to the ganglion from the internal carotid plexus (via the deep petrosal nerve). Sensory fibers reach the ganglion via pterygopalatine branches of the maxillary nerve (CN V_2). Secretomotor postsynaptic parasympathetic and vasoconstrictive postsynaptic sympathetic fibers are distributed to the lacrimal, nasal, palatine, and pharyngeal glands. Similarly, sensory fibers are distributed to the mucosa of the nasal cavity, palate, and uppermost pharynx.

CLINICAL BOX

PTERYGOPALATINE FOSSA

Transantral Approach to Pterygopalatine Fossa

Surgical access to the deeply placed pterygopalatine fossa is gained through the maxillary sinus. After elevating the upper lip, the maxillary gingiva and anterior wall of the sinus are traversed to enter the sinus. The posterior wall is then chipped away as needed to open the anterior wall of the pterygopalatine fossa. In the case of chronic *epistaxis* (nosebleed), the third part of the maxillary artery may be ligated in the fossa to control the bleeding.

The Bottom Line: Pterygopalatine Fossa

The pterygopalatine fossa is a major distributing center for branches of the maxillary nerve and the pterygopalatine (third) part of the maxillary artery. ● It is located between, and has communications with, the infratemporal fossa, nasal cavity, orbit, middle cranial fossa, pharyngeal vault, maxillary sinus, and oral cavity (palate). ● The contents of the pterygopalatine fossa are the maxillary nerve (CN V_2), the parasympathetic pterygopalatine ganglion, the third part of the maxillary artery and accompanying veins, and a surrounding fatty matrix.

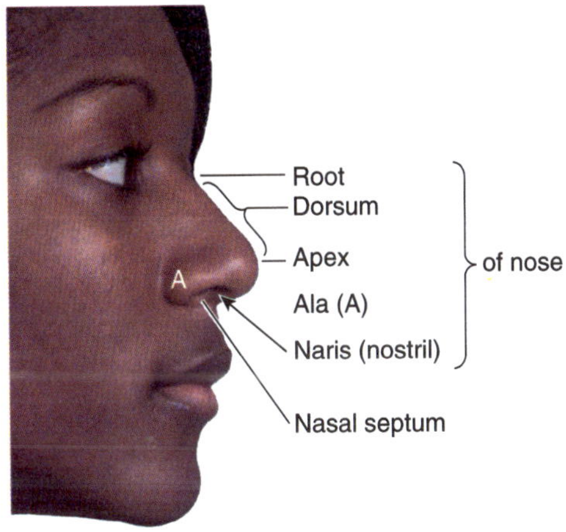

(A) Lateral view

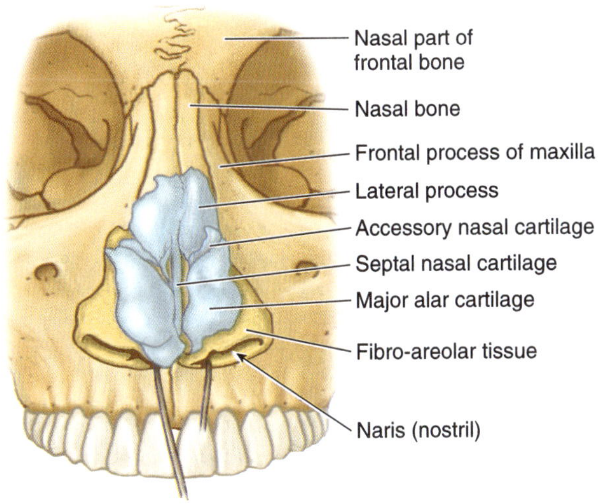

(B) Anterior view

FIGURE 8.104. External nose. A. The surface anatomy of the nose is shown. The nose is attached to the forehead by the root of the nose. The rounded border between the apex and the root is the dorsum of the nose. **B.** The cartilages of the nose are retracted inferiorly to expose the sesamoid cartilages. The lateral nasal cartilages are fixed by sutures to the nasal bones and are continuous with the septal nasal cartilage.

NOSE

The **nose** is the part of the respiratory tract superior to the hard palate and contains the peripheral organ of smell. It includes the external nose and nasal cavity, which is divided into right and left cavities by the *nasal septum* (Fig. 8.104A). The functions of the nose include olfaction (smelling), respiration (breathing), filtration of dust, humidification of inspired air, and reception and elimination of secretions from the paranasal sinuses and nasolacrimal ducts.

External Nose

The **external nose** is the visible portion that projects from the face. Its skeleton is mainly cartilaginous (Fig. 8.104B). Noses vary considerably in size and shape, mainly because of differences in these cartilages. The **dorsum of the nose** extends from the **root of the nose** to the **apex** (tip) **of the nose**. The inferior surface of the nose is pierced by two piriform (L. pear-shaped) openings, the **nares** (nostrils, anterior nasal apertures), which are bound laterally by the **alae** (wings) **of the nose**. The superior bony part of the nose, including its root, is covered by thin skin.

The skin over the cartilages of the nose is covered with thicker skin, which contains many sebaceous glands. The skin extends into the **vestibule of the nose** (Fig. 8.106A), where it has a variable number of stiff hairs (*vibrissae*). Because they are usually moist, these hairs filter dust particles from air entering the nasal cavity. The junction of the skin and mucous membrane is beyond the hair-bearing area.

SKELETON OF EXTERNAL NOSE

The supporting skeleton of the nose is composed of bone and hyaline cartilage. The **bony part of the nose** (Figs. 8.104B and 8.105) consists of the *nasal bones, frontal processes of the maxillae*, the *nasal part of the frontal bone* and its *nasal spine*, and the bony parts of the nasal septum. The **cartilaginous part of the nose** consists of five main cartilages: two lateral cartilages, two alar cartilages, and one septal cartilage. The U-shaped **alar cartilages** are free and movable. They dilate or constrict the nares when the muscles acting on the nose contract.

NASAL SEPTUM

The *nasal septum* divides the chamber of the nose into two *nasal cavities*. The septum has a bony part and a soft mobile cartilaginous part. The main components of the nasal septum are the **perpendicular plate of the ethmoid**, the vomer, and the septal cartilage. The thin perpendicular plate of the ethmoid bone, forming the superior part of the nasal septum, descends from the *cribriform plate* and is continued superior to this plate as the *crista galli*. The **vomer**, a thin flat bone, forms the postero-inferior part of the nasal septum,

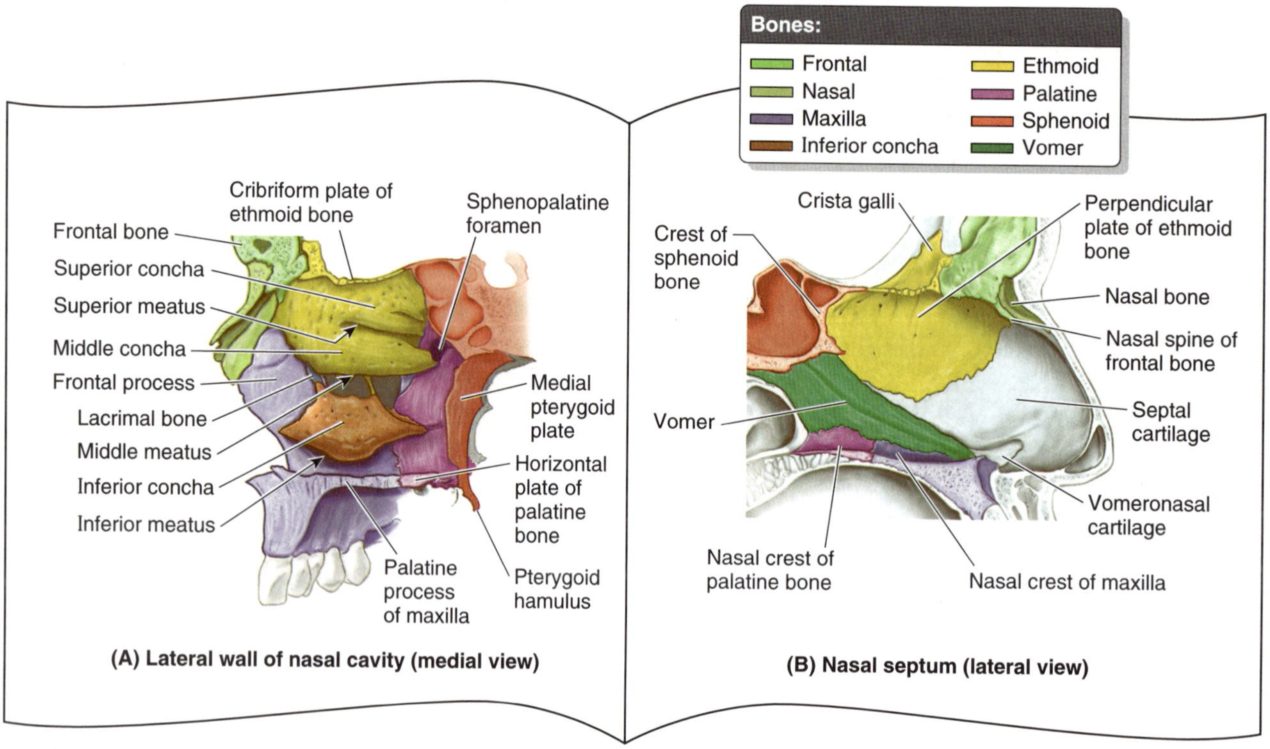

FIGURE 8.105. Lateral and medial (septal) walls of right side of nasal cavity. The walls are separated and shown as adjacent pages of a book. The medial view shows the right lateral wall of the nasal cavity, and the lateral view shows the nasal septum. The nasal septum has a hard (bony) part located deeply (posteriorly) where it is protected and a soft or mobile part located superficially (anteriorly) mostly in the more vulnerable external nose.

with some contribution from the nasal crests of the maxillary and palatine bones. The **septal cartilage** has a tongue-and-groove articulation with the edges of the bony septum.

Nasal Cavities

The term *nasal cavity* refers to either the entire cavity or to the right or left half, depending on the context. The nasal cavity is entered anteriorly through the nares (nostrils). It opens posteriorly into the *nasopharynx* through the *choanae* (Fig. 8.9). Mucosa lines the nasal cavity, except for the *nasal vestibule*, which is lined with skin (Fig. 8.106A).

The **nasal mucosa** is firmly bound to the periosteum and perichondrium of the supporting bones and cartilages of the nose. The mucosa is continuous with the lining of all the chambers with which the nasal cavities communicate: the nasopharynx posteriorly, the paranasal sinuses superiorly and laterally, and the lacrimal sac and conjunctiva superiorly. The inferior two thirds of the nasal mucosa is the respiratory area, and the superior one third is the olfactory area (Fig. 8.109B). Air passing over the **respiratory area** is warmed and moistened before it passes through the rest of the upper respiratory tract to the lungs. The **olfactory area** contains the
N43.3 peripheral organ of smell; sniffing draws air to the area. For microanatomy of olfactory epithelium, refer *diFiore's Atlas of Histology with Functional Correlations*, 1st South Asian Edition, Chapter 17, Respiratory System, p. 436.

BOUNDARIES OF NASAL CAVITIES

The nasal cavities have a roof, floor, and medial and lateral AN37.1
walls:

- The *roof of the nasal cavities* is curved and narrow, except at its posterior end, where the hollow *body of the sphenoid* forms the roof. It is divided into three parts (frontonasal, ethmoidal, and sphenoidal) named from the bones forming each part (Fig. 8.105).
- The *floor of the nasal cavities* is wider than the roof and is formed by the *palatine processes of the maxilla* and the *horizontal plates of the palatine bone*.
- The *medial wall of the nasal cavities* is formed by the nasal septum.
- The *lateral walls of the nasal cavities* are irregular owing to three bony plates, the *nasal conchae*, which project inferiorly, somewhat like louvers (Figs. 8.105A, 8.106, and 8.111).

FEATURES OF NASAL CAVITIES

The **nasal conchae** (superior, middle, and inferior) curve inferomedially, hanging like louvers or short curtains from the lateral wall. The conchae (L. shells) or turbinates of many mammals (especially running mammals and those existing in extreme environments) are highly convoluted, scroll-like structures that offer a vast surface area for heat exchange.

(continued on p. 1018)

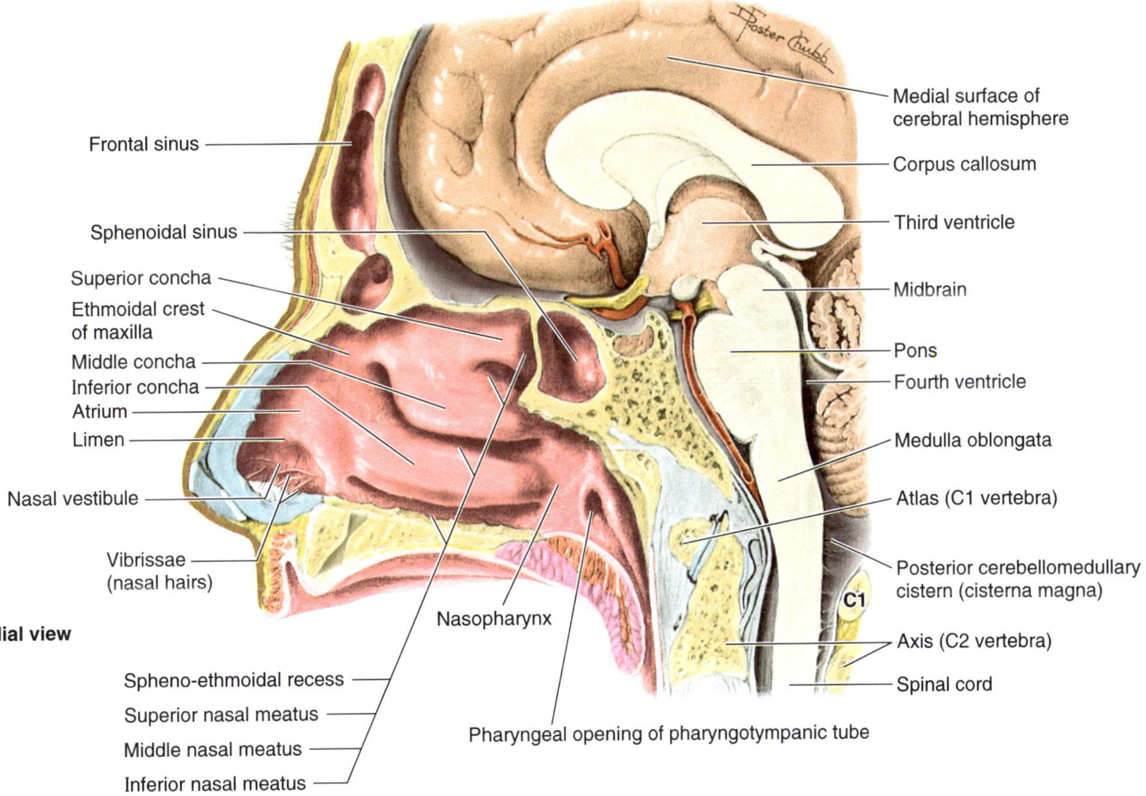

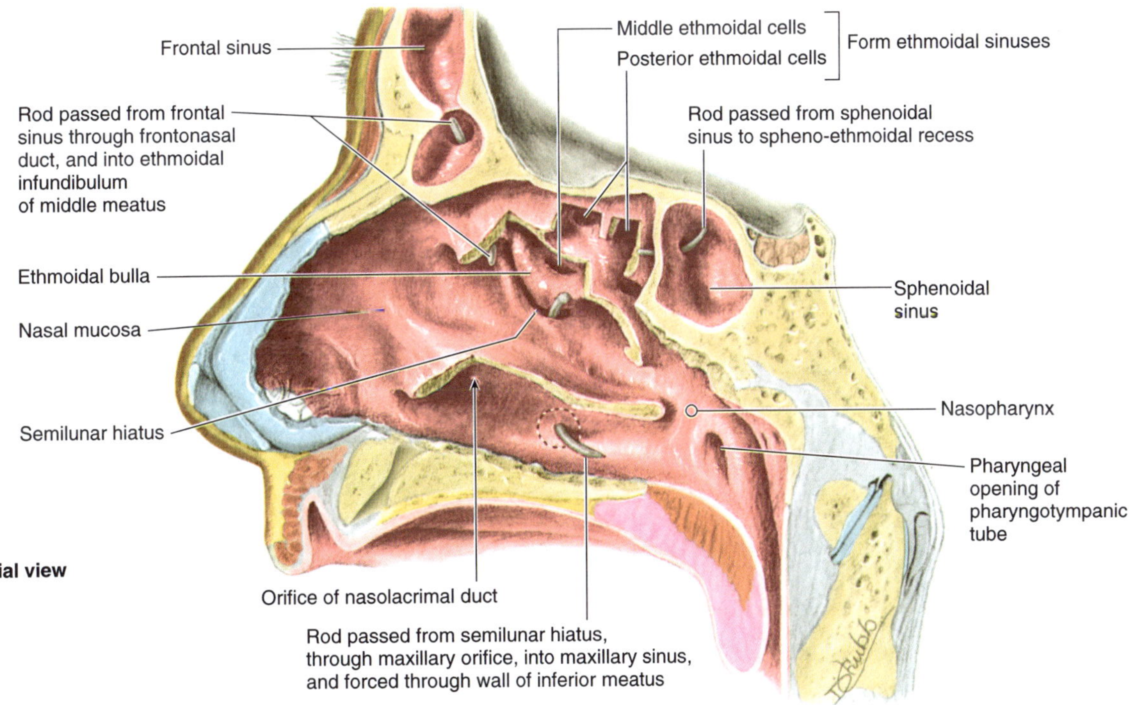

FIGURE 8.106. Lateral wall of nasal cavity of right half of head. A. The inferior and middle conchae, curving medially and inferiorly from the lateral wall, divide the wall into three nearly equal parts and cover the inferior and middle meatus, respectively. The superior concha is small and anterior to the sphenoidal sinus, and the middle concha has an angled inferior border and ends inferior to the sphenoidal sinus. The inferior concha has a slightly curved inferior border and ends inferior to the middle concha approximately 1 cm anterior to the orifice of the pharyngotympanic tube (approximately the width of the medial pterygoid plate). **B.** This dissection of the lateral wall of the nasal cavity shows the communications through the lateral wall of the nasal cavity. Parts of the superior, middle, and inferior conchae are cut away. The sphenoidal sinus occupies the body of the sphenoid bone. Its orifice, superior to the middle of its anterior wall, opens into the spheno-ethmoidal recess. The orifices of posterior, middle, and anterior ethmoidal cells open into the superior meatus, middle meatus, and semilunar hiatus, respectively.

In both humans with simple plate-like nasal conchae and animals with complex turbinates, a recess or **nasal meatus** (singular and plural; passage(s) in the nasal cavity) underlies each of the bony formations. The nasal cavity is therefore divided into five passages: a posterosuperiorly placed *spheno-ethmoidal recess*, three laterally located *nasal meatus* (superior, middle, and inferior), and a medially placed *common nasal meatus* into which the four lateral passages open. The **inferior concha** is the longest and broadest of the conchae and is formed by an independent bone (of the same name, inferior concha) covered by a mucous membrane that contains large vascular spaces that can enlarge affecting the caliber of the nasal cavity. The **middle** and **superior conchae** are medial processes of the ethmoid bone. When infected or irritated, the mucosa covering the conchae may swell rapidly, blocking the nasal passage(s) on that side.

The **spheno-ethmoidal recess**, lying superoposterior to the superior concha, receives the opening of the *sphenoidal sinus*, an air-filled cavity in the body of the sphenoid. The **superior nasal meatus** is a narrow passage between the superior and the middle nasal conchae into which the posterior ethmoidal sinuses open by one or more orifices (Fig. 8.106A). The middle nasal meatus is longer and deeper than the superior one. The anterosuperior part of this passage leads into a funnel-shaped opening, the **ethmoidal infundibulum**, through which it communicates with the frontal sinus (Fig. 8.107). The passage that leads inferiorly from each frontal sinus to the infundibulum is the *frontonasal*

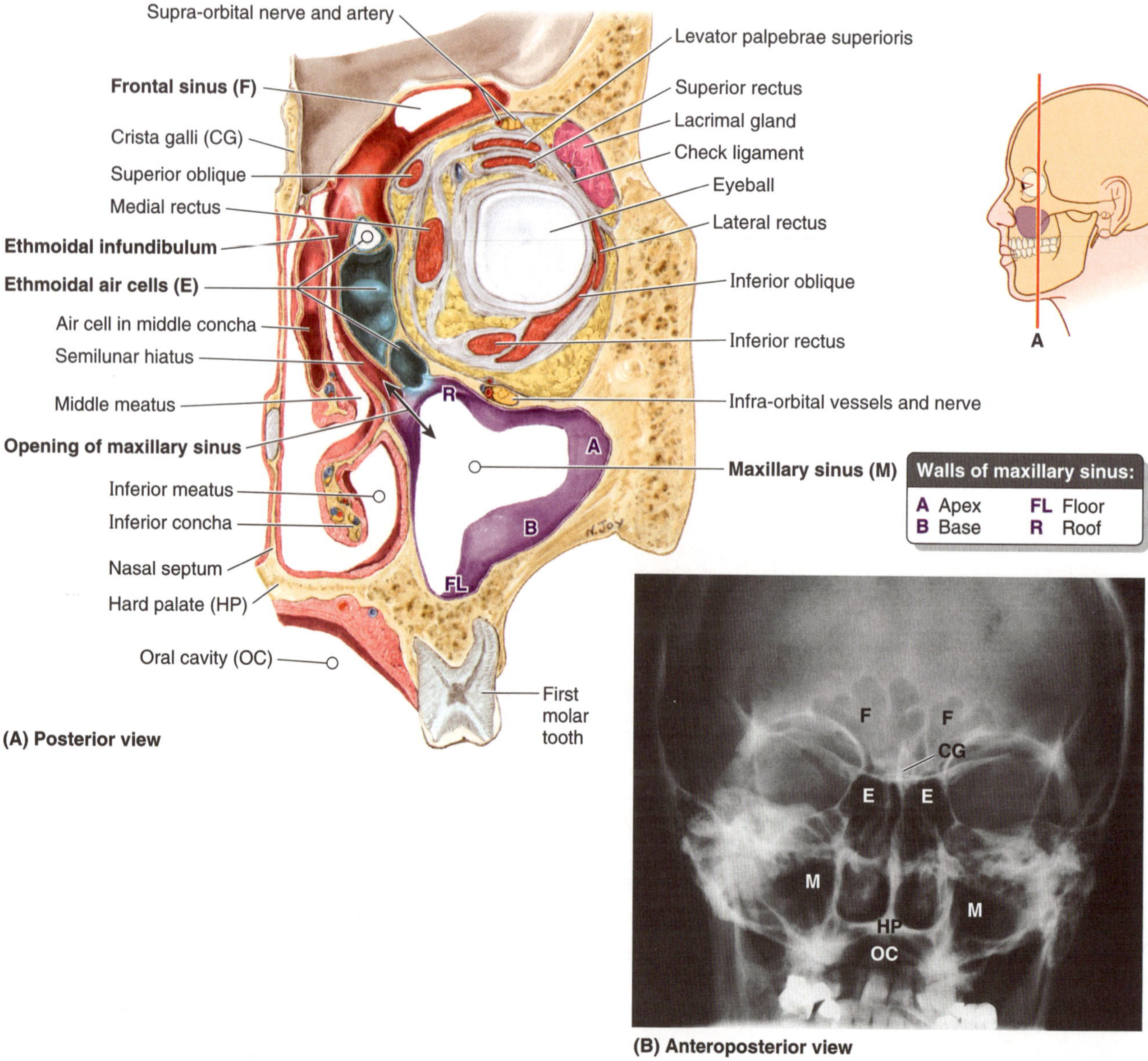

AN43.7

FIGURE 8.107. Coronal section of right half of head. A. The orientation drawing illustrates the plane of the section. Observe the relationship of the orbit, nasal cavity, and paranasal sinuses. The orbital contents, including the four recti and the fascia uniting them, form a circle (a cone when viewed in three dimensions) around the internal aspect of the posterior part (fundus) of the eyeball. **B.** Radiograph of cranium demonstrating nasal cavity and paranasal sinuses. Letters refer to structures labeled in part **A.**

duct (Fig. 8.106B). The **semilunar hiatus** (L. *hiatus semilunaris*) is a semicircular groove into which the frontal sinus opens. The **ethmoidal bulla** (L. bubble), a rounded elevation located superior to the semilunar hiatus, is visible when the middle concha is removed. The bulla is formed by middle ethmoidal cells that form the *ethmoidal sinuses*.

The **inferior nasal meatus** is a horizontal passage inferolateral to the inferior nasal concha. The *nasolacrimal duct*, which drains tears from the lacrimal sac, opens into the anterior part of this meatus (see Fig. 8.46A). The **common nasal meatus** is the medial part of the nasal cavity between the conchae and the nasal septum, into which the lateral recesses and meatus open.

Vasculature and Innervation of Nose

AN37.1 The *arterial supply of the medial and lateral walls of the nasal cavity* (Fig. 8.108) is from five sources:

1. *Anterior ethmoidal artery* (from the ophthalmic artery).
2. *Posterior ethmoidal artery* (from the ophthalmic artery).
3. *Sphenopalatine artery* (from the maxillary artery).
4. *Greater palatine artery* (from the maxillary artery).
5. *Septal branch of the superior labial artery* (from the facial artery).

The first three arteries divide into lateral and medial (septal) branches. The greater palatine artery reaches the septum via the incisive canal through the anterior hard palate. The anterior part of the nasal septum is the site of an anastomotic arterial plexus involving all five arteries supplying the septum (*Kiesselbach area*). The external nose also receives blood from first and fifth arteries listed above, plus nasal branches of the infra-orbital artery and the lateral nasal branches of the facial artery.

A rich **submucosal venous plexus**, deep to the nasal mucosa, provides *venous drainage of the nose via* the sphenopalatine, facial, and ophthalmic veins. The plexus is an important part of the body's thermoregulatory system, exchanging heat and warming air before it enters the lungs. Venous blood from the external nose drains mostly into the facial vein via the angular and lateral nasal veins (see Fig. 8.25). However, recall that it lies within the "danger area" of the face because of communications with the *cavernous (dural venous) sinus* (see the clinical box "Thrombophlebitis of Facial Vein").

Regarding the *nerve supply of the nose*, the nasal mucosa can be divided into postero-inferior and anterosuperior portions by an oblique line passing approximately through the anterior nasal spine and the spheno-ethmoidal recess (Fig. 8.109). The nerve supply of the postero-inferior portion of the nasal mucosa is chiefly from the maxillary nerve, by way of the *nasopalatine nerve* to the nasal septum, and posterior superior lateral nasal and inferior lateral nasal branches of the *greater palatine nerve* to the lateral wall. The nerve supply of the anterosuperior portion is from the ophthalmic nerve (CN V_1) by way of the **anterior** and **posterior ethmoidal nerves**, branches of the nasociliary nerve. Most of the external nose (dorsum and apex) is also supplied by CN V_1 (via the infratrochlear nerve and the external nasal branch of the

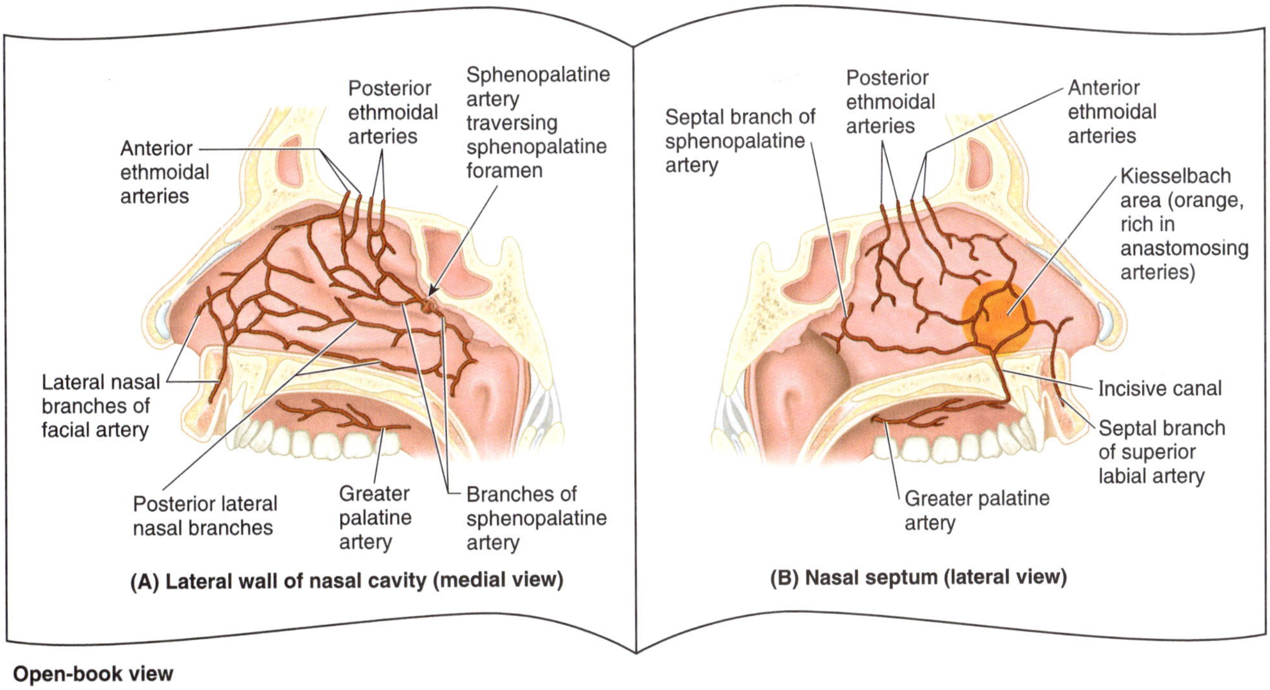

FIGURE 8.108. Arterial supply of nasal cavity. An open-book view of the lateral and medial walls of the right side of the nasal cavity is shown. The left "page" shows the lateral wall of the nasal cavity. The sphenopalatine artery (a branch of the maxillary artery) and the anterior ethmoidal artery (a branch of the ophthalmic artery) are the most important arteries to the nasal cavity. The right "page" shows the nasal septum. An anastomosis of four to five named arteries supplying the septum occurs in the antero-inferior portion of the nasal septum (Kiesselbach area, *orange*), an area commonly involved in chronic epistaxis (nosebleeds).

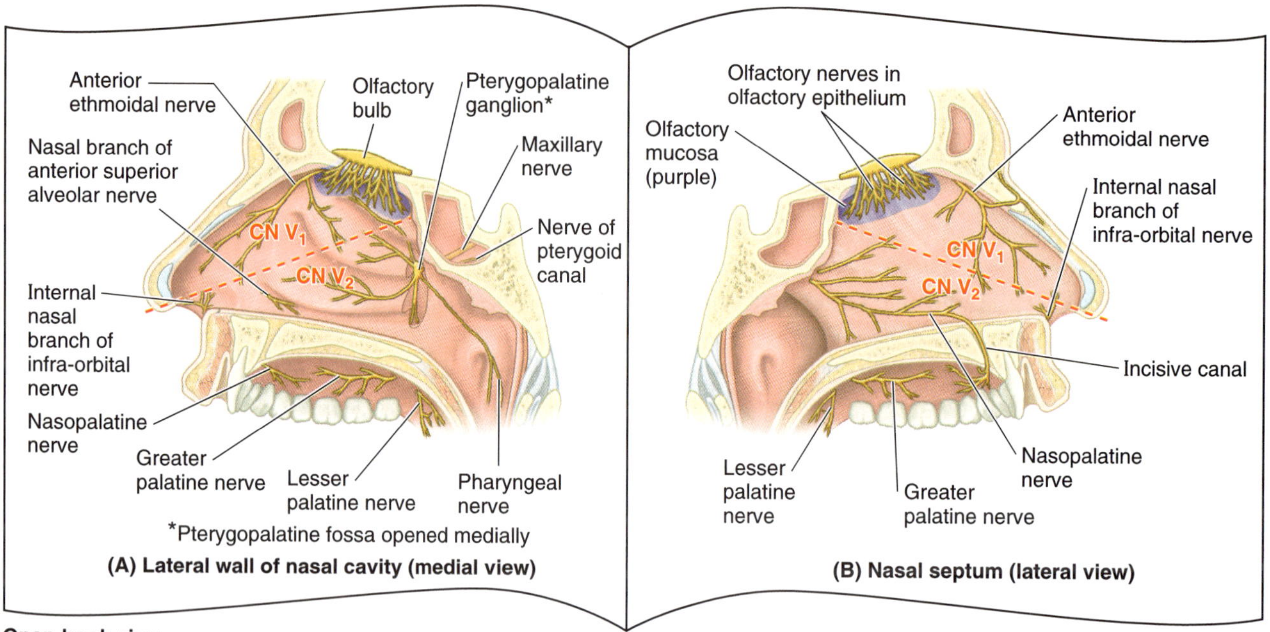

Open-book view

FIGURE 8.109. Innervation of nasal cavity. An open-book view of the lateral and medial (septal) walls of the right side of the nasal cavity is shown. A *dashed line* extrapolated approximately from the spheno-ethmoidal recess to the apex of the nose demarcates the territories of the ophthalmic (CN V_1) and maxillary (CN V_2) nerves for supplying general sensation to both the lateral wall and the nasal septum. The olfactory nerve (CN I) is distributed to the olfactory mucosa superior to the level of the superior concha on both the lateral wall and the nasal septum.

anterior ethmoidal nerve). However, the alae of the nose are supplied by the nasal branches of the infra-orbital nerve (CN V_2). The **olfactory nerves**, concerned with smell, arise from cells in the **olfactory epithelium** in the superior part of the lateral and septal walls of the nasal cavity. The central processes of these cells (forming the olfactory nerve) pass through the *cribriform plate* and end in the **olfactory bulb**, the rostral expansion of the **olfactory tract** (Fig. 8.105A).

Paranasal Sinuses

N37.2 The **paranasal sinuses** are air-filled extensions of the respiratory part of the nasal cavity into the following cranial bones: frontal, ethmoid, sphenoid, and maxilla. They are named according to the bones in which they are located. The sinuses continue to invade the surrounding bone, and marked extensions are common in the crania of older people.

FRONTAL SINUSES

The **right and left frontal sinuses** are between the outer and inner tables of the frontal bone, posterior to the superciliary arches and the root of the nose (Figs. 8.106, 8.107, and 8.110). Frontal sinuses are usually detectable in children by 7 years of age. The right and left sinuses each drain through a **frontonasal duct** into the *ethmoidal infundibulum*, which opens into the *semilunar hiatus* of the middle nasal meatus. The frontal sinuses are innervated by branches of the *supra-orbital nerves* (CN V_1).

The right and left frontal sinuses are rarely of equal size, and the septum between them is not usually situated entirely in the median plane. The frontal sinuses vary in size from approximately 5 mm to large spaces extending laterally into the greater wings of the sphenoid. Often, a frontal sinus has two parts: a vertical part in the squamous part of the frontal bone, and a horizontal part in the orbital part of the frontal bone. One or both parts may be large or small. When the supra-orbital part is large, its roof forms the floor of the anterior cranial fossa and its floor forms the roof of the orbit.

ETHMOIDAL CELLS

The **ethmoidal cells** (sinuses) are small invaginations of the mucous membrane of the middle and superior nasal meatus into the ethmoid bone between the nasal cavity and the orbit (Figs. 8.107, 8.110, and 8.111). The ethmoidal cells usually are not visible in plain radiographs before 2 years of age; however, they are recognizable in CT scans. The **anterior ethmoidal cells** drain directly or indirectly into the middle nasal meatus through the ethmoidal infundibulum. The **middle ethmoidal cells** open directly into the middle meatus and are sometimes called "bullar cells" because they form the *ethmoidal bulla*, a swelling on the superior border of the semilunar hiatus (Fig. 8.106B). The **posterior ethmoidal cells** open directly into the superior meatus. The ethmoidal cells are supplied by the anterior and posterior ethmoidal branches of the *nasociliary nerves* (CN V_1) (Figs. 8.19 and 8.109).

SPHENOIDAL SINUSES

The **sphenoidal sinuses** are located in the body of the sphenoid, but they may extend into the wings of this bone

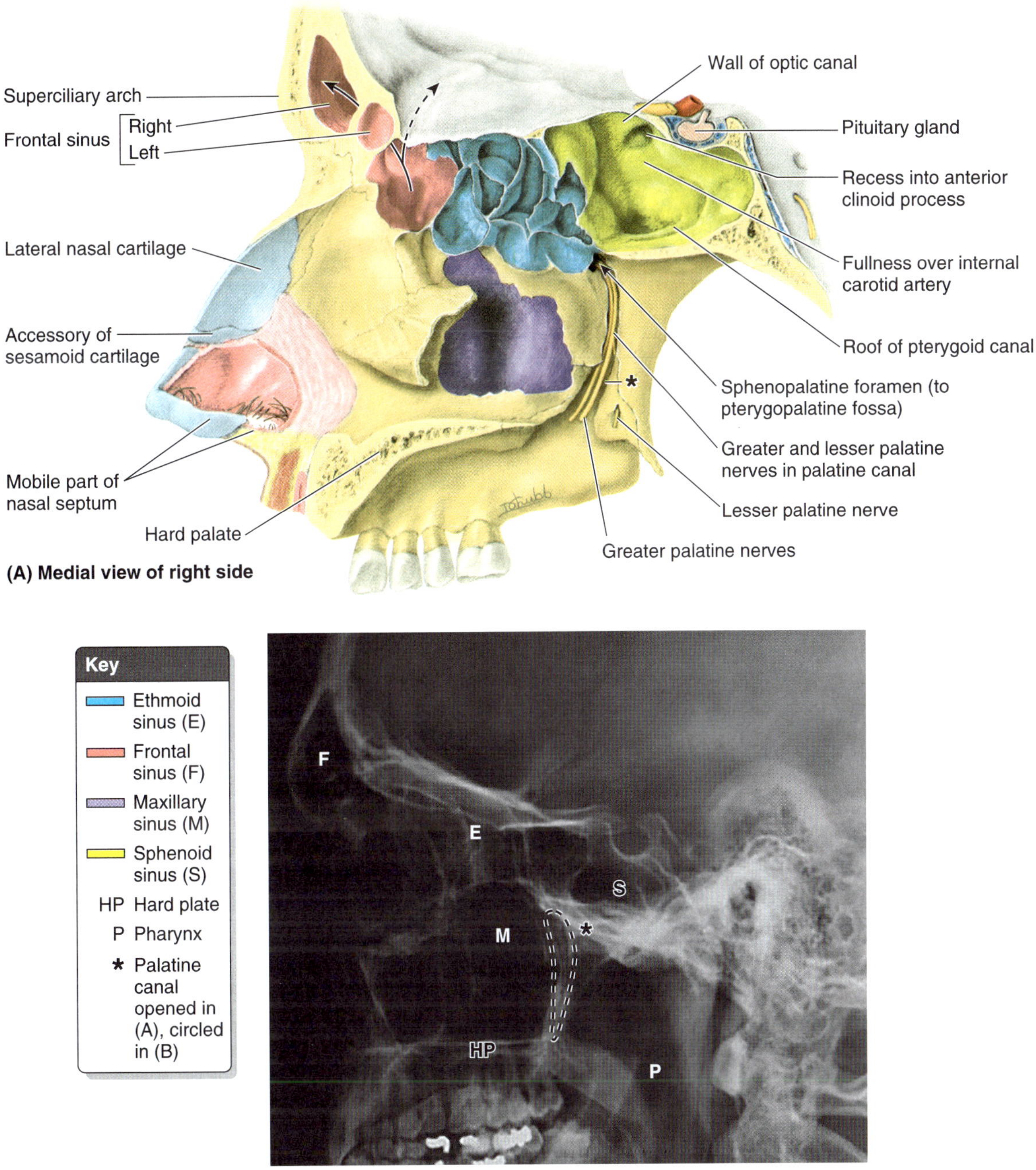

(A) Medial view of right side

(B) Left lateral radiograph

AN43.7 **FIGURE 8.110. Paranasal sinuses I. A.** The paranasal sinuses of the right side have been opened from a nasal approach and color coded. An anterior ethmoidal cell (*pink*) is invading the diploë of the frontal bone to become a frontal sinus. An offshoot (*broken arrow*) invades the orbital plate of the frontal bone. The sphenoidal sinus in this specimen is extensive, extending (1) posteriorly, inferior to the pituitary gland, to the clivus; (2) laterally, inferior to the optic nerve (CN II), into the anterior clinoid process; and (3) inferior to the pterygoid process but leaving the pterygoid canal and rising as a ridge on the floor of the sinus. The maxillary sinus is pyramidal. **B.** Radiograph of cranium demonstrating air densities (dark areas) associated with paranasal sinuses, nasal cavity, oral cavity, and pharynx. The letters are defined in part **A**.

(Figs. 8.106 and 8.110). They are unevenly divided and separated by a bony septum. Because of this extensive pneumatization (formation of air cells), the body of the sphenoid is fragile. Only thin plates of bone separate the sinuses from several important structures: the optic nerves and optic chiasm, the pituitary gland, the internal carotid arteries, and the cavernous sinuses. The sphenoidal sinuses are derived from a posterior ethmoidal cell that begins to invade the sphenoid at approximately 2 years of age. In some people, several posterior ethmoidal cells invade the sphenoid, giving rise to multiple sphenoidal sinuses that open separately into the *spheno-ethmoidal recess* (Fig. 8.106A). The posterior ethmoidal arteries and the posterior ethmoidal nerves that accompany the arteries supply the sphenoidal sinuses (Fig. 8.108).

(*continued on p.* 1023)

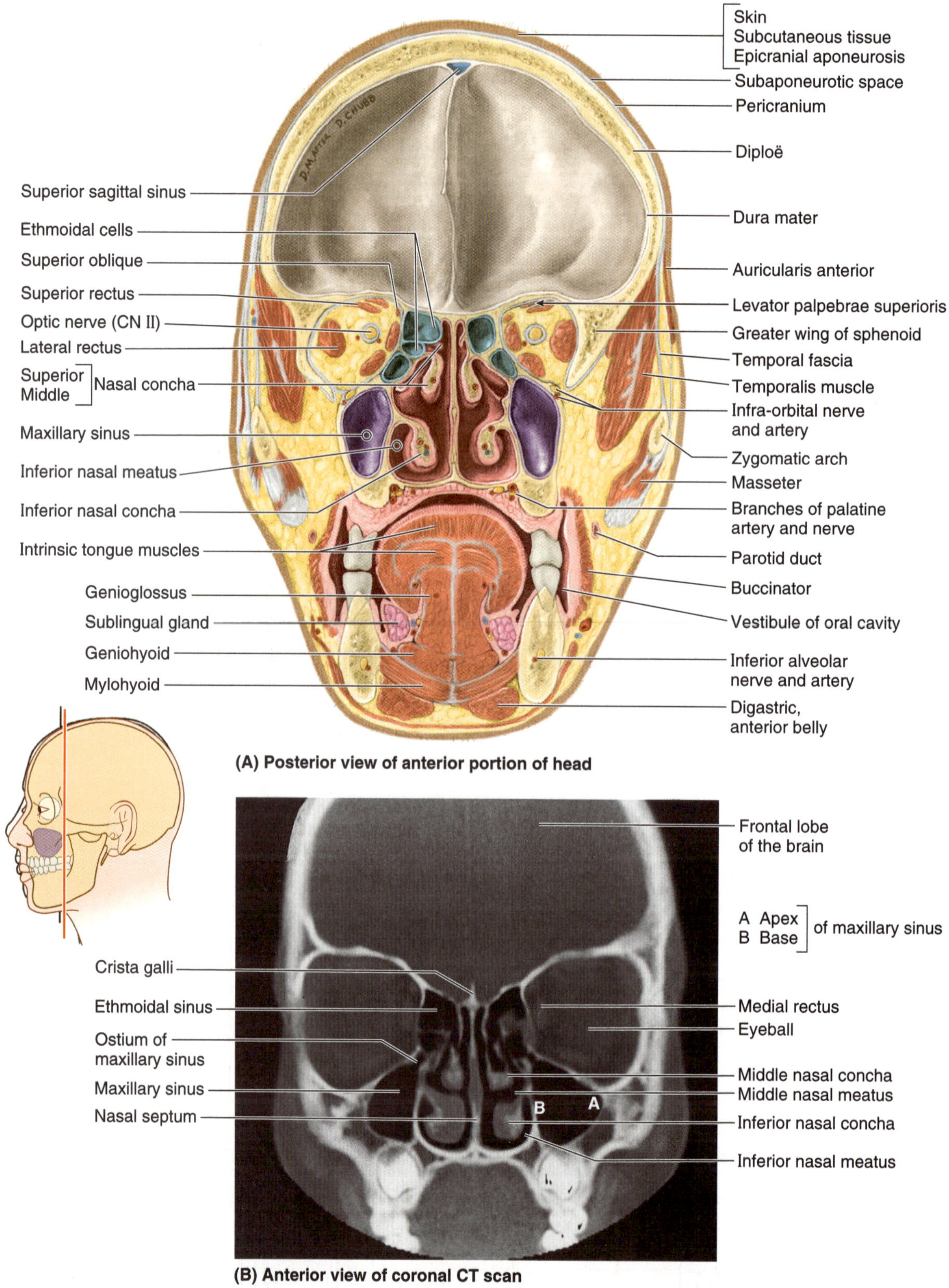

FIGURE 8.111. Paranasal sinuses II. The orientation drawing shows the plane of the section shown in both parts. **A.** The ethmoid bone occupies a central position, with its horizontal component forming the central part of the anterior cranial fossa superiorly, and the roof of the nasal cavity inferiorly. The ethmoidal cells give attachment to the superior and middle concha and form part of the medial wall of the orbit. The perpendicular plate of the ethmoid forms part of the nasal septum. The maxillary sinus forms the inferior part of the lateral wall of the nose and shares a common wall with the orbit. The middle concha shelters the semilunar hiatus into which the maxillary ostium opens (*arrow*). **B.** The CT scan demonstrates air-filled cavities shown in an anatomical section in part **A**. (Courtesy of Dr. D. Armstrong, Associate Professor of Medical Imaging, University of Toronto, Toronto, Ontario, Canada.)

MAXILLARY SINUSES

The **maxillary sinuses** are the largest of the paranasal sinuses. They occupy the bodies of the maxillae and communicate with the middle nasal meatus (Figs. 8.107, 8.110, and 8.111).

- The **apex** of the maxillary sinus extends toward and often into the zygomatic bone.
- The **base** of the maxillary sinus forms the inferior part of the lateral wall of the nasal cavity.
- The **roof** of the maxillary sinus is formed by the floor of the orbit.
- The **floor** of the maxillary sinus is formed by the alveolar part of the maxilla. The roots of the maxillary teeth, particularly the first two molars, often produce conical elevations in the floor of the sinus.

Each maxillary sinus drains by one or more openings, the **maxillary ostium** (pl. ostia), into the middle nasal meatus of the nasal cavity by way of the semilunar hiatus.

The **arterial supply of the maxillary sinus** is mainly from superior alveolar branches of the **maxillary artery** (Fig. 8.75; Table 8.12). However, branches of the *descending* and *greater palatine arteries* supply the floor of the sinus (Fig. 8.101B). **Innervation of the maxillary sinus** is from the anterior, middle, and posterior **superior alveolar nerves**, which are branches of the maxillary nerve (Fig. 8.81A).

CLINICAL BOX

THE NOSE

Nasal Fractures

Because of the prominence of the nose, fractures of the nasal bones are common in automobile accidents and contact sports (unless face guards are worn). Fractures usually result in deformation of the nose, particularly when a lateral force is applied by someone's elbow, for example; *epistaxis* (nosebleed) usually occurs. In severe fractures, disruption of the bones and cartilages results in displacement of the nose. When the injury results from a direct blow, the cribriform plate of the ethmoid bone may also be fractured.

Deviation of Nasal Septum

The nasal septum is usually deviated to one side or the other (Fig. B8.41). This could be the result of a birth injury, but more often the deviation

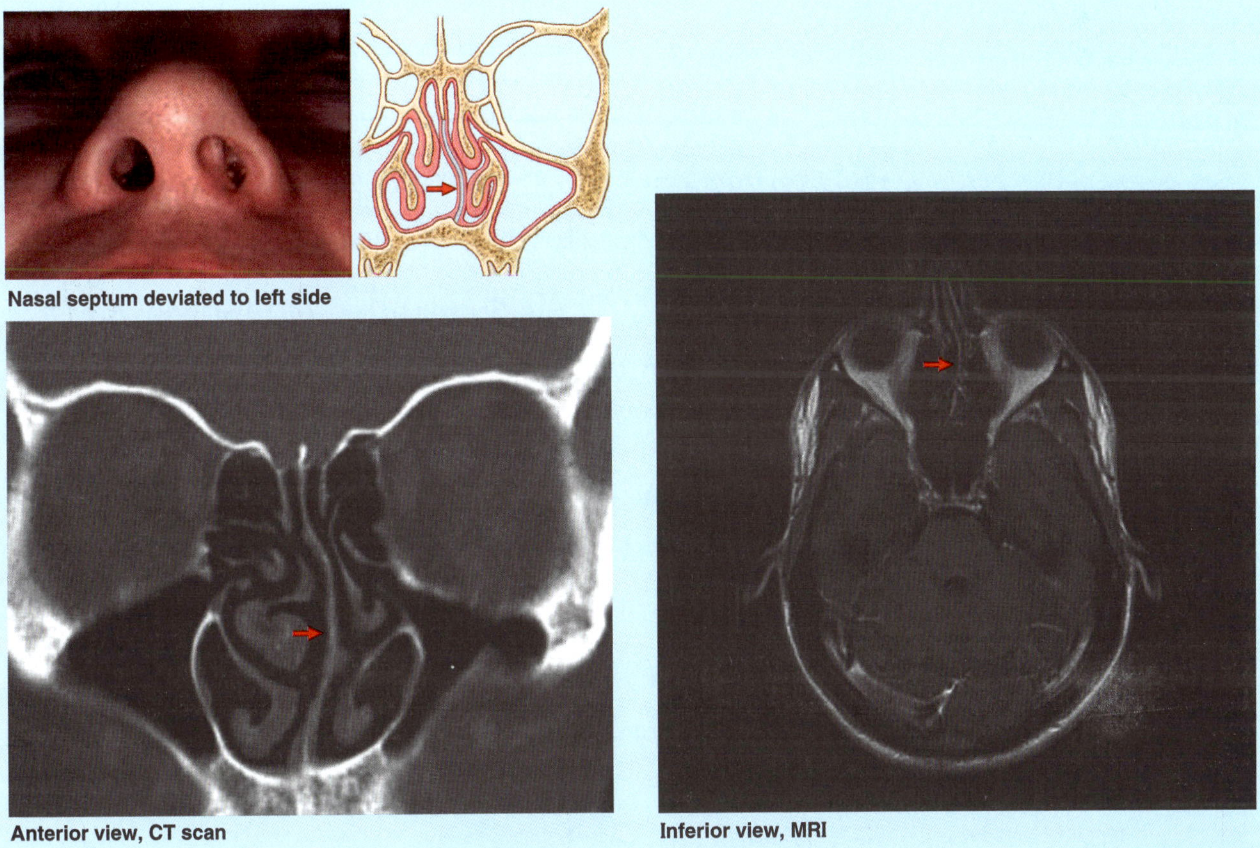

FIGURE B8.41. Deviated nasal septum.

occurs during adolescence and adulthood from trauma (e.g., during a fist fight). Sometimes, the deviation is so severe that the nasal septum is in contact with the lateral wall of the nasal cavity and often obstructs breathing or exacerbates snoring. The deviation can be corrected surgically.

Rhinitis

The nasal mucosa becomes swollen and inflamed (*rhinitis*) during severe upper respiratory infections and allergic reactions (e.g., hay fever). Swelling of the mucosa occurs readily because of its vascularity. Infections of the nasal cavities may spread to the

- anterior cranial fossa through the cribriform plate.
- nasopharynx and retropharyngeal soft tissues.
- middle ear through the *pharyngotympanic tube* (auditory tube), which connects the tympanic cavity and nasopharynx.
- paranasal sinuses.
- lacrimal apparatus and conjunctiva.

Epistaxis

Epistaxis (nosebleed) is relatively common because of the rich blood supply to the nasal mucosa. In most cases, the cause of nosebleed is trauma and the bleeding is from an area in the anterior third of the nose (Kiesselbach area—Fig. 8.108B). Epistaxis is also associated with infections and hypertension. Spurting of blood from the nose results from rupture of arteries. Mild epistaxis may also result from nose picking, which tears veins in the vestibule of the nose.

Sinusitis

AN37.3 Because the paranasal sinuses are continuous with the nasal cavities through apertures that open into them, infection may spread from the nasal cavities, producing inflammation and swelling of the mucosa of the sinuses (*sinusitis*) and local pain. Sometimes, several sinuses are inflamed (*pansinusitis*), and the swelling of the mucosa may block one or more openings of the sinuses into the nasal cavities.

Infection of Ethmoidal Cells

If nasal drainage is blocked, infections of the ethmoidal cells may break through the fragile medial wall of the orbit. Severe infections from this source may cause blindness because some posterior ethmoidal cells lie close to the optic canal, which gives passage to the optic nerve and ophthalmic artery. Spread of infection from these cells could also affect the dural sheath of the optic nerve, causing *optic neuritis*.

Infection of Maxillary Sinuses

The maxillary sinuses are the most commonly infected, probably because their ostia (openings) are commonly small and are located high on their superomedial walls (Fig. 8.111). When the mucous membrane of the sinus is congested, the maxillary ostia are often obstructed. Because of the high location of the ostia, when the head is erect, it is impossible for the sinuses to drain until they are full. Because the ostia of the right and left sinuses lie on the medial sides (i.e., are directed toward each other), when lying on one's side only the upper sinus (e.g., the right sinus if lying on the left side) drains. A cold or allergy involving both sinuses can result in nights of rolling from side to side in an attempt to keep the sinuses drained. A maxillary sinus can be cannulated and drained by passing a cannula from the naris through the maxillary ostium into the sinus.

Relationship of Teeth to Maxillary Sinus

The close proximity of the three maxillary molar teeth to the floor of the maxillary sinus poses potentially serious problems. During removal of a maxillary molar tooth, a fracture of a root of the tooth may occur. If proper retrieval methods are not used, a piece of the root may be driven superiorly into the maxillary sinus creating a communication between the oral cavity and the sinus. This may result in a sinus infection. Because the superior alveolar nerves (branches of the maxillary nerve) supply both the maxillary teeth and the mucous membrane of the maxillary sinuses, inflammation of the mucosa of the sinus is frequently accompanied by a sensation of toothache in the molar teeth.

Transillumination of Sinuses

Transillumination of the maxillary sinuses is performed in a darkened room. A bright light is placed in the patient's mouth on one side of the hard palate or firmly against the cheek (an in Fig. B8.42A). The light passes through the maxillary sinus and appears as a crescent-shaped, dull glow inferior to the orbit. If a sinus contains excess fluid, a mass, or a thickened mucosa, the glow is decreased. The frontal sinuses can also be transilluminated by directing the light superiorly under the medial aspect of the eyebrow, normally producing a glow superior to the orbit (Fig. B8.42B). Because of the great variation in the development of the sinuses, the pattern and extent of sinus illumination differs from person to person (Bickley, 2016).

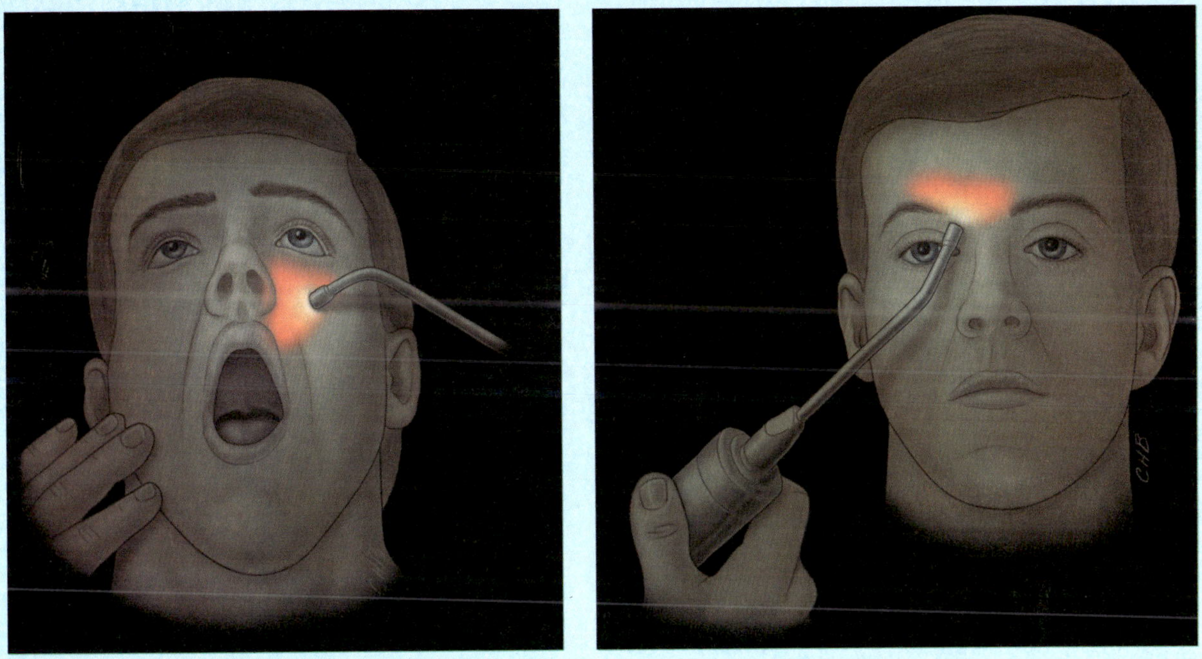

(A) Transillumination of maxillary sinus

(B) Transillumination of frontal sinus

FIGURE B8.42. Transillumination of paranasal sinuses.

The Bottom Line: Nose

The nose is the ventilation system that traverses the head, enabling the flow of air between the external environment and the lower respiratory system (lungs). • As air is drawn in through the nose, its chemistry is sampled (smell and taste augmentation), and it is warmed, humidified, and filtered for the lungs. As it exits, heat and moisture are released with it. • The nose also provides a drainage route for mucus and lacrimal fluid.

Skeleton of nose: Opening anteriorly via the nares, the nasal cavity is subdivided by a median nasal septum. • The protruding external nose and anterior septum benefit from the flexibility provided by a cartilaginous skeleton, reducing the potential for nasal fractures. • Except for the septum and floor, the walls of the nasal cavity are highly pneumatized by the paranasal sinuses, and its lateral walls bear conchae.

Nasal cavities: Both the sinuses and conchae increase the secretory surface area for exchange of moisture and heat. • Essentially, all surfaces are covered with thick, vascular, secretory mucosa, the anterosuperior portion of which (including that of most of the paranasal sinuses) is supplied by the ophthalmic artery and nerve (CN V_1) and the postero-inferior portion (including that of the maxillary sinus) by the maxillary artery and nerve (CN V_2). • The mucosa of the roof and adjacent areas of walls and septum also receive special sensory innervation from the olfactory nerve (CN I). • Posteriorly, the nasal cavity is continuous with the nasopharynx via the choanae; the soft palate serves as a valve or gate controlling access to and from the nasal passageway. • The bone and mucosa of the lateral walls of this passageway are perforated by openings of the nasolacrimal ducts, the paranasal sinuses and the pharyngotympanic tube. • Only the bone is perforated by the pterygopalatine foramen, providing passage of neurovascular structures into the nasal mucosa.

Paranasal sinuses: The paranasal sinuses are named for the bones they occupy. • The maxillary sinus is the largest. • Most sinuses open into the middle nasal meatus, but the sphenoidal sinuses enter the spheno-ethmoidal recess.

EAR

The **ear**—the organ of hearing and equilibrium (balance)—is divided into the external, middle, and internal ear (Fig. 8.112). The external ear and middle ear are mainly concerned with the transfer of sound to the internal ear, which contains the organ for equilibrium as well as for hearing. The *tympanic membrane* separates the external ear from the middle ear. The *pharyngotympanic tube* joins the middle ear to the nasopharynx.

External Ear

N40.1 The **external ear** is composed of the shell-like *auricle (pinna)*, which collects sound, and the *external acoustic meatus* (ear canal), which conducts sound to the tympanic membrane.

AURICLE

The **auricle** (L. *auris*, ear) is composed of an irregularly shaped plate of elastic cartilage that is covered by thin skin (Fig. 8.113). The auricle has several depressions and elevations. The **concha of the auricle** is the deepest depression. The elevated margin of the auricle is the **helix**. The other depressions and elevations are identified in Figure 8.113. The noncartilaginous **lobule** (lobe) consists of fibrous tissue, fat, and blood vessels. It is easily pierced for taking small blood samples and inserting earrings. The **tragus** (G. *tragos*, goat; alluding to the hairs that tend to grow from this formation, like a goat's beard) is a tongue-like projection overlapping the opening of the external acoustic meatus. The **arterial supply** to the auricle is derived mainly from the *posterior auricular* and *superficial temporal arteries* (Fig. 8.114A).

The main **nerves to the skin of the auricle** are the great auricular and auriculotemporal nerves. The **great auricular nerve** supplies the cranial (medial) surface (commonly called the "back of the ear") and the posterior part (*helix, antihelix*, and *lobule*) of the lateral surface ("front of ear"). The *auriculotemporal nerve*, a branch of CN V_3, supplies the skin of the anterior aspect of the lateral surface of the auricle, including the *rim of the concha, crus of the helix*, and *tragus* (Figs. 8.112 and 8.114A). The skin of the concha is mostly innervated by the *auricular branch of the vagus*, with minor contribution by the facial nerve.

The **lymphatic drainage** of the auricle is as follows: the lateral surface of the superior half of the auricle drains to the *superficial parotid lymph nodes* (Fig. 8.114B); the cranial surface of the superior half of the auricle drains to the **mastoid lymph nodes** and *deep cervical lymph nodes*; and the

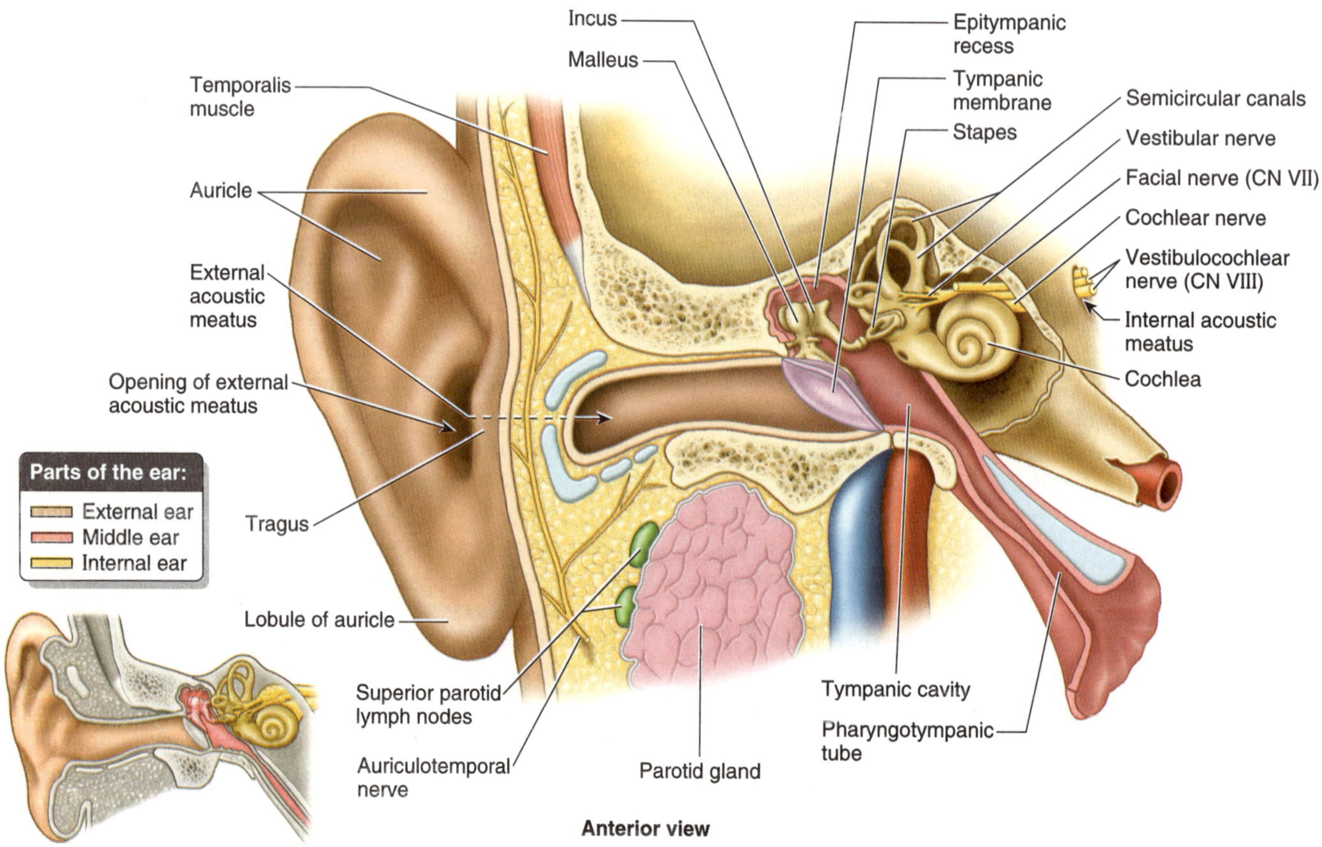

FIGURE 8.112. Parts of ear. A coronal section of the ear, with an accompanying orientation figure, demonstrates that the ear has three parts: external, middle, and internal. The external ear consists of the auricle and external acoustic meatus. The middle ear is an air space in which the auditory ossicles are located. The internal ear contains the membranous labyrinth; its chief divisions are the cochlear labyrinth and the vestibular labyrinth.

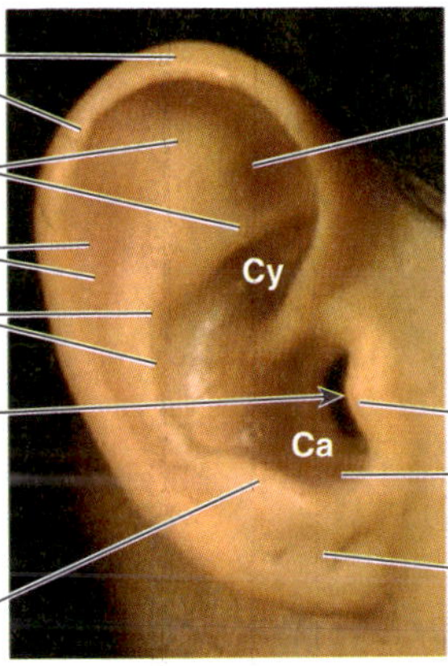

FIGURE 8.113. External ear. The parts of the auricle commonly used in clinical descriptions are labeled. The external ear includes the auricle and external acoustic meatus.

remainder of the auricle, including the lobule, drains into the **superficial cervical lymph nodes**.

EXTERNAL ACOUSTIC MEATUS AND TYMPANIC MEMBRANE

The **external acoustic meatus** is an ear canal that leads inward through the tympanic part of the temporal bone from the auricle to the tympanic membrane, a distance of 2–3 cm in adults (Fig. 8.112). The lateral third of this slightly S-shaped canal is cartilaginous and is lined with skin that is continuous with the auricular skin. The medial two thirds of the meatus is bony and lined with thin skin that is continuous with the external layer of the tympanic membrane. The ceruminous and sebaceous glands in the subcutaneous tissue of the cartilaginous part of the meatus produce *cerumen* (earwax).

The **tympanic membrane**, approximately 1 cm in diameter, is a thin, oval semitransparent membrane at the medial end of the external acoustic meatus (Figs. 8.112 and 8.115). This membrane forms a partition between the external acoustic meatus and the tympanic cavity of the middle ear. The tympanic membrane is covered with thin skin externally and mucous membrane of the middle ear internally. Viewed through an *otoscope*, the tympanic membrane has a concavity toward the external acoustic meatus with a shallow, cone-like central depression, the peak of which is the **umbo** (Fig. 8.115A) (see the clinical box "Otoscopic Examination"). The central axis of the tympanic membrane passes perpendicularly through the umbo like the handle of an umbrella, running anteriorly and inferiorly as it runs laterally. Thus, the tympanic membrane is oriented like a mini radar or satellite dish positioned to receive signals coming from the ground in front and to the side of the head.

Superior to the lateral process of the *malleus* (one of the small ear bones, or *auditory ossicles*, of the middle ear), the membrane is thin and is called the pars **flaccida** (flaccid part). It lacks the radial and circular fibers present in the remainder of the membrane, called the **pars tensa** (tense part). The flaccid part forms the lateral wall of the superior recess of the tympanic cavity.

The tympanic membrane moves in response to air vibrations that pass to it through the external acoustic meatus. Movements of the membrane are transmitted by the auditory ossicles through the middle ear to the internal ear (Fig. 8.112).

The skin of the superior and anterior walls of the external acoustic meatus and the supero-anterior two thirds of the external surface of the tympanic membrane are supplied mainly by the *auriculotemporal nerve* (Fig. 8.114A), a branch of CN V_3. The skin of the posterior and inferior walls of the meatus and postero-inferior third of the external surface of the tympanic membrane are supplied by the *auricular branch of the vagus* (CN X). The internal surface of the tympanic membrane is supplied by the *glossopharyngeal nerve* (CN IX).

Middle Ear

The **tympanic cavity** or **cavity of the middle ear** is the narrow air-filled chamber in the petrous part of the temporal bone (Figs. 8.112 and 8.116). The cavity has two parts: the **tympanic cavity proper**, the space directly internal to the tympanic membrane, and the **epitympanic recess**, the space superior to the membrane. The tympanic cavity is connected anteromedially with the nasopharynx by the *pharyngotympanic tube* and posterosuperiorly with the mastoid cells through the *mastoid antrum* (Figs. 8.116A and 8.117). The tympanic cavity is lined with mucous membrane that is continuous with the lining of the pharyngotympanic tube, mastoid cells, and mastoid antrum. AN40

The contents of the middle ear include the following:

- Auditory ossicles (malleus, incus, and stapes).
- Stapedius and tensor tympani muscles.
- Chorda tympani nerve, a branch of CN VII (Fig. 8.117).
- Tympanic plexus of nerves.

WALLS OF TYMPANIC CAVITY

The middle ear is shaped like a red blood cell or a narrow box with concave sides (Fig. 8.117B). It has six walls:

1. The **tegmental wall (roof)** is formed by a thin plate of bone, the tegmen tympani, which separates the tympanic cavity from the dura mater on the floor of the middle cranial fossa (Fig. 8.117A).
2. The **jugular wall (floor)** is formed by a layer of bone that separates the tympanic cavity from the superior bulb of the internal jugular vein (Fig. 8.117A, B).
3. The **membranous (lateral) wall** is formed almost entirely by the peaked convexity of the *tympanic membrane*; superiorly, it is formed by the lateral bony wall of the *epitympanic recess*. The handle of the malleus is attached to the tympanic membrane, and its head extends into the epitympanic recess.
4. The **labyrinthine (medial) wall (medial wall)** separates the tympanic cavity from the internal ear. It also features the *promontory of the labyrinthine wall*, formed by the initial part (basal turn) of the cochlea, and the *oval* and *round windows*, which, in a dry cranium, communicate with the internal ear.

(*continued on p.* 1030)

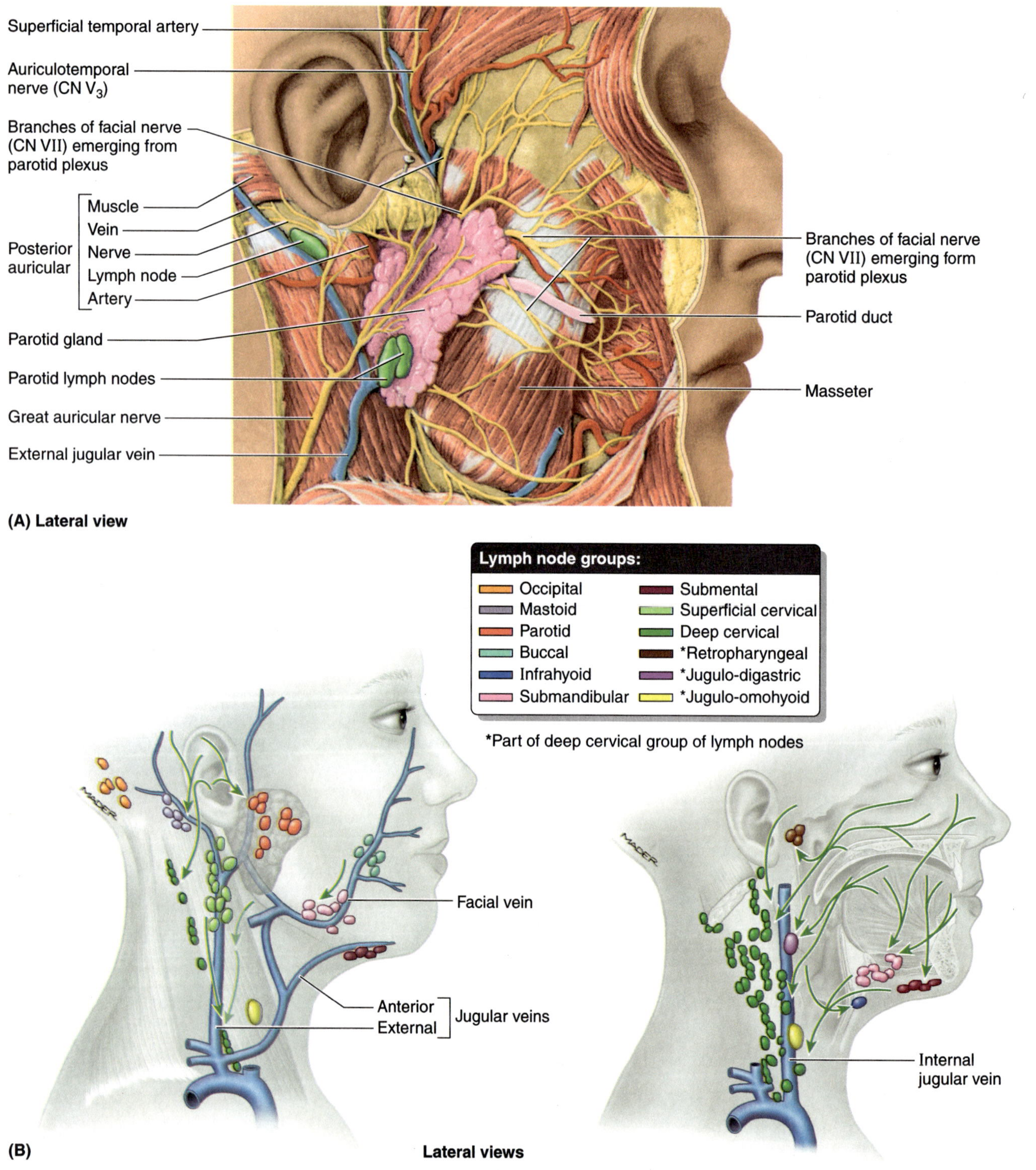

FIGURE 8.114. Dissection of face and lymphatic drainage of head. A. The posterior auricular and superficial temporal arteries and veins and the great auricular and auriculotemporal nerves provide the circulation and innervation of the external ear. **B.** Lymphatic drainage is to the parotid lymph nodes and the mastoid and superficial cervical lymph nodes, all which drain to the deep cervical nodes.

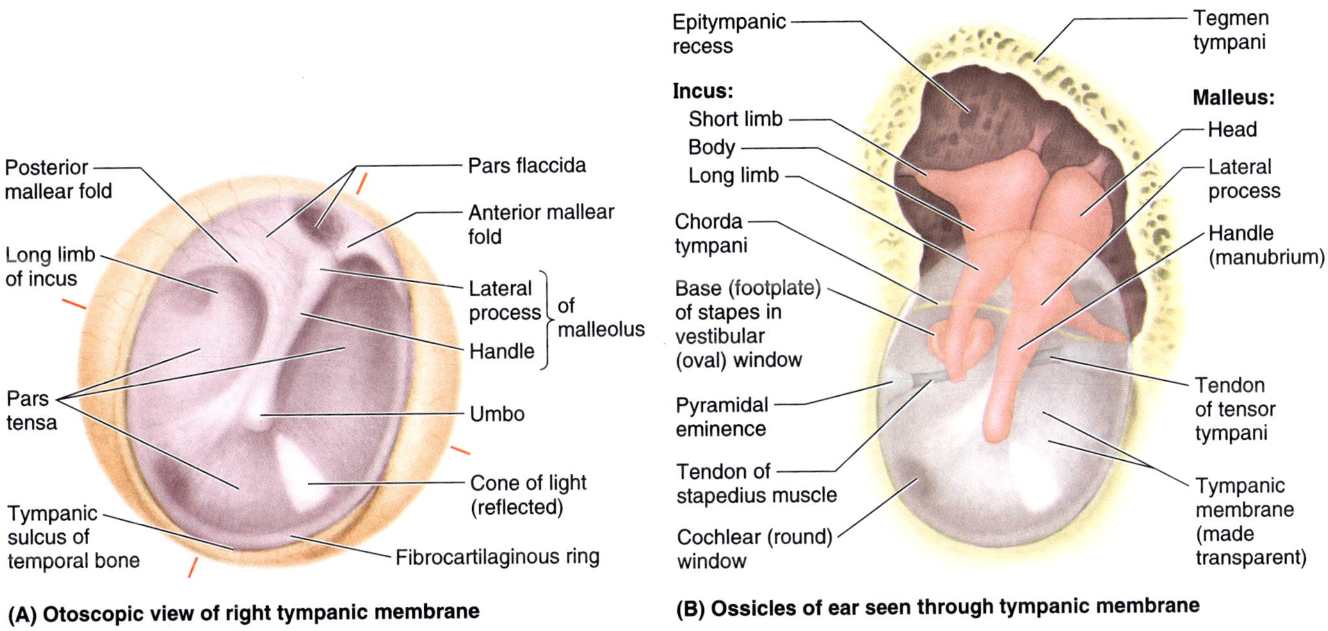

FIGURE 8.115. Tympanic membrane and lateral approach to tympanic cavity. A. An otoscopic view of the right tympanic membrane is demonstrated. The *cone of light* is a reflection of the light of the otoscope. **B.** The tympanic membrane has been rendered semitransparent and the lateral wall of the epitympanic recess has been removed to demonstrate the ossicles of the middle ear in situ.

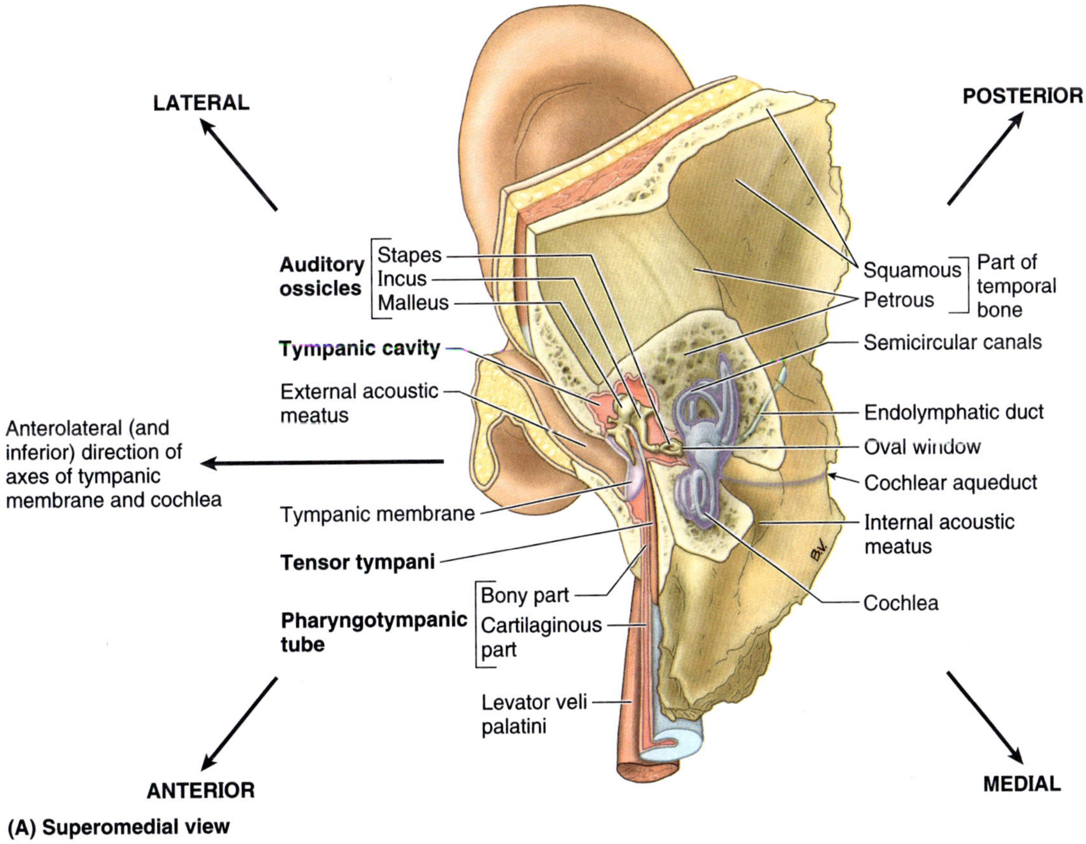

FIGURE 8.116. General scheme and orientation of components of ear. A. The ear is shown in situ. The external acoustic meatus runs lateral to medial. The axis of the tympanic membrane and the axis about which the cochlea winds runs inferiorly and anteriorly as it proceeds laterally. The long axes of the bony and membranous labyrinths and of the pharyngotympanic tube and parallel tensor tympani and levator palatini muscles lie perpendicular to those of the tympanic membrane and cochlea (i.e., they run inferiorly and anteriorly as they proceed medially).

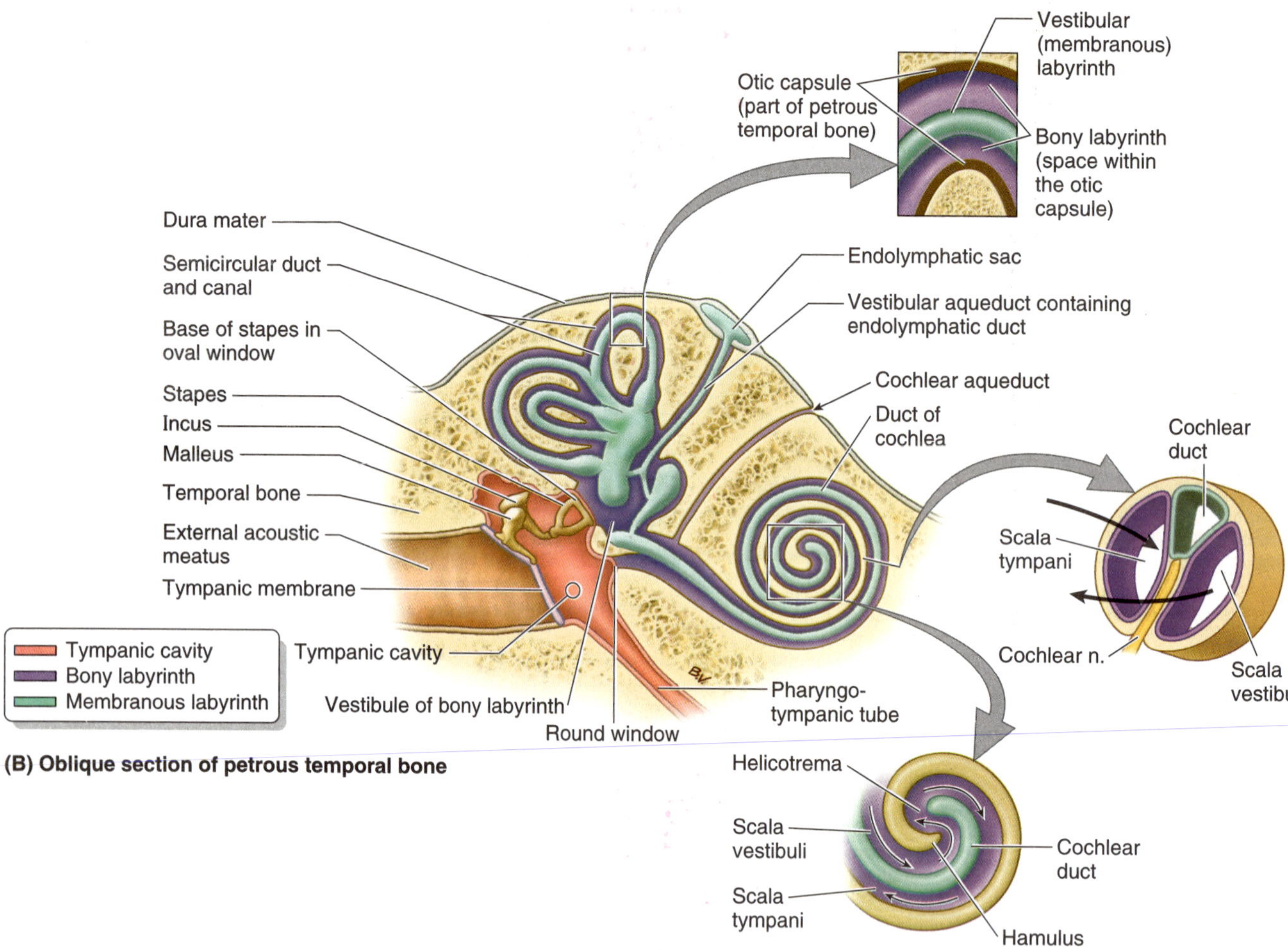

(B) Oblique section of petrous temporal bone

FIGURE 8.116. (Continued) B. The middle and internal parts of the ear are shown. The middle ear lies between the tympanic membrane and the internal ear. Three auditory ossicles stretch from the lateral to the medial wall of the tympanic cavity. The pharyngotympanic tube is a communication between the anterior wall of the tympanic cavity and the lateral wall of the nasopharynx. The internal ear is composed of a closed system of membranous tubes and bulbs, the membranous labyrinth, which is filled with a fluid called endolymph (*orange*) and bathed in surrounding fluid called perilymph (*purple*).

5. The **mastoid wall (posterior wall)** features an opening in its superior part, the **aditus (L. access) to the mastoid antrum**, connecting the tympanic cavity to the mastoid cells. The canal for the facial nerve descends between the posterior wall and the antrum, medial to the aditus.
6. The anterior **carotid wall** separates the tympanic cavity from the carotid canal; superiorly, it has the **opening of the pharyngotympanic tube** and the **canal for the tensor tympani**.
7. The **mastoid antrum** is a cavity in the mastoid process of the temporal bone (Fig. 8.117A). The antrum (L. from G., cave), like the tympanic cavity, is separated from the middle cranial fossa by a thin plate of the temporal bone, called the **tegmen tympani**. This structure forms the *tegmental wall* (roof) for the ear cavities and is also part of the floor of the lateral part of the middle cranial fossa. The mastoid antrum is the common cavity into which the mastoid cells open. The antrum and mastoid cells are lined by mucous membrane that is continuous with the lining of the middle ear. Antero-inferiorly, the antrum is related to the canal for the facial nerve.

PHARYNGOTYMPANIC TUBE

AN40.2

The **pharyngotympanic tube (auditory tube)** connects the tympanic cavity to the nasopharynx (upper or nasal part of the pharynx), where it opens posterior to the inferior nasal meatus (Fig. 8.116). The posterolateral third of the tube is bony, and the remainder is cartilaginous. The pharyngotympanic tube is lined by mucous membrane that is continuous posteriorly with that of the tympanic cavity and anteriorly with that of the nasopharynx.

The *function of the pharyngotympanic tube* is to equalize pressure in the middle ear with the atmospheric pressure, thereby allowing free movement of the tympanic membrane. By allowing air to enter and leave the tympanic cavity, this tube balances the pressure on both sides of the membrane. Because the walls of the cartilaginous part of the tube are normally in apposition, the tube must be actively opened. It is opened by a combination of the expanding girth of the belly of the *levator veli palatine*, as it contracts longitudinally, pushing against one wall and the *tensor veli palatini* pulling on the other. Because these are muscles of the soft palate,

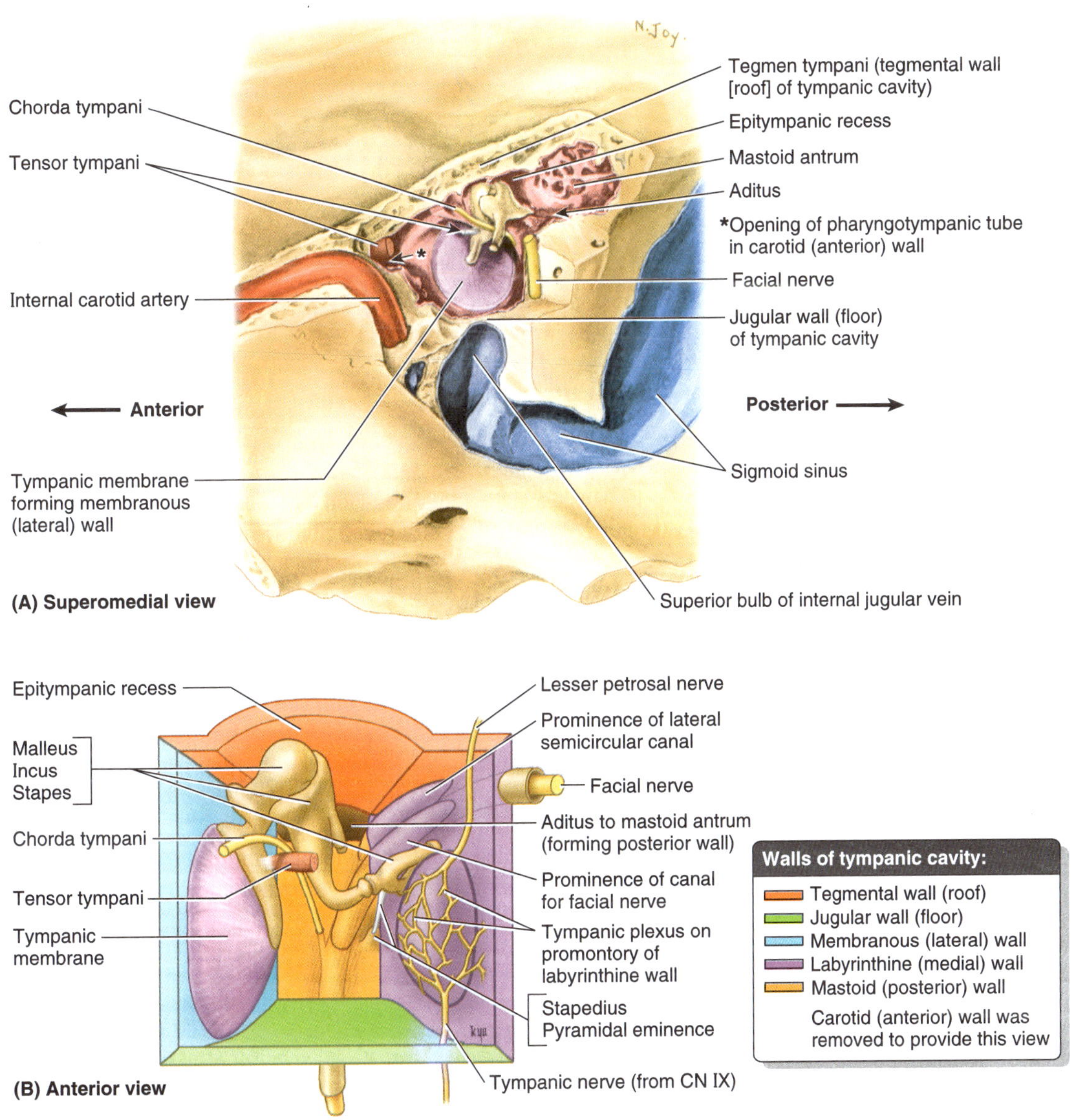

FIGURE 8.117. Walls of tympanic cavity. A. This specimen was dissected with a drill from the medial aspect. The *tegmen tympani*, forming the roof of the tympanic cavity and the mastoid antrum, is fairly thick in this specimen; usually, it is extremely thin. The internal carotid artery is the main relation of the anterior wall, the internal jugular vein is the main relation of the floor, and the facial nerve (CN VII) is a main feature of the posterior wall. The chorda tympani passes between the malleus and the incus. **B.** In this view of the middle ear, the carotid (anterior) wall of the tympanic cavity has been removed. The tympanic membrane forms most of the membranous (lateral) wall; superior to it is the epitympanic recess, in which are housed the larger parts of the malleus and incus. Branches of the tympanic plexus provide innervation to the mucosa of the middle ear and adjacent pharyngotympanic tube. However, one branch, the lesser petrosal nerve, is conveying presynaptic parasympathetic fibers to the otic ganglion for secretomotor innervation of the parotid gland.

equalizing pressure ("popping the eardrums") is commonly associated with activities such as yawning and swallowing.

The *arteries of the pharyngotympanic tube* are derived from the *ascending pharyngeal artery*, a branch of the external carotid artery, and the *middle meningeal artery* and *artery of the pterygoid canal*, branches of the maxillary artery (Fig. 8.118; Table 8.12).

The *veins of the pharyngotympanic tube* drain into the pterygoid venous plexus. The **lymphatic drainage** of the tube is to the *deep cervical lymph nodes* (Fig. 8.114B).

The **nerves of the pharyngotympanic tube** arise from the *tympanic plexus* (Fig. 8.117B), which is formed by fibers of the glossopharyngeal nerve (CN IX). Anteriorly, the tube also receives fibers from the *pterygopalatine ganglion* (Fig. 8.109A).

AUDITORY OSSICLES

The **auditory ossicles** form a mobile *chain of small bones* across the tympanic cavity from the tympanic membrane to the **oval window** (L. *fenestra vestibuli*), an oval opening on the labyrinthine wall of the tympanic cavity leading to the *vestibule of the bony labyrinth* (Figs. 8.116B and 8.119A). These ossicles are the first bones to be fully ossified during development and are essentially mature at birth. The bone

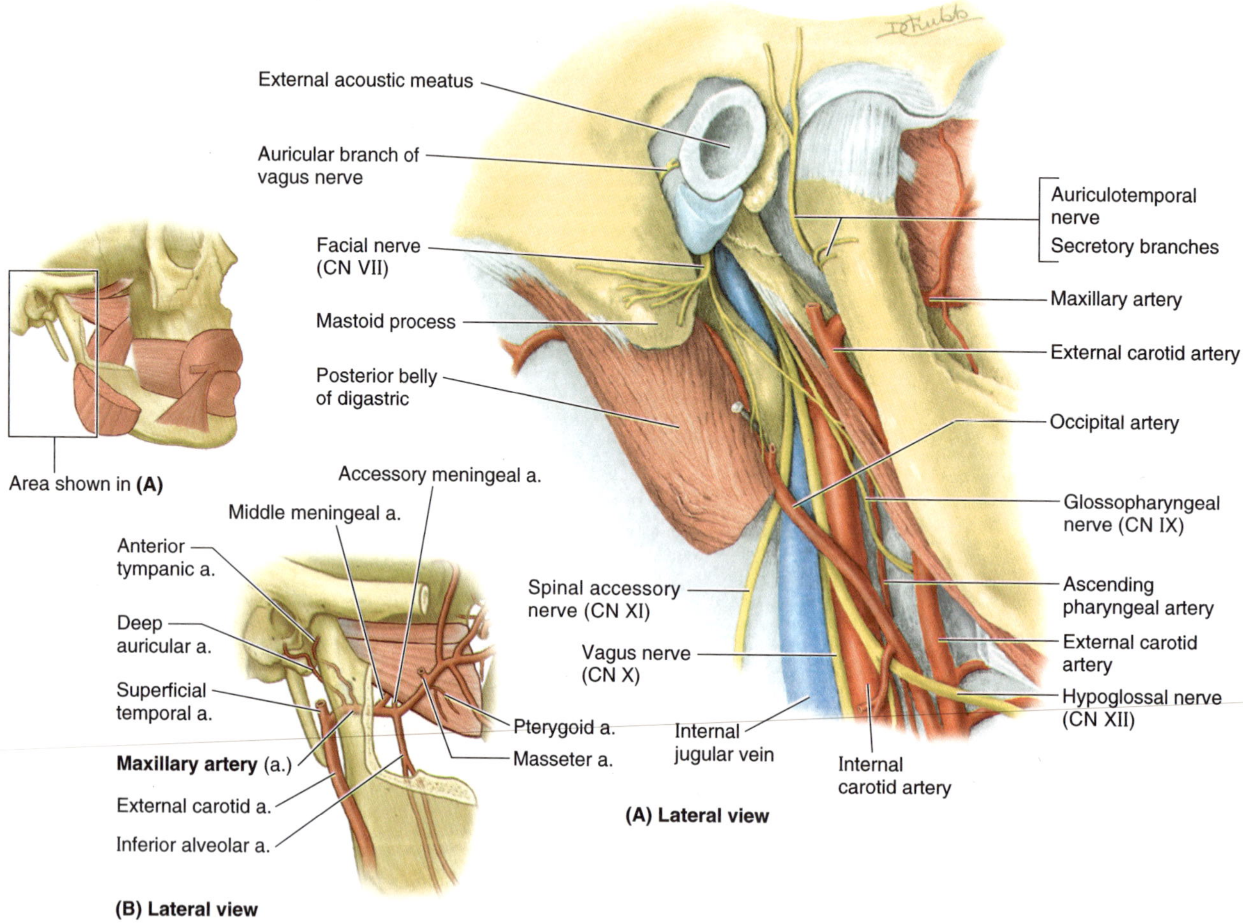

FIGURE 8.118. Neurovascular structures in vicinity of external and middle ear. A. In this dissection of structures deep to parotid bed, the facial nerve (CN VII), the posterior belly of the digastric muscle, and the nerve to it are retracted. The deeply placed ascending pharyngeal artery is the only medial branch of the external carotid artery. It supplies the pharynx, palatine tonsil, pharyngotympanic tube, and the medial wall of the tympanic cavity before it terminates by sending meningeal branches to the cranial cavity. **B.** Maxillary artery and its branches. The branches of the first (mandibular) part supply the external acoustic meatus and tympanic membrane. The middle meningeal artery sends branches to the pharyngotympanic tube before entering the cranium through the foramen spinosum.

from which they are formed is exceptionally dense (hard). The ossicles are covered with the mucous membrane lining the tympanic cavity; but unlike other bones, they lack a surrounding layer of osteogenic periosteum.

Malleus. The **malleus** (L. a hammer) attaches to the tympanic membrane. The rounded superior **head of the malleus** lies in the epitympanic recess (Fig. 8.119B). The **neck of the malleus** lies against the flaccid part of the tympanic membrane, and the **handle of the malleus** is embedded in the tympanic membrane, with its tip at the umbo; thus, the malleus moves with the membrane. The head of the malleus articulates with the incus; the tendon of the tensor tympani inserts into its handle near the neck. The *chorda tympani* crosses the medial surface of the neck of the malleus. The malleus functions as a lever, with the longer of its two processes and its handle attached to the tympanic membrane.

Incus. The **incus** (L. an anvil) is located between the malleus and the stapes and articulates with them. It has a **body** and two limbs. Its large body lies in the epitympanic recess (Fig. 8.119A), where it articulates with the head of the malleus (Fig. 8.119C). The **long limb** lies parallel to the handle of the malleus, and its interior end articulates with the stapes by way of the **lenticular process**, a medially directed projection. The **short limb** is connected by a ligament to the posterior wall of the tympanic cavity.

Stapes. The **stapes** (L. stirrup) is the smallest ossicle. It has a head, two limbs, and a base (Fig. 8.119D). Its head, directed laterally, articulates with the incus (Fig. 8.119A). The **base** (footplate) of the stapes fits into the *oval window* on the medial wall of the tympanic cavity. The oval base is attached to the margins of the oval window. The base of the stapes is considerably smaller than the tympanic membrane; as a result, the vibratory force of the stapes is increased approximately 10 times over that of the tympanic membrane. Consequently, the auditory ossicles increase the force but decrease the amplitude of the vibrations transmitted from the tympanic membrane through the ossicles to the internal ear (see Fig. 8.123).

Muscles Associated with Auditory Ossicles. Two muscles dampen or resist movements of the auditory ossicles; one also dampens movements (vibration) of the

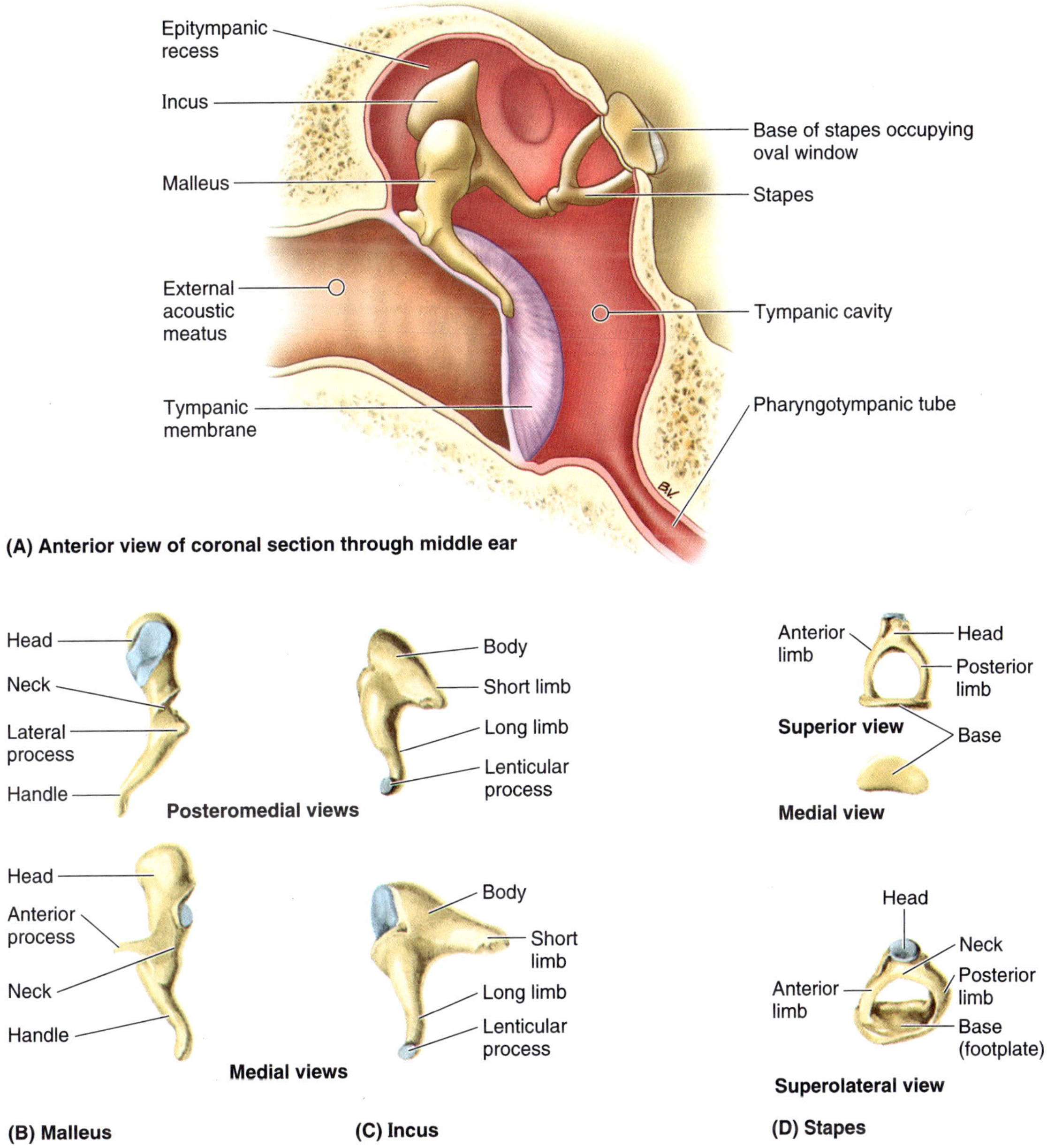

FIGURE 8.119. Auditory ossicles. A. The ossicles are shown in situ. **B–D.** The isolated ossicles are shown.

tympanic membrane. The **tensor tympani** is a short muscle that arises from the superior surface of the cartilaginous part of the pharyngotympanic tube, the greater wing of the sphenoid, and the petrous part of the temporal bone (Figs. 8.116A and 8.117). The muscle inserts into the handle of the malleus and pulls the handle medially, which tenses the tympanic membrane, reducing the amplitude of its oscillations. This action tends to prevent damage to the internal ear when one is exposed to loud sounds. The tensor tympani is supplied by the mandibular nerve (CN V_3).

The **stapedius** is a tiny muscle inside the **pyramidal eminence** (pyramid), a hollow, cone-shaped prominence on the posterior wall of the tympanic cavity (Figs. 8.115B and 8.117B). The tendon of the stapedius enters the tympanic cavity by emerging from a pinpoint foramen in the apex of the eminence and inserts on the neck of the stapes. The stapedius pulls the stapes posteriorly and tilts its base in the *oval window*, thereby tightening the anular ligament and reducing the oscillatory range. It also prevents excessive movement of the stapes. The nerve to the stapedius arises from the facial nerve (CN VII).

Internal Ear

The **internal ear** contains the **vestibulocochlear organ** concerned with the reception of sound and the maintenance of balance. Buried in the petrous part of the temporal bone (Figs. 8.116 and 8.120A), the internal ear consists of

(*continued on p.* 1035)

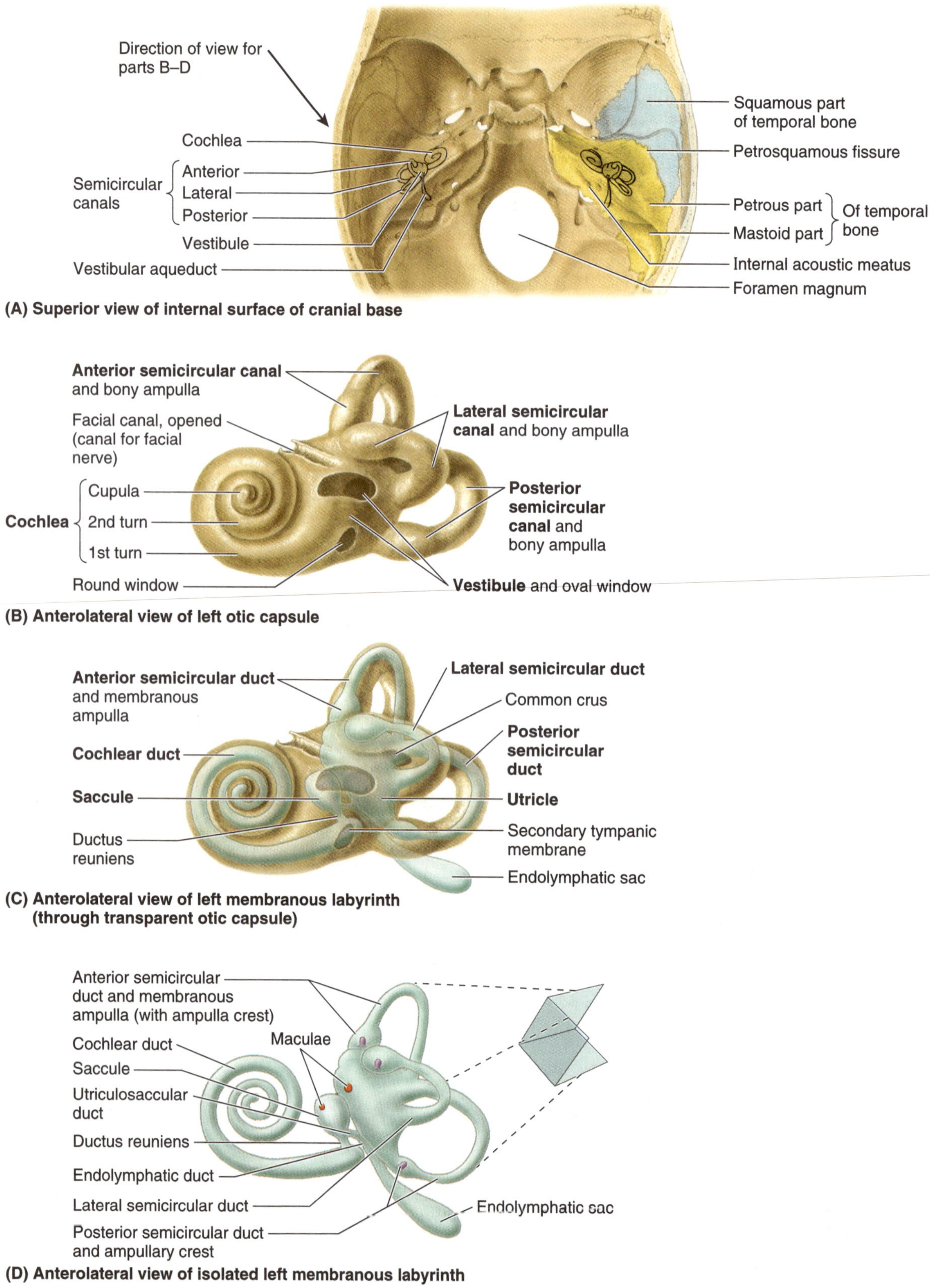

FIGURE 8.120. Bony and membranous labyrinths of internal ear. A. This view of the interior of the base of the cranium shows the temporal bone and the location of the bony labyrinth. **B.** The walls of the bony labyrinth have been carved out of the petrous temporal bone. **C.** A similar view of the bony labyrinth occupied by perilymph and the membranous labyrinth is shown. **D.** The membranous labyrinth, shown after removal from the bony labyrinth, is a closed system of ducts and chambers filled with endolymph and bathed by perilymph. It has three parts: the cochlear duct, which occupies the cochlea; the saccule and utricle, which occupy the vestibule; and the three semicircular ducts, which occupy the semicircular canals. The utricle communicates with the saccule through the utriculosaccular duct. The lateral semicircular duct lies in the horizontal plane and is more horizontal than it appears in this drawing.

the sacs and ducts of the membranous labyrinth. The *membranous labyrinth*, containing *endolymph*, is suspended within the perilymph-filled *bony labyrinth*, either by delicate filaments similar to the filaments of arachnoid mater that traverse the subarachnoid space or by the substantial spiral ligament. It does not float. These fluids are involved in stimulating the end organs for balance and hearing, respectively.

BONY LABYRINTH

The **bony labyrinth** is a series of cavities (cochlea, vestibule, and semicircular canals) contained within the **otic capsule** of the petrous part of the temporal bone (Figs. 8.116A and 8.120B). The otic capsule is made of bone that is denser than the remainder of the petrous temporal bone and can be isolated (carved) from it using a dental drill. The otic capsule is often erroneously illustrated and identified as being the bony labyrinth. However, *the bony labyrinth is the fluid-filled space*, which is surrounded by the otic capsule. Thus, the bony labyrinth is most accurately represented by a cast of the otic capsule after removal of the surrounding bone.

Cochlea. The cochlea is the shell-shaped part of the bony labyrinth that contains the **cochlear duct** (Fig. 8.120C) and is the part of the internal ear concerned with hearing. The **spiral canal of the cochlea** begins at the vestibule and makes 2.5 turns around a bony core, the **modiolus** (Fig. 8.121), the cone-shaped core of spongy bone about which the spiral canal of the cochlea turns. The modiolus contains canals for blood vessels and for distribution of the branches of the cochlear nerve. The apex of the cone-shaped modiolus, like the axis of the tympanic membrane, is directed laterally, anteriorly, and inferiorly. The large basal turn of the cochlea produces the *promontory of the labyrinthine wall* of the tympanic cavity (Fig. 8.117B). At the basal turn, the bony labyrinth communicates with the subarachnoid space superior to the jugular foramen through the **cochlear aqueduct** (Fig. 8.116B). It also features the **round window** (L. *fenestra cochleae*), closed by the **secondary tympanic membrane** (Fig. 8.120B, C).

Vestibule of Bony Labyrinth. The **vestibule of the bony labyrinth** is a small oval chamber (approximately 5 mm long) that contains the **utricle** and **saccule** (Fig. 8.120C) and parts of the balancing apparatus (vestibular labyrinth). The vestibule features the *oval window* on its lateral wall, occupied by the base of the stapes. The vestibule is continuous with the bony cochlea anteriorly, the semicircular canals posteriorly, and the posterior cranial fossa by the **vestibular aqueduct** (Fig. 8.116B). The aqueduct extends to the posterior surface of the petrous part of the temporal bone, where it opens posterolateral to the *internal acoustic meatus* (Fig. 8.120A). The vestibular aqueduct transmits the endolymphatic duct (Figs. 8.116B and 8.120D) and two small blood vessels.

Semicircular Canals. The **semicircular canals (anterior, posterior, and lateral)** communicate with the vestibule of the bony labyrinth (Fig. 8.120B). The canals lie posterosuperior to the vestibule into which they open; they are set at right angles to each other. The canals occupy three planes in space. Each semicircular canal forms approximately two thirds of a circle and is approximately 1.5 mm in diameter, except at one end where there is a swelling, the **bony ampulla**. The canals have only five openings into the vestibule because the anterior and posterior canals have one limb common to both. Lodged within the canals are the *semicircular ducts* (Fig. 8.120C, D).

MEMBRANOUS LABYRINTH

The **membranous labyrinth** consists of a series of communicating sacs and ducts that are suspended in the bony labyrinth (Fig. 8.120C). The labyrinth contains **endolymph**, a watery fluid similar in composition to intracellular fluid, therefore differing in composition from the surrounding **perilymph** (which is like extracellular fluid) that fills the remainder of the bony labyrinth. The membranous labyrinth—composed of two functional divisions, (1) the *vestibular labyrinth* and (2) the *cochlear labyrinth*—consists of more parts than does the bony labyrinth:

1. **Vestibular labyrinth**, concerned with equilibrium, is composed of
   - the utricle and saccule, two small communicating sacs occupying the vestibule of the bony labyrinth.
   - the utriculosaccular duct, connecting the utricle and saccule.
   - three semicircular ducts, occupying the semicircular canals.
   - the endolymphatic duct, ending at the endolymphatic sac.
2. **Cochlear labyrinth**, concerned with hearing, is composed of the cochlear duct occupying the spiral canal of the cochlea.

The two divisions of the membranous labyrinth are connected via the **ductus reuniens**, extending between the saccule and the cochlear duct.

The **semicircular ducts** open into the utricle through five openings, reflective of the way the surrounding semicircular canals open into the vestibule. The utricle communicates with the saccule through the **utriculosaccular duct**, from which the *endolymphatic duct* arises (Fig. 8.120D).

The utricle and saccule have specialized areas of sensory epithelium called **maculae**. The **macula of the utricle** (L. *macula utriculi*) is in the floor of the utricle, parallel with the base of the cranium, whereas the **macula of the saccule** (L. *macula sacculi*) is vertically placed on the medial wall of the saccule. The maculae are sensitive to gravity and linear acceleration or deceleration. **Hair cells** (nonneuronal mechanoreceptors stimulated by the deflection of sensory hairs, or stereocilia) **in the maculae** are innervated by fibers of the vestibular division of the vestibulocochlear nerve (CN VIII), the **vestibular nerve**. The cell bodies of the primary sensory

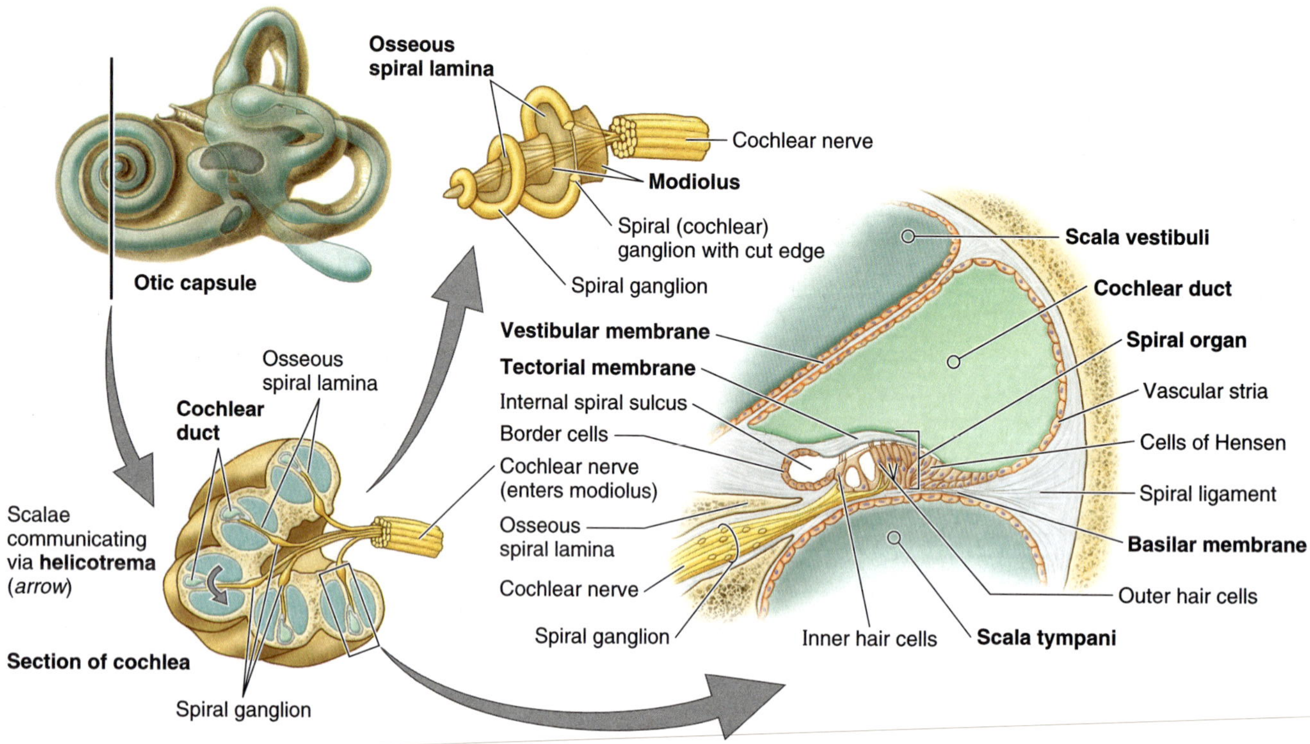

FIGURE 8.121. Structure of cochlea. The cochlea has been sectioned along the axis about which the cochlea winds (see *orientation FIGURE*). An isolated, cone-like, bony core of the cochlea, the modiolus, is shown after the turns of the cochlea are removed, leaving only the spiral lamina winding around it like the thread of a screw. Details of the area enclosed in the rectangle are also shown.

neurons are in the **vestibular ganglion** (Fig. 8.122) in the internal acoustic meatus.

The *endolymphatic duct* traverses the *vestibular aqueduct* (Fig. 8.116B) and emerges through the bone of the posterior cranial fossa, where it expands into a blind pouch, the **endolymphatic sac** (Figs. 8.116B, 8.120C, and 8.122). The endolymphatic sac is located between the two layers of dura mater on the posterior surface of the petrous part of the temporal bone. The sac is a storage reservoir for excess endolymph, formed by the blood capillaries in the membranous labyrinth.

The **spiral ligament**, a spiral thickening of the periosteal lining of the cochlear canal, secures the *cochlear duct* to the spiral canal of the cochlea (Fig. 8.121). The vestibular labyrinth is suspended by delicate filaments that traverse the perilymph.

Semicircular Ducts. Each semicircular duct has an **ampulla** at one end containing a sensory area, the **ampullary crest** (L. *crista ampullari*) (Fig. 8.122). The crests are sensors rotational acceleration or deceleration of the head, recording movements of the endolymph in the ampulla

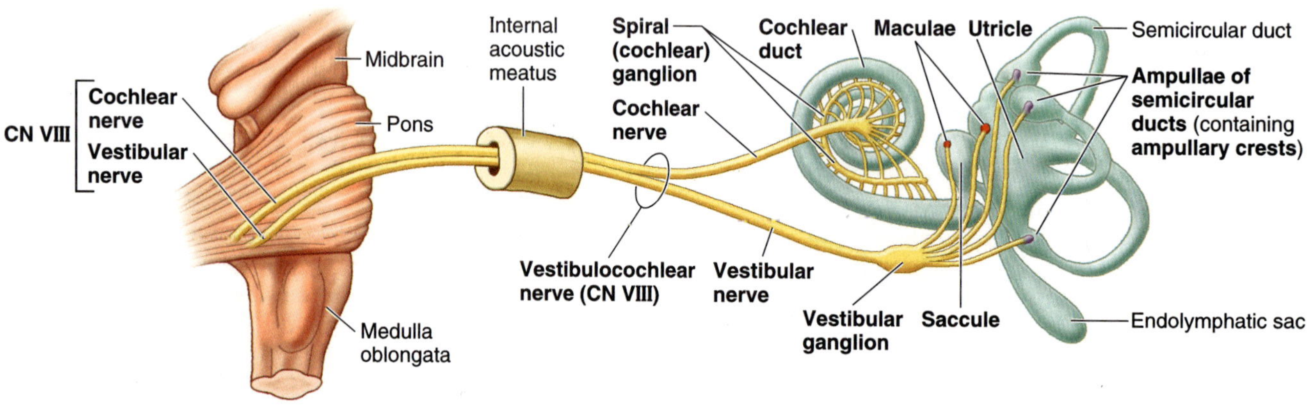

FIGURE 8.122. Vestibulocochlear nerve. CN VIII has two parts: the cochlear nerve (the nerve of hearing) and the vestibular nerve (the nerve of balance). The cell bodies of the sensory fibers that make up the two parts of this nerve constitute the spiral and vestibular ganglia.

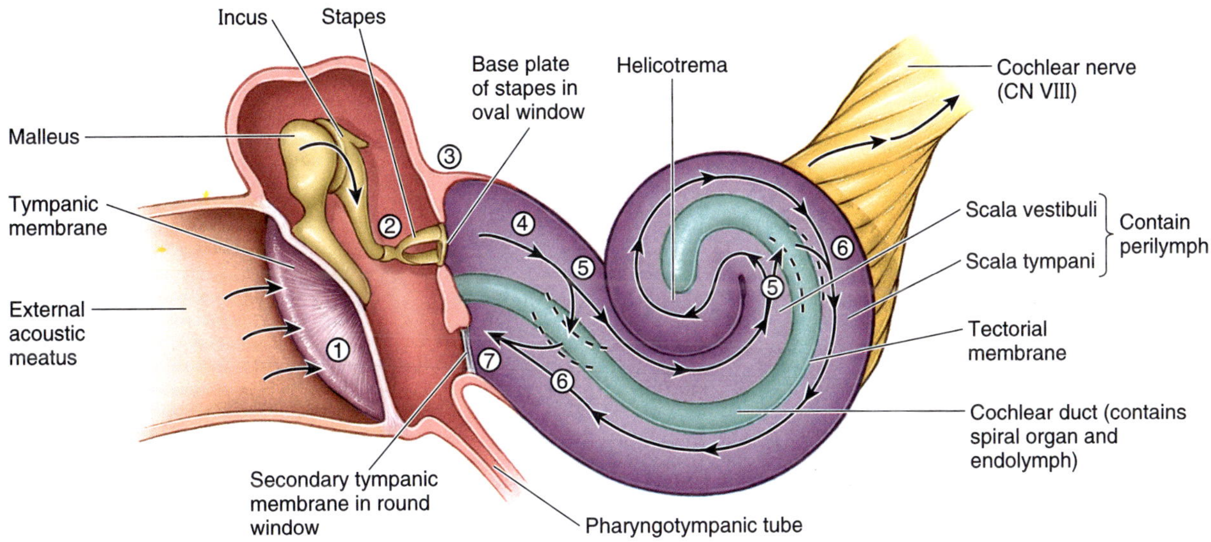

FIGURE 8.123. Sound transmission through the ear. The cochlea is depicted schematically as if consisting of a single coil to demonstrate the transmission of sound stimuli through the ear. *1*, Sound waves entering the external ear strike the tympanic membrane, causing it to vibrate. *2*, Vibrations initiated at the tympanic membrane are transmitted through the ossicles of the middle ear and their articulations. *3*, The base of the stapes vibrates with increased strength and decreased amplitude in the oval window. *4*, Vibrations of the base of the stapes create pressure waves in the perilymph of the scala vestibuli. *5*, Pressure waves in the scala vestibuli cause displacement of the basilar membrane of the cochlear duct. Short waves (high pitch) cause displacement near the oval window. Longer waves (low pitch) cause more distant displacement, nearer to the helicotrema at the apex of the cochlea. Movement of the basilar membrane bends the hair cells of the spiral organ. Neurotransmitter is released, stimulating action potentials conveyed by the cochlear nerve to the brain. *6*, Vibrations are transferred across the cochlear duct to the perilymph of the scala tympani. *7*, Pressure waves in the perilymph are dissipated (dampened) by the secondary tympanic membrane at the round window into the air of the tympanic cavity.

resulting from rotation of the head in the plane of the duct. The **hair cells of the crests**, like those of the maculae, stimulate primary sensory neurons of the vestibular nerve, whose cell bodies are also in the vestibular ganglion.

Cochlear Duct. The **cochlear duct** is a spiral tube, closed at one end and triangular in cross section. The duct is firmly suspended across the cochlear canal between the *spiral ligament* on the external wall of the cochlear canal (Fig. 8.121) and the **osseous spiral lamina** of the modiolus. Spanning the spiral canal in this manner, the endolymph-filled cochlear duct divides the perilymph-filled spiral canal into two channels that are continuous at the apex of the cochlea at the **helicotrema**, a semilunar communication at the apex of the cochlea.

Waves of hydraulic pressure created in the perilymph of the vestibule by the vibrations of the base of the stapes ascend to the apex of the cochlea by one channel, the scala vestibuli (Fig. 8.123). The pressure waves then pass through the helicotrema and descend back to the basal turn of the cochlea by the other channel, the **scala tympani**. Here, the pressure waves again become vibrations, this time of the *secondary tympanic membrane* in the round window, and the energy initially received by the (primary) tympanic membrane is finally dissipated into the air of the tympanic cavity.

The roof of the cochlear duct is formed by the **vestibular membrane**. The floor of the duct is also formed by part of the duct, the **basilar membrane**, plus the outer edge of the osseous spiral lamina. The receptor of auditory stimuli is the **spiral organ** (of Corti), situated on the basilar membrane (Fig. 8.121). It is overlaid by the gelatinous **tectorial membrane**.

The spiral organ contains hair cells, the tips of which are embedded in the tectorial membrane. The organ is stimulated to respond by deformation of the cochlear duct induced by the hydraulic pressure waves in the perilymph, which ascend and descend in the surrounding scalae vestibuli and tympani. The hair cells of the spiral organ are innervated by the cochlear division of the vestibulocochlear nerve (CN VIII), the **cochlear nerve**. The cell bodies of the primary sensory neurons are in the spiral (cochlear) ganglion, located at the root of the spiral lamina of the cochlea.

For microanatomy of cochlea-organ of corti, refer *diFiore's Atlas of Histology with Functional Correlations*, 1st South Asian Edition, Chapter 22, Organs of Special Senses: Visual Auditory Systems, p. 645. AN43.3

INTERNAL ACOUSTIC MEATUS

The **internal acoustic meatus** is a narrow canal that runs laterally for approximately 1 cm within the petrous part of the temporal bone (Fig. 8.120A). The **internal acoustic meatus opening** is in the posteromedial part of this bone, in line with the external acoustic meatus. The internal acoustic meatus is closed laterally by a thin, perforated plate of bone that separates it from the internal ear. Through this plate pass the facial nerve (CN VII), the vestibulocochlear nerve (CN VIII) and its divisions, and blood vessels. The vestibulocochlear nerve divides near the lateral end of the internal acoustic meatus into two parts: a cochlear nerve and a vestibular nerve (Fig. 8.122).

8

CLINICAL BOX

EAR

External Ear Injury

Bleeding within the auricle resulting from trauma may produce an *auricular hematoma*. A localized collection of blood forms between the perichondrium and auricular cartilage, causing distortion of the contours of the auricle. As the hematoma enlarges, it compromises the blood supply to the cartilage. If untreated (e.g., by aspiration of blood), fibrosis (formation of fibrous tissue) develops in the overlying skin, forming a deformed auricle (e.g., the cauliflower or boxer's ear of some professional boxers and wrestlers).

Otoscopic Examination

Examination of the external acoustic meatus and tympanic membrane begins by straightening the meatus. In adults, the helix is grasped and pulled posterosuperiorly (up, out, and back). These movements reduce the curvature of the external acoustic meatus, facilitating insertion of the *otoscope* (Fig. B8.43A). The meatus is relatively short in infants; therefore, extra care must be exercised to prevent injury to the tympanic membrane. The meatus is straightened in infants by pulling the auricle inferoposteriorly (down and back). The examination also provides a clue to tenderness, which can indicate inflammation of the auricle and/or the meatus.

The tympanic membrane is normally translucent and pearly gray (Fig. B8.43B). The handle of the malleus is usually visible near the center of the membrane (the umbo). From the umbo at the inferior end of the handle, a bright *cone of light* is reflected from the otoscope's illuminator. This *light reflex* is visible radiating antero-inferiorly in the healthy ear.

Acute Otitis Externa

AN40.

Otitis externa is an inflammation of the external acoustic meatus. The infection often develops in swimmers who do not dry their meatus (ear canals) after swimming and/or use ear drops. The inflammation may also be the result of a bacterial infection of the skin lining the meatus. The affected individual complains of itching and pain in the external ear. Pulling the auricle or applying pressure on the tragus increases the pain.

Otitis Media

AN40.

An earache and a bulging red tympanic membrane may indicate there is pus or fluid in the middle ear, which is a sign of *otitis media* (Fig. B8.44A). Infection of the middle ear is often secondary to upper respiratory infections. Inflammation and swelling of the mucous membrane lining the tympanic cavity may cause partial or complete blockage of the pharyngotympanic tube (Fig. 8.112). The tympanic membrane becomes red and bulges, and the person may complain of "ear popping" or crackling. An amber-colored bloody fluid may be observed through the tympanic membrane. If untreated, otitis media may produce impaired hearing owing to scarring of the auditory ossicles, limiting their ability to move in response to sound.

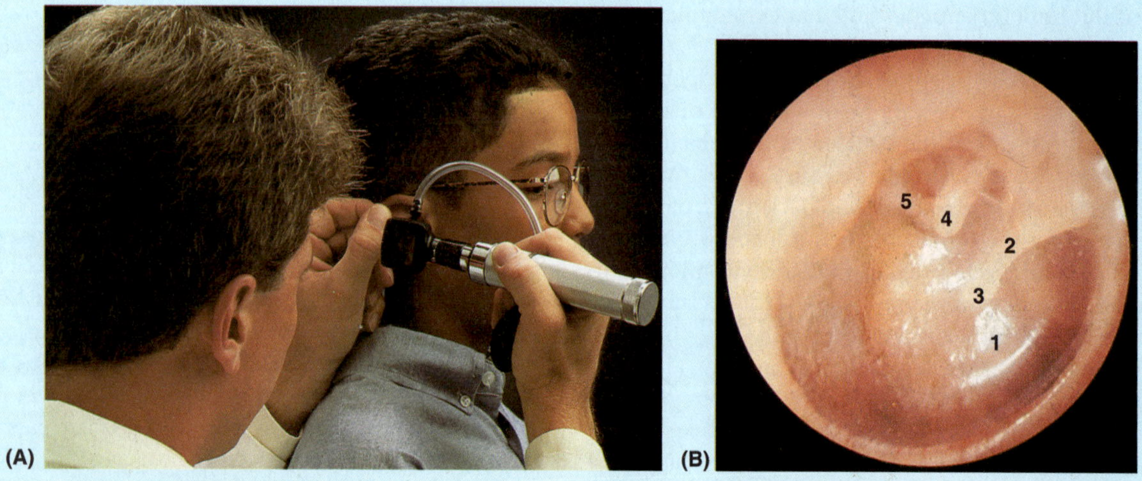

FIGURE B8.43. **A.** Otoscopic examination. **B.** Normal tympanic membrane. *1*, cone of light; *2*, handle of malleus; *3*, umbo; *4*, long limb of incus; *5*, posterior limb of stapes.

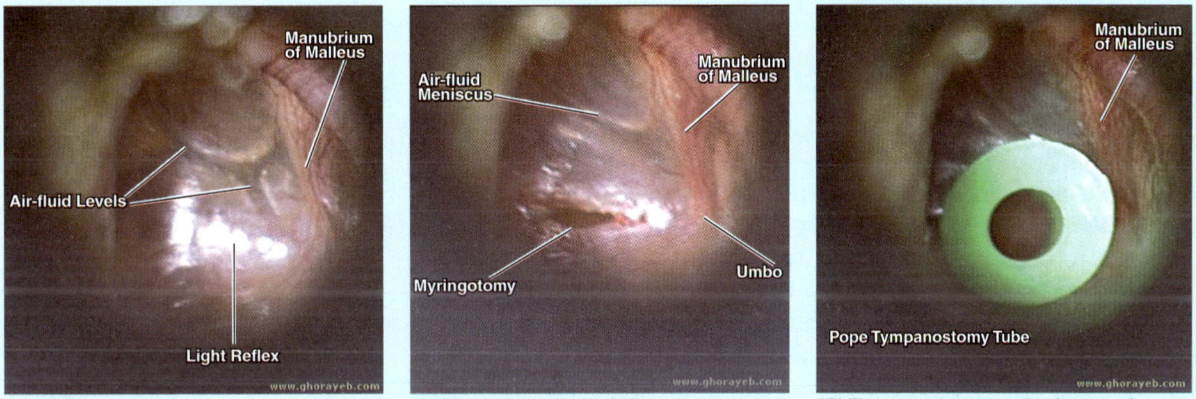

(A) Otitis media (B) Myringotomy incision (C) Tympanostomy tube inserted

(A–C) Otoscopic views

FIGURE B8.44. Otitis media and surgical treatment.

Perforation of Tympanic Membrane

AN40.5 Perforation of the tympanic membrane ("ruptured eardrum") may result from otitis media and is one of several causes of middle ear deafness. Perforation may also result from foreign bodies in the external acoustic meatus, trauma, or excessive pressure (e.g., during scuba diving). Minor ruptures of the tympanic membrane often heal spontaneously. Large ruptures usually require surgical repair. Because the superior half of the tympanic membrane is much more vascular than the inferior half, incisions to release pus from a middle ear abscess (*myringotomy*), for example, are made postero-inferiorly through the membrane (Fig. B8.44B). This incision also avoids injury to the chorda tympani nerve and auditory ossicles. In persons with chronic middle ear infections, myringotomy may be followed by insertion of *tympanostomy or pressure-equalization* (PE) *tubes* in the incision to enable drainage of effusion and ventilation of pressure (Fig. B8.44C).

Mastoiditis

Infections of the mastoid antrum and mastoid cells (*mastoiditis*) result from a middle ear infection that causes inflammation of the mastoid process (Fig. B8.45). Infections may spread superiorly into the middle cranial fossa through the petrosquamous fissure in children and cause *osteomyelitis* (bone infection) of the tegmen tympani. Since the advent of antibiotics, mastoiditis is uncommon. During operations for mastoiditis, surgeons are conscious of the course of the facial nerve to avoid injuring it. One point of access to the tympanic cavity is through the mastoid antrum. In children, only a thin plate of bone must be removed from the lateral wall of the antrum to expose the tympanic cavity. In adults, bone must be penetrated for 15 mm or more. At present, most mastoidectomies are endaural (i.e., performed through the posterior wall of the external acoustic meatus).

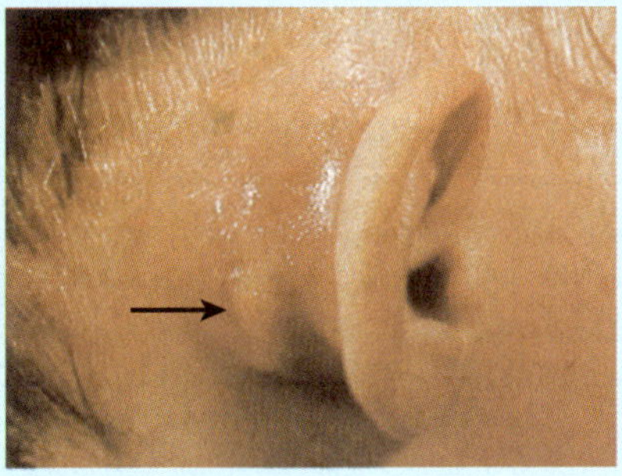

FIGURE B8.45. Mastoiditis (ruptured retro-auricular abscess).

Blockage of Pharyngotympanic Tube

The pharyngotympanic tube forms a route for an infection to pass from the nasopharynx to the tympanic cavity. This tube is easily blocked by swelling of its mucous membrane, even as a result of mild infections (e.g., a cold), because the walls of its cartilaginous part are normally already in apposition. When the pharyngotympanic tube is occluded, residual air in the tympanic cavity is usually absorbed into the mucosal blood vessels, resulting in lower pressure in the tympanic cavity, retraction of the tympanic membrane, and interference with its free movement. Finally, hearing is affected.

Paralysis of Stapedius

The tympanic muscles have a protective action in that they dampen large vibrations of the tympanic membrane resulting from loud noises. Paralysis of the stapedius (e.g., resulting from a lesion of the facial nerve) is associated with excessive acuteness of hearing, called *hyperacusis* or *hyperacusia*. This condition results from uninhibited movements of the stapes.

Motion Sickness

The maculae of the membranous labyrinth are primarily static organs, which have small dense particles (*otoliths*) embedded among hair cells. Under the influence of gravity, the otoliths cause bending of the hair cells, which stimulate the vestibular nerve, and provide awareness of the position of the head in space; the hairs also respond to quick tilting movements and to linear acceleration and deceleration. *Motion sickness* results from discordance between vestibular and visual stimulation.

Dizziness and Hearing Loss

Injuries of the peripheral auditory system cause three major symptoms: *hearing loss* (usually conductive hearing loss), *vertigo* (dizziness) when the injury involves the semicircular ducts, and *tinnitus* (buzzing or ringing) when the injury is localized in the cochlear duct. Tinnitus and hearing loss may result from lesions anywhere in the peripheral or central auditory pathways. The two types of hearing loss are as follows:

- *Conductive hearing loss*: resulting from anything in the external or middle ear that interferes with conduction of sound or movement of the oval or round windows. People with this type of hearing loss often speak with a soft voice because, to them, their own voices sound louder than background sounds. This type of hearing loss may be improved surgically or by use of a hearing aid device.
- *Sensorineural hearing loss*: resulting from defects in the pathway from the cochlea to the brain: defects of the cochlea, cochlear nerve, brainstem, or cortical connections. *Cochlear implants* are one approach employed to restore sound perception when the hair cells of the spiral organ have been damaged (Fig. B8.46). Sounds received by a small external microphone are transmitted to an implanted receiver that sends electrical impulses to the cochlea, stimulating the cochlear nerve. Hearing remains relatively crude, but it enables perception of rhythm and intensity of sounds.

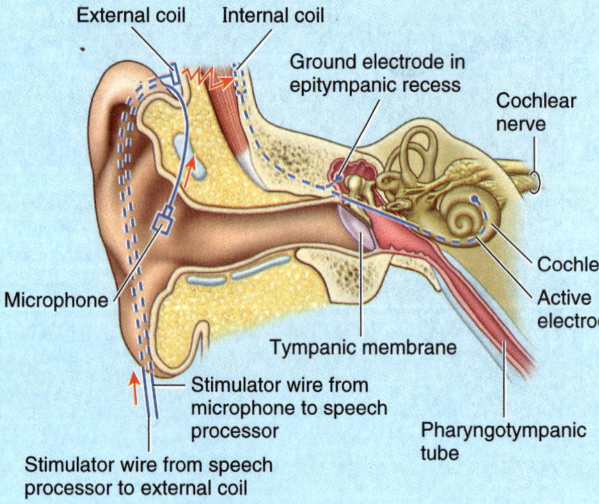

FIGURE B8.46. Cochlear implant.

Ménière Syndrome

Ménière syndrome is related to excess endolymph production or *blockage of the endolymphatic duct* (Fig. 8.116B) and is characterized by recurrent attacks of tinnitus, hearing loss, and vertigo. These symptoms are accompanied by a sense of pressure in the ear, distortion of sounds, and sensitivity to noises (Storper, 2016). A characteristic sign is ballooning of the cochlear duct, utricle, and saccule caused by an increase in endolymphatic volume.

High-Tone Deafness

Persistent exposure to excessively loud sounds causes degenerative changes in the spiral organ, resulting in high-tone deafness. This type of hearing loss commonly occurs in workers who are exposed to loud noises and do not wear protective earmuffs (e.g., individuals working for long periods around jet engines).

Otic Barotrauma

Injury caused to the ear by an imbalance in pressure between ambient (surrounding) air and the air in the middle ear is called *otic barotrauma*. This type of injury usually occurs in fliers and divers.

The Bottom Line: Ear

The ear is divided into external, middle, and internal parts. • All three parts are concerned with the sense of hearing, but the internal ear also has a vestibular function. • The external ear is a funnel-like conduit for airborne sound waves to reach the middle ear. • The protruding auricle and lateral part of the external acoustic meatus have an elastic cartilage skeleton that allows flexibility. • The primary sensory innervation of the external ear is provided by CN V

continued on next page

The Bottom Line (continued)

and CN X. • The tympanic membrane responds to airborne sound waves, converting them to vibrations transmitted by the solid medium of the ossicles of the middle ear. • Because its entire lateral wall is formed by a thin membrane, the middle ear (tympanic cavity) is a pressure-sensitive space, ventilated by means of the pharyngotympanic tube. • The mucosa lining both the cavity and tube is innervated by CN IX. • At the oval window, between the middle and internal ears, the solid medium vibrations of the ossicles are converted to fluid-borne sonar waves. • The internal ear consists of a delicate and complex membranous labyrinth filled with fluid that resembles intracellular fluid (endolymph), suspended within a bony cave otherwise occupied by extracellular fluid (perilymph). • Although much larger and slightly less complex, the architecture of the bony labyrinth is a reflection of that of the membranous labyrinth. • The posterior portion of the bony labyrinth takes the form of three semicircular canals and ducts; the ampulla of each of the ducts contains an ampullary crest that is sensitive to motion of the head. • The central bony vestibule contains a membranous utricle and saccule, each provided with a macula to monitor the position of the head relative to the line of gravitational pull. • The neuroepithelial crests and maculae are innervated by the vestibular portion of CN VIII. • The anterior portion of the internal ear contains a membranous cochlear duct, suspended between two limbs of continuous pathway for the sonar waves that are conducted by the perilymph; the duct and perilymphatic channels spiral through the 2.5 turns of the bony cochlea. • Deformation of the spiral organ within the cochlear duct by the sonar waves stimulates impulses conducted by the cochlear part of CN VIII for the sense of hearing.

8

Multiple-Choice Questions

1. **All of the following are true about the location of otic ganglion EXCEPT:**
   a. Inferior to foramen ovale
   b. Lateral to mandibular nerve
   c. Lateral to tensor veli palatini
   d. Anterior to the middle meningeal artery

   (Ref: Page 980)

2. **Which of the following is NOT true about dura mater?**
   a. It is the thick outermost layer of cranial meninges
   b. It has external periosteal and inner meningeal layers
   c. Dural venous sinuses lie below the meningeal layer
   d. It is supplied by the trigeminal nerve

   (Ref: Page 922)

3. **Foramen ovale transmits all the following structures EXCEPT:**
   a. Lesser petrosal nerve
   b. Maxillary nerve
   c. Mandibular nerve
   d. Motor root of the trigeminal nerve

   (Ref: Page 891)

4. **Which of the following structures is seen inside the cavernous sinus?**
   a. Maxillary division of V nerve
   b. Mandibular division of V nerve
   c. Trochlear nerve
   d. Internal carotid artery

   (Ref: Page 927)

5. **All of the following bones are parts of the inferior wall of orbit EXCEPT:**
   a. Ethmoid
   b. Maxillary
   c. Palatine
   d. Zygomatic

   (Ref: Page 948)

6. **Lacrimation is affected due to damage to which of the following nerves?**
   a. Nasociliary nerve
   b. Greater petrosal nerve
   c. Trigeminal nerve
   d. Anterior ethmoidal nerve

   (Ref: Page 950)

7. **The pharyngeal branch of vagus supplies all the following muscles of soft palate EXCEPT:**
   a. Palatoglossus
   b. Levator veli palatini
   c. Tensor veli palatini
   d. Palatopharyngeus

   (Ref: Page 997)

8. **Dilator pupillae is supplied by:**
   a. Oculomotor nerve
   b. Sympathetic fibers from the fronto-orbital branch of V nerve
   c. Preganglionic parasympathetic fibers from the Edinger–Westphal nucleus
   d. Postganglionic sympathetic fibers from the superior cervical ganglion

   (Ref: Page 963)

9. Posterior ethmoidal air sinuses open into:

a. Hiatus semilunaris
b. Ethmoidal bulla
c. Superior meatus
d. Sphenoethmoidal recess

(Ref: Page 1018)

10. Which quadrant of the tympanic membrane is preferred for making surgical incision during myringotomy?

a. Anterosuperior
b. Anteroinferior
c. Posterosuperior
d. Posteroinferior

(Ref: Page 1039)

11. All of the following are true about the boundaries of pterygopalatine fossa EXCEPT:

a. Anteriorly—maxilla
b. Posteriorly—pterygoid process
c. Medially—perpendicular plate of ethmoid
d. Superiorly—greater wing of sphenoid

(Ref: Page 1011)

12. The openings in the posterior wall of pterygopalatine fossa are all of the following EXCEPT:

a. Pharyngeal canal
b. Sphenopalatine foramen
c. Foramen rotundum
d. Pterygoid canal

(Ref: Page 1013)

13. Dural border hemorrhage results from injury to:

a. Middle meningeal artery
b. Internal carotid artery
c. Middle meningeal vein
d. Cerebral vein

(Ref: Page 934)

14. The site of choice for cisternal puncture in infants is:

a. Pontine
b. Chiasmatic
c. Cerebellomedullary
d. Interpeduncular

(Ref: Page 943)

15. All of the following are branches of the basilar artery EXCEPT:

a. Anterior inferior cerebellar
b. Posterior cerebral
c. Posterior inferior cerebellar
d. Superior cerebellar

(Ref: Page 942)

16. In an X-ray with fracture of base of skull, the fracture line passes through the left foramen ovale. Which of the following nerves is likely to be injured in this case?

a. Ophthalmic nerve
b. Oculomotor nerve
c. Maxillary nerve
d. Mandibular nerve

(Ref: Page 891)

17. Tractotomy of spinal tract of CN V was performed in a 56-year-old female patient with intractable trigeminal neuralgia. After surgery, she complaints of loss of sensation on one side of face except over the angle of mandible. This is because this region is supplied by:

a. Auriculotemporal nerve
b. Lesser occipital nerve
c. Greater auricular nerve
d. Zygomaticotemporal nerve

(Ref: Page 909)

18. Forehead is the preferred site for tepid sponging as it is a site of anastomosis between the branches of external and internal carotid arteries. Which branch of internal carotid artery anastomoses in this site?

a. Angular artery
b. Supra-orbital artery
c. Superficial temporal artery
d. Posterior auricular artery

(Ref: Page 913)

19. A needle passed through the anterior fontanelle of a fetus has to pierce through which of the following layer of meninges to reach the superior sagittal sinus?

a. Periosteal layer of dura mater
b. Meningeal layer of dura mater
c. Arachnoid mater
d. Pia mater

(Ref: Page 924)

20. Carotid angiogram of a patient shows an aneurysm of internal carotid artery within the cavernous sinus compressing a structure just inferolateral to it. Name the structure compressed.

a. Optic nerve
b. Oculomotor nerve
c. Trochlear nerve
d. Abducent nerve

(Ref: Page 927)

21. A fracture in which of the following can present with CSF otorrhea?

a. Floor of anterior cranial fossa
b. Floor of middle cranial fossa
c. Floor of posterior cranial fossa
d. Floor of pituitary fossa

(Ref: Page 1027)

22. An ophthalmologist instructs a patient to read down a page with the gaze of both eyes directed medially. Which extraocular muscle is he testing?

a. Medial rectus
b. Inferior rectus
c. Superior oblique
d. Inferior oblique

(Ref: Page 960)

23. Infiltration of anesthetic drug inferomedial to the lower third molar tooth will block which of the following nerves?

a. Lingual nerve
b. Inferior alveolar nerve
c. Glossopharyngeal nerve
d. Hypoglossal nerve

(Ref: Page 980)

24. A canula to drain maxillary sinus is inserted through the maxillary ostium located in which of the following sites?

a. Superior nasal meatus
b. Middle nasal meatus
c. Sphenoethmoidal recess
d. Ethmoidal infundibulum

(Ref: Page 1023)

25. A 15-year-old swimmer with chronic otitis media presents with loss of taste sensation. Which of the following nerves is affected?

a. Lingual nerve
b. Hypoglossal nerve
c. Chordatympani nerve
d. Vagus nerve

(Ref: Page 1032)

Answer Keys for MCQs

1. **b** 2. **c** 3. **b** 4. **d** 5. **a** 6. **b** 7. **c** 8. **d** 9. **c** 10. **d** 11. **c** 12. **b**
13. **d** 14. **c** 15. **c** 16. **d** 17. **c** 18. **b** 19. **a** 20. **d** 21. **b** 22. **c** 23. **a** 24. **b**
25. **c**.

Refer to *Appendix* A at the end of the book for *Student Case Study Questions and Answers* of Volume 3.

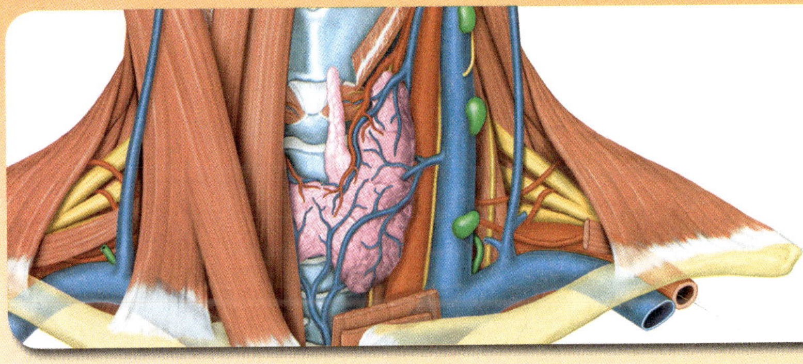

Neck

9

OVERVIEW / 1047

BONES OF NECK / 1047

Cervical Vertebrae / 1047

Hyoid Bone / 1049

CLINICAL BOX: Bones of Neck / 1050

FASCIA OF NECK / 1050

Cervical Subcutaneous Tissue and Platysma / 1050

Deep Cervical Fascia / 1052

CLINICAL BOX: Cervical Fascia / 1053

SUPERFICIAL STRUCTURES OF NECK: CERVICAL REGIONS / 1054

Sternocleidomastoid Region / 1054

TABLE 9.1. Cervical Regions/Triangles and Contents / 1055

TABLE 9.2. Cutaneous and Superficial Muscles of Neck / 1056

Posterior Cervical Region / 1057

Lateral Cervical Region / 1057

Anterior Cervical Region / 1064

TABLE 9.3. Muscles of Anterior Cervical Region (Extrinsic Muscles of Larynx) / 1067

Surface Anatomy of Cervical Regions and Triangles of Neck / 1070

CLINICAL BOX: Superficial Structures of Neck: Cervical Regions / 1072

DEEP STRUCTURES OF NECK / 1077

Prevertebral Muscles / 1077

Root of Neck / 1077

TABLE 9.4. Prevertebral Muscles / 1077

CLINICAL BOX: Deep Structures of Neck / 1082

VISCERA OF NECK / 1083

Endocrine Layer of Cervical Viscera / 1083

Respiratory Layer of Cervical Viscera / 1087

TABLE 9.5. Muscles of Larynx / 1093

Alimentary Layer of Cervical Viscera / 1097

TABLE 9.6. Muscles of Pharynx / 1102

Surface Anatomy of Endocrine and Respiratory Layers of Cervical Viscera / 1104

LYMPHATICS OF NECK / 1105

CLINICAL BOX: Viscera and Lymphatics of Neck / 1106

Multiple-Choice Questions / 1117

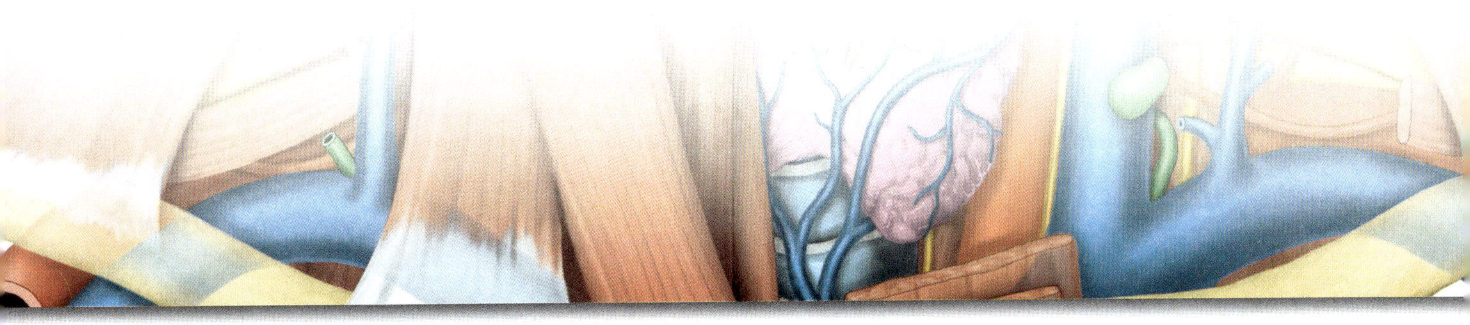

CLINICAL BOX KEY

Anatomical Variations | Diagnostic Procedures | Life Cycle | Surgical Procedures | Trauma | Pathology

Competencies Covered in the Chapter

AN25.4 Describe embryological basis of tracheo-oesophageal fistula / 1114

AN26.5 Describe features of typical and atypical cervical vertebrae (atlas and axis) / 1047, 1049

AN26.7 Describe the features of the 7th cervical vertebra / 1049

AN29.1 Describe and demonstrate attachments, nerve supply, relations and actions of sternocleidomastoid / 1054, 1056

AN29.3 Explain anatomical basis of wry neck / 1072

AN29.4 Describe and demonstrate attachments of inferior belly of omohyoid / 1067

AN29.4 Describe and demonstrate attachments of scalenus anterior, scalenus medius, and levator scapulae / 1077, 1078

AN31.3 Describe anatomical basis of Horner's syndrome / 1082

AN32.1 Describe boundaries and subdivisions of anterior triangle / 1055

AN32.2 Describe and demonstrate boundaries and contents of muscular, carotid, digastric and submental triangles / 1055, 1064

AN35.1 Describe the parts, extent, attachments, modifications of deep cervical fascia / 1052

AN35.2 Describe and demonstrate location, parts, borders, surfaces, relations and blood supply of thyroid gland / 1083

AN35.3 Demonstrate and describe the origin, parts, course and branches of subclavian artery / 1079

AN35.4 Describe and demonstrate origin, course, relations, tributaries and termination of internal jugular and brachiocephalic veins / 1060, 1069

AN35.5 Describe and demonstrate extent, drainage, and applied anatomy of cervical lymph nodes / 1062, 1105

AN35.6 Describe and demonstrate the extent, formation, relation and branches of cervical sympathetic chain / 1082

AN35.7 Describe the course and branches of IX and XII nerve in the neck / 1070

AN35.7 Describe the course and branches of X nerve in the neck / 1080

AN35.7 Describe the course and branches of XI nerve in the neck / 1060

AN35.8 Describe the anatomically relevant clinical features of thyroid swellings / 1108

AN35.10 Describe the fascial spaces of neck / 1052

AN36.1 Describe the morphology, relations, blood supply, and applied anatomy of palatine tonsil / 1100

AN36.2 Describe the components and functions of Waldeyer's lymphatic ring / 1103

AN36.3 Describe the boundaries and clinical significance of pyriform fossa / 1101

AN36.3 Describe the clinical significance of pyriform fossa / 1113

AN36.4 Describe the anatomical basis of tonsillitis, tonsillectomy, adenoids and peri-tonsillar abscess / 1113

AN38.1 Describe the morphology, identify structure of the wall, nerve supply, blood supply and actions of intrinsic and extrinsic muscles of the larynx / 1087

AN38.3 Describe anatomical basis of recurrent laryngeal nerve injury / 1109

AN43.2 Identify, describe and draw the microanatomy of thyroid gland / 1085

AN43.2 Identify, describe, and draw the microanatomy of parathyroid gland / 1086

AN43.4 Describe the development and developmental basis of congenital anomalies of thyroid gland / 1107

AN43.4 Describe the development and developmental basis of congenital anomalies of branchial apparatus / 1113

AN43.5 Demonstrate palpation of carotid arteries / 1072, 1075

AN43.5 Demonstrate palpation of internal jugular venous pulse / 1076

AN43.5 Demonstrate the location of hyoid bone, thyroid cartilage, and cricoid cartilage with their vertebral levels / 1104

AN43.6 Demonstrate surface projection of common carotid artery, internal jugular vein, subclavian vein, external jugular vein, and accessory nerve / 1070

AN43.6 Demonstrate surface projection of thyroid gland / 1104

AN43.7 Identify the anatomical structures in plain X-ray cervical spine—lateral view / 1048

OVERVIEW

The **neck** is the transitional area between the base of the cranium superiorly and the clavicles inferiorly. The neck joins the head to the trunk and limbs, serving as a major conduit for structures passing between them. In addition, several important organs with unique functions are located here: the larynx and the thyroid and parathyroid glands, for example.

The neck is relatively slender to allow the flexibility necessary to position the head to maximize the efficiency of its sensory organs (mainly the eyeballs but also the ears, mouth, and nose). Thus, many important structures are crowded together in the neck, such as muscles, glands, arteries, veins, nerves, lymphatics, trachea, esophagus, and vertebrae. Consequently, the neck is a well-known region of vulnerability. Furthermore, several vital structures, including the trachea, esophagus, and thyroid gland, lack the bony protection afforded other parts of the systems to which these structures belong.

The main arterial blood flow to the head and neck (the *carotid arteries*) and the principal venous drainage (the *jugular veins*) lie anterolaterally in the neck (Fig. 9.1). Carotid/jugular blood vessels are the major structures commonly injured in penetrating wounds of the neck. The *brachial plexuses of nerves* originate in the neck and pass inferolaterally to enter the axillae and continue into and supply the upper limbs.

In the middle of the anterior aspect of the neck is the *thyroid cartilage*, the largest of the cartilages of the larynx, and the trachea. Lymph from structures in the head and neck drains into cervical lymph nodes.

BONES OF NECK

The skeleton of the neck is formed by the cervical vertebrae, hyoid bone, manubrium of the sternum, and clavicles (Figs. 9.2 and 9.3). These bones are parts of the axial skeleton except the clavicles, which are part of the appendicular skeleton.

Cervical Vertebrae

AN26.

Seven *cervical vertebrae* form the cervical region of the vertebral column, which encloses the spinal cord and meninges. The stacked, centrally placed vertebral bodies support the head, and the intervertebral (IV) articulations—especially the craniovertebral joints at its superior end—provide the flexibility necessary to allow positioning of the head.

The cervical vertebrae, cervical IV joints, and movement of the cervical region of the vertebral column are described

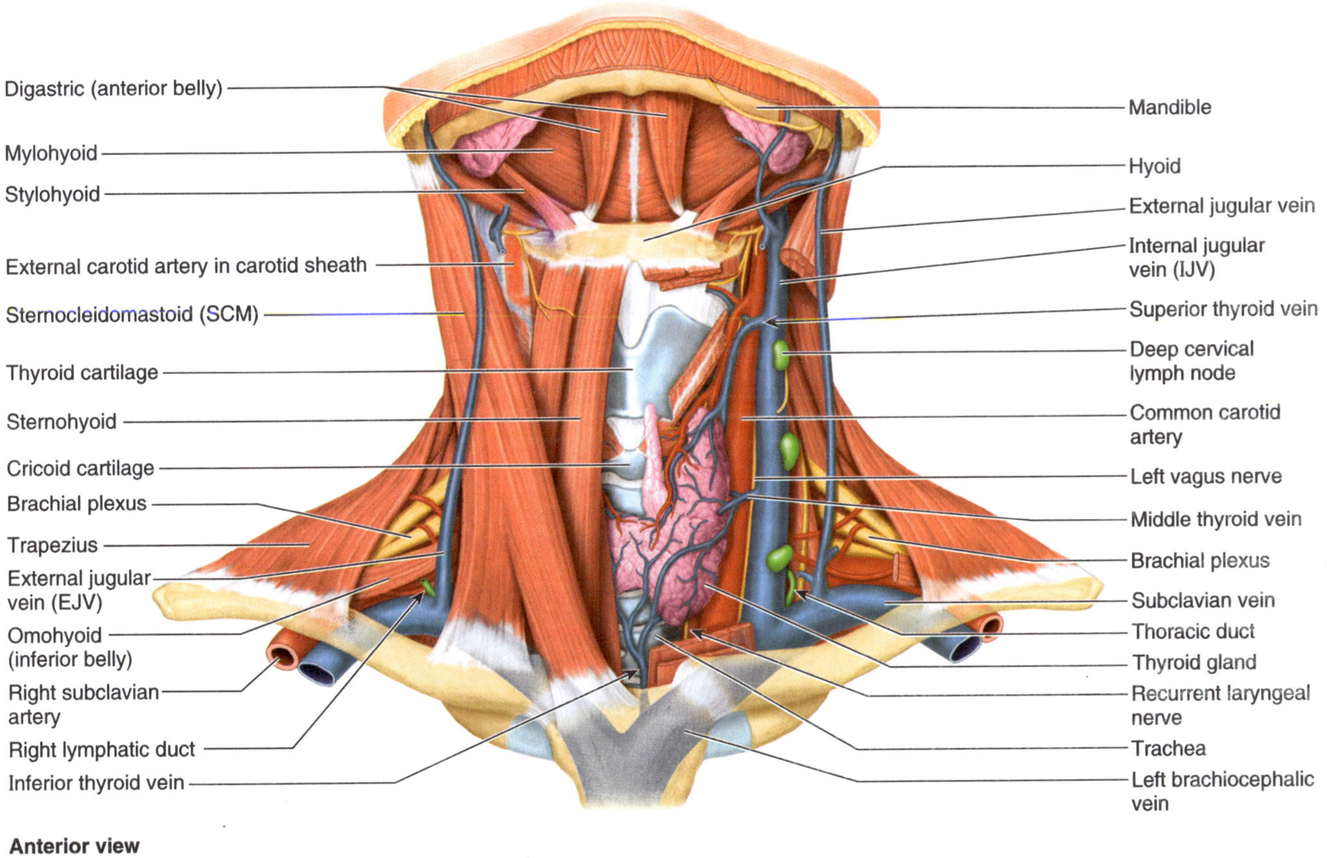

FIGURE 9.1. Dissection of anterior neck. The fascia has been removed and the muscles on the left side have been reflected to show the hyoid bone, thyroid gland, and structures related to the carotid sheath: carotid artery, internal jugular vein (IJV), vagus nerve (CN X), and deep cervical lymph nodes.

(continued on p. 1049)

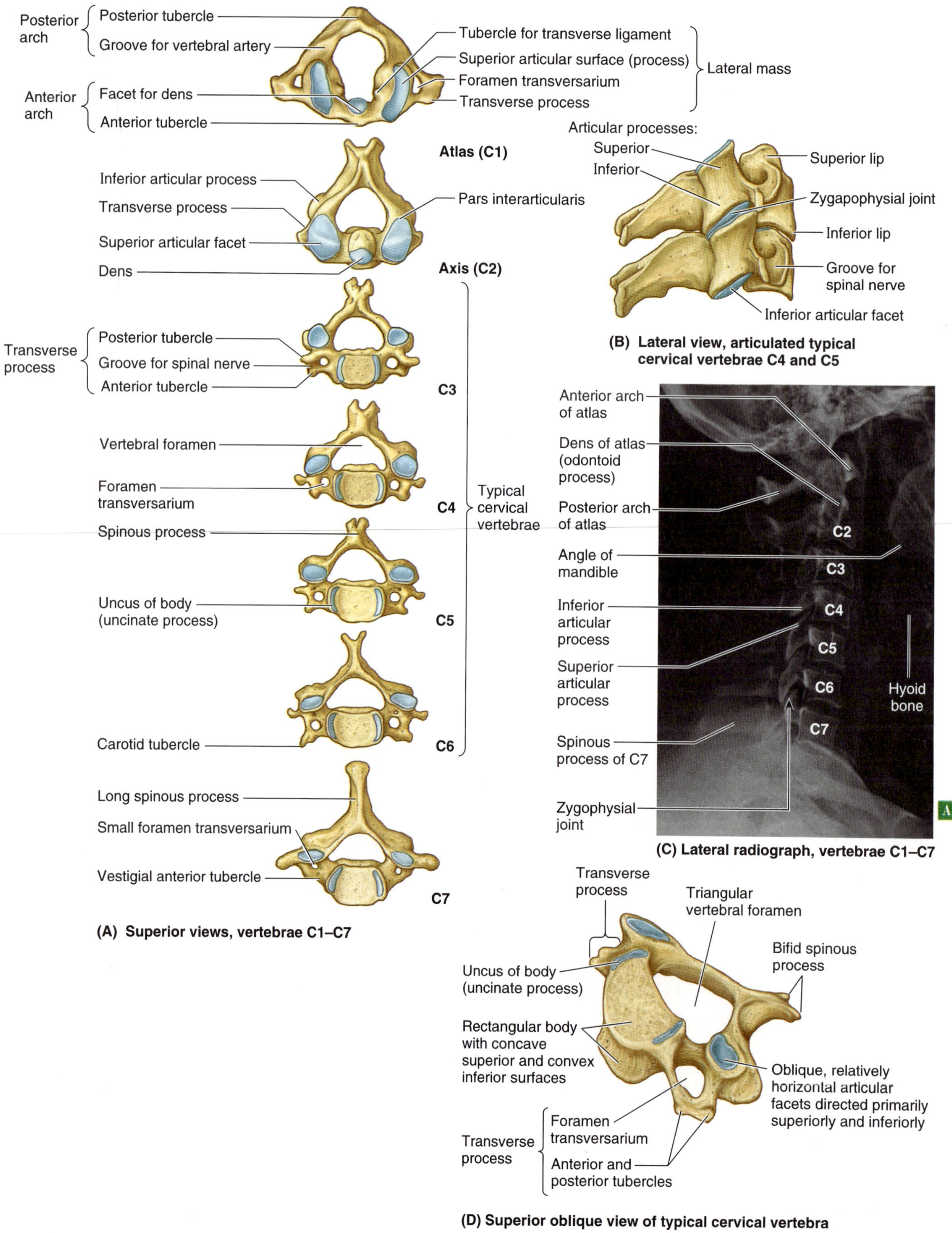

FIGURE 9.2. Cervical vertebrae. A. The 3rd–6th vertebrae are "typical" cervical vertebrae; the 1st, 2nd, and 7th are "atypical." **B, C.** Illustration and radiograph of articulated cervical vertebrae. **D.** Typical cervical vertebra demonstrating a rectangular body with articular unci (uncinate processes) on its lateral aspects, a triangular vertebral foramen, a bifid spinous process, and foramina transversaria.

AN43.7

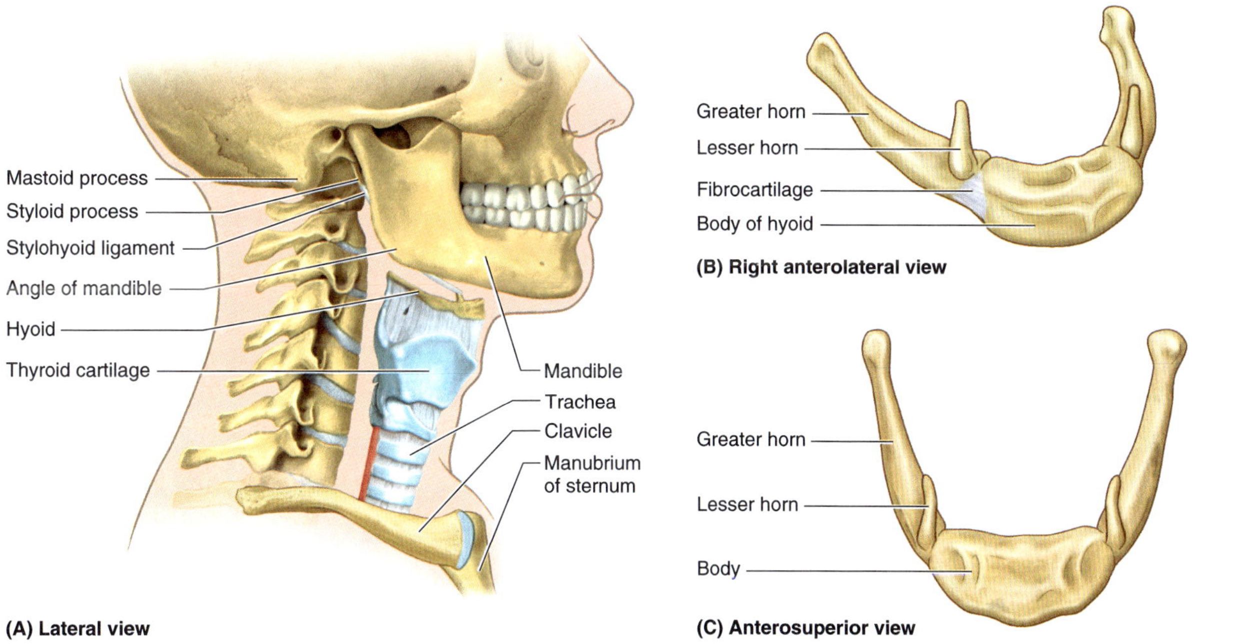

FIGURE 9.3. Bones and cartilages of neck. A. The bony and cartilaginous landmarks of the neck are the vertebrae, mastoid and styloid processes, angles of the mandible, hyoid bone, thyroid cartilage, clavicle, and manubrium of the sternum. **B, C.** The hyoid bone and its features are demonstrated.

with the back (Chapter 2, Back). Therefore, only a brief review follows.

The four *typical cervical vertebrae (3rd–6th)* have the following characteristics (Fig. 9.2A, D):

- The vertebral body is small and longer from side to side than anteroposteriorly; the superior surface is concave, and the inferior surface is convex.
- The vertebral foramen is large and triangular.
- The transverse processes of all cervical vertebrae (typical or atypical) include **foramina transversaria** for the vertebral vessels (the vertebral veins and, except for vertebra C7, the vertebral arteries).
- The superior facets of the articular processes are directed superoposteriorly, and the inferior facets are directed inferoposteriorly.
- Their spinous processes are short and, in individuals of European heritage, bifid.

AN26.5 AN26.7 There are three *atypical cervical vertebrae (C1, C2, and C7)* (Fig. 9.2A):

1. The *C1 vertebra or atlas*: a ring-like, kidney-shaped bone lacking a spinous process or body and consisting of two lateral masses connected by anterior and posterior arches. Its concave superior articular facets receive the occipital condyles.
2. The *C2 vertebra or axis*: a peg-like *den* (odontoid process) projects superiorly from its body.
3. The *vertebra prominens (C7)*: so-named because of its long spinous process, which is not bifid. Its transverse processes are large, but its foramina transversaria are small.

Hyoid Bone

The mobile **hyoid bone** (or simply, the **hyoid**) lies in the anterior part of the neck at the level of the C3 vertebra in the angle between the mandible and the thyroid cartilage (Fig. 9.3). The hyoid is suspended by muscles that connect it to the mandible, styloid processes, thyroid cartilage, manubrium of the sternum, and scapulae.

The hyoid is unique among bones for its isolation from the remainder of the skeleton. The U-shaped hyoid derives its name from the Greek word *hyoeidçs*, meaning "shaped like the letter upsilon," the 20th letter in the Greek alphabet. The hyoid does not articulate with any other bone. It is suspended from the styloid processes of the temporal bones by the *stylohyoid ligaments* (Fig. 9.3A) and is firmly bound to the thyroid cartilage. The hyoid consists of a body and greater and lesser horns (L. *cornua*). Functionally, the hyoid serves as an attachment for anterior neck muscles and a prop to keep the airway open.

The **body of the hyoid**, its middle part, faces anteriorly and is approximately 2.5 cm wide and 1 cm thick (Fig. 9.3B, C). Its anterior convex surface projects anterosuperiorly; its posterior concave surface projects postero-inferiorly. Each end of its body is united to a **greater horn** that projects posterosuperiorly and laterally from the body. In young people, the greater horns are united to the body by fibrocartilage. In older people, the horns are usually united by bone. Each **lesser horn** is a small bony projection from the superior part of the body of the hyoid near its union with the greater horn. It is connected to the body of the hyoid by fibrous tissue and sometimes to the greater horn by a synovial joint. The lesser horn projects superoposteriorly toward the styloid process; it may be partly or completely cartilaginous in some adults.

CLINICAL BOX

BONES OF NECK

Cervical Pain

Cervical pain (neck pain) has several causes, including inflamed lymph nodes, muscle strain, and protruding intervertebral (IV) discs. Enlarged cervical lymph nodes may indicate a malignant tumor in the head; however, the primary cancer may be in the thorax or abdomen because the neck connects the head to the trunk (e.g., lung cancer may metastasize through the neck to the cranium). Most chronic cervical pain is caused by bony abnormalities (e.g., *cervical osteoarthritis*) or by trauma. Cervical pain is usually affected by movement of the head and neck, and it may be exaggerated during coughing or sneezing, for example.

Injuries of Cervical Vertebral Column

Fractures and dislocations of the cervical vertebra may injure the spinal cord and/or the vertebral arteries and sympathetic plexuses passing through the foramina transversaria. See the clinical boxes "Dislocation of Cervical Vertebrae," "Fracture and Dislocation of Atlas," and "Fracture and Dislocation of Axis" in Chapter 2, Back.

Fracture of Hyoid Bone

Fracture of the hyoid (or of the styloid processes of the temporal bone; see Chapter 8, Head) occurs in people who are manually strangled by compression of the throat. This results in depression of the body of the hyoid onto the thyroid cartilage. Inability to elevate the hyoid and move it anteriorly beneath the tongue makes swallowing and maintenance of the separation of the alimentary and respiratory tracts difficult and may result in *aspiration pneumonia*.

FASCIA OF NECK

Structures in the neck are surrounded by a layer of subcutaneous tissue (superficial fascia) and are compartmentalized by layers of deep cervical fascia. The fascial planes determine the direction an infection may spread in the neck.

Cervical Subcutaneous Tissue and Platysma

The **cervical subcutaneous tissue** (superficial cervical fascia) is a layer of fatty connective tissue that lies between the dermis of the skin and the investing layer of deep cervical fascia (Fig. 9.4A). The cervical subcutaneous tissue is usually thinner than in other regions, especially anteriorly. It contains cutaneous nerves, blood and lymphatic vessels, superficial lymph nodes, and variable amounts of fat. Anterolaterally, it contains the platysma (Fig. 9.4B).

PLATYSMA

The **platysma** (G. flat plate) is a broad, thin sheet of muscle in the subcutaneous tissue of the neck (Figs. 9.4B and 9.5). Like other facial and scalp muscles, the platysma develops from a continuous sheet of musculature derived from mesenchyme in the 2nd pharyngeal arch of the embryo and is supplied by branches of the facial nerve, CN VII. The external jugular vein (EJV), descending from the angle of the mandible to the middle of the clavicle (see Fig. 9.1), and the main cutaneous nerves of the neck are deep to the platysma.

The platysma covers the anterolateral aspect of the neck. Its fibers arise in the deep fascia covering the superior parts of the deltoid and pectoralis major muscles and sweep superomedially over the clavicle to the inferior border of the mandible. The anterior borders of the two muscles decussate over the chin and blend with the facial muscles. Inferiorly, the fibers diverge, leaving a gap anterior to the larynx and trachea (Fig. 9.5). Much variation exists in terms of the continuity (completeness) of this muscular sheet, which often occurs as isolated slips. The platysma is supplied by the cervical branch of CN VII.

The Bottom Line: Bones of Neck

Cervical vertebrae: The neck is a movable "connecting stalk" with a segmented axial skeleton. • The stacked, centrally placed vertebral bodies support the head. • The IV articulations—especially the craniovertebral joints at its superior end—provide the flexibility necessary to allow positioning of the head to maximize the use of its sensory organs. • Multiple processes of the vertebrae provide both the attachments and the leverage necessary to move the head into and maintain those positions. • The foramina of the cervical vertebrae provide protective passage for the spinal cord and the vertebral arteries that nourish the bones and are a major component of the brain's blood supply. • The vertebrae provide little protection for other structures of the neck.

Hyoid bone: Unique in terms of its isolation from the rest of the skeleton, the U-shaped hyoid is suspended between the body of the mandible superiorly and the manubrium of the sternum inferiorly. • The hyoid provides a movable base for the tongue and attachment for the middle part of the pharynx. • The hyoid also maintains the patency of the pharynx, required for swallowing and respiration.

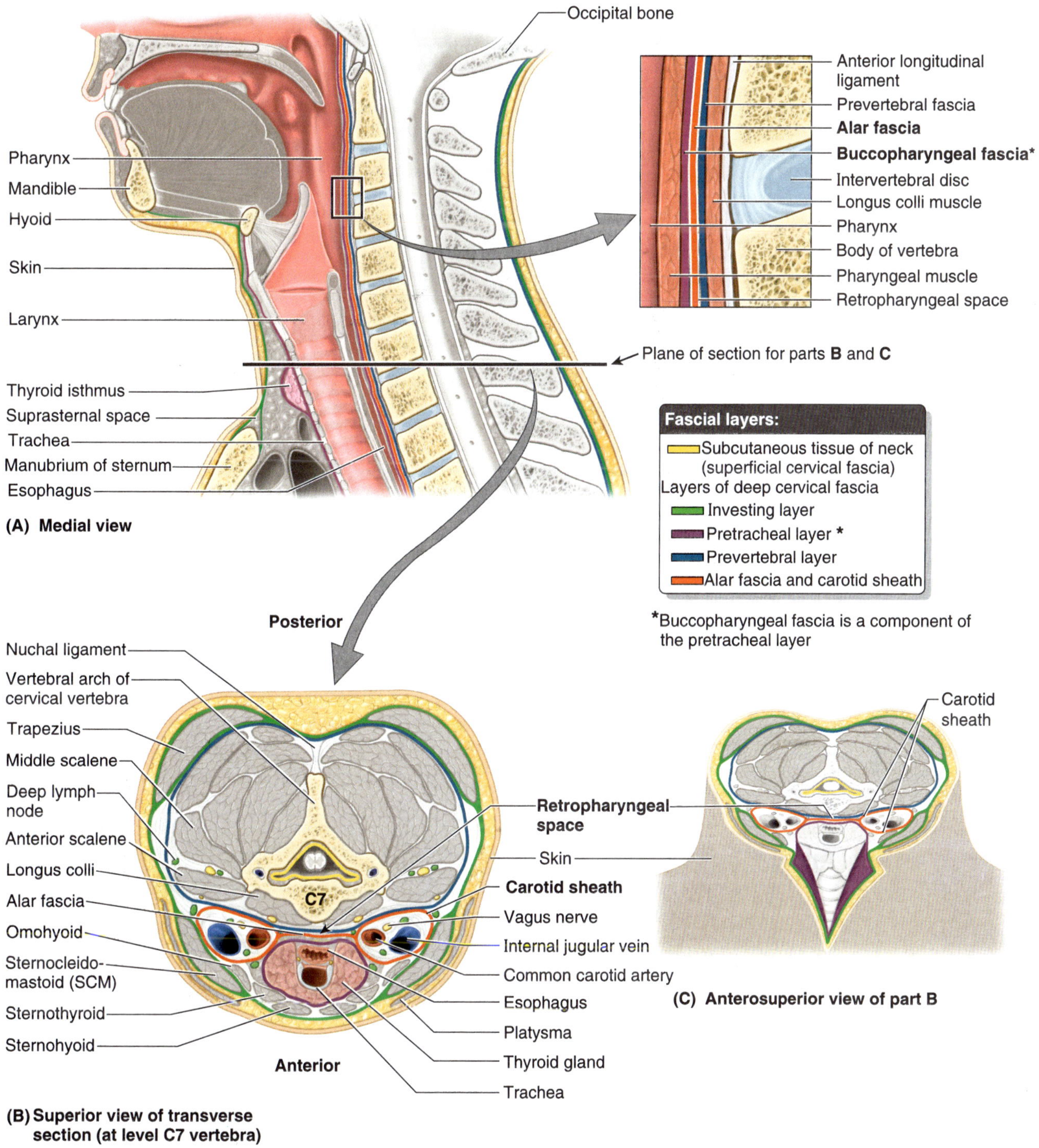

FIGURE 9.4. Sections of head and neck demonstrating cervical fascia. A. The right half of the head and neck have been sectioned in the median plane. The *detail* illustrates the fascia in the retropharyngeal region. **B.** This transverse section of the neck passes through the isthmus of the thyroid gland at the C7 vertebral level, as indicated in part **(A)**. The outermost layer of deep cervical fascia, the investing layer, splits to enclose the trapezius and sternocleidomastoid (SCM) at the four corners of the neck. The investing layer and its embedded muscles surround two main fascial columns. The pretracheal (visceral) layer encloses muscles and viscera in the anterior neck; the prevertebral (musculoskeletal) layer encircles the vertebral column and associated muscles. The carotid sheaths are neurovascular conduits related to both fascial columns. **C.** The fascial compartments of the neck are shown to demonstrate an anterior midline approach to the thyroid gland. Although the larynx, trachea, and thyroid gland are nearly subcutaneous in the midline, two layers of deep cervical fascia (the investing and pretracheal layers) must be incised to reach them.

Acting from its superior attachment to the mandible, *the platysma tenses the skin*, producing vertical skin ridges and releasing pressure on the superficial veins (Table 9.2). Men commonly use actions of the platysma when shaving their necks and when easing tight collars. Acting from its inferior attachment, the platysma helps depress the mandible and draw the corners of the mouth inferiorly, as in a grimace. As a muscle of facial expression, the platysma serves to convey tension or stress.

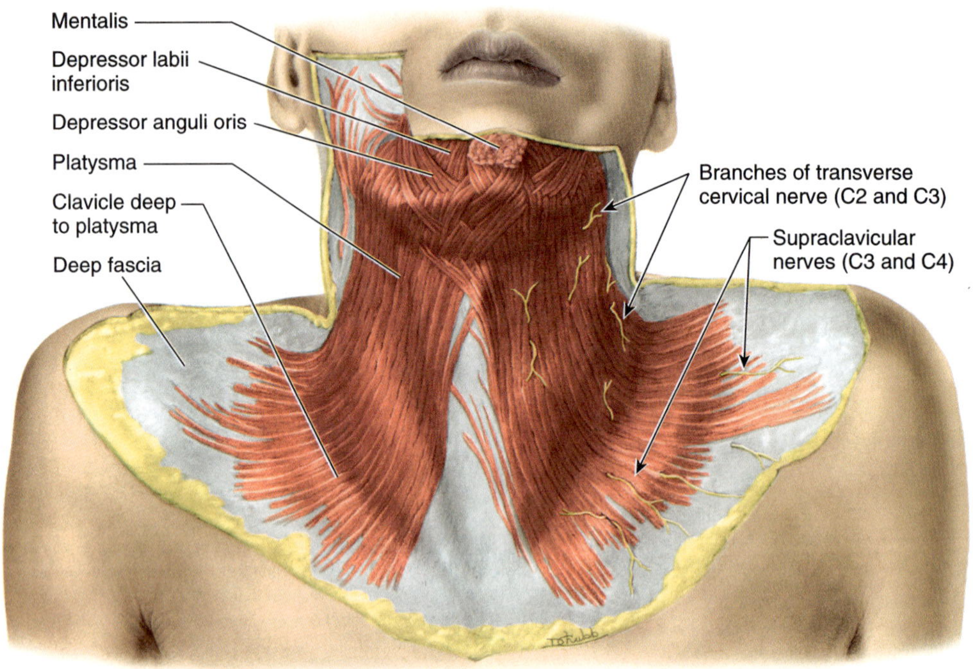

FIGURE 9.5. Platysma. The thin platysma muscle spreads subcutaneously like a sheet, passes over the clavicles, and is pierced by cutaneous nerves. Much variation is present in the continuity of this muscular sheet.

Deep Cervical Fascia

N35.1 N35.10 The **deep cervical fascia** consists of three fascial layers (sheaths): *investing*, *pretracheal*, and *prevertebral* (Fig. 9.4A, B). These layers support the cervical viscera (e.g., thyroid gland), muscles, vessels, and deep lymph nodes. The deep cervical fascia also condenses around the common carotid arteries, internal jugular veins (IJVs), and vagus nerves to form the *carotid sheath* (Fig. 9.4B, C).

These three fascial layers form natural cleavage planes through which tissues may be separated during surgery, and they limit the spread of abscesses (collections of pus) resulting from infections. The deep cervical fascial layers also afford the slipperiness that allows structures in the neck to move and pass over one another without difficulty, for example, when swallowing and turning the head and neck.

INVESTING LAYER OF DEEP CERVICAL FASCIA

The **investing layer of deep cervical fascia**, the most superficial deep fascial layer, surrounds the entire neck deep to the skin and subcutaneous tissue. At the "four corners" of the neck, it splits into superficial and deep layers to enclose (invest) the *trapezius* and *sternocleidomastoid (SCM) muscles* (Fig. 9.4B, C). These muscles are derived from the same embryonic sheet of muscle and are innervated by the same nerve (CN XI). They have essentially continuous attachments to the cranial base superiorly and to the scapular spine, acromion, and clavicle inferiorly.

Superiorly, the investing layer of deep cervical fascia attaches to the

- superior nuchal lines of the occipital bone.
- mastoid processes of the temporal bones.
- zygomatic arches.
- inferior border of the mandible.
- hyoid bone.
- spinous processes of the cervical vertebrae.

Just inferior to its attachment to the mandible, the investing layer of deep fascia splits to enclose the submandibular gland; posterior to the mandible, it splits to form the fibrous capsule of the parotid gland. The *stylomandibular ligament* is a thickened modification of this fascial layer (see Fig. 8.71).

Inferiorly, the investing layer of deep cervical fascia attaches to the manubrium of the sternum, clavicles, and acromions and spines of the scapulae. The investing layer of deep cervical fascia is continuous posteriorly with the periosteum covering the C7 spinous process and with the *nuchal ligament* (L. *ligamentum nuchae*), a triangular membrane that forms a median fibrous septum between the muscles of the two sides of the neck (Fig. 9.4B).

Inferiorly between the sternal heads of the SCMs and just superior to the manubrium, the investing layer of deep cervical fascia remains divided into two layers to enclose the SCM; one layer attaches to the anterior and the other to the posterior surface of the manubrium. A **suprasternal space** lies between these layers (Fig. 9.4A). It encloses the inferior ends of the anterior jugular veins, the *jugular venous arch*, fat, and a few deep lymph nodes.

PRETRACHEAL LAYER OF DEEP CERVICAL FASCIA

The thin **pretracheal layer of deep cervical fascia** is limited to the anterior part of the neck (Fig. 9.4). It extends inferiorly from the hyoid into the thorax, where it blends with the fibrous pericardium covering the heart. The pretracheal layer of fascia includes a thin *muscular part*, which encloses the infrahyoid muscles, and a *visceral part*, which encloses the thyroid gland, trachea, and esophagus, and is continuous posteriorly and superiorly with the **buccopharyngeal fascia** of the pharynx. The pretracheal layer of deep fascia blends laterally with the carotid sheaths. Superior to the hyoid, a thickening of the pretracheal fascia forms a pulley or trochlea through which the *intermediate tendon of the digastric muscle* passes, suspending the hyoid. By wrapping around the lateral border of the intermediate tendon of the omohyoid, the pretracheal layer also tethers the two-bellied *omohyoid muscle*, redirecting the course of the muscle between the bellies.

PREVERTEBRAL LAYER OF DEEP CERVICAL FASCIA

The **prevertebral layer of deep cervical fascia** forms a tubular sheath for the vertebral column and the muscles associated with it, such as the *longus colli* and *longus capitis* anteriorly, the scalenes laterally, and the *deep cervical muscles* posteriorly (Fig. 8.4A, B).

The prevertebral layer of deep fascia is fixed to the cranial base superiorly. Inferiorly, it blends with the *endothoracic fascia* peripherally and fuses with the *anterior longitudinal ligament* centrally at approximately the T3 vertebra (see Chapter 2, Back) (Fig. 9.4A). The prevertebral fascia extends laterally as the *axillary sheath* (Chapter 3, Upper Limb), which surrounds the axillary vessels and brachial plexus. The cervical parts of the sympathetic trunks are embedded in the prevertebral layer of deep cervical fascia.

Carotid Sheath. The **carotid sheath** is a tubular fascial investment that extends from the cranial base to the root of the neck. This sheath blends anteriorly with the investing and pretracheal layers of fascia and posteriorly with the prevertebral layer of fascia (Figs. 9.4B, C and 9.6). The carotid sheath contains the

- common and internal carotid arteries.
- internal jugular vein.
- vagus nerve (CN X).
- some deep cervical lymph nodes.
- carotid sinus nerve.
- sympathetic nerve fibers (carotid peri-arterial plexuses).

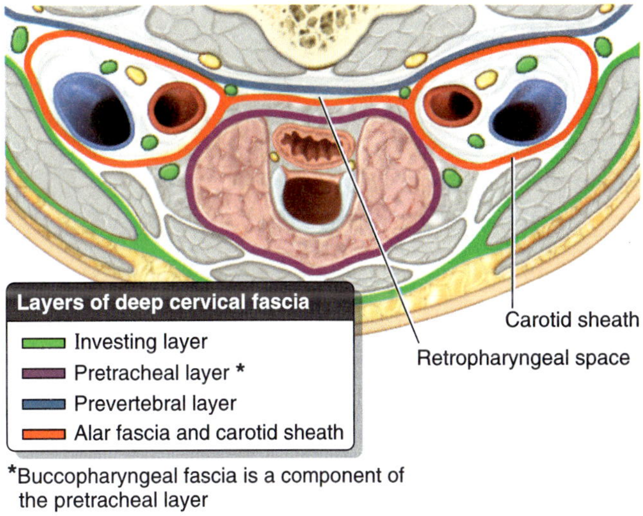

FIGURE 9.6. Carotid sheath.

The carotid sheath communicates with the mediastinum of the thorax inferiorly and extends to the cranial base (basiocciput) superiorly. These communications represent potential pathways for the spread of infection and extravasated blood.

Retropharyngeal Space. The **retropharyngeal space** is the largest and most important interfascial space in the neck (Fig. 9.6). It is a potential space that consists of loose connective tissue between the superior part of the prevertebral layer of deep cervical fascia and the buccopharyngeal fascia surrounding the pharynx superficially. Inferiorly, the buccopharyngeal fascia is continuous with the pretracheal layer of deep cervical fascia.

The **alar fascia** forms a further subdivision of the retropharyngeal space. This thin layer is attached along the midline of the buccopharyngeal fascia from the cranium to the level of the C7 vertebra. From this attachment, it extends laterally and terminates in the carotid sheath. The retropharyngeal space permits movement of the pharynx, esophagus, larynx, and trachea relative to the vertebral column during swallowing. This space is closed superiorly by the cranial base and on each side by the carotid sheath. It opens inferiorly into the superior mediastinum (see Chapter 4, Thorax).

9

CLINICAL BOX

CERVICAL FASCIA

Paralysis of Platysma

Paralysis of the platysma, resulting from injury to the cervical branch of the facial nerve (see Fig. 8.16B), causes the skin to fall away from the neck in slack folds. Consequently, during surgical dissections of the neck, extra care is necessary to preserve the cervical branch of the facial nerve. When suturing wounds of the neck, surgeons carefully suture the skin and edges of the platysma. If this is not done, the skin wound will be distracted (pulled in different directions) by the contracting platysma muscle fibers, and a disfiguring scar may develop.

Spread of Infections in Neck

The investing layer of deep cervical fascia helps prevent the *spread of abscesses (purulent infections)* caused by tissue destruction. If an infection occurs between the investing layer of deep cervical fascia and the muscular part of the pretracheal fascia surrounding the infrahyoid muscles, the infection will usually not spread beyond the superior edge of the manubrium of the sternum. If, however, the infection occurs between the investing fascia and the visceral part of pretracheal fascia, it can spread into the thoracic cavity anterior to the pericardium.

Pus from an abscess posterior to the prevertebral layer of deep cervical fascia may extend laterally in the neck and form a swelling posterior to the SCM. The pus may perforate the prevertebral layer of deep cervical fascia and enter the retropharyngeal space, producing a bulge in the pharynx (*retropharyngeal abscess*). This abscess may cause difficulty in swallowing (*dysphagia*) and speaking (*dysarthria*).

Infections in the head may also spread inferiorly posterior to the esophagus and enter the posterior mediastinum, or it may spread anterior to the trachea and enter the anterior mediastinum. Infections in the retropharyngeal space may also extend inferiorly into the superior mediastinum. Similarly, air from a ruptured trachea, bronchus, or esophagus (*pneumomediastinum*) can pass superiorly in the neck.

The Bottom Line: Fascia of Neck

Cervical subcutaneous tissue and platysma: The subcutaneous tissue (superficial cervical fascia) is usually thinner in the neck than in other regions, especially anteriorly. • It contains the platysma, a muscle of facial expression.

Deep cervical fascia: Like deep fascia elsewhere, the function of the deep cervical fascia is (1) to provide containment of muscles and viscera in compartments with varying degrees of rigidity, (2) to provide the slipperiness that allows structures to slide over each other, and (3) to serve as a conduit for the passage of neurovascular structures. • Two major fascial compartments of the neck are separated by the retropharyngeal space. • Anteriorly, the pretracheal fascia surrounds the cervical viscera and extrinsic musculature associated with it (suprahyoid and infrahyoid muscles). • Posteriorly, the prevertebral fascia surrounds the musculoskeletal elements of the neck associated with and including the cervical vertebrae. • These two fascial compartments are contained within the third and most superficial layer of deep cervical fascia, the investing layer, which includes the superficial muscles (trapezius and SCM). • The investing fascia attaches to the cranium superiorly and the pectoral girdle inferiorly. • Lying anterolateral at the common junctions of these three layers are the major neurovascular conduits, the carotid sheaths. • The superior and inferior boundaries and continuities of these fascial layers, compartments, and interfascial spaces establish pathways for the spread of infection, fluid, gas, or tumors.

SUPERFICIAL STRUCTURES OF NECK: CERVICAL REGIONS

To allow clear communication regarding the location of structures, injuries, or pathologies, the neck is divided into regions (Fig. 9.7; Table 9.1). Between the cranium (mandible anteriorly and occipital bone posteriorly) and clavicles, the neck is divided into four major regions based on the usually visible and/or palpable borders of the large and relatively superficial SCM and trapezius muscles, which are contained within the outermost (investing) layer of deep cervical fascia.

AN29.1 Sternocleidomastoid Region

The **sternocleidomastoid (SCM) muscle** is a key muscular landmark in the neck, forming the **sternocleidomastoid region**. The SCM visibly divides each side of the neck into the *anterior* and *lateral cervical regions* (anterior and posterior triangles). The SCM is a broad, strap-like muscle that has two heads: the rounded tendon of the **sternal head** attaches to the manubrium, and the thick, fleshy **clavicular head** attaches to the superior surface of the medial third of the clavicle (Figs. 9.7 and 9.8; Table 9.2).

The two heads of the SCM are separated inferiorly by a space, visible superficially as a small triangular depression, the **lesser supraclavicular fossa** (Fig. 9.7B). The heads join superiorly as they pass obliquely upward toward the cranium. The superior attachment of the SCM is the mastoid process of the temporal bone and the superior nuchal line of the occipital bone. The investing layer of deep cervical fascia splits to form a sheath for the SCM (Fig. 9.4B).

The SCMs produce movement at the craniovertebral joints, the cervical intervertebral joints, or at both (Fig. 9.8; Table 9.2). The cranial attachments of the SCMs lie posterior to the axis of the atlanto-occipital (AO) joints. Starting from the anatomical position, with tonic contraction maintaining the position of the cervical vertebral column, bilateral

(*continued on p.* 1057)

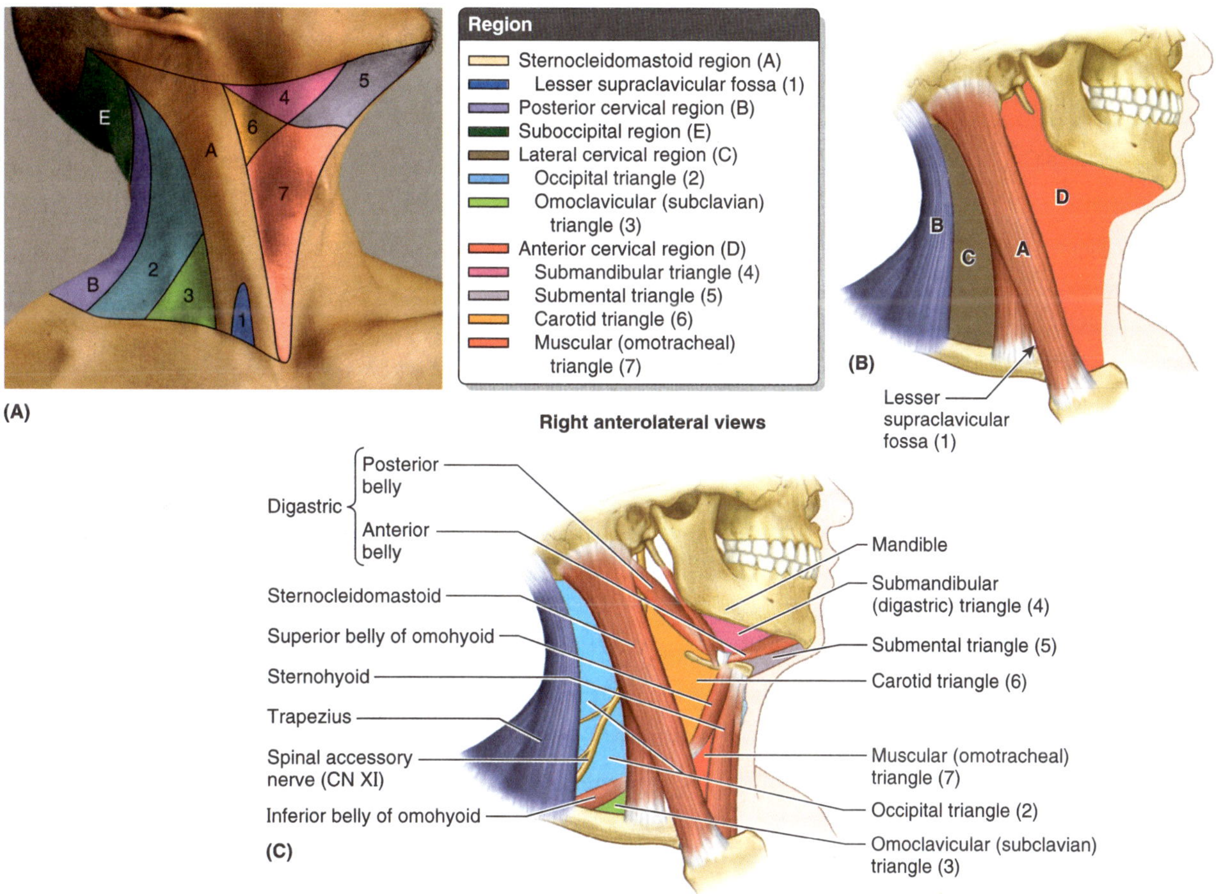

AN32.1 **FIGURE 9.7.** Cervical regions and triangles.

TABLE 9.1. CERVICAL REGIONS/TRIANGLES AND CONTENTS

Region[a]	Main Contents and Underlying Structures
Sternocleidomastoid region (A)	Sternocleidomastoid muscle; superior part of external jugular vein; greater auricular nerve; transverse cervical nerve
Lesser supraclavicular fossa (1)	Inferior part of internal jugular vein
Posterior cervical region (B)	Trapezius muscle; cutaneous branches of posterior rami of cervical spinal nerves; suboccipital region or triangle (E) lies deep to superior part of this region
Lateral cervical region (posterior triangle) (C)	
Occipital triangle (2)	Part of external jugular vein; posterior branches of cervical plexus of nerves; spinal accessory nerve (CN XI)[b]; trunks of brachial plexus; cervicodorsal trunk; cervical lymph node
Omoclavicular (subclavian) triangle (3)	Subclavian artery (third part); part of subclavian vein (sometimes); suprascapular artery; supraclavicular lymph nodes
AN32.2 **Anterior cervical region (anterior triangle)** (D)	
Submandibular (digastric) triangle (4)	Submandibular gland almost fills triangle; submandibular lymph nodes; hypoglossal nerve (CN XII); mylohyoid nerve; parts of facial artery and vein
Submental triangle (5)	Submental lymph nodes and small veins that unite to form anterior jugular vein
Carotid triangle (6)	Carotid sheath containing common carotid artery and its branches; internal jugular vein and its tributaries; vagus nerve; external carotid artery and some of its branches; hypoglossal nerve (CN XII) and superior root of ansa cervicalis; spinal accessory nerve (CN XI)[b]; thyroid gland, larynx, and pharynx; deep cervical lymph nodes; branches of cervical plexus
Muscular (omotracheal) triangle (7)	Sternothyroid and sternohyoid muscles; thyroid and parathyroid glands

[a]Letters and numbers in parentheses refer to Figure 9.7A, B.
[b]The spinal accessory nerve (CN XI) refers to the traditional "spinal root of CN XI." The traditional "cranial root" is now considered part of the vagus nerve (CN X) (Lachman et al., 2002).

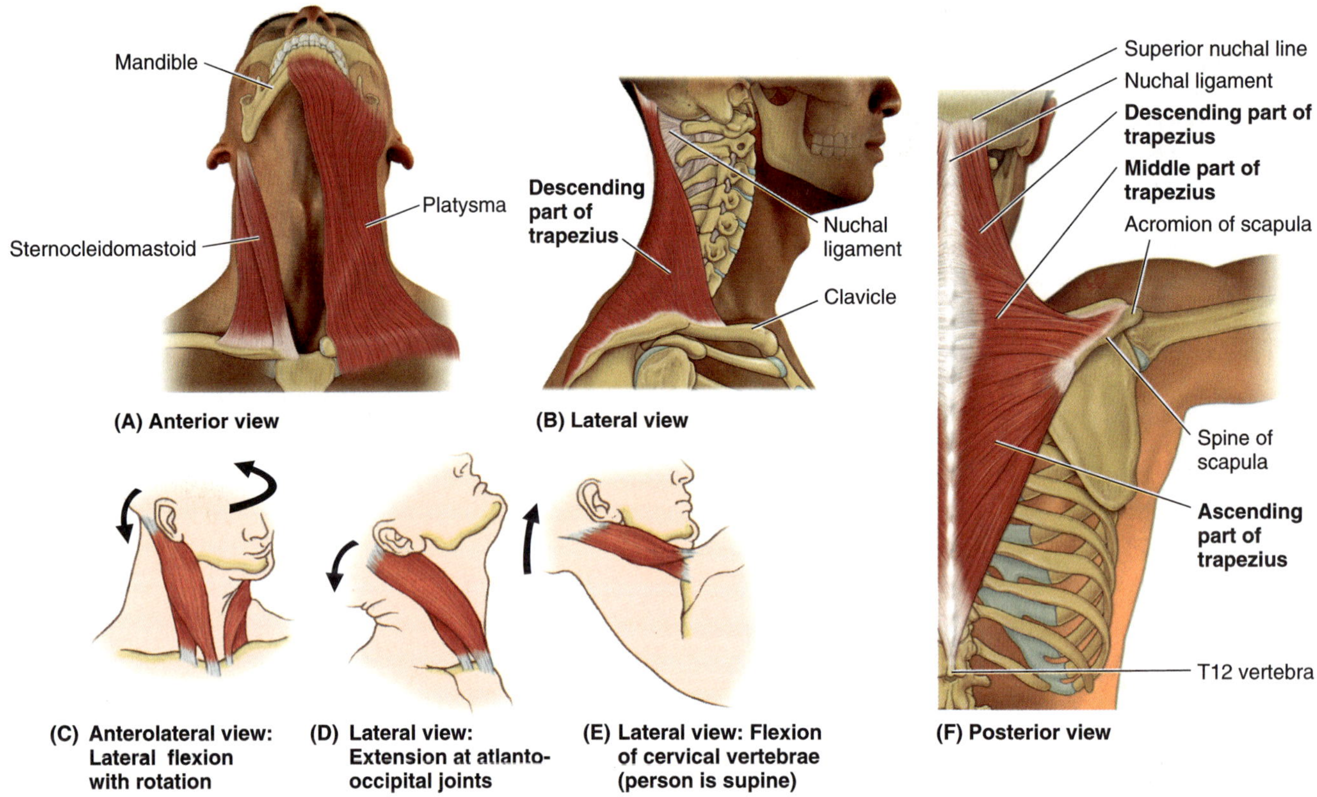

FIGURE 9.8. Muscles of neck.

TABLE 9.2. CUTANEOUS AND SUPERFICIAL MUSCLES OF NECK

Muscle	Superior/Medial Attachment	Inferior/Lateral Attachment	Innervation	Main Action(s)
Platysma	Inferior border of mandible, skin, and subcutaneous tissues of lower face	Fascia covering superior parts of pectoralis major and deltoid muscles	Cervical branch of facial nerve (CN VII)	Draws corners of mouth inferiorly and widens it as in expressions of sadness and fright; draws skin of neck superiorly when teeth are clenched
N29.1 **Sternocleidomastoid (SCM)**	Lateral surface of mastoid process of temporal bone and lateral half of superior nuchal line	*Sternal head*: anterior surface of manubrium of sternum *Clavicular head*: superior surface of medial third of clavicle	Spinal accessory nerve (CN XI, motor); C3 and C4 nerves (pain and proprioception)	*Unilateral contraction*: tilts head to same side (i.e., laterally flexes neck) and rotates it so face is turned superiorly toward opposite side (Fig. 9.6C) *Bilateral contraction*: (1) extends neck at atlanto-occipital joints (Fig. 9.6D), (2) flexes cervical vertebrae so that chin approaches manubrium (Fig. 9.6E), or (3) extends superior cervical vertebrae while flexing inferior vertebrae so chin is thrust forward with head kept level With cervical vertebrae fixed, may elevate manubrium and medial ends of clavicles, assisting pump-handle action of deep respiration (see Chapter 4, Thorax)
Trapezius	Medial third of superior nuchal line, external occipital protuberance, nuchal ligament, spinous processes of C7–T12 vertebrae, and lumbar and sacral spinous processes	Lateral third of clavicle, acromion, and spine of scapula	Spinal accessory nerve (CN XI; motor); C3 and C4 nerves (pain and proprioception)	Elevates, retracts, and rotates scapulae superiorly *Descending (superior) fibers*: elevate scapulae/shoulders, maintain level of shoulders against gravity or resistance *Transverse (middle) fibers*: retract scapulae *Ascending (inferior) fibers*: depress scapulae/shoulders *Descending and ascending fibers together*: rotate spinous process of scapulae superiorly With shoulders fixed, *bilateral contraction* extends neck; *unilateral contraction* produces lateral flexion to same side

contraction of the SCMs (especially their more posterior fibers) will cause extension of the head at the AO joints, elevating the chin (Fig. 9.8D).

Acting bilaterally, the SCMs can also flex the neck. They can do this in two different ways:

1. If initially the head is flexed anteriorly at the AO joints by the prevertebral muscles (and/or the suprahyoid and infrahyoid muscles) against resistance, the SCMs (especially the anterior fibers) flex the entire cervical vertebral column so that the chin approaches the manubrium (Fig. 9.8E). However, gravity is usually the prime mover for this movement when standing erect.
2. Acting antagonistically with the extensors of the neck (i.e., the deep cervical muscles), bilateral contraction of the SCMs can flex the lower neck while producing limited extension at the AO joint and upper neck, protruding the chin while keeping the head level. Such flexion movements also occur when lifting the head off the ground while lying supine (with gravity providing the resistance in place of the deep cervical muscles).

It is probable that most of the time smaller synergistic muscles and/or eccentric contraction (controlled relaxation of the muscle, gradually yielding to gravity) are involved in initiating flexion or extension, with the SCMs providing the power and range of movement once initiated.

Acting unilaterally, the SCM laterally flexes the neck (bends the neck sideways) and rotates the head so the ear approaches the shoulder of the ipsilateral (same) side while elevating and rotating the chin toward the contralateral (opposite) side. If the head and neck are fixed, *bilateral contraction* of the SCMs elevates the clavicles and manubrium and thus the anterior ribs. In this way, the SCMs act as accessory muscles of respiration in assisting production of the pump-handle movement of the thoracic wall.

To test the SCM, the head is turned to the opposite side against resistance (hand against chin). If it is acting normally, the SCM can be seen and palpated.

Posterior Cervical Region

The region posterior to the anterior borders of (i.e., corresponding to the area of) the trapezius is the **posterior cervical region** (Fig. 9.7; Table 9.1). The *suboccipital region* is deep to the superior part of this region (see Fig. 9.8). The **trapezius** is a large, flat triangular muscle that covers the posterolateral aspect of the neck and thorax (Fig. 9.8F). The trapezius is a

- superficial muscle of the back (see Chapter 2, Back).
- posterior axio-appendicular muscle that acts on the pectoral girdle (see Chapter 3, Upper Limb).
- cervical muscle that can produce movement of the cranium.

The trapezius attaches the pectoral girdle to the cranium and the vertebral column and assists in suspending it. Its attachments, nerve supply, and main actions are described in Table 9.2. The skin of the posterior cervical region is innervated in a segmental pattern by the posterior rami of cervical spinal nerves that pierce, but do not innervate, the trapezius (see Fig. 2.28).

To test the trapezius, the shoulder is shrugged against resistance. If the muscle is acting normally, its superior border can be seen and palpated. If the trapezius is paralyzed, the shoulder droops; however, the combined actions of the levator scapulae and superior fibers of the serratus anterior help support the shoulder and may compensate for the paralysis to some degree (see Chapter 3, Upper Limb).

Lateral Cervical Region

The **lateral cervical region** (posterior triangle) is bounded (Figs. 9.7 and 9.9)

- anteriorly by the posterior border of the SCM.
- posteriorly by the anterior border of the trapezius.
- Inferiorly by the middle third of the clavicle between the trapezius and the SCM.
- by an *apex*, where the SCM and trapezius meet on the superior nuchal line of the occipital bone.
- by a *roof*, formed by the investing layer of deep cervical fascia.
- by a *floor*, formed by muscles covered by the prevertebral layer of deep cervical fascia.

The lateral cervical region wraps around the lateral surface of the neck like a spiral. The region is covered by skin and subcutaneous tissue containing the platysma.

MUSCLES IN LATERAL CERVICAL REGION

The floor of the lateral cervical region is usually formed by the prevertebral fascia overlying four muscles (Figs. 9.9 and 9.10): splenius capitis, levator scapulae, middle scalene (L. *scalenus medius*), and posterior scalene (L. *scalenus posterior*). Sometimes the inferior part of the anterior scalene (L. *scalenus anterior*) appears in the inferomedial angle of the lateral cervical region, where it is usually hidden by the SCM. An occasional offshoot of the anterior scalene, the *smallest scalene* (L. *scalenus minimus*), passes posterior to the subclavian artery to attach to the 1st rib (Agur and Dalley, 2017).

For a more precise localization of structures, the lateral cervical region is divided into a large occipital triangle superiorly and a small omoclavicular triangle inferiorly by the *inferior belly of the omohyoid* (Fig. 9.7; Table 9.1).

- The **occipital triangle** is so called because the *occipital artery* appears in its apex (Figs. 9.8 and 9.9; see Fig. 9.13). The most important nerve crossing the occipital triangle is the *spinal accessory nerve* (CN XI).
- The **omoclavicular** (subclavian) **triangle** is indicated on the surface of the neck by the *supraclavicular fossa*. The inferior part of the EJV crosses this triangle superficially; the *subclavian artery* lies deep in it (Fig. 9.11; see Fig. 9.13).

(continued on p. 1059)

9

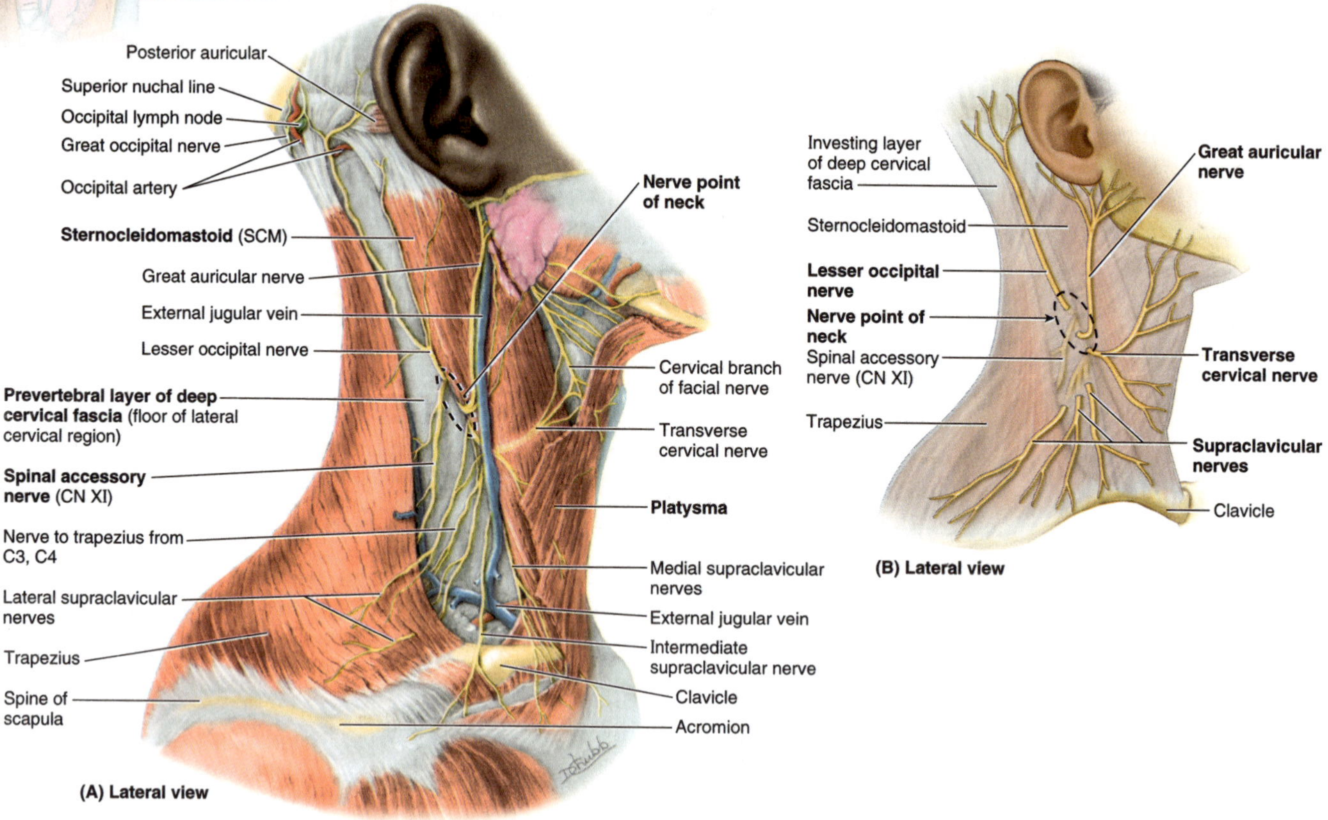

FIGURE 9.9. Superficial dissection of lateral cervical region. The subcutaneous tissue and the investing layer of deep fascia have been removed, sparing most of the platysma and the cutaneous nerves. Between the trapezius (in the posterior cervical region) and the SCM, the prevertebral layer of deep cervical fascia forms the floor of the lateral cervical region. The spinal accessory nerve (CN XI) is the only motor nerve superficial to this fascia.

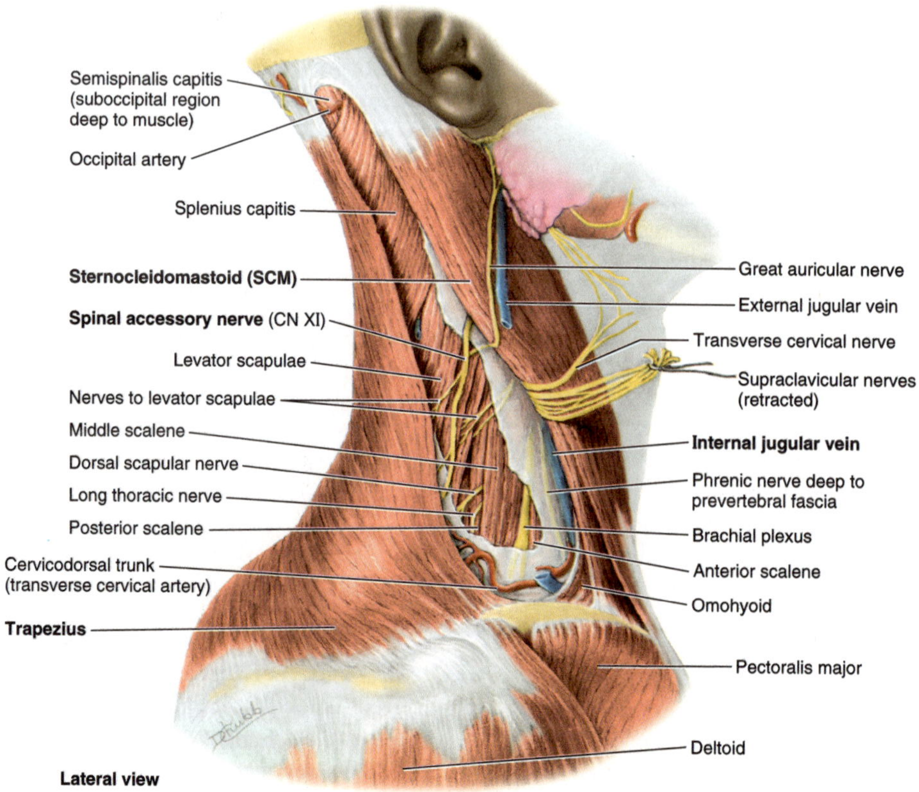

FIGURE 9.10. Deep dissection of lateral cervical region. The investing layer of the deep cervical fascia has been removed. Although the spinal accessory nerve (CN XI) is superficial to it, the brachial plexus and motor nerves of the cervical plexus run deep to the prevertebral layer of deep cervical fascia that covers the floor of the triangle.

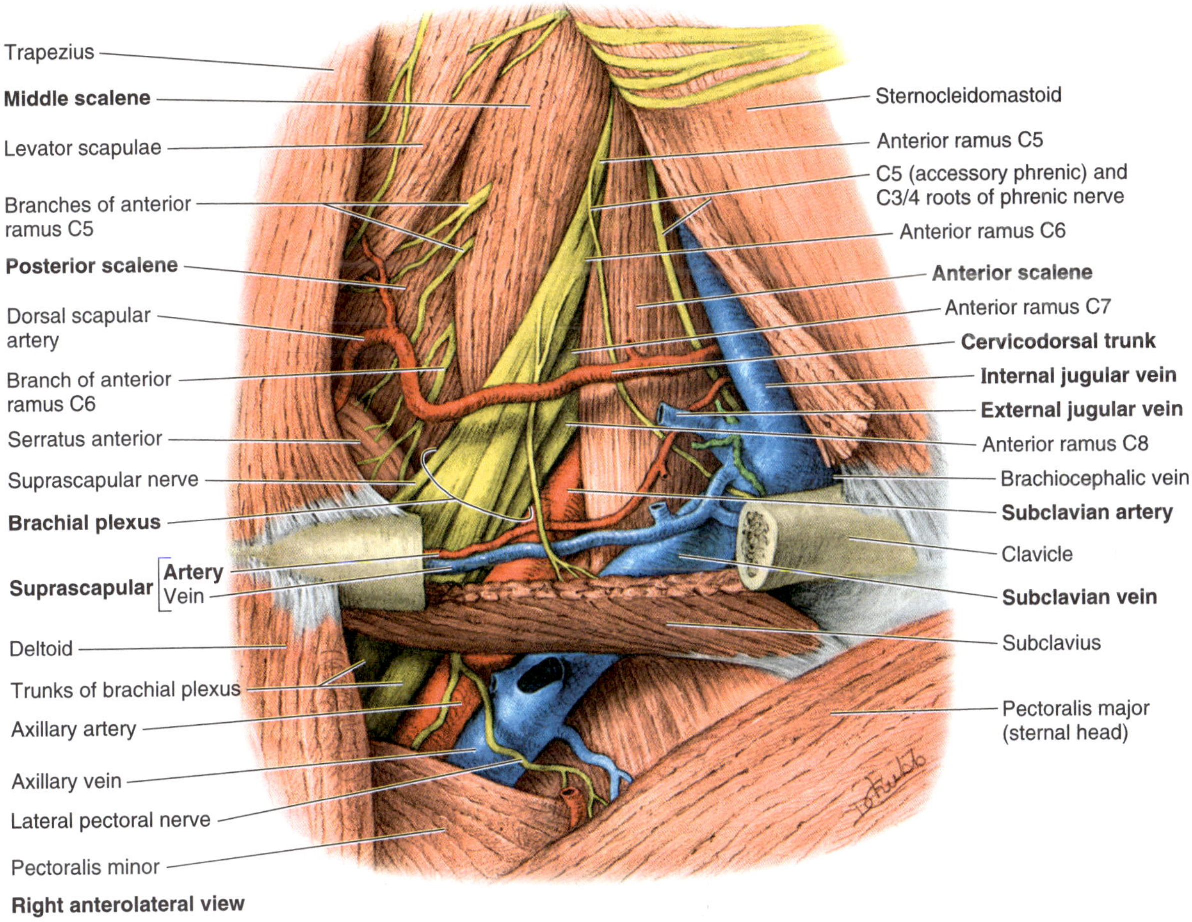

FIGURE 9.11. Deeper dissection of inferior part of lateral cervical region. All fascia, the omohyoid muscle, and the clavicular head of the pectoralis major have been removed to reveal the subclavian vein and third part of the subclavian artery. The internal jugular vein, deep to the SCM, is not in the lateral cervical region but is close to it. The brachial plexus of nerves and subclavian vessels pass to the upper limb, the name of the vessels changing to *axillary* inferior to the clavicle at the lateral border of the 1st rib.

These vessels are separated by the investing layer of deep cervical fascia. Because the third part of the subclavian artery is located in this region, the omoclavicular triangle is often called the subclavian triangle (Fig. 9.7).

ARTERIES IN LATERAL CERVICAL REGION

The arteries in the lateral cervical region include the lateral branches of the thyrocervical trunk, the third part of the subclavian artery, and part of the occipital artery (Figs. 9.10 to 9.12). The *thyrocervical trunk*, a branch of the subclavian artery, most commonly gives rise to a suprascapular artery and a cervicodorsal trunk from its lateral aspect; its terminal branches are the ascending cervical and inferior thyroid artery.

The **suprascapular artery** passes inferolaterally across the anterior scalene muscle and phrenic nerve (Fig. 9.11). It then crosses the third part of the subclavian artery and the cords of the brachial plexus to pass posterior to the clavicle to supply muscles on the posterior aspect of the scapula. Alternately, the suprascapular artery may arise directly from the third part of the subclavian artery.

Also, arising laterally, the **cervicodorsal trunk** (Weiglein et al., 2005), sometimes known as the transverse cervical artery, further bifurcates into the *superficial cervical artery* (superficial branch of transverse cervical artery) and the *dorsal scapular artery* (deep branch of transverse cervical artery). These branches run superficially and laterally across the phrenic nerve and anterior scalene muscle, 2–3 cm superior to the clavicle. They then cross or pass through the *trunks of the brachial plexus*, supplying branches to their *vasa nervorum* (blood vessels of nerves). The **superficial cervical artery** passes deep (anterior) to the trapezius accompanying the spinal accessory nerve (CN XI). The **dorsal scapular artery** may arise independently, directly from the third (or, less often, the second) part of the subclavian artery. When it is a branch of the subclavian, the dorsal scapular artery passes laterally through the trunks of the brachial plexus, anterior to the middle scalene. Regardless of its origin, its distal portion runs deep to the levator scapulae and rhomboid muscles, supplying both and participating in the arterial anastomoses around the scapula (Chapter 3, Upper Limb). The *occipital artery*, a branch of the external carotid artery, enters the

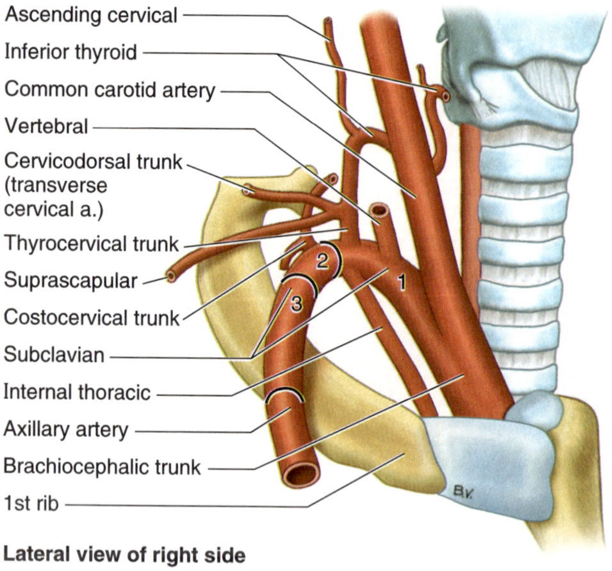

FIGURE 9.12. Subclavian artery: its parts and branches. There are three parts of the subclavian artery: medial (*1*), posterior (*2*), and lateral (*3*) to the anterior scalene muscle. The cervicodorsal trunk (transverse cervical artery) and suprascapular artery occasionally arise directly (or via a common trunk) from the second or third parts of the subclavian artery instead of directly from the thyrocervical trunk via a common trunk, as shown here, or independently.

lateral cervical region at its apex and ascends over the head to supply the posterior half of the scalp (Fig. 9.10).

The **subclavian artery** supplies blood to the upper limb. The third part begins approximately a finger's breadth superior to the clavicle, opposite the lateral border of the anterior scalene muscle. It is hidden in the inferior part of the lateral cervical region, posterosuperior to the subclavian vein. The third part of the artery is the longest and most superficial part. It lies on the 1st rib, and its pulsations can be felt by applying deep pressure in the omoclavicular triangle. The artery is in contact with the 1st rib as it passes posterior to the anterior scalene muscle; consequently, compression of the subclavian artery against this rib can control bleeding in the upper limb. The inferior trunk of the brachial plexus lies directly posterior to the third part of the artery. The branches that occasionally arise from the third part (suprascapular artery, dorsal scapular artery) are aberrant forms of more typical patterns in which they arise elsewhere (from the thyrocervical trunk via a cervicodorsal trunk).

VEINS IN LATERAL CERVICAL REGION

The **external jugular vein (EJV)** begins near the angle of the mandible (just inferior to the auricle) by the union of the posterior division of the *retromandibular vein* with the *posterior auricular vein* (Fig. 9.13). The EJV crosses the SCM obliquely, deep to the platysma, and enters the antero-inferior part of the lateral cervical region (Fig. 9.8). It then pierces the investing layer of deep cervical fascia, which forms the roof of this region, at the posterior border of the SCM. The EJV descends to the inferior part of the lateral cervical region and terminates in the subclavian vein (Figs. 9.11 and 9.13). It drains most of the scalp and side of the face.

The **subclavian vein**, the major venous channel draining AN35.4
the upper limb, curves through the inferior part of the lateral cervical region. It passes anterior to the anterior scalene muscle and phrenic nerve and unites at the medial border of the muscle with the IJV to form the **brachiocephalic vein**, posterior to the medial end of the clavicle. Just superior to the clavicle, the EJV receives the *cervicodorsal*, *suprascapular*, and *anterior jugular veins*.

NERVES OF LATERAL CERVICAL REGION

The **spinal accessory nerve (CN XI)** passes deep to the AN35.7
SCM, supplying it before entering the lateral cervical region

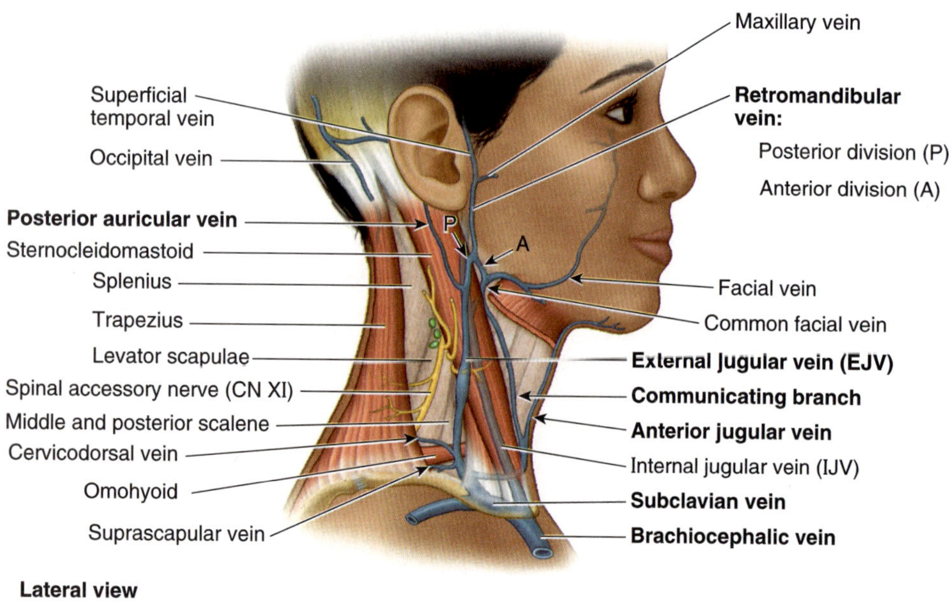

FIGURE 9.13. Superficial veins of neck. The superficial temporal and maxillary veins merge, forming the retromandibular vein, the posterior division of which unites with the posterior auricular vein to form the EJV. The facial vein receives the anterior division of the retromandibular vein before emptying into the internal jugular vein, deep to the SCM. The anterior jugular veins may lie superficial or deep to the investing layer of the deep cervical fascia.

at or inferior to the junction of the superior and middle thirds of the posterior border of the SCM (Figs. 9.9 and 9.10). The nerve passes postero-inferiorly, within or deep to the investing layer of deep cervical fascia, running on the levator scapulae from which it is separated by the prevertebral layer of fascia. CN XI then disappears deep to the anterior border of the trapezius at the junction of its superior two thirds with its inferior one third.

The **roots of the brachial plexus** (anterior rami of C5–C8 and T1) appear between the anterior and the middle scalene muscles (Fig. 9.11). The five rami unite to form the *three trunks of the brachial plexus*, which descend inferolaterally through the lateral cervical region. The plexus then passes between the 1st rib, clavicle, and superior border of the scapula (the *cervico-axillary canal*) to enter the axilla, providing innervation for most of the upper limb (see Chapter 3, Upper Limb).

The **suprascapular nerve**, which arises from the superior trunk of the *brachial plexus* (not cervical plexus), runs laterally across the lateral cervical region to supply the supraspinatus and infraspinatus muscles on the posterior aspect of the scapula. It also sends articular branches to the glenohumeral joint.

The *anterior rami of C1–C4* make up the **roots of the cervical plexus** (Fig. 9.14). The **cervical plexus** consists of an irregular series of (primary) nerve loops and the branches that arise from the loops. Each participating ramus, except the first, divides into ascending and descending branches that unite with the branches of the adjacent spinal nerve to form the loops. The cervical plexus lies anteromedial to the levator scapulae and middle scalene muscles and deep to the SCM. The superficial branches of the plexus that initially pass posteriorly are cutaneous (sensory) branches (Fig. 9.14A, C, D). The deep branches passing anteromedially are motor branches, including the *roots of the phrenic nerve* (to the diaphragm) and the *ansa cervicalis* (Fig. 9.14A, B).

The **superior root of the ansa cervicalis**, conveying fibers from spinal nerves C1 and C2, briefly joins and then descends from the hypoglossal nerve (CN XII) as it traverses the lateral cervical region (Fig. 9.14A, B). The **inferior root of the ansa cervicalis** arises from a loop between spinal nerves C2 and C3. The superior and inferior roots of the ansa cervicalis unite, forming a secondary loop, the **ansa cervicalis**, consisting of fibers from the C1–C3 spinal nerves, which branch from the secondary loop to supply the infrahyoid muscles, including the *omohyoid*, *sternothyroid*, and *sternohyoid* (Figs. 9.14A, 9.15A, and 9.16). The fourth infrahyoid muscle, the *thyrohyoid*, receives C1 fibers, which descend independently from the hypoglossal nerve, distal to the superior root of the ansa cervicalis (**nerve to thyrohyoid**) (Figs. 9.14A, B and 9.15B).

Cutaneous branches of the cervical plexus emerge around the middle of the posterior border of the SCM, often called the **nerve point of the neck** (Fig. 9.9), and supply the skin of the neck, superolateral thoracic wall, and scalp between the auricle and the external occipital protuberance (Fig. 9.14A, C, D). Close to their origin, the roots of the cervical plexus receive gray rami communicantes, most of which descend from the large *superior cervical ganglion* in the superior part of the neck.

Branches of cervical plexus arising from the nerve loop between the anterior rami of C2 and C3 are the

- **lesser occipital nerve** (C2): supplies the skin of the neck and scalp posterosuperior to the auricle.
- **great auricular nerve** (C2 and C3): ascends vertically across the oblique SCM to the inferior pole of the parotid gland, where it divides to supply the skin over—and the sheath surrounding—the gland, the mastoid process, and both surfaces of the auricle and an area of skin extending from the angle of the mandible to the mastoid process.
- **transverse cervical nerve** (C2 and C3): supplies the skin covering the anterior cervical region. It curves around the middle of the posterior border of the SCM inferior to the great auricular nerve and passes anteriorly and horizontally across it deep to the EJV and platysma, dividing into superior and inferior branches.

The branches of the cervical plexus arising from the nerve loop formed between the anterior rami of C3–C4 are the

- **supraclavicular nerves** (C3 and C4): emerge as a common trunk under cover of the SCM, sending small branches to the skin of the neck that cross the clavicle and supply the skin over the shoulder.

In addition to the ansa cervicalis and phrenic nerves arising from the loops of the plexus, **deep motor branches of the cervical plexus** include branches arising from the roots that supply the rhomboids (dorsal scapular nerve; C4 and C5), serratus anterior (long thoracic nerve; C5–C7), and nearby prevertebral muscles.

The **phrenic nerves** originate chiefly from the C4 nerve but receive contributions from the C3 and C5 nerves (Figs. 9.11 and 9.14A, B). The phrenic nerves contain motor, sensory, and sympathetic nerve fibers. These nerves provide the sole motor supply to the diaphragm as well as sensation to its central part. In the thorax, each phrenic nerve supplies the mediastinal pleura and pericardium (see Chapter 4, Thorax). Receiving variable communicating fibers in the neck from the cervical sympathetic ganglia or their branches, each phrenic nerve forms at the superior part of the lateral border of the anterior scalene muscle at the level of the superior border of the thyroid cartilage. The phrenic nerve descends obliquely with the IJV across the anterior scalene, deep to the prevertebral layer of deep cervical fascia and the transverse cervical and suprascapular arteries.

On the left, the phrenic nerve crosses anterior to the first part of the subclavian artery; *on the right*, it lies on the anterior scalene muscle and crosses anterior to the second part of the subclavian artery. On both sides, the phrenic nerve runs posterior to the subclavian vein and anterior to the internal thoracic artery as it enters the thorax.

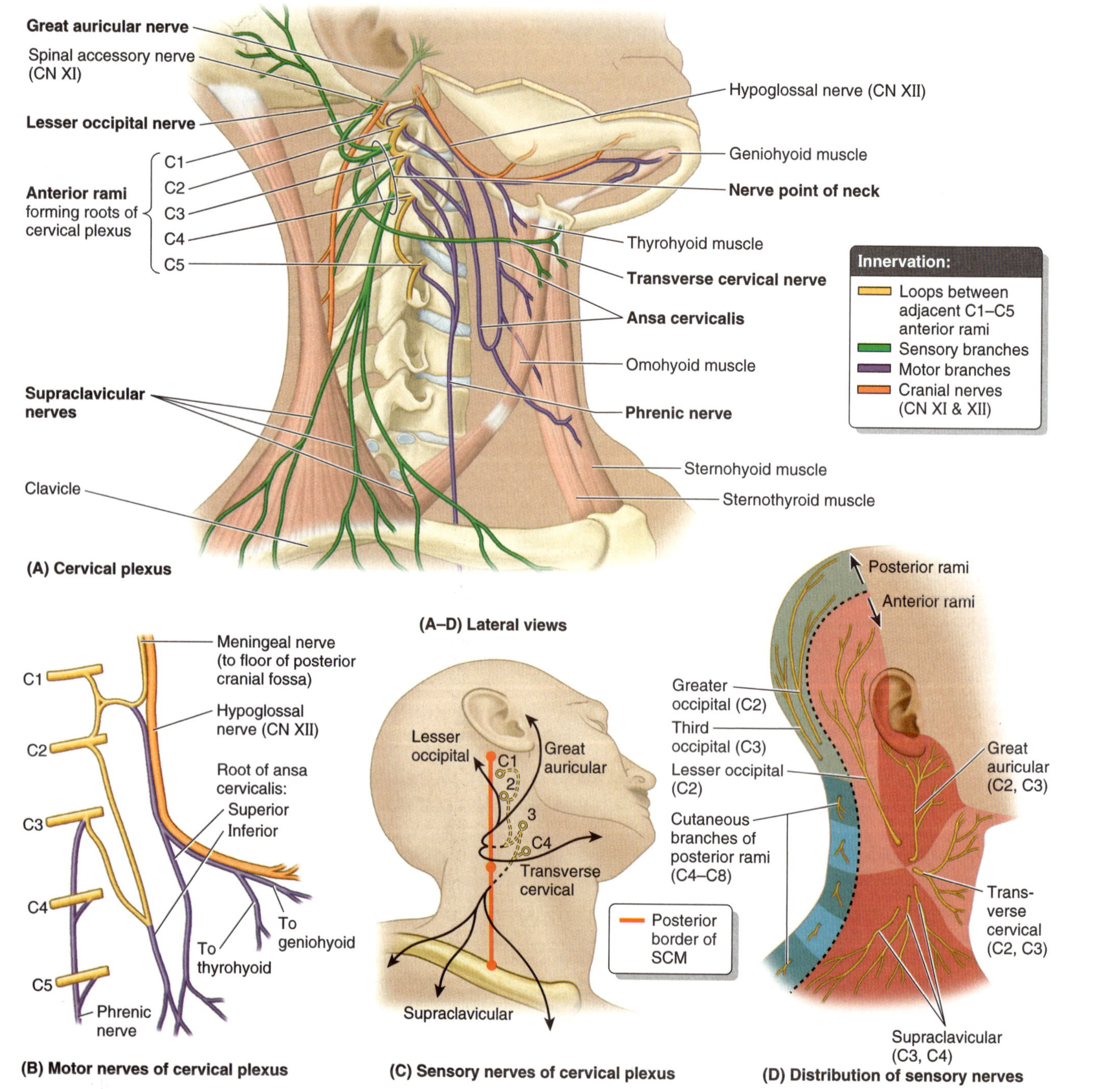

FIGURE 9.14. Cervical plexus of nerves. A–C. The plexus consists of nerve loops formed between the adjacent anterior rami of the first four cervical nerves and the receiving gray rami communicantes from the superior cervical sympathetic ganglion (not shown here) (Fig. 9.25A). Motor **(B)** and sensory nerves **(C)** arise from the loops of the plexus. The ansa cervicalis **(A, B)** is a second-level loop, the superior limb of which arises from the loop between the C1 and the C2 vertebrae but travels initially with the hypoglossal nerve (CN XII), which is not part of the cervical plexus. **D.** The areas of skin innervated by the sensory (cutaneous) nerves of the cervical plexus (derived from anterior rami) and by the posterior rami of cervical spinal nerves are shown.

The contribution of the C5 nerve to the phrenic nerve may be derived from an **accessory phrenic nerve** (Fig. 9.11). Frequently, it is a branch of the nerve to the subclavius. If present, the accessory phrenic nerve lies lateral to the main nerve and descends posterior and sometimes anterior to the subclavian vein. The accessory phrenic nerve joins the phrenic nerve either in the root of the neck or in the thorax.

LYMPH NODES IN LATERAL CERVICAL REGION

Lymph from superficial tissues in the lateral cervical region enters the **superficial cervical lymph nodes** that lie along the EJV superficial to the SCM. Efferent vessels from these nodes drain into the **deep cervical lymph nodes**, which form a chain along the course of the IJV embedded in the fascia of the carotid sheath (Figs. 9.4B and 9.15A). AN35.5

(*continued on p.* 1064)

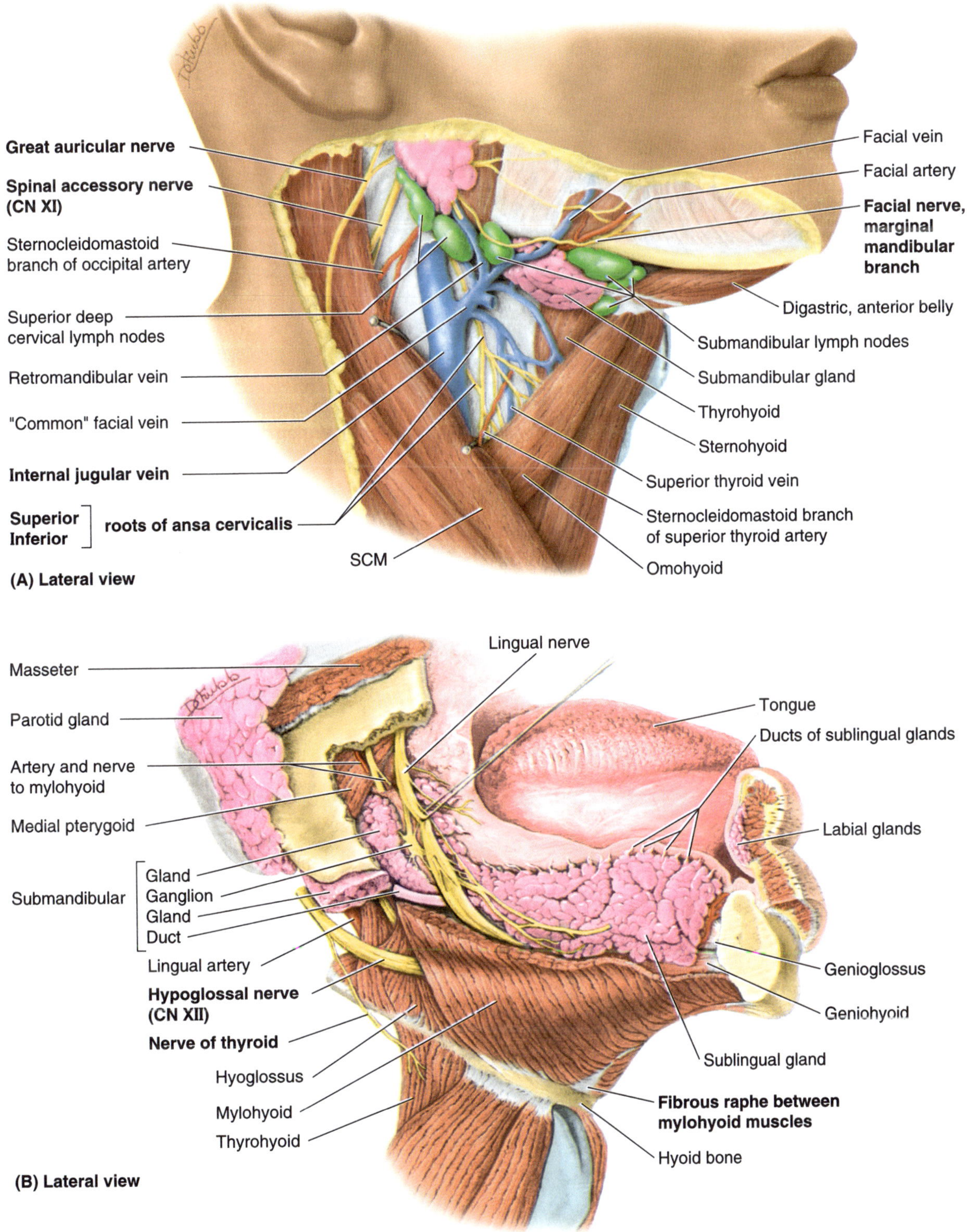

FIGURE 9.15. Dissections of anterior cervical and suprahyoid regions. A. This superficial dissection of the neck displays the submandibular gland and lymph nodes. **B.** In this dissection of the suprahyoid region, the right half of the mandible and the superior part of the mylohyoid muscle have been removed. The cut surface of the mylohyoid becomes progressively thinner as it is traced anteriorly.

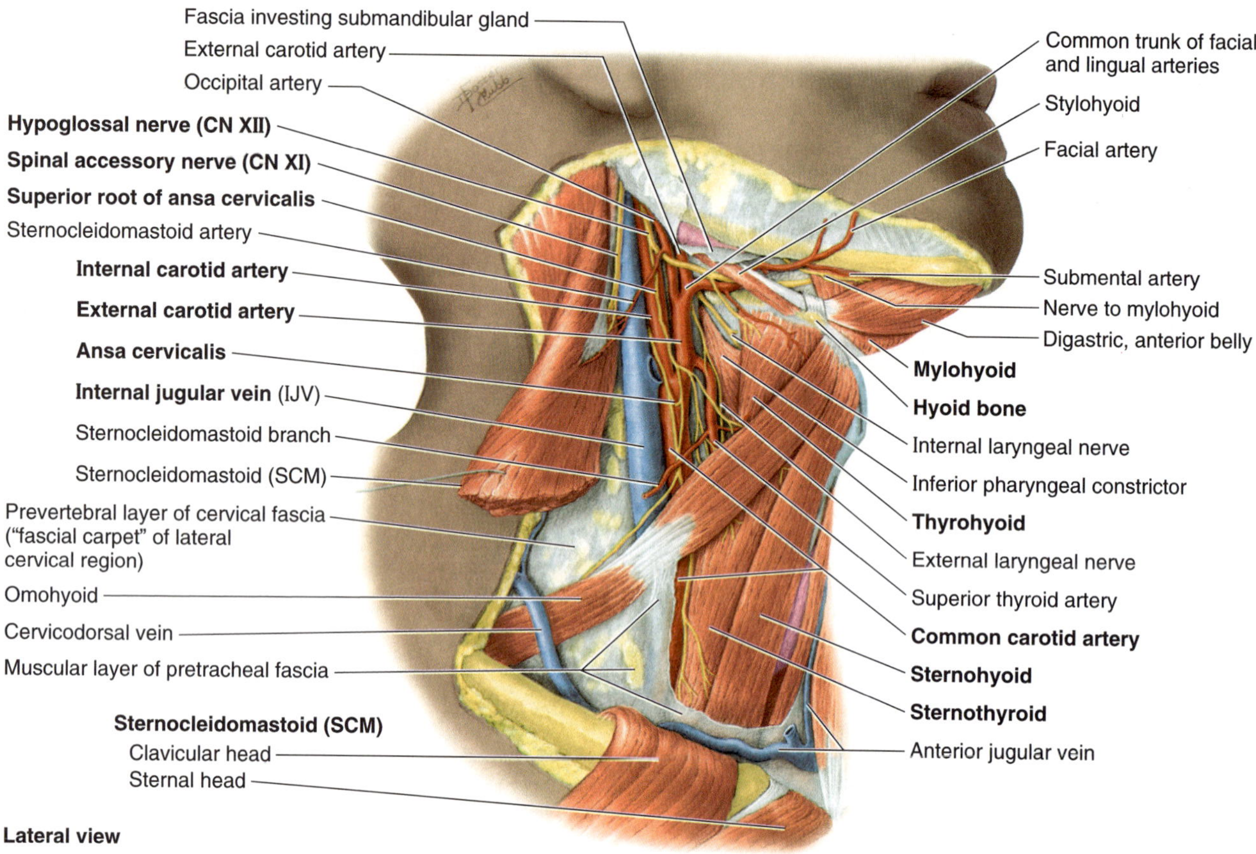

FIGURE 9.16. Deep dissection of anterior cervical region. The common facial vein and its tributaries have been removed, revealing arteries and nerves, including the ansa cervicalis and its branches to the infrahyoid muscles. The facial and lingual arteries in this person arise by a common trunk that passes deep to the stylohyoid and digastric muscles to enter the submandibular triangle.

Anterior Cervical Region

N32.2 The **anterior cervical region** (anterior triangle) (Table 9.1) has the following:

- An *anterior boundary* formed by the median line of the neck.
- A *posterior boundary* formed by the anterior border of the SCM.
- A *superior boundary* formed by the inferior border of the mandible.
- An *apex* located at the jugular notch in the manubrium.
- A *roof* formed by subcutaneous tissue containing the platysma.
- A *floor* formed by the pharynx, larynx, and thyroid gland.

For more precise localization of structures, the anterior cervical region is subdivided into four smaller triangles by the digastric and omohyoid muscles: the unpaired submental triangle and three small paired triangles—submandibular, carotid, and muscular.

The **submental triangle**, inferior to the chin, is a suprahyoid area bounded inferiorly by the body of the hyoid and laterally by the right and left anterior bellies of the digastric muscles. The floor of the submental triangle is formed by the two mylohyoid muscles, which meet in a median **fibrous raphe** (Fig. 9.15B). The apex of the submental triangle is at the *mandibular symphysis*, the site of union of the halves of the mandible during infancy. The base of the submental triangle is formed by the hyoid (Fig. 9.17). This triangle contains several small **submental lymph nodes** and small veins that unite to form the *anterior jugular vein* (Fig. 9.17).

The **submandibular triangle** is a glandular area between the inferior border of the mandible and the anterior and posterior bellies of the digastric muscle (Fig. 9.7A, C; see also Fig. 9.12). The floor of the submandibular triangle is formed by the mylohyoid and hyoglossus muscles and the middle pharyngeal constrictor. The **submandibular gland** nearly fills this triangle (Fig. 9.15A). (Because of its functional association with the mouth as well as its anatomical association with the floor of the mouth, the gland is discussed in Chapter 8, Head.)

Submandibular lymph nodes lie on each side of the submandibular gland and along the inferior border of the mandible (Fig. 9.15A). The *hypoglossal nerve* (CN XII) provides motor innervation to the intrinsic and extrinsic muscles of the tongue. It passes into the submandibular triangle, as does the *nerve to the mylohyoid* (a branch of CN V_3, which also supplies the anterior belly of the digastric), parts of the *facial artery* and vein, and the *submental artery* (a branch of the facial artery) (Figs. 9.15 and 9.16).

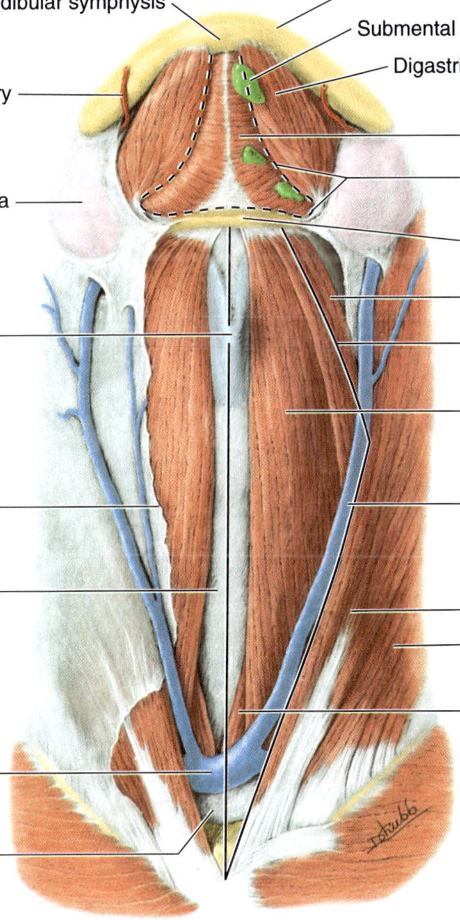

FIGURE 9.17. Superficial dissection of anterior cervical region. The submental triangle is bounded inferiorly by the body of the hyoid and laterally by the right and left anterior bellies of the digastric muscles. The floor of this triangle is formed by the two mylohyoid muscles and the raphe between them (not distinct here; see Fig. 9.15B). The muscular triangle is bounded by the superior belly of the omohyoid, the anterior border of the SCM and the midline.

The **carotid triangle** is a vascular area bounded by the superior belly of the omohyoid, the posterior belly of the digastric, and the anterior border of the SCM (Figs. 9.7, 9.15A and 9.16). This triangle is important because the *common carotid artery* ascends into it. Its pulse can be auscultated or palpated by compressing it lightly against the transverse processes of the cervical vertebrae. At the level of the superior border of the thyroid cartilage, the common carotid artery divides into the *internal* and *external carotid arteries* (Figs. 9.16, 9.18; see Fig. 9.20). Located within the carotid triangle are the following:

- **Carotid sinus**: a dilation of the proximal part of the internal carotid artery (Fig. 9.18), which may involve the common carotid artery. Innervated principally by the glossopharyngeal nerve (CN IX) through the **carotid sinus nerve** as well as by the vagus nerve (CN X), it is a *baroreceptor* (pressoreceptor) that reacts to changes in arterial blood pressure.
- **Carotid body**: a small, reddish brown ovoid mass of tissue in life that lies in a septum on the medial (deep) side of the bifurcation of the common carotid artery in close relation to the carotid sinus. Supplied mainly by the carotid sinus

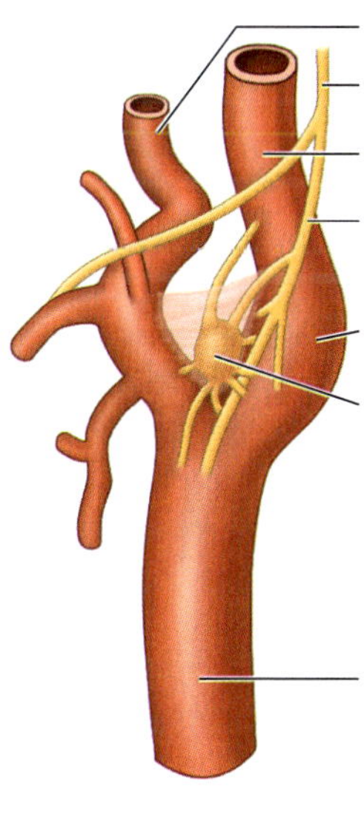

FIGURE 9.18. Carotid body and carotid sinus. This small epithelioid body lies within the bifurcation of the common carotid artery. The carotid sinus and the associated network of sensory fibers of the glossopharyngeal nerve (CN IX) are also shown.

nerve (CN IX) and by CN X, it is a *chemoreceptor* that monitors the level of oxygen in the blood. It is stimulated by low levels of oxygen and initiates a reflex that increases the rate and depth of respiration, cardiac rate, and blood pressure.

The neurovascular structures in the carotid triangle are surrounded by the *carotid sheath*: the carotid arteries medially, the *IJV* laterally, and the *vagus nerve* posteriorly (Fig. 9.4B, C). Superiorly, the common carotid is replaced by the internal carotid artery. The *ansa cervicalis* usually lies on (or is embedded in) the anterolateral aspect of the sheath (Fig. 9.16). Many *deep cervical lymph nodes* lie along the carotid sheath and the IJV.

The **muscular triangle** is bounded by the superior belly of the omohyoid muscle, the anterior border of the SCM, and the median plane of the neck (Figs. 9.7 and 9.17). This triangle contains the *infrahyoid muscles* and viscera (e.g., the thyroid and parathyroid glands).

MUSCLES IN ANTERIOR CERVICAL REGION

In the anterolateral part of the neck, the *hyoid* provides attachments for the suprahyoid muscles superior to it and the infrahyoid muscles inferior to it. These **hyoid muscles** steady or move the hyoid and larynx (Figs. 9.16, 9.17, and 9.19). For descriptive purposes, they are divided into suprahyoid and infrahyoid muscles, the attachments, innervation, and main actions of which are presented in Table 9.3.

The **suprahyoid muscles** are superior to the hyoid and connect it to the cranium (Figs. 9.15A, 9.16, 9.17 and 9.19; Table 9.3). The suprahyoid group of muscles includes the *mylohyoid, geniohyoid, stylohyoid, and digastric muscles*. As a group, these muscles constitute the substance of the floor of the mouth, supporting the hyoid in providing a base from which the tongue functions and elevating the hyoid and larynx in relation to swallowing and tone production. Each **digastric muscle** has two bellies, joined by an **intermediate tendon** that descends toward the hyoid. A **fibrous sling** derived from the pretracheal layer of deep cervical fascia allows the tendon to slide anteriorly and posteriorly as it connects this tendon to the body and greater horn of the hyoid.

The difference in nerve supply between the anterior and the posterior bellies of the digastric muscles results from their different embryological origin from the 1st and 2nd pharyngeal arches, respectively. CN V supplies derivatives of the 1st arch, and CN VII supplies those of the 2nd arch.

The **infrahyoid muscles**, often called *strap muscles* because of their ribbon-like appearance, are inferior to the hyoid (Figs. 9.16 and 9.19; Table 9.3). These four muscles anchor the hyoid, sternum, clavicle, and scapula and depress the hyoid and larynx during swallowing and speaking. They also work with the suprahyoid muscles to steady the hyoid, providing a firm base for the tongue. The infrahyoid group of muscles are arranged in two planes: a *superficial plane*, made up of the sternohyoid and omohyoid, and a *deep plane*, composed of the sternothyroid and thyrohyoid.

Like the digastric, the omohyoid has two bellies (superior and inferior) united by an *intermediate tendon*. The fascial sling for the intermediate tendon connects to the clavicle.

The **sternothyroid** is wider than the **sternohyoid**, under which it lies. The sternothyroid covers the lateral lobe of the thyroid gland. Its attachment to the *oblique line* of the lamina of the thyroid cartilage immediately superior to the gland limits upward extension of an enlarged thyroid (see the clinical box "Enlargement of Thyroid Gland" later in this chapter). The **thyrohyoid** appears to be the continuation of the sternothyroid muscle, running superiorly from the oblique line of the thyroid cartilage to the hyoid.

ARTERIES IN ANTERIOR CERVICAL REGION

The anterior cervical region contains the **carotid system of arteries**, consisting of the common carotid artery and its terminal branches, the internal and external carotid arteries. It also contains the IJV, its tributaries, and the anterior jugular veins (Figs. 9.20 and 9.21). The common carotid artery and one of its terminal branches, the *external carotid artery*, are the main arterial vessels in the carotid triangle. Branches of the external carotid (e.g., the superior thyroid artery) also originate in the carotid triangle. Each *common carotid artery* ascends within the *carotid sheath* with the IJV and vagus nerve to the level of the superior border of the thyroid cartilage. Here, each common carotid artery terminates by dividing into the internal and external carotid arteries. The *internal carotid artery* has no branches in the neck; the external carotid has several.

The **right common carotid artery** begins at the bifurcation of the *brachiocephalic trunk*. The right subclavian artery is the other branch of this trunk. From the arch of the aorta, the **left common carotid artery** ascends into the neck. Consequently, the left common carotid has a course of approximately 2 cm in the superior mediastinum before entering the neck.

The **internal carotid arteries** are direct continuations of the common carotids superior to the origin of the external carotid artery, at the level of the superior border of the thyroid cartilage. The proximal part of each internal carotid artery is the site of the *carotid sinus* (Figs. 9.18 and 9.20). The *carotid body* is located in the cleft between the internal and the external carotid arteries. The internal carotid arteries enter the cranium through the *carotid canals* in the petrous parts of the temporal bones and become the main arteries of the brain and structures in the orbits (see Chapter 8, Head). No named branches arise from the internal carotid arteries in the neck.

The **external carotid arteries** supply most structures external to the cranium; the orbit and the part of the forehead and scalp supplied by the supra-orbital artery are the major exceptions. There is some deep distribution as well (e.g., via the middle meningeal artery). Each external carotid artery runs posterosuperiorly to the region between the neck of the mandible and the lobule of the auricle, where it is embedded in the parotid gland, and terminates by dividing into two branches, the *maxillary artery* and the *superficial*

(*continued on p.* 1069)

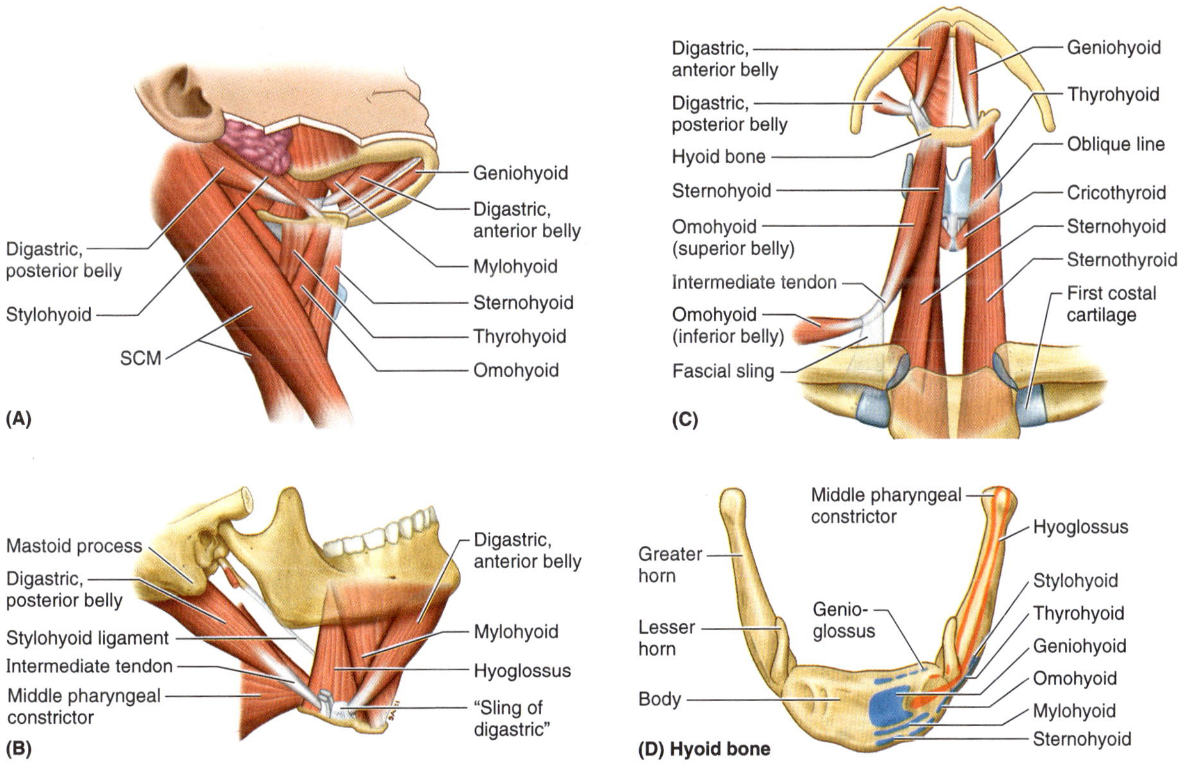

FIGURE 9.19. Muscles of anterior cervical region.

TABLE 9.3. MUSCLES OF ANTERIOR CERVICAL REGION (EXTRINSIC MUSCLES OF LARYNX)

Muscle	Origin	Insertion	Innervation	Main Action(s)
Suprahyoid muscles				
Mylohyoid	Mylohyoid line of mandible	Mylohyoid raphe and body of hyoid	Nerve to mylohyoid, a branch of inferior alveolar nerve (from mandibular nerve, CN V_3)	Elevates hyoid, floor of mouth, and tongue during swallowing and speaking
Geniohyoid	Inferior mental spine of mandible	Body of hyoid	C1 via hypoglossal nerve (CN XII)	Pulls hyoid anterosuperiorly; shortens floor of mouth; widens pharynx
Stylohyoid	Styloid process of temporal bone		Stylohyoid (preparotid) branch of facial nerve (CN VII)	Elevates and retracts hyoid, thus elongating floor of mouth
Digastric	*Anterior belly*: digastric fossa of mandible	Intermediate tendon to body and greater horn of hyoid	Nerve to mylohyoid, a branch of inferior alveolar nerve	Working with infrahyoid muscles, depresses mandible against resistance; elevates and steadies hyoid during swallowing and speaking
	Posterior belly: mastoid notch of temporal bone		Digastric (preparotid) branch of facial nerve (CN VII)	
Infrahyoid muscles				
Sternohyoid	Manubrium of sternum and medial end of clavicle	Body of hyoid	C1–C3 by a branch of ansa cervicalis	Depresses hyoid after elevation during swallowing
AN29.4 **Omohyoid**	Superior border of scapula near suprascapular notch	Inferior border of hyoid		Depresses, retracts, and steadies hyoid
Sternothyroid	Posterior surface of manubrium of sternum	Oblique line of thyroid cartilage	C2 and C3 by a branch of ansa cervicalis	Depresses hyoid and larynx
Thyrohyoid	Oblique line of thyroid cartilage	Inferior border of body and greater horn of hyoid	C1 via hypoglossal nerve (CN XII)	Depresses hyoid and elevates larynx

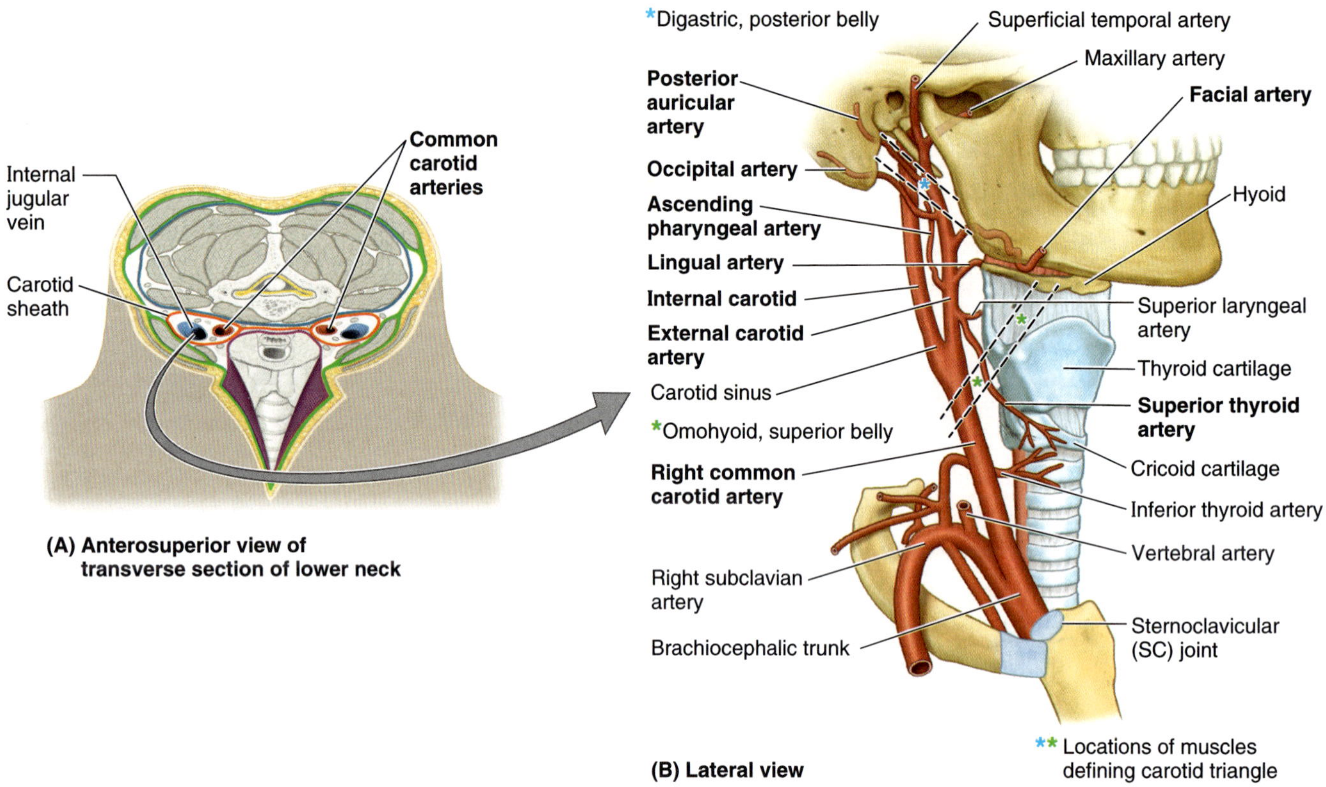

FIGURE 9.20. **Subclavian and carotid arteries and their branches. A.** The positions of the carotid sheaths are demonstrated. **B.** The muscles (posterior belly of the digastric and omohyoid muscles) indicate the superior and inferior boundaries of the carotid triangle.

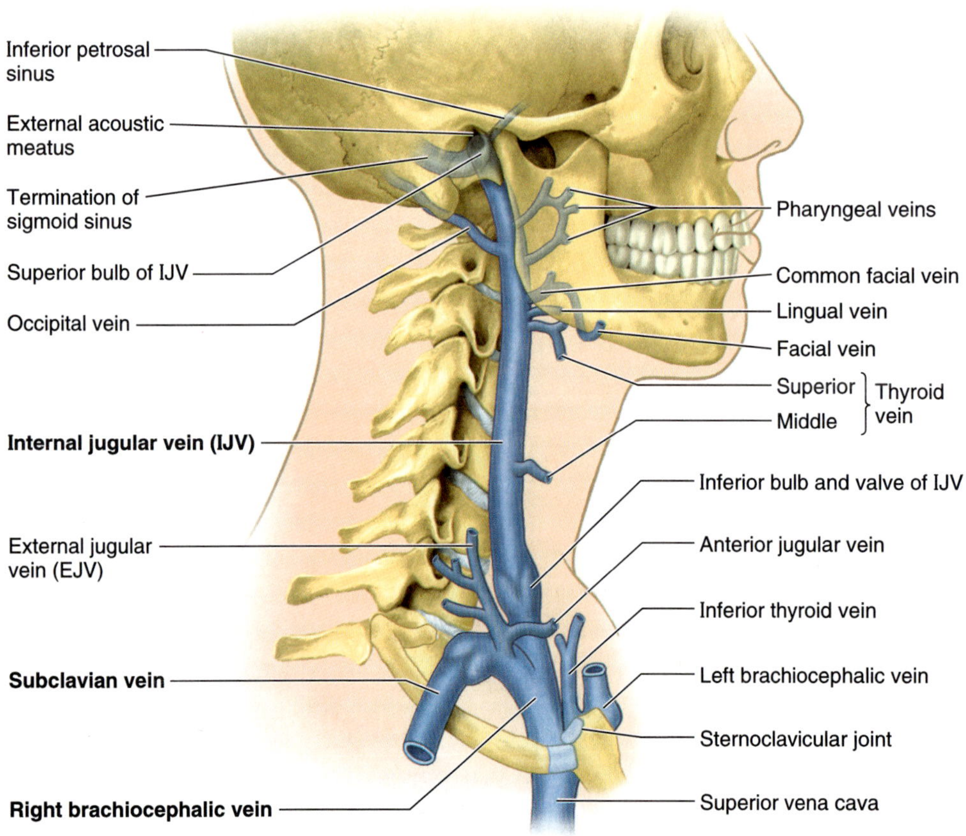

FIGURE 9.21. **Internal jugular vein.** The IJV is the main venous structure in the neck. It originates as a continuation of the S-shaped sigmoid (dural venous) sinus. As it descends in the neck, it is contained in the carotid sheath. It terminates at the T1 vertebral level, superior to the sternoclavicular joint, by uniting with the subclavian vein to form the brachiocephalic vein. A large valve near its termination prevents reflux of blood into the vein.

temporal artery (Fig. 9.20). Before these terminal branches, six arteries arise from the external carotid artery:

1. **Ascending pharyngeal artery**: arises as the first or second branch of the external carotid artery and is its only medial branch. It ascends on the pharynx deep (medial) to the internal carotid artery and sends branches to the pharynx, prevertebral muscles, middle ear, and cranial meninges.
2. **Occipital artery**: arises from the posterior aspect of the external carotid artery, superior to the origin of the facial artery. It passes posteriorly, immediately medial and parallel to the attachment of the posterior belly of the digastric muscle in the **occipital groove** in the temporal bone, and ends by dividing into numerous branches in the posterior part of the scalp. During its course, it passes superficial to the internal carotid artery and CN IX–XI.
3. **Posterior auricular artery**: a small posterior branch of the external carotid artery, which is usually the last preterminal branch. It ascends posteriorly between the external acoustic meatus and mastoid process to supply the adjacent muscles, parotid gland, facial nerve, and structures in the temporal bone, auricle, and scalp.
4. **Superior thyroid artery**: the most inferior of the three anterior branches of the external carotid artery, runs antero-inferiorly deep to the infrahyoid muscles to reach the thyroid gland. In addition to supplying this gland, it gives off branches to the infrahyoid muscles and SCM and gives rise to the *superior laryngeal artery*, supplying the larynx.
5. **Lingual artery**: arises from the anterior aspect of the external carotid artery, where it lies on the middle pharyngeal constrictor. It arches supero-anteriorly and passes deep to the hypoglossal nerve (CN XII), the stylohyoid muscle, and the posterior belly of the digastric muscle. It disappears deep to the hyoglossus muscle, giving branches to the posterior tongue. It then turns superiorly at the anterior border of this muscle, bifurcating into the deep lingual and sublingual arteries.
6. **Facial artery**: arises anteriorly from the external carotid artery, either in common with the lingual artery or immediately superior to it (Figs. 9.16 and 9.20). After giving rise to the *ascending palatine artery* and a *tonsillar artery*, the facial artery passes superiorly under cover of the digastric and stylohyoid muscles and the angle of the mandible. It loops anteriorly and enters a deep groove in and supplies the submandibular gland. It then gives rise to the *submental artery* to the floor of the mouth and hooks around the middle of the inferior border of the mandible to enter the face.

Memory device for the six branches of the external carotid artery: 1, 2, and 3—one branch arises medially (ascending pharyngeal), two branches arise posteriorly (occipital and posterior auricular), and three branches arise anteriorly (superior thyroid, lingual, and facial).

VEINS IN ANTERIOR CERVICAL REGION

Most veins in the anterior cervical region are tributaries of the IJV, typically the largest vein in the neck (Figs. 9.16 and 9.21). The IJV drains blood from the brain, anterior face, cervical viscera, and deep muscles of the neck. It commences at the *jugular foramen* in the posterior cranial fossa as the direct continuation of the sigmoid sinus (see Chapter 8, Head). AN35.

From a dilation at its origin, the **superior bulb of the IJV**, the vein descends in the *carotid sheath* (Fig. 9.20A), accompanying the internal carotid artery superior to the carotid bifurcation and the common carotid artery and vagus nerve inferiorly (see Fig. 9.26). The vein lies laterally within the carotid sheath, with the nerve located posteriorly.

The *cervical sympathetic trunk* lies posterior to the carotid sheath. Although closely related, the trunk is not within the sheath; instead, it is embedded in the prevertebral layer of deep cervical fascia. The IJV leaves the anterior cervical region by passing deep to the SCM. The inferior end of the vein passes deep to the gap between the sternal and clavicular heads of this muscle. Posterior to the sternal end of the clavicle, the IJV merges with the subclavian vein to form the *brachiocephalic vein* (Fig. 9.21). The inferior end of the IJV dilates to form the **inferior bulb of the IJV**. This bulb has a bicuspid valve that permits blood to flow toward the heart while preventing backflow into the vein, as might occur if inverted (e.g., standing on one's head or when intrathoracic pressure is increased).

The tributaries of the IJV are the inferior petrosal sinus and the facial and lingual (often by a common trunk), pharyngeal, and superior and middle thyroid veins. The **occipital vein** usually drains into the *suboccipital venous plexus*, drained by the deep cervical vein and the vertebral vein, but it may drain into the IJV.

The **inferior petrosal sinus** leaves the cranium through the jugular foramen and enters the superior bulb of the IJV. The *facial vein* empties into the IJV opposite or just inferior to the level of the hyoid. The facial vein may receive the superior thyroid, lingual, or sublingual veins. The *lingual veins* form a single vein from the tongue, which empties into the IJV at the level of origin of the lingual artery. The *pharyngeal veins* arise from the venous plexus on the pharyngeal wall and empty into the IJV approximately at the level of the angle of the mandible. The superior and middle thyroid veins leave the thyroid gland and drain into the IJV.

NERVES IN ANTERIOR CERVICAL REGION

Several nerves, including branches of cranial nerves, are located in the anterior cervical region:

- **Transverse cervical nerve** (C2 and C3): supplies the skin covering the anterior cervical region. This nerve was discussed with the cervical plexus earlier in this chapter (Figs. 9.9 and 9.14A, C, D).

9

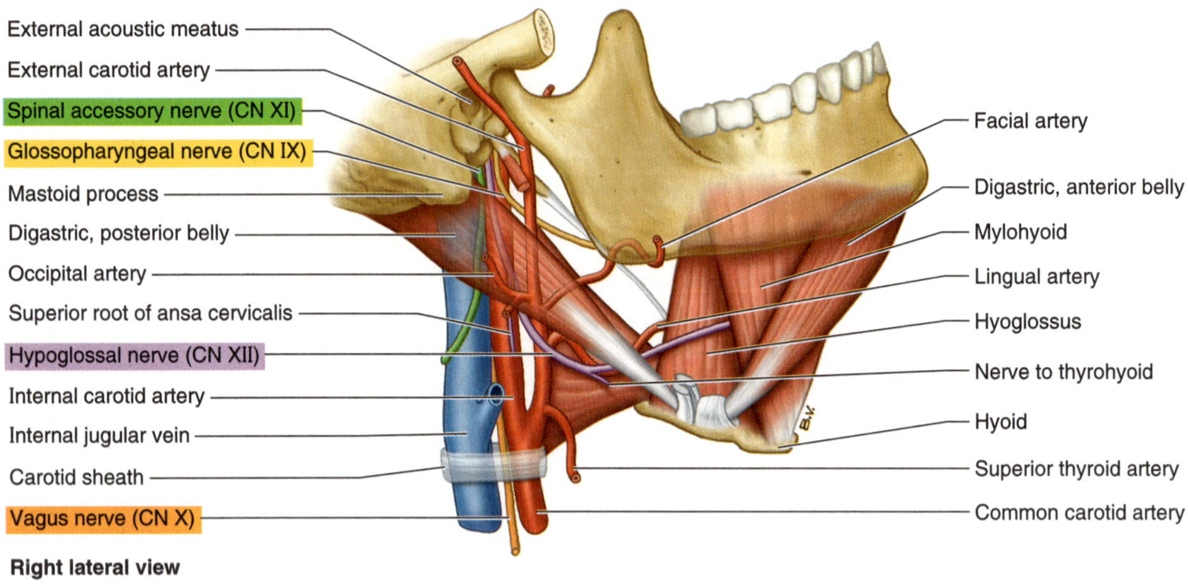

FIGURE 9.22. Relationships of nerves and vessels to suprahyoid muscles of anterior cervical region. The posterior belly of the digastric muscle, running from the mastoid process to the hyoid, holds a superficial and key position in the neck.

AN35.7
- **Hypoglossal nerve** (CN XII): the motor nerve of the tongue enters the submandibular triangle deep to the posterior belly of the digastric muscle to supply the intrinsic and four of the five extrinsic muscles of the tongue (Figs. 9.14A, 9.16, and 9.22). The nerve passes between the external carotid and jugular vessels and gives off the superior root of the ansa cervicalis and then a branch to the geniohyoid muscle (Fig. 9.14). In both cases, the branch conveys only fibers from the C1 spinal nerve, which joined its proximal part; no hypoglossal fibers are conveyed in these branches (see Chapter 10, Summary of Cranial Nerves, for details).
- Branches of the **glossopharyngeal** (CN IX) and **vagus** (CN X) nerves: in the submandibular and carotid triangles (Figs. 9.18 and 9.22). CN IX is primarily related to the tongue and pharynx. In the neck, CN X gives rise to pharyngeal, laryngeal, and cardiac branches.

Surface Anatomy of Cervical Regions and Triangles of Neck

The skin of the neck is thin and pliable. The subcutaneous tissue contains the *platysma*, a thin sheet of striated muscle that ascends to the face (Figs. 9.5 and 9.23A). Its fibers can be observed, especially in thin people, by asking them to contract the platysma muscles (e.g., by pretending to ease a tight collar).

The *SCM* is the key muscular landmark of the neck. It defines the *sternocleidomastoid region* and divides the neck into anterior and lateral cervical regions (Fig. 9.23B). This broad bulging muscle is easy to observe and palpate throughout its length as it passes superolaterally from the *sternum* and *clavicle*. Its superior attachment to the *mastoid process* is palpable posterior to the lobule of the auricle. The SCM can be made to stand out by asking the person to rotate the face toward the contralateral side and elevate the chin. In this contracted state, the anterior and posterior borders of the muscle are clearly defined.

The *jugular notch* of the manubrium forms the inferior AN43.6
boundary of the fossa between the sternal heads of the SCMs (Fig. 9.23C, D). The *suprasternal space* and *jugular venous arch* are located superior to this notch (Figs. 9.4A and 9.17). The *lesser supraclavicular fossa*, between the sternal and the clavicular heads of the SCM, overlies the inferior end of the IJV (Fig. 9.23B, D). It can be entered here by a needle or catheter (see "Internal Jugular Vein Puncture").

The *EJV* runs vertically across the SCM toward the *angle of the mandible* (Fig. 9.23D). It may be prominent, especially if distended by asking the person to take a deep breath and hold it, expiring against resistance (*Valsalva maneuver*) or by using gentle pressure on the inferior part of the vein. These actions impede venous return to the right side of the heart. The EJV is less obvious in children and middle-aged women because their subcutaneous tissues tend to be thicker than those in men.

The great auricular nerve parallels the EJV, approximately a finger's breadth posterior to the vein. Deep to the superior half of the SCM is the cervical plexus, and deep to the inferior half of the SCM are the IJV, common carotid artery, and vagus nerve in the carotid sheath.

The *trapezius*, which defines the *posterior cervical region*, can be observed and palpated by asking the person to shrug the shoulders against resistance (Fig. 9.23B–D). Superiorly, inferior to its attachment to the *external occipital protuberance*, the muscle overlies the *suboccipital region* (see Fig. 2.37).

The inferior belly of the *omohyoid muscle* can just barely be seen and palpated as it passes superomedially across the inferior part of the *lateral cervical region*. Easiest to observe

(*continued on p.* 1072)

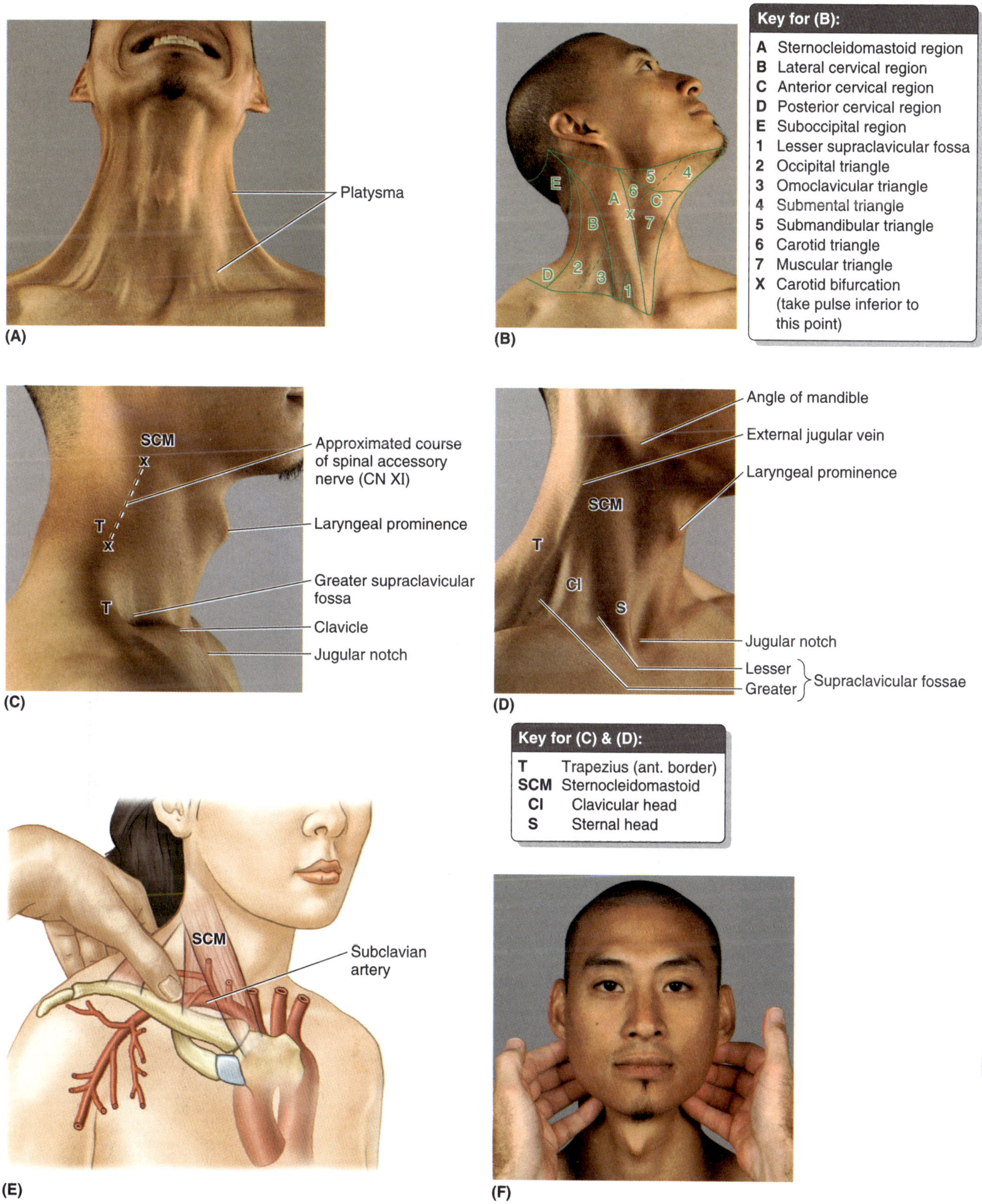

FIGURE 9.23. Surface anatomy of neck. A. Contraction of the platysma. **B.** The regions (*A–E*) and triangles (*2–7*) of the neck. **C.** The course of the spinal accessory nerve (CN XI). **D.** The landmarks of the anterolateral neck. **E.** Checking the subclavian artery pulse. **F.** Palpation of the submandibular lymph nodes.

in thin people, the omohyoid muscle can often be seen contracting when they are speaking.

Just inferior to the inferior belly of the omohyoid is the *greater supraclavicular fossa*, the depression overlying the *omoclavicular triangle* (Fig. 9.23C, D). The third part of the subclavian artery passes through this triangle before coursing posterior to the clavicle and across the 1st rib. The greater supraclavicular fossa is clinically important because **subclavian arterial pulsations** can be palpated here in most people. The course of the *subclavian artery* in the neck is represented by a curved line from the *sternoclavicular (SC) joint* to the midpoint of the clavicle. To feel subclavian pulsations, press inferoposteriorly (down and back) immediately posterior to the junction of the medial and middle thirds of the clavicle (Fig. 9.23E). This is the pressure point for the subclavian artery; firmer pressure, compressing the artery against the 1st rib, can occlude the artery when hemorrhage is occurring distally in the upper limb.

The chief contents of the larger *occipital triangle*, superior to the omohyoid muscle, are the spinal accessory nerve (CN XI); cutaneous branches of cervical nerves C2, C3, and C4; and cervical lymph nodes. Because of the vulnerability and frequency of iatrogenic injury of the spinal accessory nerve, it is important to be able to estimate the location of CN XI in the lateral cervical region. Its course can be approximated by a line that intersects the junction of the superior and middle thirds of the posterior border of the SCM and the junction of the middle and lower thirds of the anterior border of the trapezius (Fig. 9.23C).

The cervical viscera and carotid arteries and their branches are approached surgically through the *anterior cervical region*, between the anterior border of the SCM and the midline (Fig. 9.23B). Of the four smaller triangles into which this region is subdivided, the submandibular and carotid triangles are especially important clinically.

The *submandibular gland* nearly fills the *submandibular triangle*. It is palpable as a soft mass inferior to the body of the mandible, especially when the apex of the tongue is forced against the maxillary incisor teeth. The *submandibular lymph nodes* lie superficial to the gland (Fig. 9.15A). These nodes receive lymph from the face inferior to the eye and from the mouth. If enlarged, these nodes can be palpated by moving the fingertips from the angle of the mandible along its inferior border (Fig. 9.23D, F). If continued until the fingers meet under the chin, enlarged *submental lymph nodes* can be palpated in the *submental triangle* (Fig. 9.23B).

The carotid arterial system is located in the *carotid tri-* AN43.5
angle. This area is important for surgical approaches to the carotid sheath containing the common carotid artery, IJV, and vagus nerve (Figs. 9.16 and 9.22). The carotid triangle also contains the hypoglossal nerve (CN XII) and cervical sympathetic trunk. The *carotid sheath* can be marked out by a line joining the SC joint to a point midway between the mastoid process and the angle of the mandible. The **carotid pulse** can be palpated by placing the index and 3rd fingers on the thyroid cartilage and pointing them posterolaterally between the trachea and SCM. The pulse is palpable just medial to the SCM. The palpation is performed low in the neck to avoid pressure on the *carotid sinus*, which could cause a reflex drop in blood pressure and heart rate (Figs. 9.18 and 9.23B).

CLINICAL BOX

SUPERFICIAL STRUCTURES OF NECK: CERVICAL REGIONS

Congenital Torticollis

AN29.3 *Torticollis* (L. *tortus*, twisted + L. *collum*, neck) is a contraction or shortening of the cervical muscles that produces twisting of the neck and slanting of the head. The most common type of torticollis (wry neck) results from a *fibrous tissue tumor* (L. *fibromatosis colli*) that develops in the SCM before or shortly after birth. The lesion, like a normal unilateral SCM contraction, causes the head to tilt toward, and the face to turn away from, the affected side (Fig. B9.1). When torticollis occurs prenatally, the abnormal position of the infant's head usually necessitates a breech delivery.

Occasionally, the SCM is injured when an infant's head is pulled too much during a difficult birth, tearing its fibers

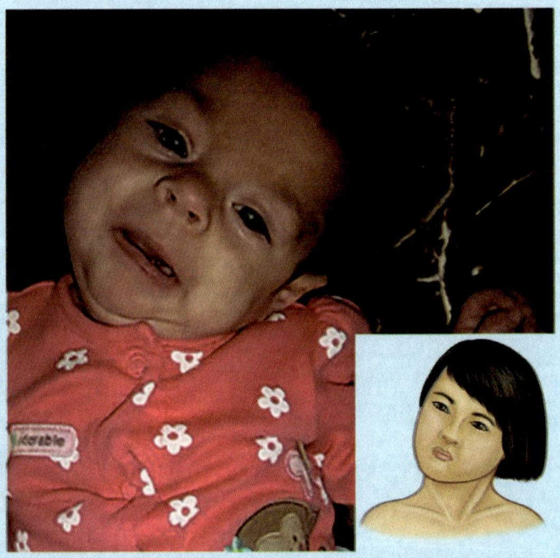

FIGURE B9.1. Congenital torticollis.

(*muscular torticollis*) (Kliegman et al., 2016). A *hematoma* (localized mass of extravasated blood) occurs that may develop into a fibrotic mass that entraps a branch of the spinal accessory nerve (CN XI) and thus denervates part of the SCM. The stiffness and twisting of the neck results from fibrosis and shortening of the SCM. Surgical release of the SCM from its inferior attachments to the manubrium and clavicle inferior to the level of CN XI may be necessary to enable the person to hold and rotate the head normally.

Spasmodic Torticollis

Cervical dystonia (abnormal tonicity of the cervical muscles), commonly known as *spasmodic torticollis*, usually begins in adulthood. It may involve any bilateral combination of lateral neck muscles, especially the SCM and trapezius. Characteristics of this disorder are sustained turning, tilting, flexing, or extending of the neck. Shifting the head laterally or anteriorly can occur involuntarily (Fahn, 2016). The shoulder is usually elevated and displaced anteriorly on the side to which the chin turns.

Subclavian Vein Puncture

The right or left subclavian vein is often the point of entry to the venous system for *central line placement*, such as a pulmonary artery catheter (PAC, also known as a Swan-Ganz or right heart catheter). Central lines are inserted to administer parenteral (venous nutritional) fluids and medications and to measure central venous pressure. In an infraclavicular subclavian vein approach, the administrator places the thumb of one hand on the middle part of the clavicle and the index finger on the jugular notch in the manubrium (Fig. B9.2). The needle punctures the skin inferior to the thumb (middle of the clavicle) and is advanced medially toward the tip of the index finger (jugular notch) until the tip enters the right venous angle, posterior to the sternoclavicular joint. Here, the internal jugular and subclavian veins merge to form the brachiocephalic vein. If the needle is not inserted carefully, it may puncture the pleura and lung, resulting in *pneumothorax*. Furthermore, if the needle is inserted too far posteriorly, it may enter the subclavian artery. When the needle has been inserted correctly, a soft, flexible catheter is inserted into the subclavian vein, using the needle as a guide.

Right Cardiac Catheterization

For *right cardiac catheterization* (to take measurements of pressures in the right chambers of the heart), puncture of the IJV can be used to introduce a catheter through the right brachiocephalic vein into the superior vena cava (SVC) and the right side of the heart. Although the preferred route is through the IJV or subclavian vein, it may be necessary in some patients to use the EJV. This vein is not ideal for catheterization because its angle of junction with the subclavian vein makes passage of the catheter difficult.

Prominence of External Jugular Vein

The EJV may serve as an "internal barometer." When venous pressure is in the normal range, the EJV is usually visible above the clavicle for only a short distance. However, when venous pressure rises (e.g., as in heart failure), the vein is prominent throughout its course along the side of the neck. Consequently, routine observation of the EJVs during physical examinations may give diagnostic signs of heart failure, SVC obstruction, enlarged supraclavicular lymph nodes, or increased intrathoracic pressure.

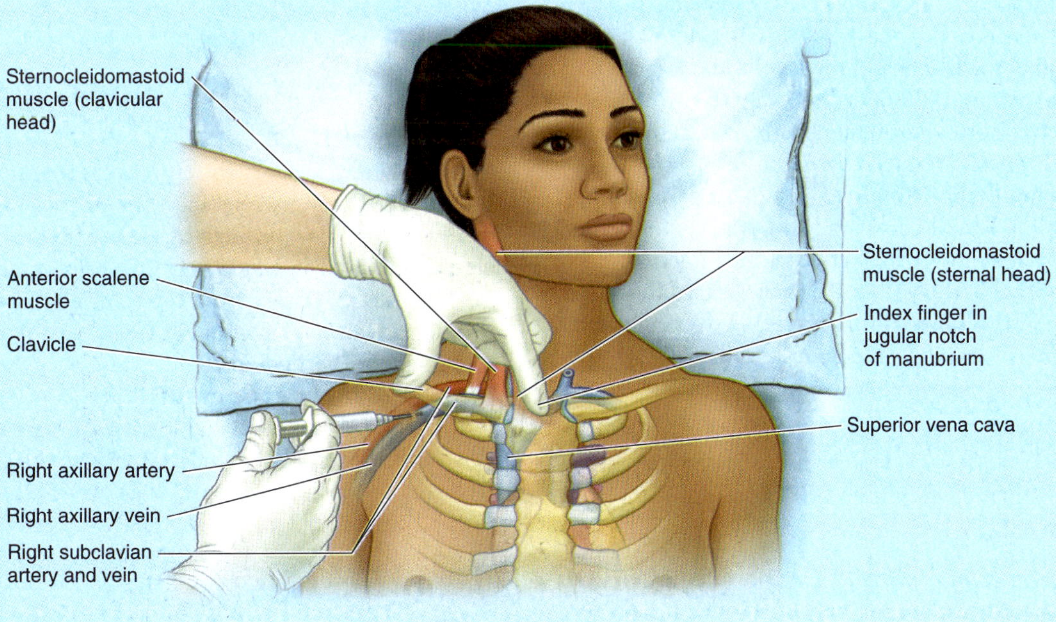

FIGURE B9.2. Subclavian vein puncture.

Severance of External Jugular Vein

If the *EJV is severed* along the posterior border of the SCM, where it pierces the roof of the lateral cervical region (e.g., by a knife slash), its lumen is held open by the tough investing layer of deep cervical fascia, and the negative intrathoracic pressure air will suck air into the vein. This action produces a churning noise in the thorax and cyanosis (a bluish discoloration of the skin and mucous membranes resulting from an excessive concentration of reduced hemoglobin in the blood). A *venous air embolism* produced in this way will fill the right side of the heart with froth, which nearly stops blood flow through it, resulting in *dyspnea* (shortness of breath). The application of firm pressure to the severed jugular vein until it can be sutured will stop the bleeding and entry of air into the blood.

Lesions of Spinal Accessory Nerve (CN XI)

Lesions of the spinal accessory nerve (CN XI) are uncommon. This nerve may be damaged by the following:

- Penetrating trauma, such as a stab or bullet wound.
- Surgical procedures in the lateral cervical region.
- Tumors at the cranial base or cancerous cervical lymph nodes.
- Fractures of the jugular foramen, where CN XI leaves the cranium.

Although contraction of one SCM turns the head to one side, a unilateral lesion of CN XI usually does not produce an abnormal position of the head. However, people with CN XI damage usually have weakness in turning the head to the opposite side against resistance. Lesions of the CN XI produce weakness and atrophy of the trapezius, impairing neck movements.

Unilateral paralysis of the trapezius is evident by the patient's inability to elevate and retract the shoulder and by difficulty in elevating the upper limb superior to the horizontal level. The normal prominence in the neck produced by the trapezius is also reduced. *Drooping of the shoulder* is an obvious sign of CN XI injury. During extensive surgical dissections in the lateral cervical region—for example, during removal of cancerous lymph nodes—the surgeon isolates CN XI to preserve it, if possible. An awareness of the superficial location of this nerve during superficial procedures in the lateral cervical region is important because CN XI is the most commonly iatrogenic nerve injury (G. *iatros*, physician or surgeon).

Severance of Phrenic Nerve, Phrenic Nerve Block, and Phrenic Nerve Crush

Severance of a phrenic nerve results in paralysis of the corresponding half of the diaphragm (see the clinical box "Paralysis of the Diaphragm" in Chapter 4, Thorax). A *phrenic nerve block* produces a short period of paralysis of the diaphragm on one side (e.g., for a lung operation). The anesthetic is injected around the nerve where it lies on the anterior surface of the middle third of the anterior scalene muscle. A surgical *phrenic nerve crush* (e.g., compressing the nerve injuriously with forceps) produces a longer period of paralysis (sometimes for weeks after surgical repair of a diaphragmatic hernia). If an accessory phrenic nerve is present, it must also be crushed to produce complete paralysis of the hemidiaphragm.

Nerve Blocks in Lateral Cervical Region

For regional anesthesia before neck surgery, a *cervical plexus block* inhibits nerve impulse conduction. The anesthetic agent is injected at several points along the posterior border of the SCM, mainly at the junction of its superior and middle thirds, the *nerve point of the neck* (Figs. 9.9 and 9.14A). Half of the diaphragm is usually paralyzed by a cervical plexus block, due to the inclusion of the phrenic nerve in the block. Therefore, this procedure is not performed on persons with pulmonary or cardiac disease. For anesthesia of the upper limb, the anesthetic agent in a *supraclavicular brachial plexus block* is injected around the supraclavicular part of the brachial plexus. The main injection site is superior to the midpoint of the clavicle.

Injury to Suprascapular Nerve

The suprascapular nerve is vulnerable to injury in fractures of the middle third of the clavicle. *Injury to the suprascapular nerve* results in loss of lateral rotation of the humerus at the glenohumeral joint. Consequently, the relaxed limb rotates medially into the *waiter's tip position* (see Chapter 3, Fig. B3.13B). The ability to initiate abduction of the limb is also affected.

Ligation of External Carotid Artery

Ligation of an external carotid artery is sometimes necessary to control bleeding from one of its relatively inaccessible branches. This procedure decreases blood flow through the artery and its branches but does not eliminate it. Blood flows in a retrograde (backward) direction into the artery from the external carotid artery on the other side through communications between its branches (e.g., those in the face and scalp) and across the midline. When the external carotid or subclavian arteries are ligated, the descending branch of the occipital artery provides the main collateral circulation, anastomosing with the vertebral and deep cervical arteries.

Surgical Dissection of Carotid Triangle

The carotid triangle provides an important surgical approach to the carotid system of arteries. It also provides access to the IJV, the vagus and hypoglossal nerves, and the cervical sympathetic trunk. Damage or compression of the vagus and/or recurrent laryngeal nerves during *surgical dissection of the carotid triangle* may produce an alteration in the voice because these nerves supply laryngeal muscles.

Carotid Occlusion and Endarterectomy

Atherosclerotic thickening of the intima of the internal carotid artery may obstruct blood flow. Symptoms resulting from this obstruction depend on the degree of obstruction and the amount of collateral blood flow to the brain and structures in the orbit from other arteries. A partial occlusion of the internal carotid may cause a *transient ischemic attack* (TIA), a sudden focal loss of neurological function (e.g., dizziness and disorientation) that disappears within 24 hours. Arterial occlusion may also cause a *minor stroke*, a loss of neurological function such as weakness or sensory loss on one side of the body that exceeds 24 hours but disappears within 3 weeks.

Obstruction of blood flow can be observed in a *Doppler color study* (Fig. B9.3A). A Doppler is a diagnostic instrument that emits an ultrasonic beam and detects its reflection from moving fluid (blood) in a manner that distinguishes the fluid from the static surrounding tissue, providing information about its pressure, velocity, and turbulence. *Carotid occlusion*, causing stenosis (narrowing) in otherwise healthy persons (Fig. B9.3B), can be relieved by opening the artery at its origin and stripping off the atherosclerotic plaque with the intima. This procedure is called *carotid endarterectomy*. After the operation, drugs that inhibit clot formation are administered until the endothelium has regrown. Because of the relations of the internal carotid artery, there is risk of cranial nerve injury during the procedure involving one or more of the following nerves: CN IX, CN X (or its branch, the superior laryngeal nerve), CN XI, or CN XII (Fig. 9.22).

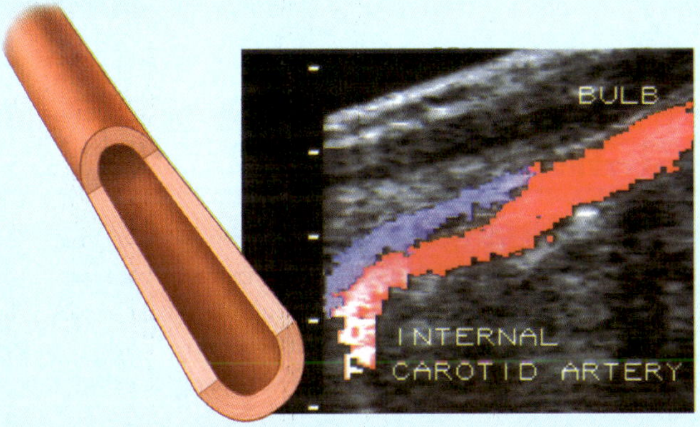

(A) Doppler color flow study of normal internal carotid artery

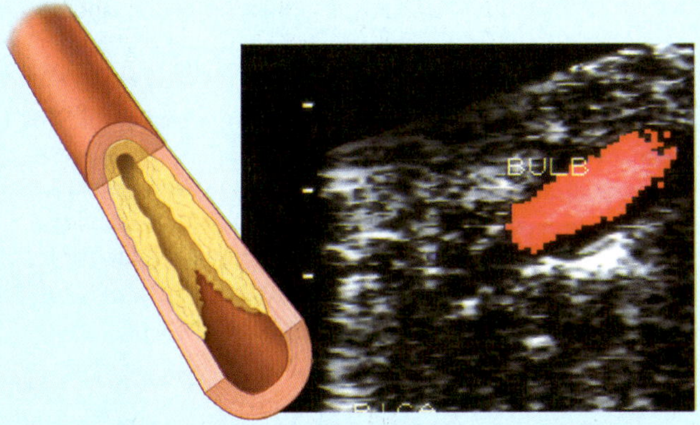

(B) Doppler color flow study of occluded carotid artery

FIGURE B9.3. Doppler study of carotid blood flow.

Carotid Pulse

The *carotid pulse* ("neck pulse") is easily felt by palpating the common carotid artery in the side of the neck, where it lies in a groove between the trachea and the infrahyoid muscles (Fig. 9.16). It is usually easily palpated just deep to the anterior border of the SCM at the level of the superior border of the thyroid cartilage. It is routinely checked during *cardiopulmonary resuscitation* (CPR). Absence of a carotid pulse indicates cardiac arrest. AN43

Carotid Sinus Hypersensitivity

In people with *carotid sinus hypersensitivity* (exceptional responsiveness of the carotid sinuses in various types of vascular disease), external pressure on the carotid artery may cause slowing of the heart rate, a fall in blood pressure, and cardiac ischemia resulting in fainting (*syncope*). In all forms of syncope, symptoms result from a sudden and critical decrease in cerebral perfusion (Shih, 2016). Consequently, this method of checking the pulse is not recommended for people with cardiac or vascular disease. Alternate sites, such as the radial artery at the wrist, should be used to check pulse rate in people with carotid sinus hypersensitivity.

Role of Carotid Bodies

The *carotid bodies* are in an ideal position to monitor the oxygen content of blood before it reaches the brain (Fig. 9.18). A decrease in PO_2 (partial pressure of oxygen), as occurs at high altitudes or in pulmonary disease, activates the aortic and carotid chemoreceptors, increasing alveolar ventilation. The carotid bodies also respond to increased carbon dioxide (CO_2) tension or free hydrogen ions in the blood. The glossopharyngeal nerve (CN IX, perhaps with involvement of the vagus nerve) conducts the information centrally, resulting in reflexive stimulation of the respiratory centers of the brain that increase the depth and rate of breathing. The pulse rate and blood pressure also increase. With increased ventilation and circulation, more oxygen is taken in and the concentration of CO_2 is reduced accordingly.

Internal Jugular Pulse

N43.5 Although pulsations are most commonly associated with arteries, *pulsations of the (IJV)* can provide information about heart activity corresponding to electrocardiogram (ECG) recordings and right atrial pressure. The IJV pulse is not palpable in the same manner as arterial pulses; however, the vein's pulsations are transmitted through the surrounding tissue and may be observed beneath the SCM superior to the medial end of the clavicle.

Because there are no valves in the brachiocephalic vein or the superior vena cava, a wave of contraction passes up these vessels to the inferior bulb of the IJV. The pulsations are especially visible when the person's head is inferior to the lower limbs *(Trendelenburg position)*. The internal jugular pulse increases considerably in conditions such as mitral valve disease (see Chapter 4, Thorax), which increases pressure in the pulmonary circulation and right side of the heart. The right IJV runs a straighter, more direct course to the right atrium than does the left; therefore, it is the one that is examined (Bickley, 2016).

Internal Jugular Vein Puncture

A needle and catheter may be inserted into the IJV for diagnostic or therapeutic purposes. The right IJV is preferable because it is usually larger and straighter. During this procedure, the clinician palpates the common carotid artery and inserts the needle into the IJV just lateral to it at a 30° angle, aiming at the apex of the triangle between the sternal and clavicular heads of the SCM, the lesser supraclavicular fossa (Fig. B9.4). The needle is then directed inferolaterally toward the ipsilateral nipple.

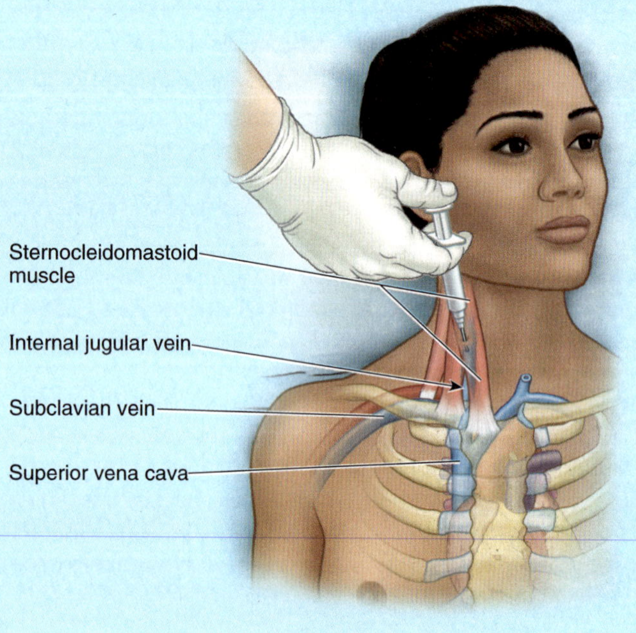

FIGURE B9.4. Internal jugular vein puncture.

The Bottom Line: Superficial Structures of Neck: Cervical Regions

Sternocleidomastoid (SCM) and trapezius: The SCM and trapezius muscles share their origins from a common embryologic source, innervation by the spinal accessory nerve (CN XI), enclosure by the investing layer of deep cervical fascia, a linear superior attachment to the cranial base, and an inferior attachment to the pectoral girdle. • Their superficial masses and palpable borders provide the basis for describing the regions of the neck. • The SCM produces multiple movements of the head and neck. • The trapezius causes multiple movements of the scapula, depending on whether the muscles act unilaterally or bilaterally, and independently or in conjunction with concentric or eccentric contraction of other muscles.

Lateral cervical region: The lateral cervical region is bounded by the SCM, trapezius, and middle third of the clavicle, with a muscular floor formed by the lateral deep cervical muscles. • It is subdivided by the diagonally placed inferior belly of the omohyoid. • Most apparent within the superior occipital triangle is the lower half of the external jugular vein. • Most important clinically is the superficially located spinal accessory nerve (CN XI). • In the inferior and much smaller omoclavicular triangle, the brachial plexus emerges between the middle and anterior scalene muscles, the latter of which is crossed anteriorly by the phrenic nerve. • Superior to the brachial plexus, and in the same plane, is the cervical plexus. • The cutaneous branches of this plexus emerge from the midpoint of the posterior border of the SCM and radiate toward the scalp, auricle, anterior neck, and shoulder.

Anterior cervical region: The anterior cervical region is inferior to the body of the mandible, extending anteriorly from the SCM to the midline. • The bellies of the digastric, the anterior belly of the omohyoid, and the hyoid subdivide the region into smaller triangles. • The submental triangle is superficial to the floor of the mouth. • The submandibular triangle, superior to the digastric bellies, is occupied by the submandibular salivary gland and submandibular lymph nodes. • The facial artery, coursing within this triangle, is palpable as it emerges from it and crosses the body of the mandible. • The carotid triangle, between the posterior belly of the digastric, superior belly of the omohyoid, and SCM, includes much of the carotid sheath and related structures, including the bifurcation of the common carotid, the carotid sinus and body, and the initial branches of the external carotid artery. • The muscular triangle is formed and occupied by the infrahyoid muscles.

DEEP STRUCTURES OF NECK

The **deep structures of the neck** are the prevertebral muscles, located posterior to the cervical viscera and anterolateral to the cervical vertebral column and the viscera extending through the superior thoracic aperture, into the *root (most inferior part) of the neck.*

Prevertebral Muscles

The anterior and lateral vertebral or **prevertebral muscles** are deep to prevertebral layer of deep cervical fascia. The **anterior vertebral muscles**, consisting of the longus colli and capitis, rectus capitis anterior, and anterior scalene muscles (Fig. 9.24A), lie directly posterior to the *retropharyngeal space* (Fig. 9.5A, B) and medial to the neurovascular plane of the cervical and brachial plexuses and subclavian artery. The **lateral vertebral muscles**, consisting of the rectus capitis lateralis, splenius capitis, levator scapulae, and middle and posterior scalene muscles, lie posterior to this neurovascular plane and (except for the highly placed rectus capitis lateralis) form the floor of the lateral cervical region. These muscles are illustrated in Figure 9.24; their attachments, innervation, and main actions are given in Table 9.4.

Root of Neck

The **root of the neck** is the junctional area between the thorax and neck (Fig. 9.25A). It is located on the cervical side of the *superior thoracic aperture*, through which pass all structures going from the thorax to the head or upper limb and vice versa (see Fig. 4.7). The inferior boundary of the

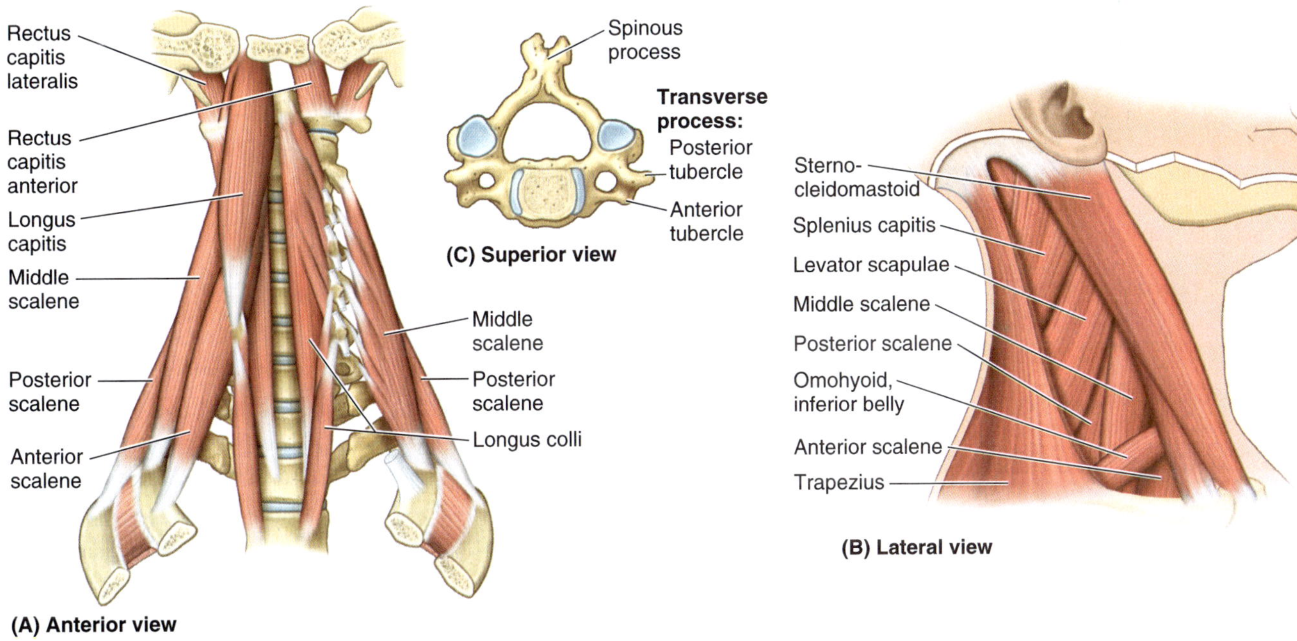

FIGURE 9.24. Prevertebral muscles.

TABLE 9.4. PREVERTEBRAL MUSCLES

Muscle	Superior Attachment	Inferior Attachment	Innervation	Main Action(s)
Anterior vertebral muscles				
Longus colli	Anterior tubercle of C1 vertebra (atlas); bodies of C1–C3 and transverse processes of C3–C6 vertebrae	Bodies of C5–T3 vertebrae; transverse processes of C3–C5 vertebrae	Anterior rami of C2–C6 spinal nerves	Flexes neck with rotation (torsion) to opposite side if acting unilaterally[a]
Longus capitis	Basilar part of occipital bone	Anterior tubercles of C3–C6 transverse processes	Anterior rami of C1–C3 spinal nerves	
Rectus capitis anterior	Base of cranium, just anterior to occipital condyle	Anterior surface of lateral mass of atlas (C1 vertebra)	Branches from loop between C1 and C2 spinal nerves	Flex head[b]
AN29.4 **Anterior scalene**	Transverse processes of C3–C6 vertebrae	1st rib	Cervical spinal nerves C4–C6	

(Continued)

TABLE 9.4. PREVERTEBRAL MUSCLES (Continued)

Muscle	Superior Attachment	Inferior Attachment	Innervation	Main Action(s)
Lateral vertebral muscles				
Rectus capitis lateralis	Jugular process of occipital bone	Transverse process of atlas (C1 vertebra)	Branches from loop between C1 and C2 spinal nerves	Flexes head and helps stabilize it[b]
Splenius capitis	Inferior half of nuchal ligament and spinous processes of superior six thoracic vertebrae	Lateral aspect of mastoid process and lateral third of superior nuchal line	Posterior rami of middle cervical spinal nerves	Laterally flexes and rotates head and neck to same side; acting bilaterally, extends head and neck[c]
29.4 **Levator scapulae**	Posterior tubercles of transverse processes C2–C6 vertebrae	Superior part of medial border of scapula	Dorsal scapular nerve C5 and cervical spinal nerves C3 and C4	Downward rotation of scapula and tilts its glenoid cavity inferiorly by rotating scapula
Middle scalene	Posterior tubercles of transverse processes of C5–C7 vertebrae	Superior surface of 1st rib; posterior to groove for subclavian artery	Anterior rami of cervical spinal nerves	Flexes neck laterally; elevates 1st rib during forced inspiration[a]
Posterior scalene		External border of 2nd rib	Anterior rami of cervical spinal nerves C7 and C8	Flexes neck laterally; elevates 2nd rib during forced inspiration[a]

[a]Flexion of neck = anterior (or lateral) bending of cervical vertebrae C2–C7.
[b]Flexion of head = anterior (or lateral) bending of the head relative to the vertebral column at the atlanto-occipital joints.
[c]Rotation of the head occurs at the atlanto-axial joints.

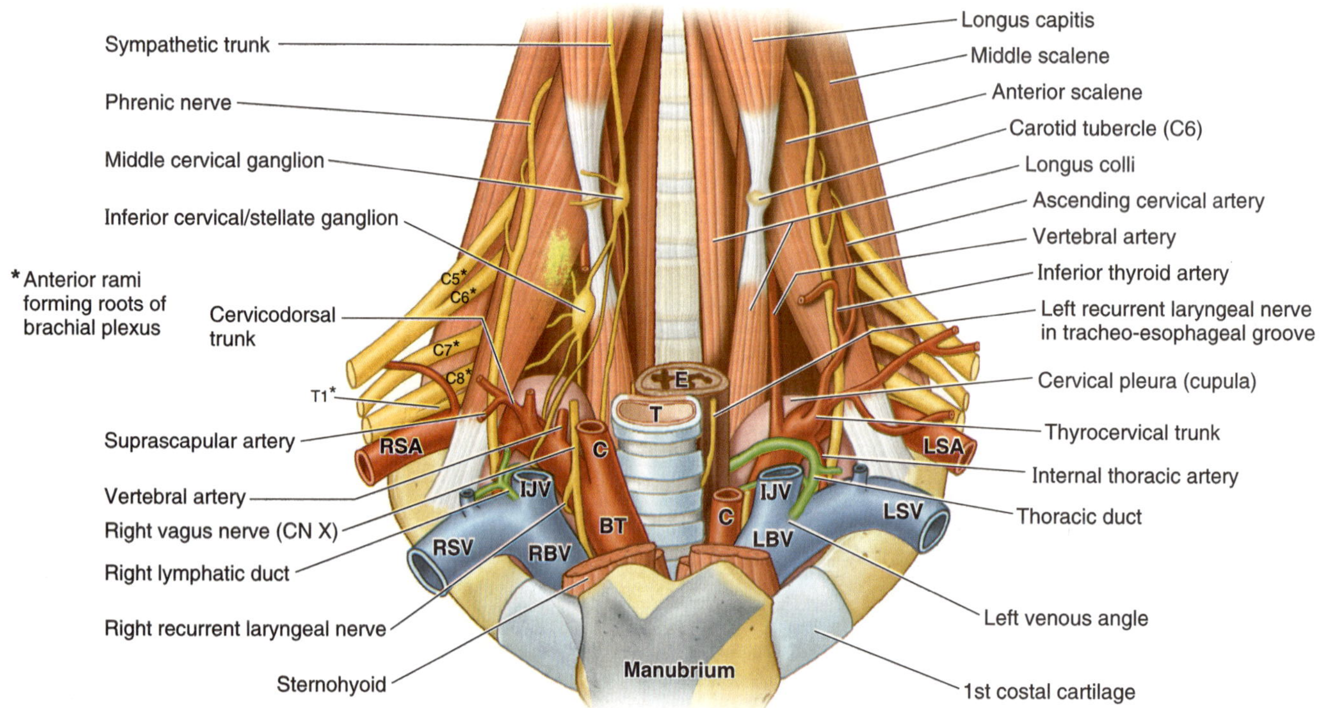

(A) Anterior view

FIGURE 9.25. Root of neck and prevertebral region. A. A dissection of the root of the neck is shown. The brachial plexus and the third part of the subclavian artery emerge between the anterior and the middle scalene muscles. The brachiocephalic veins, the first parts of the subclavian arteries, and the internal thoracic arteries arising from the subclavian arteries are closely related to the cervical pleura (cupula). The thoracic duct terminates in the root of the neck as it enters the left venous angle. BT, brachiocephalic trunk; C, common carotid; E, esophagus; IJV, internal jugular vein; LBV, left brachiocephalic vein; LSA, left subclavian artery; LSV, left subclavian vein; RBV, right brachiocephalic vein; RSA, right sub-clavian artery; RSV, right subclavian vein; T, trachea.

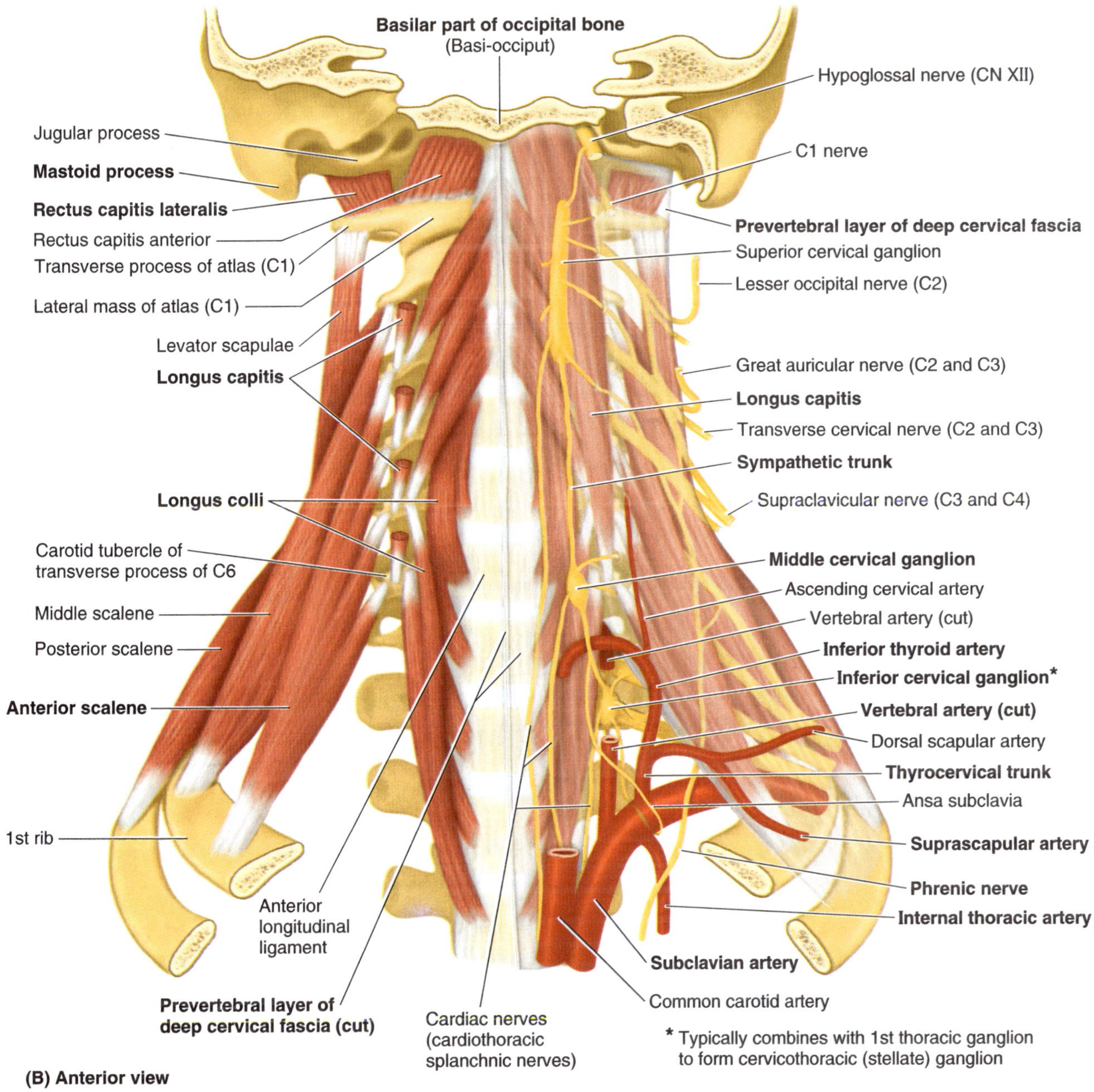

FIGURE 9.25. **(Continued) B.** In this dissection of the prevertebral region and root of the neck, the prevertebral layer of the deep cervical fascia and the arteries and nerves have been removed from the right side; the longus capitis muscle has been excised on the right side. The cervical plexus of nerves, arising from the anterior rami of C1–C4; the brachial plexus of nerves, arising from the anterior rami of C5–C8 and T1; and branches of the subclavian artery are visible on the left side.

root of the neck is the *superior thoracic aperture*, formed laterally by the 1st pair of ribs and their costal cartilages, anteriorly by the manubrium of the sternum, and posteriorly by the body of T1 vertebra. The visceral structures in the root of the neck are described in "Viscera of Neck." Only the neurovascular elements of the root of the neck are described here.

ARTERIES IN ROOT OF NECK

The *brachiocephalic trunk* is covered anteriorly by the right sternohyoid and sternothyroid muscles; it is the largest branch of the arch of the aorta (Fig. 9.26C). It arises in the midline from the beginning of the arch of the aorta, posterior to the manubrium. It passes superolaterally to the right where it divides into the right common carotid and right subclavian arteries posterior to the sternoclavicular (SC) joint. The brachiocephalic trunk usually has no preterminal branches.

The **subclavian arteries** supply the upper limbs; they also send branches to the neck and brain (Figs. 9.20B, 9.25, and 9.26). The **right subclavian artery** arises from the brachiocephalic trunk. The **left subclavian artery** arises from the arch of the aorta, about 1 cm distal to the left common carotid artery. The **left vagus nerve** runs parallel to the first part of the artery (Fig. 9.25A). Although the subclavian arteries of the two sides have different origins, their courses in the neck begin posterior to the respective SC joints as they ascend through the superior thoracic aperture and enter the root of the neck.

The subclavian arteries arch superolaterally, reaching an apex as they pass posterior to the *anterior scalene muscles*. As they begin to descend, they lie posterior to the middle of the clavicles. As the subclavian arteries cross the outer margin of the first ribs, their name changes; they become the axillary arteries. Three parts of each subclavian artery are described relative to the anterior scalene: the first part is medial to the muscle, the second part is posterior to it, and the third part is lateral to it (Figs. 9.12, 9.25B, and 9.26B, C). The cervical pleurae, apices of the lung, and sympathetic trunks lie posterior to the first part of the arteries. The third part of the subclavian artery was discussed previously in this chapter.

The branches of the subclavian arteries are as follows:

- From 1st part: *Vertebral artery, internal thoracic artery, and thyrocervical trunk.*
- From 2nd part: *Costocervical trunk.*
- From 3rd part: *Dorsal scapular artery.*

The **cervical part of the vertebral artery** arises from the first part of the subclavian artery and ascends in the pyramidal space formed between the scalene and longus colli and capitis muscles (Fig. 9.25). At the apex of this space, the artery passes deeply to course through the foramina transversaria of vertebrae C1–C6. This is the **vertebral part of the vertebral artery**. Occasionally, the vertebral artery may enter a foramen more superior than vertebra C6. In approximately 5% of people, the left vertebral artery arises from the arch of the aorta.

The **suboccipital part of the vertebral artery** courses in a groove on the posterior arch of the atlas before it enters the cranial cavity through the foramen magnum. The **cranial part of the vertebral artery** supplies branches to the medulla and spinal cord, parts of the cerebellum, and the dura of the posterior cranial fossa. At the inferior border of the pons of the brainstem, the vertebral arteries join to form the *basilar artery*, which participates in the formation of the cerebral arterial circle (see Chapter 8, Head).

The **internal thoracic artery** arises from the anteroinferior aspect of the subclavian artery and passes inferomedially into the thorax. The cervical part of the internal thoracic artery has no branches; its thoracic distribution is described in Chapter 4, Thorax (Figs. 4.14 and 4.15A).

The **thyrocervical trunk** arises from the anterosuperior aspect of the first part of the subclavian artery, near the medial border of the anterior scalene muscle (Figs. 9.25 and 9.26). It exhibits many variations in its pattern of branching, which can result in the branches arising directly from it to have different names depending on the pattern (Fig. 9.26D–G). It has four branches, the largest and most important of which is the **inferior thyroid artery**, the primary visceral artery of the neck, supplying the larynx, trachea, esophagus, and thyroid and parathyroid glands, as well as adjacent muscles (Fig. 9.26B, C; see Fig. 9.27B). The other branches of the thyrocervical trunk are the ascending cervical and suprascapular arteries and the cervicodorsal trunk (transverse cervical artery). The branches of the cervicodorsal artery were discussed previously, with the lateral cervical region. The terminal branches of the thyrocervical trunk are the inferior thyroid and ascending cervical arteries. The latter is a small artery that sends muscular branches to the lateral muscles of the upper neck and spinal branches into the intervertebral foramina.

The **costocervical trunk** arises from the posterior aspect of the second part of the subclavian artery (posterior to the anterior scalene on the right side [Fig. 9.12] and usually just medial to this muscle on the left side). The trunk passes posterosuperiorly and divides into the superior intercostal and deep cervical arteries, which supply the first two intercostal spaces and the posterior deep cervical muscles, respectively.

VEINS IN ROOT OF NECK

Two large veins terminating in the root of the neck are the EJV, draining blood received mostly from the scalp and face, and the variable **anterior jugular vein (AJV)**, usually the smallest of the jugular veins (Figs. 9.16 and 9.21). The AJV typically arises near the hyoid from the confluence of superficial submandibular veins. The AJV descends either in the subcutaneous tissue or deep to the investing layer of deep cervical fascia between the anterior median line and the anterior border of the SCM. At the root of the neck, the AJV turns laterally, posterior to the SCM, and opens into the termination of the EJV or into the subclavian vein. Superior to the manubrium, the right and left AJVs commonly unite across the midline to form the **jugular venous arch** in the suprasternal space (Fig. 9.17).

The **subclavian vein**, the continuation of the axillary vein, begins at the lateral border of the 1st rib and ends when it unites with the IJV (Fig. 9.25A). The subclavian vein passes over the 1st rib anterior to the scalene tubercle parallel to the subclavian artery, but it is separated from it by the anterior scalene muscle. It usually has only one named tributary, the EJV (Fig. 9.21).

The IJV ends posterior to the medial end of the clavicle by uniting with the subclavian vein to form the brachiocephalic vein. This union is commonly referred to as the **venous angle** and is the site where the *thoracic duct* (left side) and the *right lymphatic trunk* (right side) drain lymph collected throughout the body into the venous circulation (see Fig. 9.49). Throughout its course, the IJV is enclosed by the *carotid sheath* (Fig. 9.22).

NERVES IN ROOT OF NECK

There are three pairs of major nerves in the root of the neck: (1) vagus nerves, (2) phrenic nerves, and (3) sympathetic trunks.

AN35.7

Vagus Nerves (CN X). After its exit from the jugular foramen, each vagus nerve passes inferiorly in the neck within the posterior part of the carotid sheath in the angle between the IJV and common carotid artery (Figs. 9.22 and 9.26A, B). The **right vagus nerve** passes anterior to the first part of the subclavian artery and posterior to the brachiocephalic vein and SC joint to enter the thorax. The **left vagus nerve** descends between the left common carotid and left subclavian arteries and posterior to the SC joint to enter the thorax.

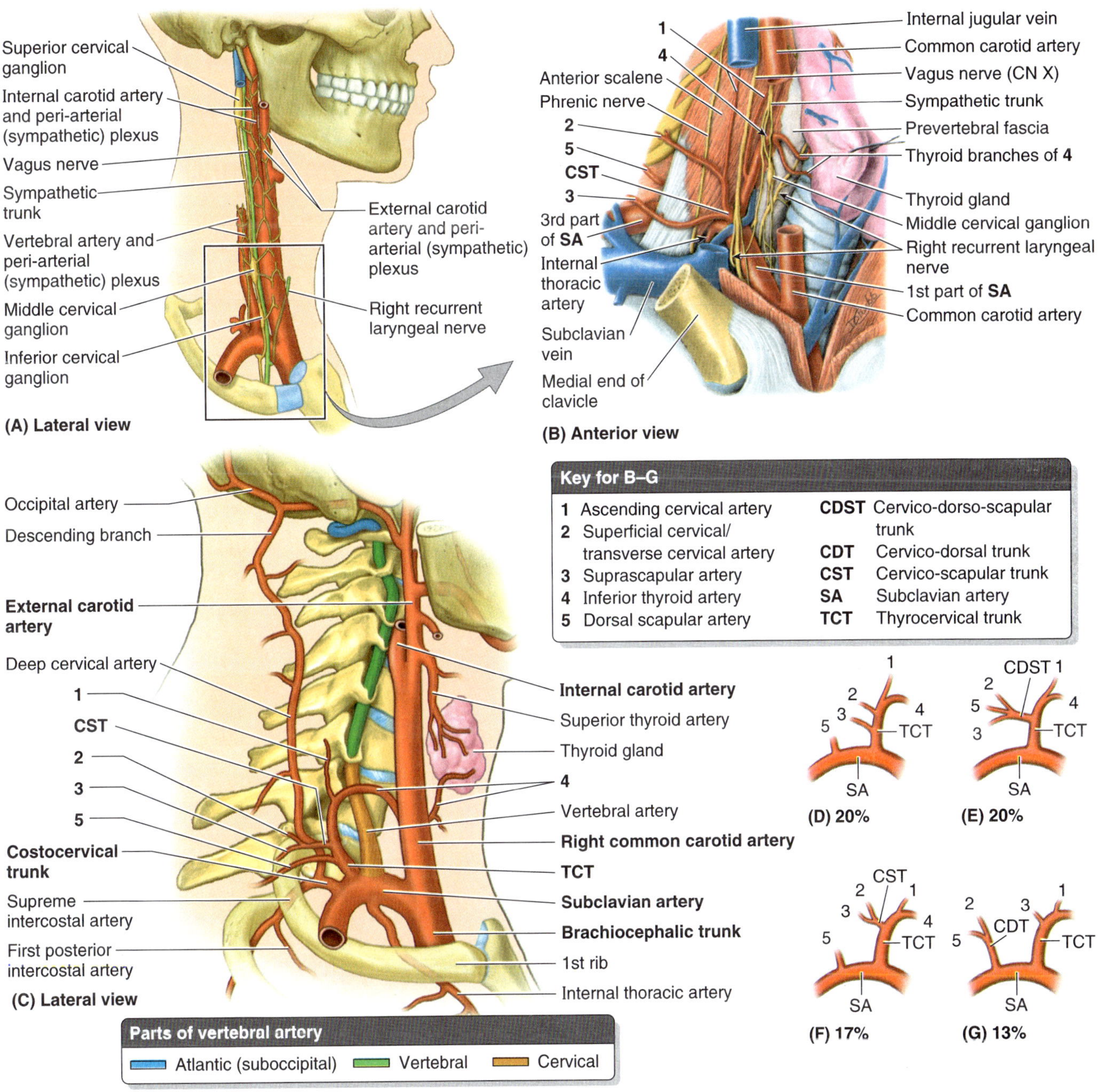

FIGURE 9.26. Nerves and arteries in neck. A. Cervical sympathetic trunk and ganglia and sympathetic peri-arterial plexuses surrounding them. **B.** Dissection of nerves and arteries. In this view of the root of the neck, the clavicle is removed, and sections are taken from the common carotid artery and IJV. The lobe of the thyroid gland is retracted to reveal the right recurrent laryngeal nerve and middle cervical (sympathetic) ganglion. **C.** Arteries of neck. The parts of the vertebral artery are color-coded, and the parts of the subclavian artery are numbered. **D–G.** Variation in branching pattern of thyrocervical trunk and aberrant origins of arteries from subclavian artery.

The **recurrent laryngeal nerves** arise from the vagus nerves in the inferior part of the neck (Fig. 9.26). The nerves of the two sides have essentially the same distribution; however, they loop around different structures and at different levels on the two sides. The **right recurrent laryngeal nerve** loops inferior to the right subclavian artery at approximately the T1–T2 vertebral level. The **left recurrent laryngeal nerve** loops inferior to the arch of the aorta at approximately the T4–T5 vertebral level. After looping, the recurrent laryngeal nerves ascend superiorly to the posteromedial aspect of the thyroid gland (Figs. 9.25, 9.26B, 9.27B, and 9.28), where they ascend in the *tracheo-esophageal groove*, supplying both trachea and esophagus and all the intrinsic muscles of the larynx except the cricothyroid.

The **cardiac branches of CN X** originate in the neck (Fig. 9.25B) as well as in the thorax and convey presynaptic parasympathetic and visceral afferent fibers to the cardiac plexus of nerves (see Chapter 4, Thorax, Fig. 4.71C).

Phrenic Nerves. The phrenic nerves are formed at the lateral borders of the anterior scalene muscles (Figs. 9.25A and 9.26B), mainly from the C4 nerve with contributions from C3 and C5. The phrenic nerves descend anterior to the anterior scalene muscles under cover of the IJVs and the SCMs. They pass under the prevertebral layer of deep cervical fascia, between the subclavian arteries and veins, and proceed to the thorax to supply the diaphragm. The phrenic nerves are important because, in addition to their sensory distribution, they provide the sole motor supply to their own half of the diaphragm (see Chapter 4, Thorax, for details).

AN35.6 **Sympathetic Trunks.** The **cervical portion of the sympathetic trunks** lie anterolateral to the vertebral column, extending superiorly to the level of the C1 vertebra or cranial base (Figs. 9.25B and 9.26). The sympathetic trunks receive no white rami communicantes in the neck (recall that white rami are only associated with spinal nerves T1–L2 or 3). The cervical portion of the trunks includes three **cervical sympathetic ganglia**: superior, middle, and inferior. These ganglia receive presynaptic fibers conveyed to the trunk by the superior thoracic spinal nerves and their associated white rami communicantes, which then ascend through the sympathetic trunk to the ganglia. After synapsing with the postsynaptic neuron in the cervical sympathetic ganglia, postsynaptic neurons send fibers to the following structures:

1. Cervical spinal nerves via *gray rami communicantes*.
2. Thoracic viscera via *cardiopulmonary splanchnic nerves*.
3. Head and viscera of the neck via *cephalic arterial branches* (rami).

The latter fibers accompany arteries as *sympathetic peri-arterial nerve plexuses*, especially the vertebral and internal and external carotid arteries (Fig. 9.26).

In approximately 80% of people, the **inferior cervical ganglion** fuses with the first thoracic ganglion to form the large **cervicothoracic ganglion** (**stellate ganglion**). This star-shaped (L. *stella*, a star) ganglion lies anterior to the transverse process of the C7 vertebra, just superior to the neck of the 1st rib on each side and posterior to the origin of the vertebral artery (Fig. 9.25B). Some postsynaptic fibers from the ganglion pass via gray rami communicantes to the anterior rami of the C7 and C8 spinal nerves (roots of the brachial plexus), and others pass to the heart via the *inferior cervical cardiac nerve* (a cardiopulmonary splanchnic nerve), which passes along the trachea to the deep *cardiac plexus*. Other fibers pass via arterial branches to contribute to the sympathetic peri-arterial nerve plexus around the vertebral artery running into the cranial cavity (Fig. 9.26A).

The **middle cervical ganglion**, the smallest of the three ganglia, is occasionally absent. When present, it lies on the anterior aspect of the inferior thyroid artery at the level of the cricoid cartilage and the transverse process of C6 vertebra, just anterior to the vertebral artery (Figs. 9.26 and 9.28). Postsynaptic fibers pass from the ganglion via gray rami communicantes to the anterior rami of the C5 and C6 spinal nerves, via a middle cervical cardiac (cardiopulmonary splanchnic) nerve to the heart and via arterial branches to form the peri-arterial plexuses to the thyroid gland.

The **superior cervical ganglion** is at the level of the C1 and C2 vertebrae (Figs. 9.25B and 9.26A). Because of its large size, it forms a good landmark for locating the sympathetic trunk, but it may need to be distinguished from a large sensory (nodose) ganglion of the vagus (CN X) when present. Postsynaptic fibers pass from it by means of cephalic arterial branches to form the internal carotid sympathetic plexus and then enter the cranial cavity (Fig. 9.26). This ganglion also sends arterial branches to the external carotid artery and gray rami to the anterior rami of the superior four cervical spinal nerves. Other postsynaptic fibers pass from it to the cardiac plexus of nerves via a **superior cervical cardiac** (cardiopulmonary splanchnic) **nerve** (see Chapter 4, Thorax).

CLINICAL BOX

DEEP STRUCTURES OF NECK

Cervicothoracic Ganglion Block

Anesthetic injected around the large cervicothoracic ganglion blocks transmission of stimuli through the cervical and superior thoracic ganglia. This *ganglion block* may relieve vascular spasms involving the brain and upper limb. It is also useful when deciding if a surgical resection of the ganglion would be beneficial to a person with excess vasoconstriction in the ipsilateral limb.

Lesion of Cervical Sympathetic Trunk

A *lesion of a cervical sympathetic trunk* in the AN31.3
neck results in a sympathetic disturbance called *Horner syndrome*, which is characterized by:

- Contraction of the pupil (*miosis*), resulting from paralysis of the dilator pupillae muscle (see Chapter 8, Head).
- Drooping of the superior eyelid (*ptosis*), resulting from paralysis of the smooth (tarsal) muscle intermingled with the striated muscle of the levator palpebrae superioris.
- Sinking in of the eye (*enophthalmos*), possibly caused by paralysis of the rudimentary smooth (orbital) muscle in the floor of the orbit.
- Vasodilation and absence of sweating on the face and neck (*anhydrosis*), caused by lack of a sympathetic (vasoconstrictive) nerve supply to the blood vessels and sweat glands.

The Bottom Line: Deep Structures of Neck

Prevertebral muscles: The prevertebral muscles, deep to the prevertebral layer of deep cervical fascia, are divided into anterior and lateral vertebral muscles by the neurovascular plane of the cervical and brachial plexuses and subclavian artery. • The anterior vertebral muscles flex the head and neck; however, this movement is normally produced by gravity in conjunction with eccentric contraction of the extensors of the neck. • Thus, the anterior vertebral muscles are called into action mainly when this movement is performed against resistance, probably initiating the movement while the strength of the movement is produced by the SCM. • The lateral vertebral muscles laterally flex the neck, participate in rotation of the neck, and fix or elevate the superior ribs during forced inspiration.

Root of the neck: The branches of the arch of the aorta bifurcate and/or traverse the root of the neck, with the branches of the subclavian artery arising here also. • The internal jugular and subclavian veins converge at the root of the neck to form the brachiocephalic veins. • The major lymphatic trunks (right lymphatic duct and thoracic duct) enter the venous angles formed by the convergence of these veins. • The phrenic and vagus nerves enter the thorax by passing anterior to the subclavian arteries and posterior to the brachiocephalic veins. • The sympathetic trunks and recurrent laryngeal nerves traverse the root of the neck posterior to the arteries, as do the visceral structures (trachea and esophagus). • The cervical portion of the sympathetic trunks includes three cervical sympathetic ganglia (inferior, middle, and superior), in which presynaptic fibers from the superior thoracic spinal cord synapse with postsynaptic neurons. • These neurons send fibers to the cervical spinal nerves, via gray rami communicantes; to the head and viscera of the neck, via cephalic arterial branches and periarterial plexuses; and to the thoracic viscera, via cardiac (cardiopulmonary splanchnic) nerves.

VISCERA OF NECK

The cervical viscera are disposed in three layers, named for their primary function (Fig. 9.27). Superficial to deep, they are as follows:

1. *Endocrine layer*: the thyroid and parathyroid glands.
2. *Respiratory layer*: the larynx and trachea.
3. *Alimentary layer*: the pharynx and esophagus.

Endocrine Layer of Cervical Viscera

The viscera of the **endocrine layer** are part of the body's endocrine system of ductless, hormone-secreting glands. The *thyroid gland* is the body's largest endocrine gland. It produces *thyroid hormone*, which controls the rate of metabolism, and *calcitonin*, a hormone controlling calcium metabolism. The *thyroid gland* affects all areas of the body except itself and the spleen, testes, and uterus. The hormone produced by the *parathyroid glands, parathormone* (PTH), controls the metabolism of phosphorus and calcium in the blood. The parathyroid glands target the skeleton, kidneys, and intestine.

THYROID GLAND

AN35.2 The **thyroid gland** lies deep to the sternothyroid and sternohyoid muscles, located anteriorly in the neck at the level of the C5–T1 vertebrae (Fig. 9.27). It consists primarily of right and left **lobes**, anterolateral to the larynx and trachea. A relatively thin **isthmus** unites the lobes over the trachea, usually anterior to the second and third tracheal rings. The thyroid gland is surrounded by a thin **fibrous capsule**, which sends septa deeply into the gland. Dense connective tissue attaches the capsule to the cricoid cartilage and superior tracheal rings. External to the capsule is a loose sheath formed by the visceral portion of the pretracheal layer of deep cervical fascia.

Arteries of Thyroid Gland. The highly vascular thyroid gland is supplied by the superior and inferior *thyroid arteries* (Figs. 9.27B and 9.28). These vessels lie between the fibrous capsule and the loose fascial sheath. Usually, the first branches of the external carotid arteries, the **superior thyroid arteries**, descend to the superior poles of the gland, pierce the pretracheal layer of deep cervical fascia, and divide into anterior and posterior branches supplying mainly the anterosuperior aspect of the gland.

The **inferior thyroid arteries**, the largest branches of the thyrocervical trunks arising from the subclavian arteries, run superomedially posterior to the carotid sheaths to reach the posterior aspect of the *thyroid gland*. They divide into several branches that pierce the pretracheal layer of the deep cervical fascia and supply the postero-inferior aspect, including the **inferior poles of the gland**. The right and left superior and inferior thyroid arteries anastomose extensively within the gland, ensuring its supply while providing potential collateral circulation between the subclavian and external carotid arteries.

In approximately 10% of people, a small, unpaired **thyroid ima artery** (L. *arteria thyroidea ima*) arises from the brachiocephalic trunk (see the clinical box "Thyroid Ima Artery"); however, it may arise from the arch of the aorta or from the right common carotid, subclavian, or internal thoracic arteries. When present, this small artery ascends on the anterior surface of the trachea, supplying small branches to it. The artery then continues to the isthmus of the thyroid gland, where it divides and supplies it.

Veins of Thyroid Gland. Three pairs of thyroid veins usually form a **thyroid plexus of veins** on the anterior surface of the thyroid gland and anterior to the trachea (Figs. 9.28 and 9.29). The **superior thyroid veins** accompany the superior

(*continued on p.* 1085)

9

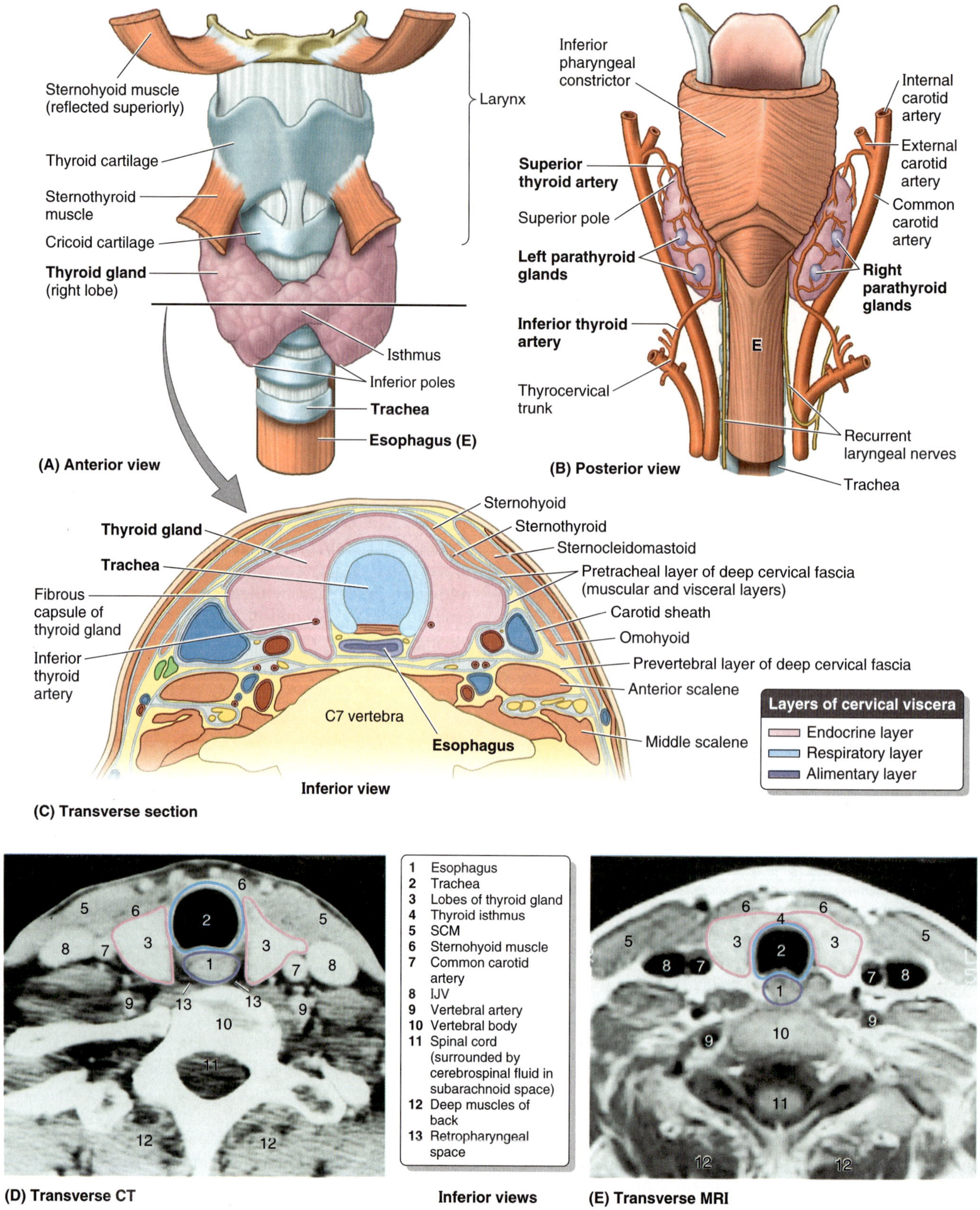

FIGURE 9.27. Relationships of thyroid gland. A. Lobes of thyroid gland. The sternothyroid muscles have been cut to expose the lobes of the normal thyroid gland. The isthmus lies anterior to the second and third tracheal rings. **B.** Parathyroid glands. They are usually embedded in the brous capsule on the posterior surface of the thyroid gland. **C.** Transverse section through thyroid isthmus. **D.** CT scan through lobes of thyroid gland. **E.** MRI through thyroid isthmus.

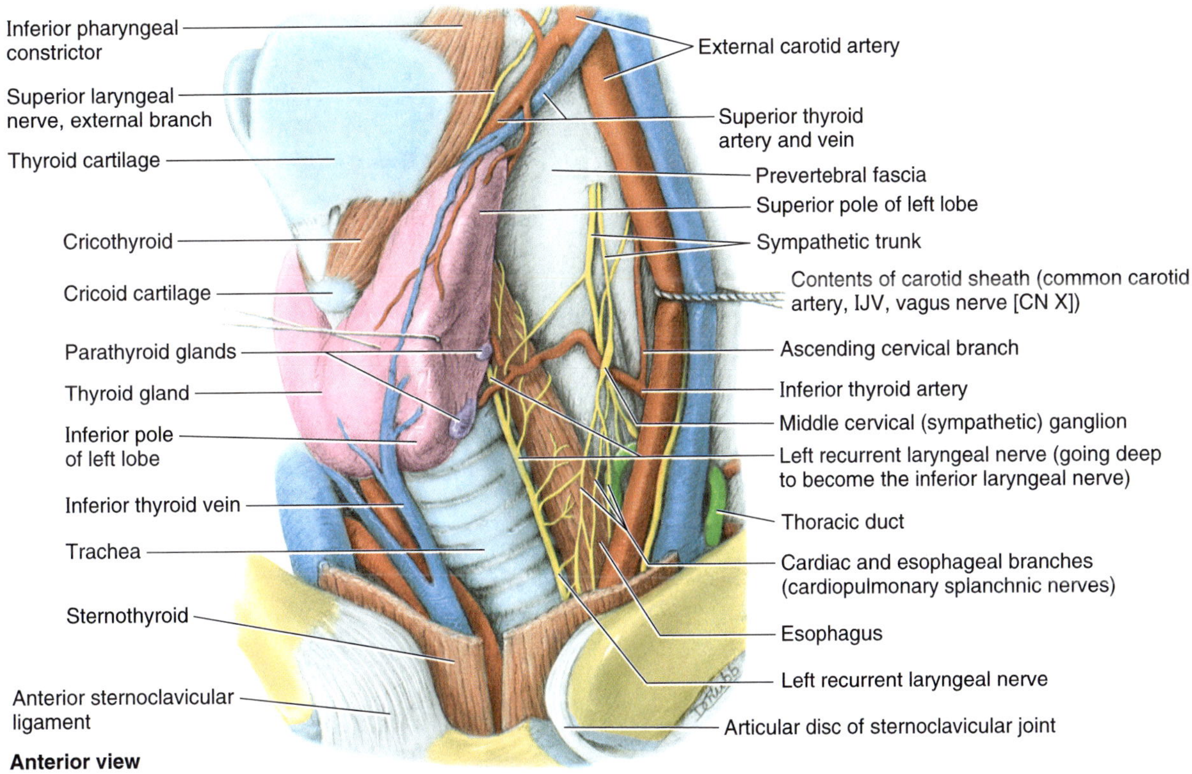

FIGURE 9.28. Dissection of left side of root of neck. The viscera (thyroid gland, trachea, and esophagus) are retracted to the right, and the contents of the left carotid sheath are retracted to the left. The middle thyroid vein, severed to allow such retraction, is not apparent. The left parathyroid glands on the posterior aspect of the left lobe of the thyroid gland are exposed. The recurrent laryngeal nerve ascends beside the trachea, in the angle between the trachea and the esophagus. The thoracic duct passes laterally, posterior to the contents of the carotid sheath as the thyrocervical trunk passes medially.

thyroid arteries; they drain the **superior poles** of the thyroid gland; the **middle thyroid veins** do not accompany but run essentially parallel courses with the inferior thyroid arteries; they drain the middle of the lobes. The usually independent **inferior thyroid veins** drain the inferior poles. The superior and middle thyroid veins drain into the IJVs; the inferior thyroid veins drain into the brachiocephalic veins posterior to the manubrium.

Lymphatic Drainage of Thyroid Gland. The lymphatic vessels of this gland run in the interlobular connective tissue, usually near the arteries; they communicate with a capsular network of lymphatic vessels. From here, the vessels pass initially to **prelaryngeal**, **pretracheal**, and **paratracheal lymph nodes**. The prelaryngeal nodes drain in turn to the superior deep cervical lymph nodes, and the pretracheal and paratracheal lymph nodes drain to the inferior deep cervical nodes (Fig. 9.30). Laterally, lymphatic vessels located along the superior thyroid veins pass directly to the inferior deep cervical lymph nodes. Some lymphatic vessels may drain into the *brachiocephalic lymph nodes* or the *thoracic duct* (Fig. 9.28).

Nerves of Thyroid Gland. The nerves of the thyroid gland are derived from the *superior, middle, and inferior cervical* (sympathetic) *ganglia* (Figs. 9.26 and 9.28). They reach the gland through the *cardiac* and *superior* and *inferior thyroid peri-arterial plexuses* that accompany the thyroid arteries. These fibers are vasomotor, not secretomotor. They cause constriction of blood vessels. Endocrine secretion from the thyroid gland is hormonally regulated by the pituitary gland.

For microanatomy of thyroid, refer *diFiore's Atlas of Histology with Functional Correlations*, 1st South Asian Edition, Chapter 19, Endocrine System, p. 512. AN43.

PARATHYROID GLANDS

The small flattened, oval **parathyroid glands** usually lie external to the thyroid capsule on the medial half of the posterior surface of each lobe of the thyroid gland, inside its sheath (Figs. 9.27B, 9.28 and 9.31A). The **superior parathyroid glands** usually lie slightly more than 1 cm superior to the point of entry of the inferior thyroid arteries into the thyroid gland. The **inferior parathyroid glands** usually lie slightly more than 1 cm inferior to the arterial entry point (Skandalakis et al., 1995). Most people have four parathyroid glands. Approximately 5% of people have more; some have only two glands. The superior parathyroid glands, more constant in position than the inferior ones, are usually at the level of the inferior border of the cricoid cartilage. The inferior parathyroid glands are usually near the inferior poles of the thyroid gland, but they may lie in various positions (Fig. 9.31B). In 1–5% of people, an inferior parathyroid gland is deep in the superior mediastinum (Norton and Wells, 1994).

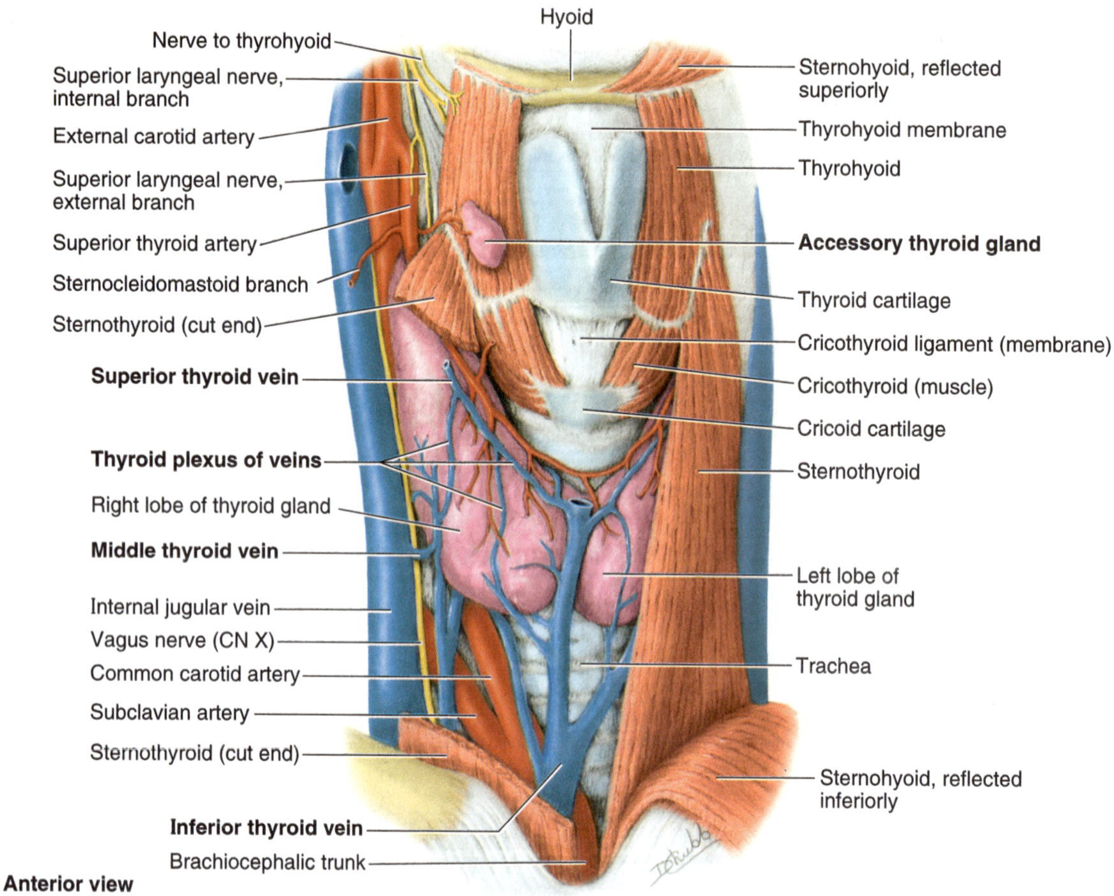

FIGURE 9.29. Thyroid gland. A dissection of the anterior aspect of the neck is shown. In this specimen, there is a small accessory thyroid gland on the right, lying on the thyrohyoid muscle, lateral to the thyroid cartilage. The superior thyroid artery is distributed primarily to the anterosuperior portion of the gland.

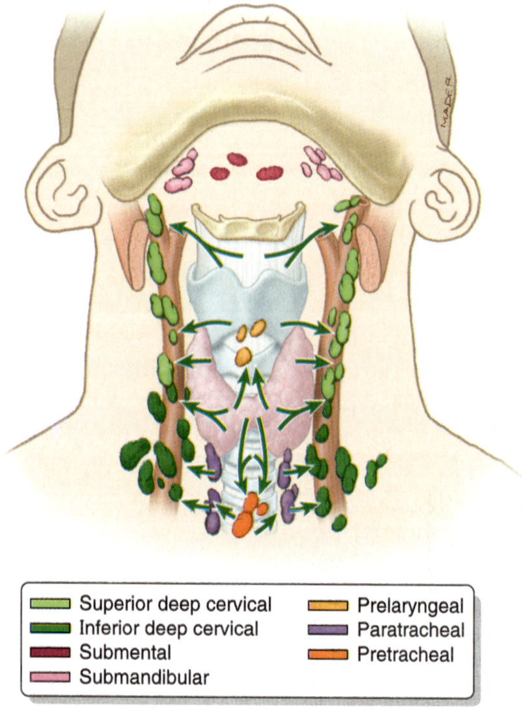

FIGURE 9.30. Lymphatic drainage of thyroid gland, larynx, and trachea. The *arrows* indicate the direction of lymph flow.

Parathyroid glands have densely packed cells for which they are quite easily recognizable from the thyroid, in contrast with the follicular structure of the thyroid. Two unique types of cells are found in the parathyroid gland namely, chief and oxyphil cells. For microanatomy of parathyroid, refer AN43.2 *diFiore's Atlas of Histology with Functional Correlations*, 1st South Asian Edition, Chapter 19, Endocrine System, p. 515.

Vessels of Parathyroid Glands. Because the *inferior thyroid arteries* provide the primary blood supply to the posterior aspect of the thyroid gland where the parathyroid glands are located, branches of these arteries usually supply these glands (Figs. 9.27B and 9.31A). However, they may also be supplied by branches from the superior thyroid arteries, thyroid ima artery, or laryngeal, tracheal, and esophageal arteries. **Parathyroid veins** drain into the *thyroid plexus of veins* of the thyroid gland and trachea (Fig. 9.29). *Lymphatic vessels* from the parathyroid glands drain with those from the thyroid gland into deep cervical lymph nodes and paratracheal lymph nodes (Fig. 9.30).

Nerves of Parathyroid Glands. The nerve supply of the parathyroid glands is abundant; it is derived from thyroid branches of the cervical (sympathetic) ganglia (Fig. 9.26). Like the nerves to the thyroid, they are vasomotor rather than secretomotor because these glands are hormonally regulated.

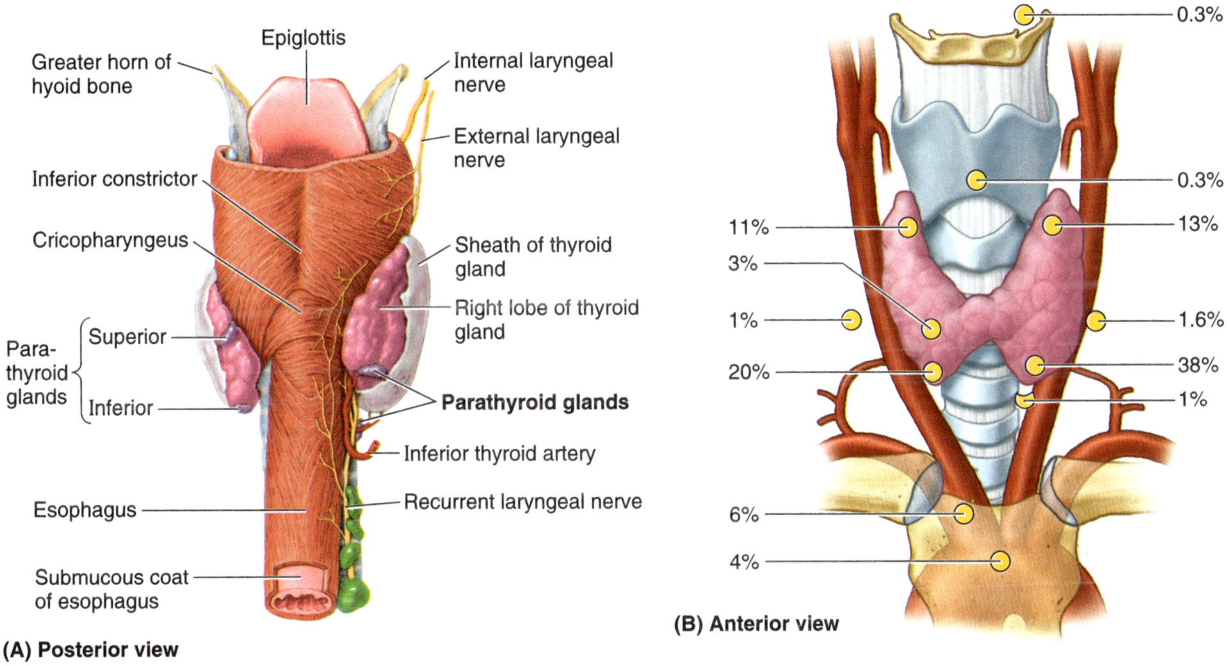

FIGURE 9.31. Thyroid and parathyroid glands. A. The thyroid sheath has been dissected from the posterior surface of the thyroid gland to reveal the three embedded parathyroid glands. Both parathyroid glands on the right side are rather low, and the inferior gland is inferior to the thyroid gland. **B.** Sites and frequencies of aberrant parathyroid glandular tissue are shown.

Respiratory Layer of Cervical Viscera

The viscera of the **respiratory layer**, the *larynx* and *trachea*, contribute to the respiratory functions of the body. The main functions of the cervical respiratory viscera are as follows:

- Routing air and food into the respiratory tract and esophagus, respectively.
- Providing a patent airway and a means of sealing it off temporarily (a "valve").
- Producing voice.

LARYNX

The **larynx** is the complex organ of voice production (the "voice box") composed of nine cartilages connected by membranes and ligaments and containing the *vocal folds* ("cords"). The larynx is located in the anterior neck at the level of the bodies of C3–C6 vertebrae (Fig. 9.32). It connects the inferior part of the pharynx (oropharynx) with the trachea. Although most commonly known for its role as the phonating mechanism for voice production, its most vital function is to

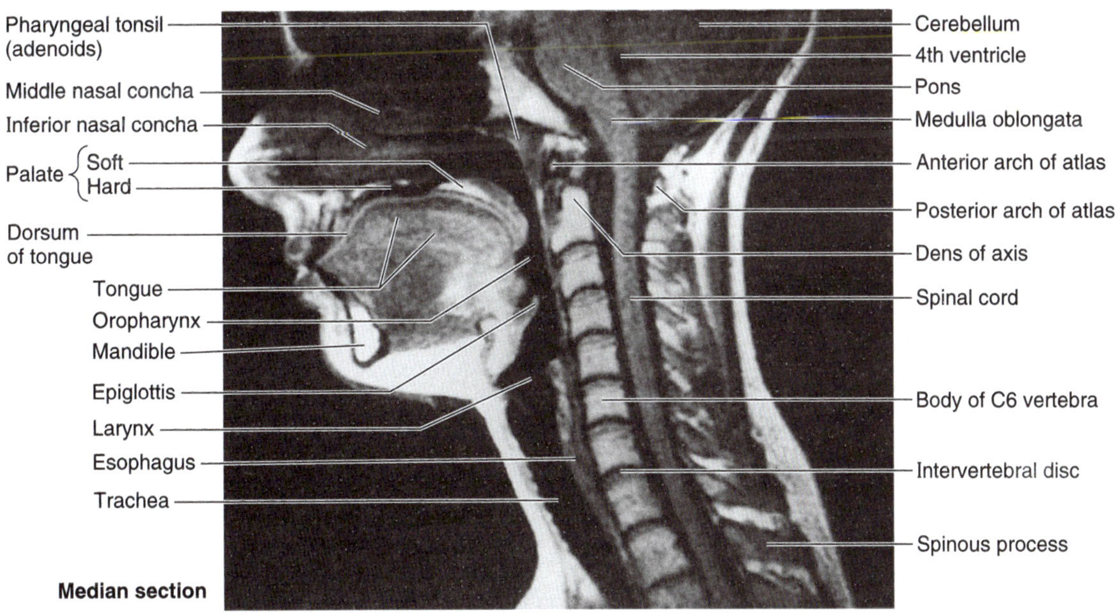

FIGURE 9.32. Median MRI of head and neck. Because the air and food passages share the oropharynx, separation of food and air must occur to continue into the trachea (anterior) and esophagus (posterior). (Courtesy of Dr. W. Kucharczyk, University Health Network, Toronto, Ontario, Canada.)

guard the air passages, especially during swallowing when it serves as the "sphincter" or "valve" of the lower respiratory tract, thus maintaining a patent airway.

Laryngeal Skeleton. The laryngeal skeleton *consists of nine cartilages*: three are single (thyroid, cricoid, and epiglottic), and three are paired (arytenoid, corniculate, and cuneiform) (Fig. 9.33A, B).

The **thyroid cartilage** is the largest of the cartilages; its superior border lies opposite the C4 vertebra. The inferior two thirds of its two plate-like **laminae** fuse anteriorly in the median plane to form the **laryngeal prominence** (Fig. 9.33A, D). This projection ("Adam's apple") is well marked in men but seldom visible in women. Superior to this prominence, the laminae diverge to form a V-shaped **superior thyroid notch**. The less distinct **inferior thyroid notch** is a shallow indentation in the middle of the inferior border of the cartilage.

The posterior border of each lamina projects superiorly as the **superior horn** and inferiorly as the **inferior horn**. The superior border and superior horns attach to the hyoid by the **thyrohyoid membrane** (Fig. 9.33A, B). The thick median part of this membrane is the **median thyrohyoid ligament**; its lateral parts are the **lateral thyrohyoid ligaments**.

The inferior horns articulate with the lateral surfaces of the cricoid cartilage at the **cricothyroid joints** (Fig. 9.33B). The main movements at these joints are rotation and gliding of the thyroid cartilage, which result in changes in the length of the vocal folds. The **cricoid cartilage** is shaped like a signet ring with its band facing anteriorly. This ring-like opening of the cartilage fits an average finger. The posterior (signet) part of the cricoid is the **lamina**, and the anterior (band) part is the **arch** (Fig. 9.33A). Although much smaller than the thyroid cartilage, the cricoid cartilage is thicker and stronger and is the only complete ring of cartilage to encircle any part of the airway. It attaches to the inferior margin of the thyroid cartilage by the **median cricothyroid ligament** and to the first tracheal ring by the **cricotracheal ligament**. Where the larynx is closest to the skin and most accessible, the median cricothyroid ligament may be felt as a soft spot during palpation inferior to the thyroid cartilage.

The **arytenoid cartilages** are paired, three-sided pyramidal cartilages that articulate with the lateral parts of the superior border of the cricoid cartilage lamina (Fig. 9.33B). Each cartilage has an apex superiorly, a vocal process anteriorly, and a large muscular process that projects laterally from its base. The **apex** bears the corniculate cartilage and attaches to the aryepiglottic fold. The **vocal process** provides the posterior attachment for the vocal ligament, and the muscular process serves as a lever to which the posterior and lateral crico-arytenoid muscles are attached. The **crico-arytenoid joints**, located between the bases of the arytenoid cartilages and the superolateral surfaces of the lamina of the cricoid cartilage (Fig. 9.33B, E), permit the arytenoid cartilages to slide toward or away from one to another, to tilt anteriorly and posteriorly, and to rotate. These movements are important in approximating, tensing, and relaxing the vocal folds.

The elastic **vocal ligaments** extend from the junction of the laminae of the thyroid cartilage anteriorly to the vocal process of the arytenoid cartilage posteriorly (Fig. 9.33E). The vocal ligaments make up the submucosal skeleton of the vocal folds. These ligaments are the thickened, free superior border of the **conus elasticus** or **cricovocal membrane**. The parts of the membrane extending laterally between the vocal folds and the superior border of the cricoid are the **lateral cricothyroid ligaments**. The fibro-elastic conus elasticus blends anteriorly with the *median cricothyroid ligament*. The conus elasticus and overlying mucosa close the tracheal inlet except for the central **rima glottidis** (opening between the vocal folds).

The **epiglottic cartilage**, consisting of elastic cartilage, gives flexibility to the **epiglottis**, a heart-shaped cartilage covered with mucous membrane (Figs. 9.33B, E and 9.35). Situated posterior to the root of the tongue and the hyoid and anterior to the **laryngeal inlet**, the epiglottic cartilage forms the superior part of the anterior wall and the superior margin of the inlet. Its broad superior end is free. Its tapered inferior end, the **stalk of the epiglottis**, is attached to the angle formed by the thyroid laminae by the **thyro-epiglottic ligament** (Fig. 9.33E). The **hyo-epiglottic ligament** attaches the anterior surface of the epiglottic cartilage to the hyoid (Fig. 9.34). The **quadrangular membrane** (Figs. 9.33B and 9.35) is a thin, submucosal sheet of connective tissue that extends between the lateral aspects of the arytenoid and epiglottic cartilages. Its free inferior margin constitutes the **vestibular ligament**, which is covered loosely by mucosa to form the **vestibular fold** (Fig. 9.35). This fold lies superior to the vocal fold and extends from the thyroid cartilage to the arytenoid cartilage. The free superior margin of the quadrangular membrane forms the **aryepiglottic ligament**, which is covered with mucosa to form the **aryepiglottic fold**. The **corniculate** and **cuneiform cartilages** appear as small nodules in the posterior part of the aryepiglottic folds. The corniculate cartilages attach to the apices of the arytenoid cartilages; the cuneiform cartilages do not directly attach to other cartilages. The quadrangular membrane and conus elasticus are the superior and inferior parts of the submucosal **fibro-elastic membrane of the larynx**.

Interior of Larynx. The **laryngeal cavity** extends from the *laryngeal inlet*, through which it communicates with the *laryngopharynx*, to the level of the inferior border of the cricoid cartilage. Here, the laryngeal cavity is continuous with the cavity of the trachea (Figs. 9.35 and 9.36A, B). The laryngeal cavity includes the

- **laryngeal vestibule**: between the laryngeal inlet and the vestibular folds.
- **middle part of the laryngeal cavity**: the central cavity (airway) between the vestibular and vocal folds.
- **laryngeal ventricle**: recesses extending laterally from the middle part of the laryngeal cavity between vestibular and vocal folds. The **laryngeal saccule** is a blind pocket opening into each ventricle that is lined with mucosal glands.
- **infraglottic cavity**: the inferior cavity of the larynx between the vocal folds and the inferior border of the cricoid cartilage, where it is continuous with the lumen of the trachea.

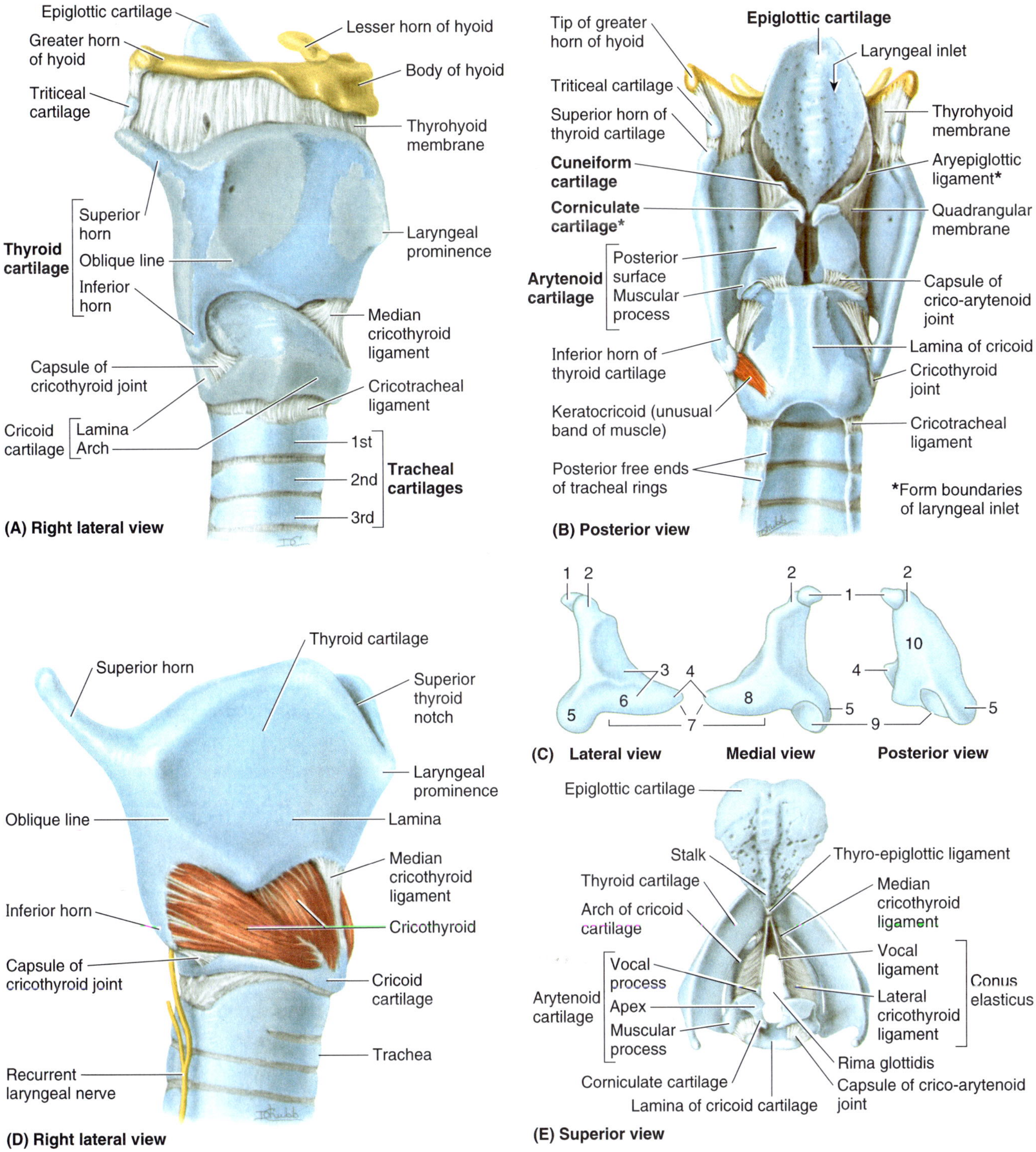

FIGURE 9.33. Skeleton of larynx. A. Although firmly connected to it, the hyoid is not part of the larynx. The larynx extends vertically from the tip of the heart-shaped epiglottis to the inferior border of the cricoid cartilage. **B.** The thyroid cartilage shields the smaller cartilages of the larynx, and the hyoid shields the superior part of the epiglottic cartilage. **C.** Three views of an isolated arytenoid cartilage are shown. *1*, Corniculate cartilage; *2*, apex of arytenoid cartilage; *3*, anterolateral surface; *4*, vocal process (projects anteriorly, provides attachment for vocal ligament); *5*, muscular process (projects laterally, for attachment of posterior and lateral crico-arytenoid muscles); *6*, oblong fovea (for attachment of thyro-arytenoid muscle); *7*, base; *8*, medial surface; *9*, articular surface; *10*, posterior surface. **D.** The thyroid cartilage and cricothyroid muscle are shown. This muscle produces movement at the cricothyroid joint. **E.** The epiglottic cartilage is pitted for mucous glands, and its stalk is attached by the thyro-epiglottic ligament to the angle of the thyroid cartilage superior to the vocal ligaments. The vocal ligament, which forms the skeleton of the vocal fold, extends from the vocal process of the arytenoid cartilage to the "angle" of the thyroid cartilage, and there joins its fellow inferior to the thyro-epiglottic ligament.

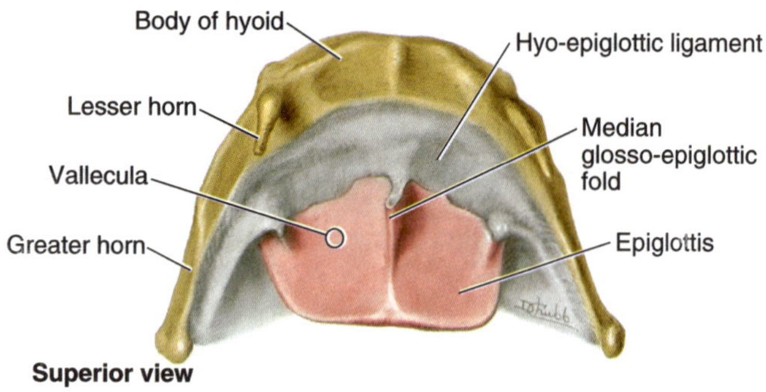

FIGURE 9.34. Epiglottis and hyo-epiglottic ligament. The epiglottis is a leaf-shaped plate of elastic fibrocartilage, which is covered with mucous membrane (*pink*) and is attached anteriorly to the hyoid by the hyo-epiglottic ligament (*gray*). The epiglottis serves as a diverter valve over the superior aperture of the larynx during swallowing.

The **vocal folds** control sound production (Figs. 9.36 and 9.37). The apex of each wedge-shaped fold projects medially into the laryngeal cavity. Each vocal fold contains a

- *vocal ligament*, consisting of thickened elastic tissue that is the medial free edge of the conus elasticus (Figs. 9.33E, 9.35 and 9.36A).
- *vocalis muscle*, composed of exceptionally fine muscle fibers immediately lateral to and terminating at intervals relative to the length of the vocal ligaments (Fig. 9.36A).

The vocal folds are the sharp-edged folds of mucous membrane overlying and incorporating the vocal ligaments and the thyro-arytenoid muscles. They are the source of the sounds (tone) that come from the larynx. These folds produce audible vibrations when their free margins are closely (but not tightly) apposed during phonation, and air is forcibly expired intermittently (Fig. 9.37C). The vocal folds also serve as the main inspiratory sphincter of the larynx when they are tightly closed. Complete adduction of the folds forms an effective sphincter that prevents entry of air.

The **glottis** (the vocal apparatus of the larynx) makes up the vocal folds and processes, together with the **rima glottidis**, the aperture between the vocal folds (Fig. 9.36C). The shape of the rima (L. slit) varies according to the position of the vocal folds (Fig. 9.37). During ordinary breathing, the rima is narrow and wedge shaped; during forced respiration, it is wide and trapezoidal in shape. The rima glottidis is slit-like when the vocal folds are closely approximated during phonation. Variation in the tension and length of the vocal folds, in the width of the rima glottidis, and in the intensity of the expiratory effort produces changes in the pitch of the voice. The lower range of pitch of the voice of postpubertal males results from the greater length of the vocal folds.

The *vestibular folds*, extending between the thyroid and the arytenoid cartilages (Figs. 9.35 and 9.36), play little or no part in voice production; they are protective in function.

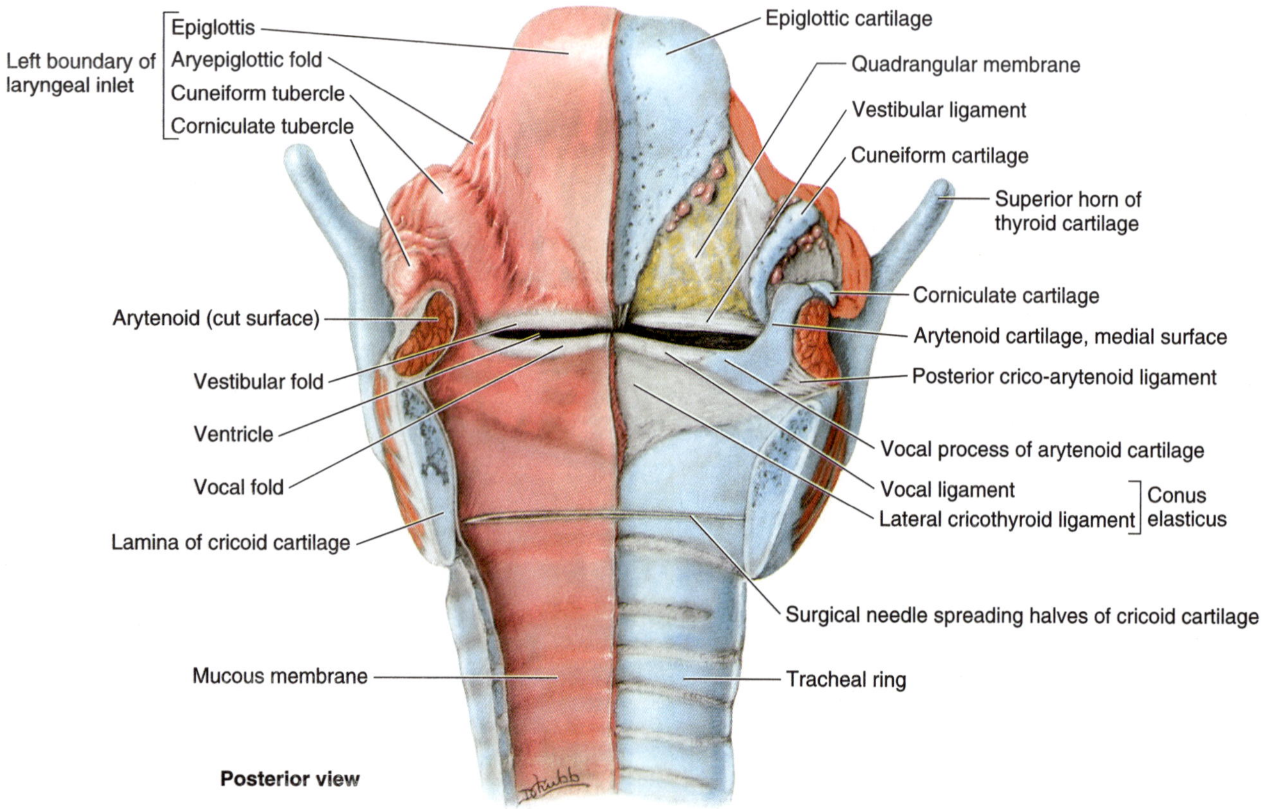

FIGURE 9.35. Interior of larynx. The posterior wall of the larynx is split in the median plane, and the two sides are spread apart and held in place by a surgical needle. On the left side, the mucous membrane is intact. On the right side, the mucous and submucous coats are peeled off, and the skeletal coat—consisting of cartilages, ligaments, and the fibro-elastic membrane—is uncovered.

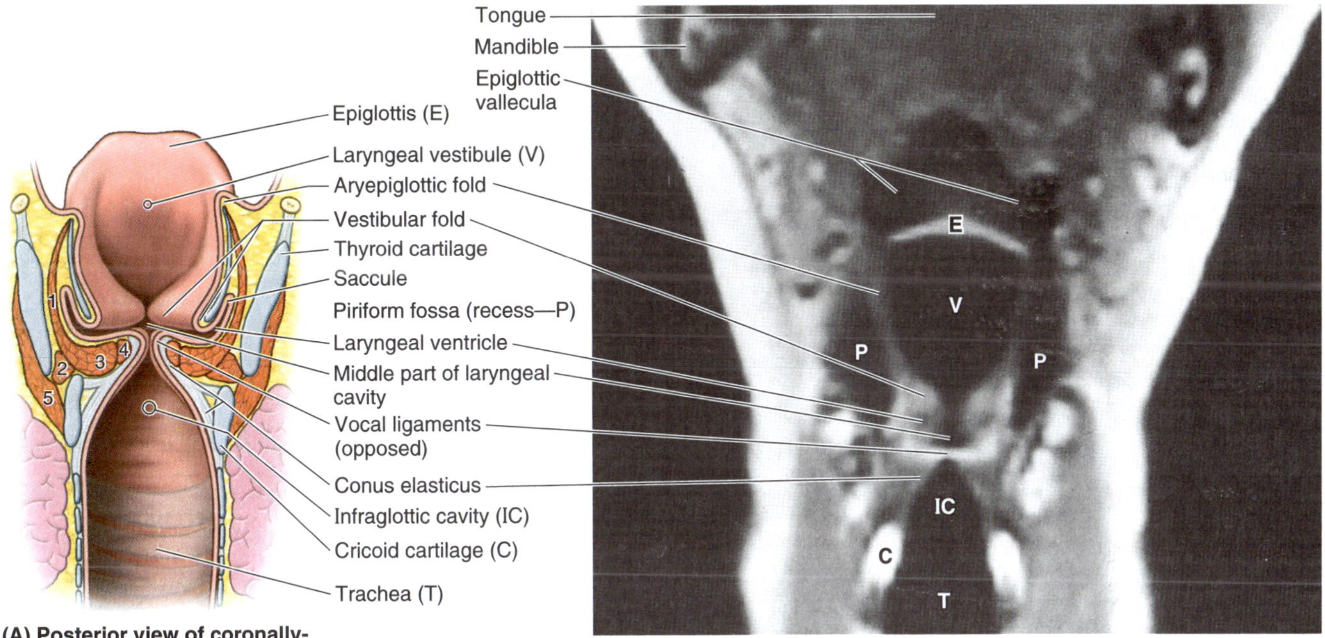

(A) Posterior view of coronally-sectioned larynx

(B) Coronal MRI study (Plane indicated in Fig. 9.42B)

Key for (A):

1 Aryepiglottic muscle
2 Lateral crico-arytenoid
3 Thyro-arytenoid
4 Vocalis
5 Cricothyroid

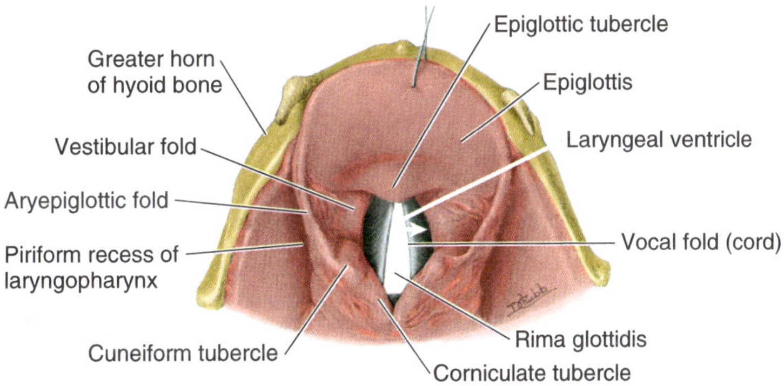

(C) Posterosuperior view, looking antero-inferiorly through laryngeal vestibule and rima glottidis

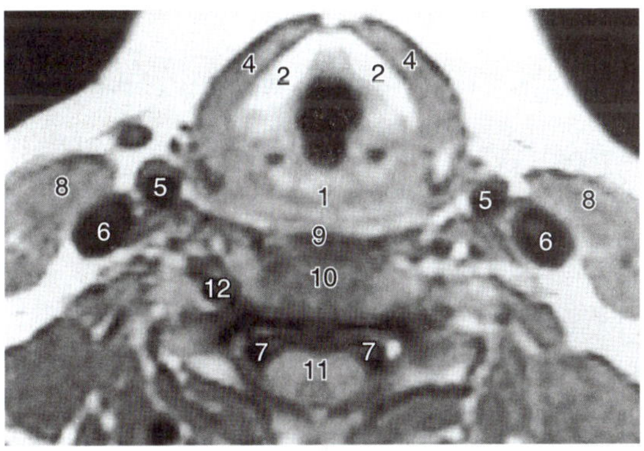

1 Esophagus
2 Thyroid cartilage
3 Lamina of cricoid cartilage
4 Sternothyroid and sternohyoid muscles
5 Common carotid artery
6 IJV
7 Anterior root of spinal nerve
8 SCM
9 Inferior pharyngeal constrictor
10 Vertebral body
11 Spinal cord
12 Vertebral artery

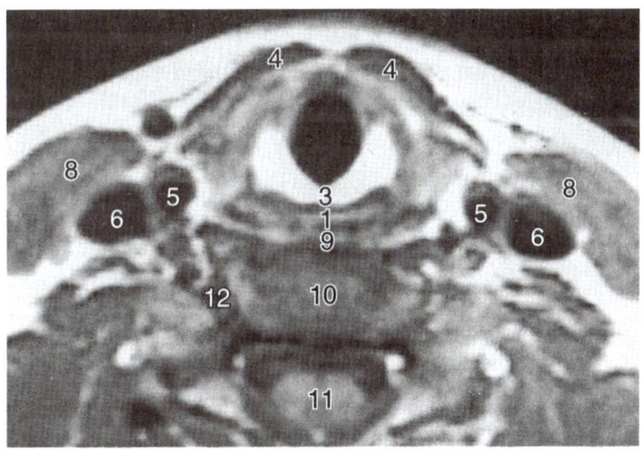

(D) Transverse MRI study of layrnx transecting thyroid cartilage

(E) Transverse MRI study of larynx transecting cricoid cartilage

FIGURE 9.36. Folds and compartments of larynx. A. This coronal section shows the compartments of the larynx: the vestibule, middle compartment with left and right ventricles, and the infraglottic cavity. **B.** This MRI study shows the epiglottic valleculae of the oropharynx, piriform fossae of the laryngopharynx, and vestibular and vocal folds of the larynx. **C.** The rima glottidis (the space between the vocal folds) is visible through the laryngeal inlet and vestibule. The laryngeal inlet is bounded (1) anteriorly by the free curved edge of the epiglottis; (2) posteriorly by the arytenoid cartilages, the corniculate cartilages that cap them, and the interarytenoid fold that unites them; and (3) on each side by the aryepiglottic fold that contains the superior end of the cuneiform cartilage. **D, E.** The planes of these transverse studies, oriented in the same direction as part **(C)**, pass superior **(D)** and inferior **(E)** to the rima glottidis. (MRI studies courtesy of Dr. W. Kucharczyk, University Health Network, Toronto, Ontario, Canada.)

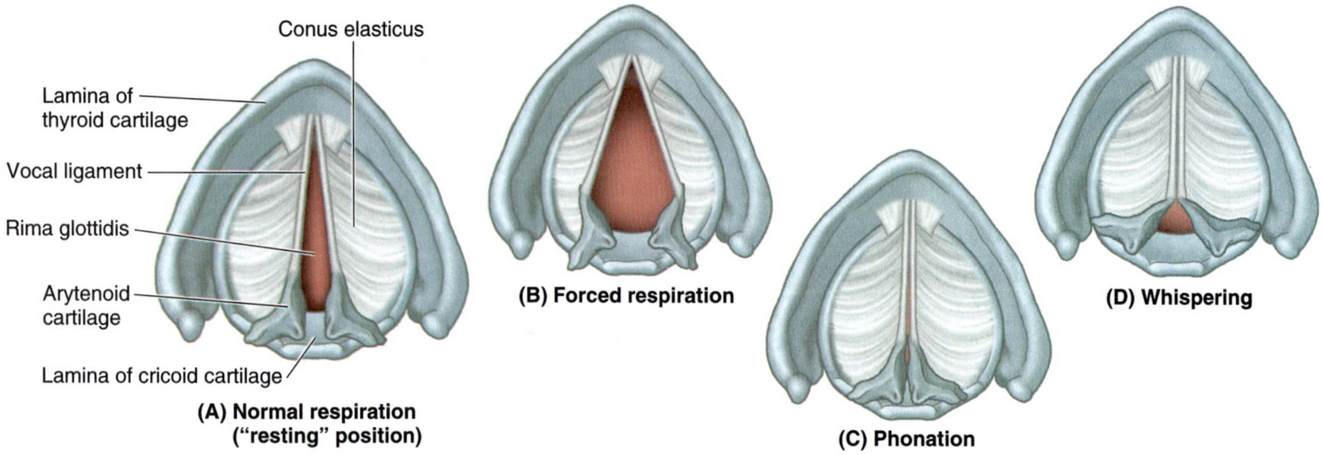

FIGURE 9.37. Variations in shape of rima glottidis. A. The shape of the rima glottidis, the aperture between the vocal folds, varies according to the position of the vocal folds. During normal respiration, the laryngeal muscles are relaxed and the rima glottidis assumes a narrow, slit-like position. **B.** During a deep inhalation, the vocal ligaments are abducted by contraction of the posterior crico-arytenoid muscles, opening the rima glottidis widely into an inverted kite shape. **C.** During phonation, the arytenoid muscles adduct the arytenoid cartilages at the same time that the lateral crico-arytenoid muscles moderately adduct. Air forced between the adducted vocal ligaments produces tone. Stronger contraction of the same muscles seals the rima glottidis (Valsalva maneuver). **D.** During whispering, the vocal ligaments are strongly adducted by the lateral crico-arytenoid muscles, but the relaxed arytenoid muscles allow air to pass between the arytenoid cartilages (intercartilaginous part of rima glottidis), which is modified into toneless speech. No tone is produced.

They consist of two thick folds of mucous membrane enclosing the *vestibular ligaments*. The space between these ligaments is the **rima vestibuli**. The lateral recesses between the vocal and the vestibular folds are the *laryngeal ventricles*.

Laryngeal Muscles. The laryngeal muscles are divided into extrinsic and intrinsic groups:

- **Extrinsic laryngeal muscles** *move the larynx as a whole* (Fig. 9.19; Table 9.3). The *infrahyoid muscles* are depressors of the hyoid and larynx, whereas the *suprahyoid muscles* (and the *stylopharyngeus*, a pharyngeal muscle discussed later in this chapter) are elevators of the hyoid and larynx.
- **Intrinsic laryngeal muscles** move the *laryngeal components*, altering the length and tension of the vocal folds and the size and shape of the rima glottidis (Fig. 9.37). All but one of the intrinsic muscles of the larynx are supplied by the *recurrent laryngeal nerve* (Figs. 9.38, 9.40, and 9.41), a branch of CN X. The cricothyroid is supplied by the external laryngeal nerve, one of the two terminal branches of the *superior laryngeal nerve*.

The actions of the intrinsic laryngeal muscles are easiest to understand when they are considered as functional groups: adductors and abductors, sphincters, and tensors and relaxers. The intrinsic muscles are illustrated in situ in Figures 9.36A, 9.38 and 9.39; their attachments, innervation, and main actions are summarized in Table 9.5.

- *Adductors and abductors*: These muscles move the vocal folds to open and close the rima glottidis. The principal adductors are the **lateral crico-arytenoid muscles**, which pull the muscular processes anteriorly, rotating the arytenoid cartilages so that their vocal processes swing medially. When this action is combined with that of the **transverse** and **oblique arytenoid muscles**, which pull the arytenoid cartilages together, air pushed through the rima glottidis causes vibrations of the vocal ligaments (phonation). When the vocal ligaments are adducted, but the transverse arytenoid muscles do not act, the arytenoid

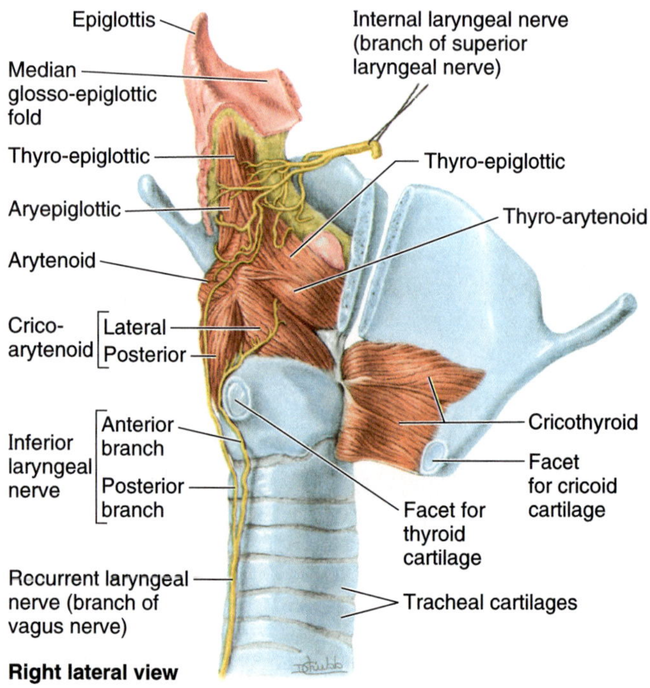

FIGURE 9.38. Muscles and nerves of larynx and cricothyroid joint. The thyroid cartilage is sawn through to the right of the median plane. The cricothyroid joint is disarticulated, and the right lamina of the thyroid cartilage is turned anteriorly (like opening a book), stripping the cricothyroid muscles off the arch of the cricoid cartilage.

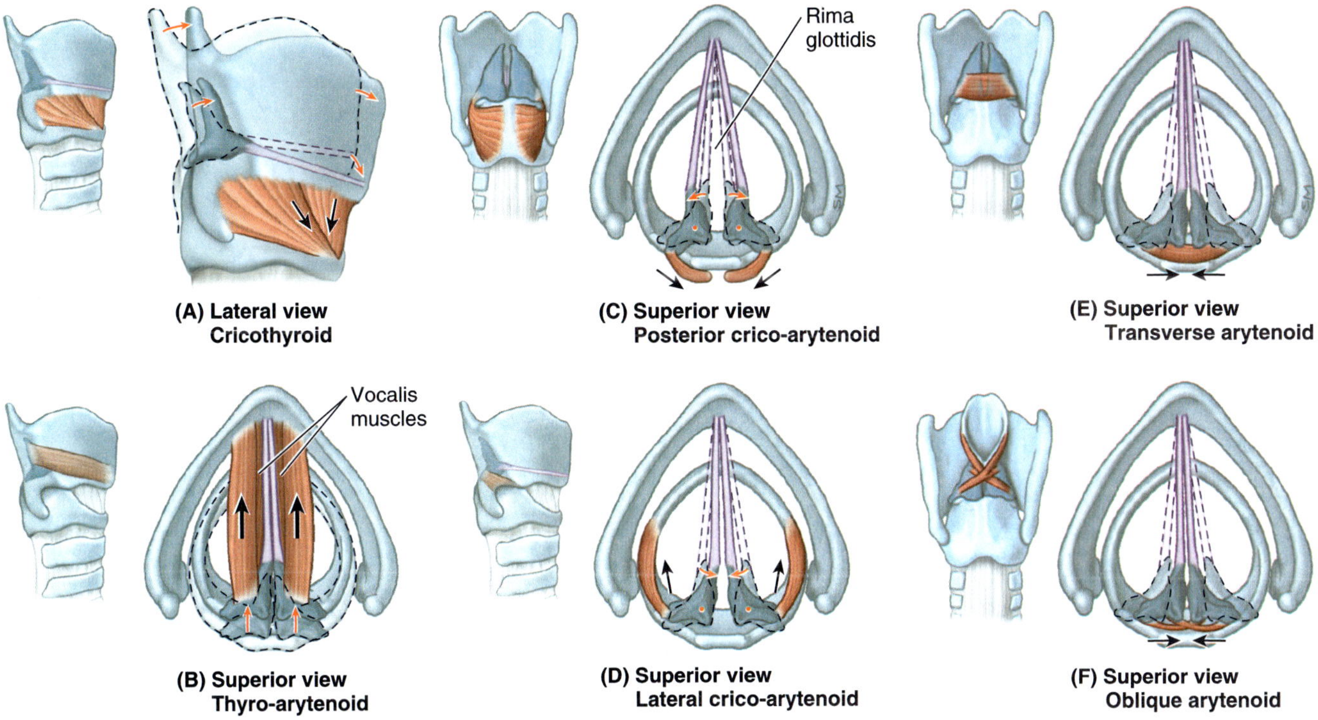

FIGURE 9.39. Muscles of larynx.

TABLE 9.5. MUSCLES OF LARYNX

Muscle	Origin	Insertion	Innervation	Main Action(s)
Cricothyroid	Anterolateral part of cricoid cartilage	Inferior margin and inferior horn of thyroid cartilage	External laryngeal nerve (from CN X)	Stretches and tenses vocal ligament
Thyro-arytenoid[a]	Lower half of posterior aspect of angle of thyroid laminae and cricothyroid ligament	Anterolateral arytenoid surface		Relaxes vocal ligament
Posterior crico-arytenoid	Posterior surface of lamina of cricoid cartilage	Vocal process of arytenoid cartilage		Abducts vocal folds
Lateral crico-arytenoid	Arch of cricoid cartilage		Inferior laryngeal nerve (terminal part of recurrent laryngeal nerve, from CN X—see Fig. 9.38)	Adducts vocal folds (interligamentous portion)
Transverse and oblique arytenoids[b]	One arytenoid cartilage	Contralateral arytenoid cartilage		Adduct arytenoid cartilages (adducting intercartilaginous portion of vocal folds, closing posterior rima glottidis)
Vocalis[c]	Lateral surface of vocal process of arytenoid cartilage	Ipsilateral vocal ligament		Relaxes posterior vocal ligament while maintaining (or increasing) tension of anterior part

[a]Superior fibers of the thyro-arytenoid muscles pass into the aryepiglottic fold, and some of them reach the epiglottic cartilage. These fibers constitute the thyro-epiglottic muscle, which widens the laryngeal inlet.
[b]Some fibers of the oblique arytenoid muscles continue as aryepiglottic muscles (Fig. 9.40).
[c]This slender muscle slip lies medial to and is composed of fibers finer than those of the thyro-arytenoid muscle.

cartilages remain apart and air may bypass the ligaments. This is the position of whispering when the breath is modified into voice in the absence of tone. The sole abductors are the **posterior crico-arytenoid muscles**, which pull the muscular processes posteriorly, rotating the vocal processes laterally and thus widening the rima glottidis.

- *Sphincters*: The combined actions of most of the muscles of the laryngeal inlet result in a sphincteric action that closes the laryngeal inlet as a protective mechanism during swallowing. Contraction of the *lateral crico-arytenoids, transverse* and *oblique arytenoids*, and *aryepiglottic muscles* brings the aryepiglottic folds together and pulls the arytenoid cartilages toward the epiglottis. This action occurs reflexively in response to the presence of liquid or particles approaching or within the laryngeal vestibule. It is perhaps our strongest reflex, diminishing only after loss of consciousness, as in drowning.

- *Tensors*: The principal tensors are the **cricothyroid muscles**, which tilt or pull the prominence or angle of the thyroid cartilage anteriorly and inferiorly toward the arch of the cricoid cartilage. This increases the distance between the thyroid prominence and the arytenoid cartilages. Because the anterior ends of the vocal ligaments attach to the posterior aspect of the prominence, the vocal ligaments elongate and tighten, raising the pitch of the voice.
- *Relaxers*: The principal muscles in this group are the **thyro-arytenoid muscles**, which pull the arytenoid cartilages anteriorly, toward the thyroid angle (prominence), thereby relaxing the vocal ligaments to lower the pitch of the voice.

The **vocalis muscles** lie medial to the thyro-arytenoid muscles and lateral to the vocal ligaments within the vocal folds. The vocalis muscles produce minute adjustments of the vocal ligaments, selectively tensing and relaxing the anterior and posterior parts, respectively, of the vocal folds during animated speech and singing.

Arteries of Larynx. The laryngeal arteries, branches of the superior and inferior thyroid arteries, supply the larynx (Fig. 9.40). The **superior laryngeal artery** accompanies the internal branch of the superior laryngeal nerve through the thyrohyoid membrane and branches to supply the internal surface of the larynx. The **cricothyroid artery**, a small branch of the superior thyroid artery, supplies the cricothyroid muscle. The **inferior laryngeal artery**, a branch of the inferior thyroid artery, accompanies the *inferior laryngeal nerve* (terminal part of the recurrent laryngeal nerve) and supplies the mucous membrane and muscles in the inferior part of the larynx.

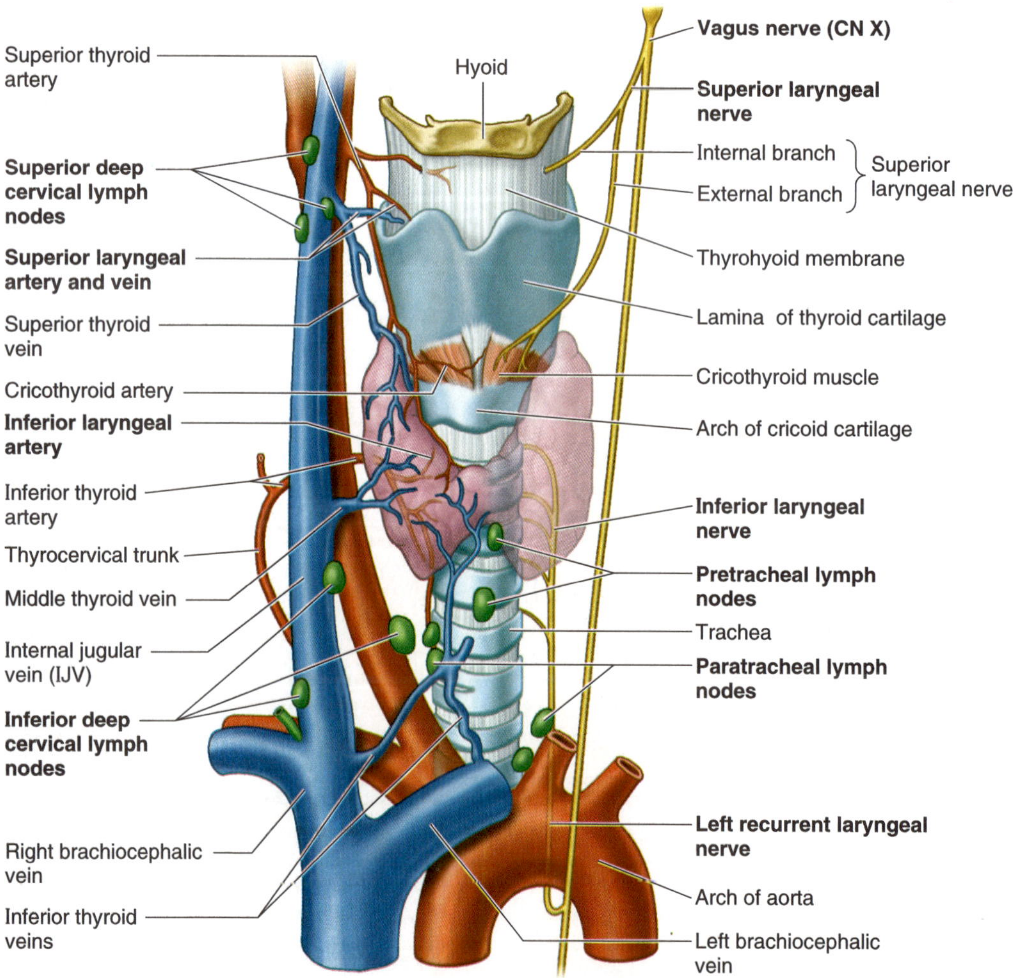

FIGURE 9.40. Vessels, nerves, and lymph nodes of larynx. The superior and inferior thyroid arteries give rise to the superior and inferior laryngeal arteries, respectively; they anastomose with each other. The laryngeal nerves are derived from the vagus (CN X) through the internal and external branches of the superior laryngeal nerve and the inferior laryngeal nerve from the recurrent laryngeal nerve. The left recurrent laryngeal nerve passes inferior to the arch of the aorta.

Veins of Larynx. The laryngeal veins accompany the laryngeal arteries. The **superior laryngeal vein** usually joins the superior thyroid vein and through it drains into the IJV (Fig. 9.40). The **inferior laryngeal vein** joins the inferior thyroid vein or the venous plexus of veins on the anterior aspect of the trachea, which empties into the left brachiocephalic vein.

Lymphatics of Larynx. The laryngeal lymphatic vessels superior to the vocal folds accompany the superior laryngeal artery through the thyrohyoid membrane and drain into the **superior deep cervical lymph nodes**. The lymphatic vessels inferior to the vocal folds drain into the *pretracheal* or *paratracheal lymph nodes*, which drain into the **inferior deep cervical lymph nodes** (Fig. 9.40).

Nerves of Larynx. The nerves of the larynx are the superior and inferior laryngeal branches of the vagus nerves (CN X). The **superior laryngeal nerve** arises from the **inferior vagal ganglion** at the superior end of the carotid triangle (Figs. 9.40 and 9.41). The nerve divides into two terminal branches within the carotid sheath: the internal laryngeal nerve (sensory and autonomic) and the external laryngeal nerve (motor).

The **internal laryngeal nerve**, the larger of the terminal branches of the superior laryngeal nerve, pierces the thyrohyoid membrane with the superior laryngeal artery, supplying sensory fibers to the laryngeal mucous membrane of the laryngeal vestibule and middle laryngeal cavity, including the superior surface of the vocal folds. The **external laryngeal nerve**, the smaller terminal branch of the superior laryngeal nerve, descends posterior to the sternothyroid muscle in company with the superior thyroid artery. At first, the external laryngeal nerve lies on the inferior pharyngeal constrictor; it then pierces the muscle, contributing to its innervation (with the pharyngeal plexus), and continues to supply the cricothyroid muscle.

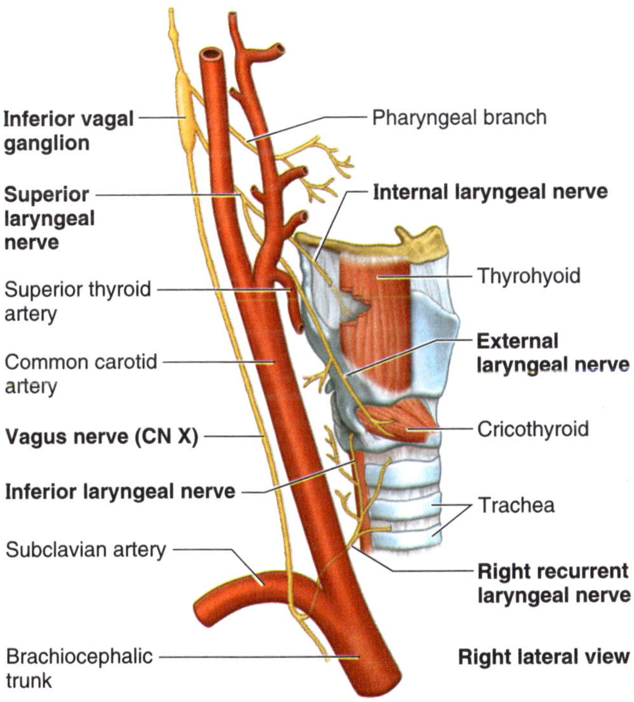

FIGURE 9.41. Laryngeal branches of right vagus nerve (CN X). The nerves of the larynx are the internal and external branches of the superior laryngeal nerve and the inferior laryngeal nerve from the recurrent laryngeal nerve. The right recurrent laryngeal nerve passes inferior to the right subclavian artery.

The **inferior laryngeal nerve**, the continuation of the recurrent laryngeal nerve (a branch of the vagus nerve), enters the larynx by passing deep to the inferior border of the inferior pharyngeal constrictor and medial to the lamina of the thyroid cartilage (Figs. 9.38, 9.40, and 9.41). It divides into anterior and posterior branches, which accompany the inferior laryngeal artery into the larynx. The anterior branch supplies the lateral crico-arytenoid, thyro-arytenoid, vocalis, aryepiglottic, and thyro-epiglottic muscles. The posterior branch supplies the posterior crico-arytenoid and transverse and oblique arytenoid muscles. Because it supplies all the intrinsic muscles except the cricothyroid, the inferior laryngeal nerve is the primary motor nerve of the larynx. However, it also provides sensory fibers to the mucosa of the infraglottic cavity.

TRACHEA

The **trachea**, extending from the larynx into the thorax, terminates inferiorly as it divides into right and left main bronchi. It transports air to and from the lungs, and its epithelium propels debris-laden mucus toward the pharynx for expulsion from the mouth. The trachea is a fibrocartilaginous tube, supported by incomplete cartilaginous **tracheal cartilages** (rings), that occupies a median position in the neck (Fig. 9.38). The tracheal cartilages keep the trachea patent; they are deficient posteriorly where the trachea is adjacent to the esophagus. The posterior gaps in the tracheal rings are spanned by the involuntary **trachealis muscle**, smooth muscle connecting the ends of the rings (Fig. 9.42). Hence, the posterior wall of the trachea is flat.

In adults, the trachea is approximately 2.5 cm in diameter, whereas in infants, it has the diameter of a pencil. The trachea extends from the inferior end of the larynx at the level of the C6 vertebra. It ends at the level of the sternal angle or the T4–T5 IV disc, where it divides into the right and left main bronchi (see Chapter 4, Thorax).

Lateral to the trachea are the common carotid arteries and the lobes of the thyroid gland (Fig. 9.40). Inferior to the isthmus of the thyroid gland are the jugular venous arch and the inferior thyroid veins (Figs. 9.17 and 9.29). The brachiocephalic trunk is related to the right side of the trachea in the root of the neck. Deviation of the trachea from the midline, apparent superficially or radiographically, often signals the presence of a pathological process. Tracheal trauma often affects the closely adherent esophagus.

(continued on p.1097)

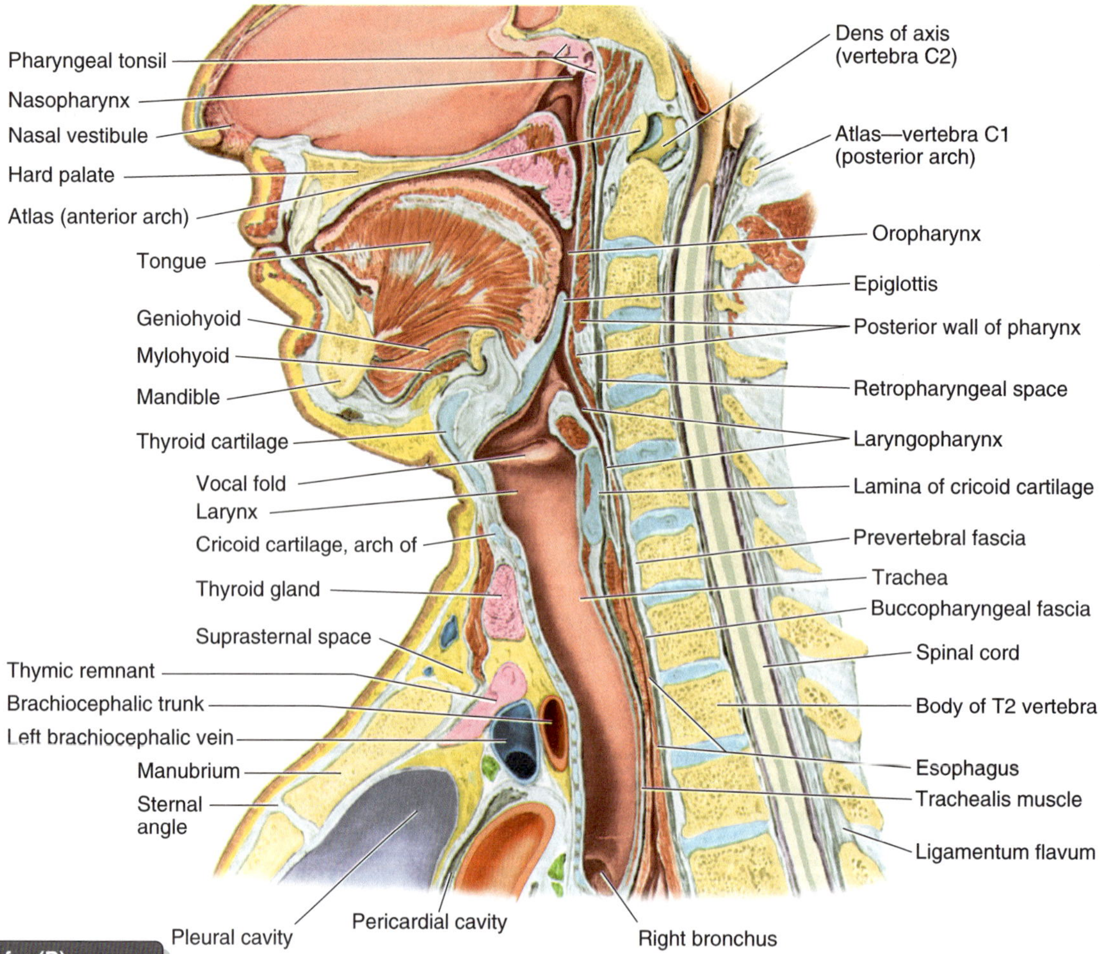

Key for (B):
Plane of coronal MRI study in Fig. 9.36B

(A) Medial view of right half of bisected head and neck (median section)

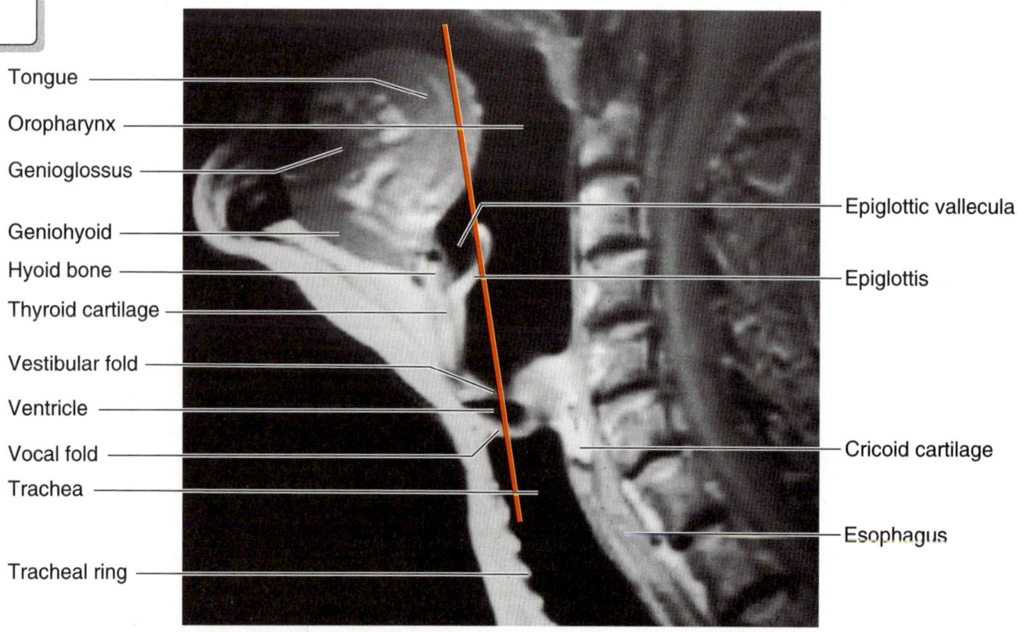

(B) Parasagittal MRI study of pharynx, larynx, and trachea

FIGURE 9.42. Median sections of head and neck. A. The pharynx extends from the cranial base to the level of the cricoid cartilage (body of C6 vertebra or the C6–C7 IV disc, as shown here), where it is continuous with the esophagus. **B.** This sagittal section does not demonstrate the continuities of the upper respiratory tract because the soft palate is elevated, closing off the nasopharynx, and the plane of section passes through the vestibular and vocal folds to the side of the rima glottidis. (Part **B**, Courtesy of Dr. W. Kucharczyk, University Health Network, Toronto, Ontario, Canada.)

Alimentary Layer of Cervical Viscera

In the alimentary layer, cervical viscera take part in the digestive functions of the body. Although the pharynx conducts air to the larynx, trachea, and lungs, the pharyngeal constrictors direct (and the *epiglottis* deflects) food to the esophagus. The esophagus, also involved in food propulsion, is the beginning of the *alimentary canal* (digestive tract).

PHARYNX

The **pharynx** is the superior expanded part of the alimentary system posterior to the nasal and oral cavities, extending inferiorly past the larynx (Figs. 9.42, 9.43 and 9.44A). The pharynx extends from the *cranial base* to the inferior border of the cricoid cartilage anteriorly and the inferior border of the C6 vertebra posteriorly. The pharynx is widest (approximately 5 cm) opposite the hyoid and narrowest (approximately 1.5 cm) at its inferior end, where it is continuous with the esophagus. The flat posterior wall of the pharynx lies against the prevertebral layer of deep cervical fascia.

Interior of Pharynx. The pharynx is divided into three parts:

1. *Nasopharynx*: posterior to the nose and superior to the soft palate.
2. *Oropharynx*: posterior to the mouth.
3. *Laryngopharynx*: posterior to the larynx.

The **nasopharynx** has a respiratory function; it is the posterior extension of the nasal cavities (Figs. 9.42 to 9.44). The nose opens into the nasopharynx through two **choanae** (paired openings between the nasal cavity and the nasopharynx). The roof and posterior wall of the nasopharynx form a continuous surface that lies inferior to the body of the sphenoid bone and the basilar part of the occipital bone (Figs. 9.43 and 9.44A).

The abundant lymphoid tissue in the pharynx forms an incomplete *tonsillar ring* around the superior part of the

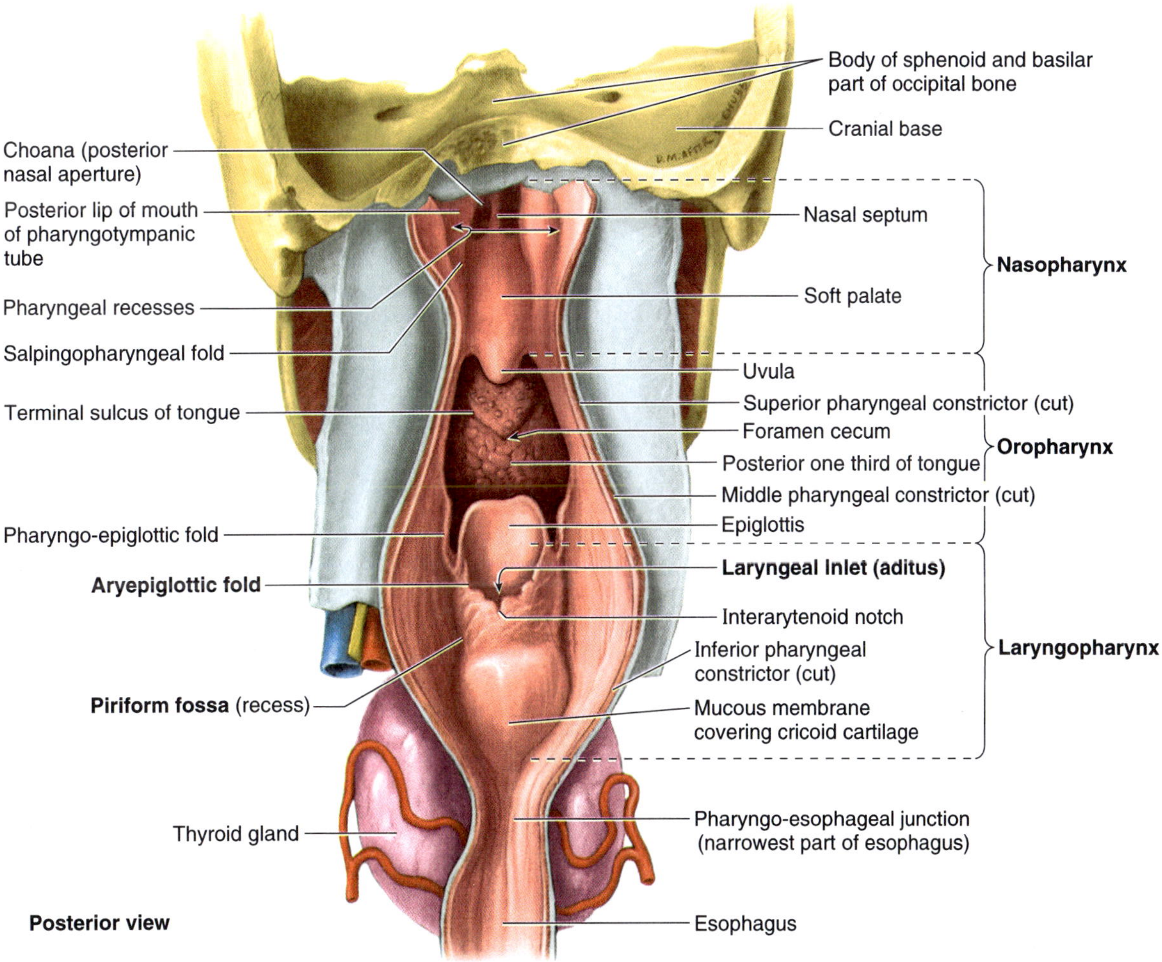

FIGURE 9.43. Anterior wall of pharynx. In this dissection, the posterior wall has been incised along the midline and spread apart. Openings in the anterior wall communicate with the nasal, oral, and laryngeal cavities. On each side of the laryngeal inlet, separated from it by the aryepiglottic fold, a piriform fossa (recess) is formed by the invagination of the larynx into the anterior wall of the laryngopharynx.

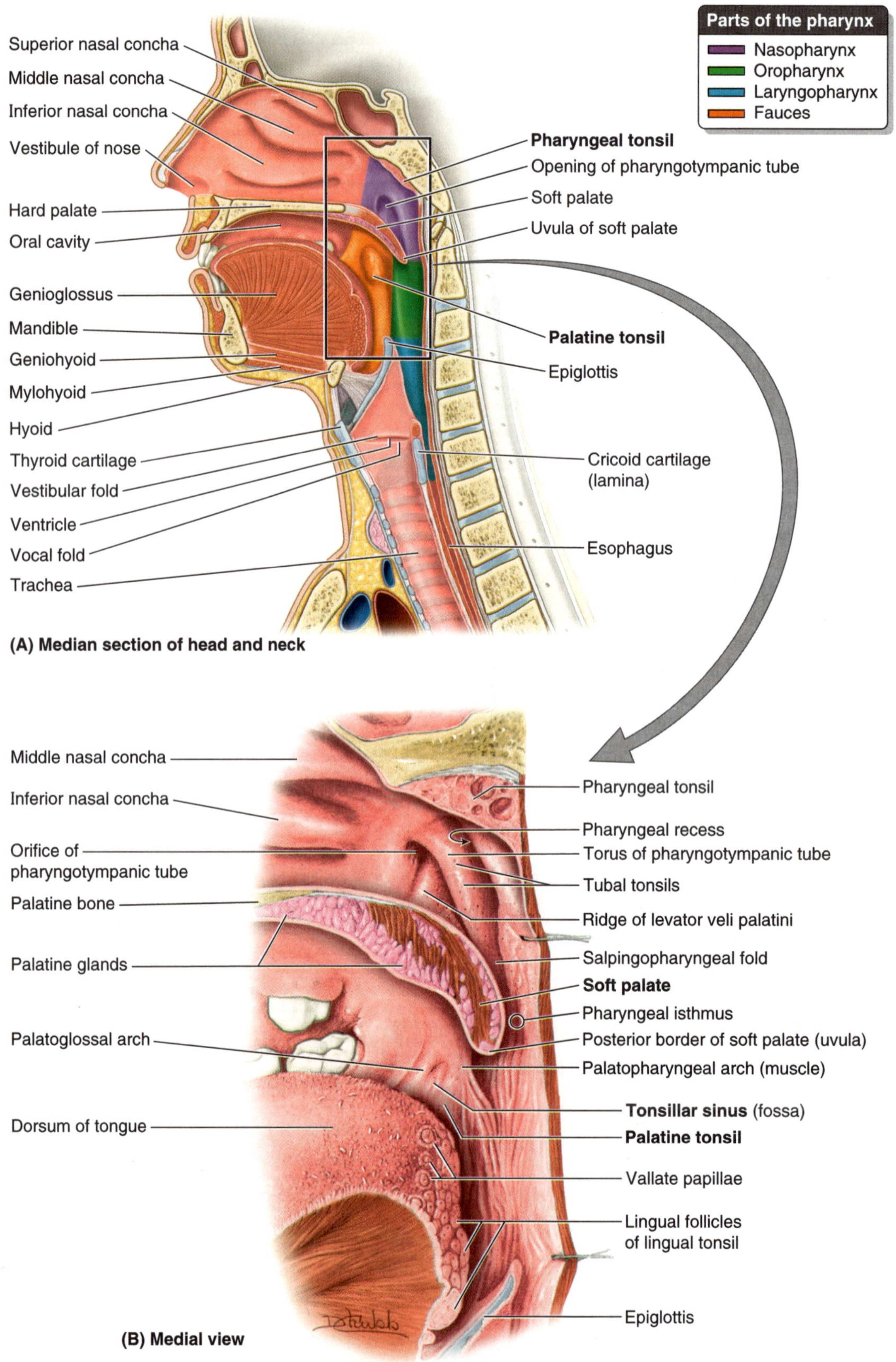

FIGURE 9.44. Internal aspect of lateral wall of pharynx. A. The upper respiratory passages and alimentary canal in the right half of a bisected head and neck are shown. The *rectangle* indicates the location of the section shown in part **B. B.** A closer view of the nasopharynx and oropharynx, which are separated anteriorly by the soft palate, is provided. The posterior border of the soft palate forms the anterior margin of the pharyngeal isthmus through which the two spaces communicate posteriorly.

pharynx (see Fig. 9.49). The lymphoid tissue is aggregated in certain regions to form masses called tonsils. The **pharyngeal tonsil** (commonly called the adenoid when enlarged) is in the mucous membrane of the roof and posterior wall of the nasopharynx (Figs. 9.42A and 9.44). Extending inferiorly from the medial end of the pharyngotympanic tube is a vertical fold of mucous membrane, the **salpingopharyngeal fold** (Figs. 9.43 and 9.44B). It covers the salpingopharyngeus muscle, which opens the pharyngeal orifice of the pharyngotympanic tube during swallowing. The collection of lymphoid tissue in the submucosa of the pharynx near the nasopharyngeal opening, or orifice of the pharyngotympanic tube, is the **tubal tonsils** (Fig. 9.44B). Posterior to the **torus of the pharyngotympanic tube** and the salpingopharyngeal fold is a slit-like lateral projection of the pharynx, the **pharyngeal recess**, which extends laterally and posteriorly.

The **oropharynx** has a digestive function. It is bounded by the soft palate superiorly, the base of the tongue inferiorly, and the palatoglossal and palatopharyngeal arches laterally (Figs. 9.44 and 9.45A). It extends from the soft palate to the superior border of the epiglottis.

Deglutition (swallowing) is the complex process that transfers a food bolus from the mouth through the pharynx and esophagus into the stomach. Solid food is masticated (chewed) and mixed with saliva to form a soft bolus (mass) that is easier to swallow. Deglutition occurs in three stages:

- **Stage 1**: voluntary; the bolus is compressed against the palate and pushed from the mouth into the oropharynx, mainly by movements of the muscles of the tongue and soft palate (Fig. 9.46A, B).
- **Stage 2**: involuntary and rapid; the soft palate is elevated, sealing off the nasopharynx from the oropharynx and laryngopharynx (Fig. 9.46C). The pharynx widens and shortens to receive the bolus of food as the suprahyoid muscles and longitudinal pharyngeal muscles contract, elevating the larynx.
- **Stage 3**: involuntary; sequential contraction of all three pharyngeal constrictor muscles creates a peristaltic ridge that forces the food bolus inferiorly into the esophagus (Fig. 9.46B–D).

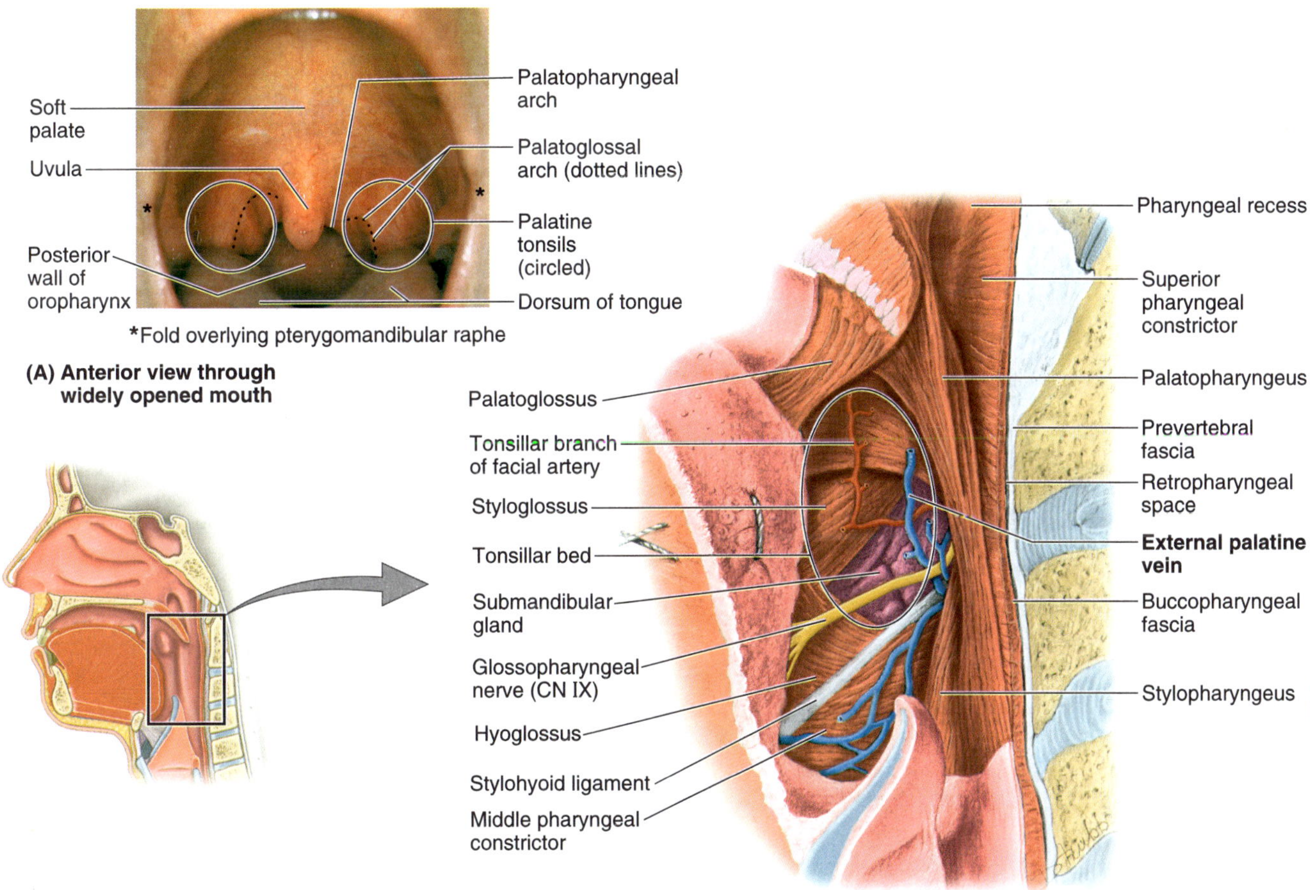

(B) Lateral view

FIGURE 9.45. Oral cavity and tonsillar bed. A. The oral cavity and palatine tonsils in a young child, with the mouth wide open and the tongue protruding as far as possible. The uvula is a muscular projection from the posterior edge of the soft palate. **B.** In this deep dissection of the tonsillar bed, the palatine tonsil has been removed. The tongue is pulled anteriorly, and the inferior (lingual) attachment of the superior pharyngeal constrictor muscle is cut away.

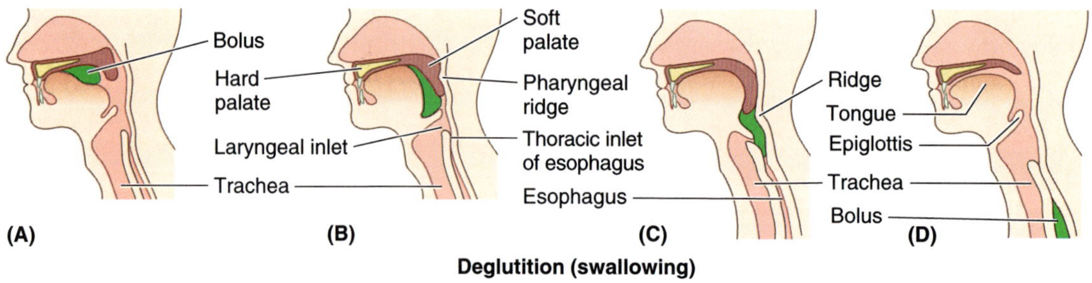

FIGURE 9.46. **Deglutition. A.** The bolus of food is squeezed to the back of the mouth by pushing the tongue against the palate. **B.** The nasopharynx is sealed off and the larynx is elevated, enlarging the pharynx to receive food. **C.** The pharyngeal sphincters contract sequentially, creating a "peristaltic ridge," squeezing food into the esophagus. The epiglottis deflects the bolus from but does not close the inlet to the larynx and trachea. **D.** The bolus of food moves down the esophagus by peristaltic contractions.

N36.1 The **palatine tonsils** are collections of lymphoid tissue on each side of the oropharynx in the interval between the palatine arches (Figs. 9.44 and 9.45A). The tonsil does not fill the **tonsillar sinus** (fossa) between the palatoglossal and palatopharyngeal arches in adults. The submucosal **tonsillar bed**, in which the palatine tonsil lies, is between these arches (Fig. 9.45B). The tonsillar bed is formed by the superior pharyngeal constrictor and the thin, fibrous sheet of **pharyngobasilar fascia** (Fig. 9.47A, B). This fascia blends with the periosteum of the cranial base and defines the limits of the pharyngeal wall in its superior part.

The **laryngopharynx** lies posterior to the larynx (Figs. 9.42A and 9.44A), extending from the superior border of the epiglottis and the pharyngo-epiglottic folds to the inferior border of the cricoid cartilage, where it narrows and becomes continuous with the esophagus. Posteriorly, the laryngopharynx is related to the bodies of the C4–C6 vertebrae. Its posterior and lateral walls are formed by the *middle*

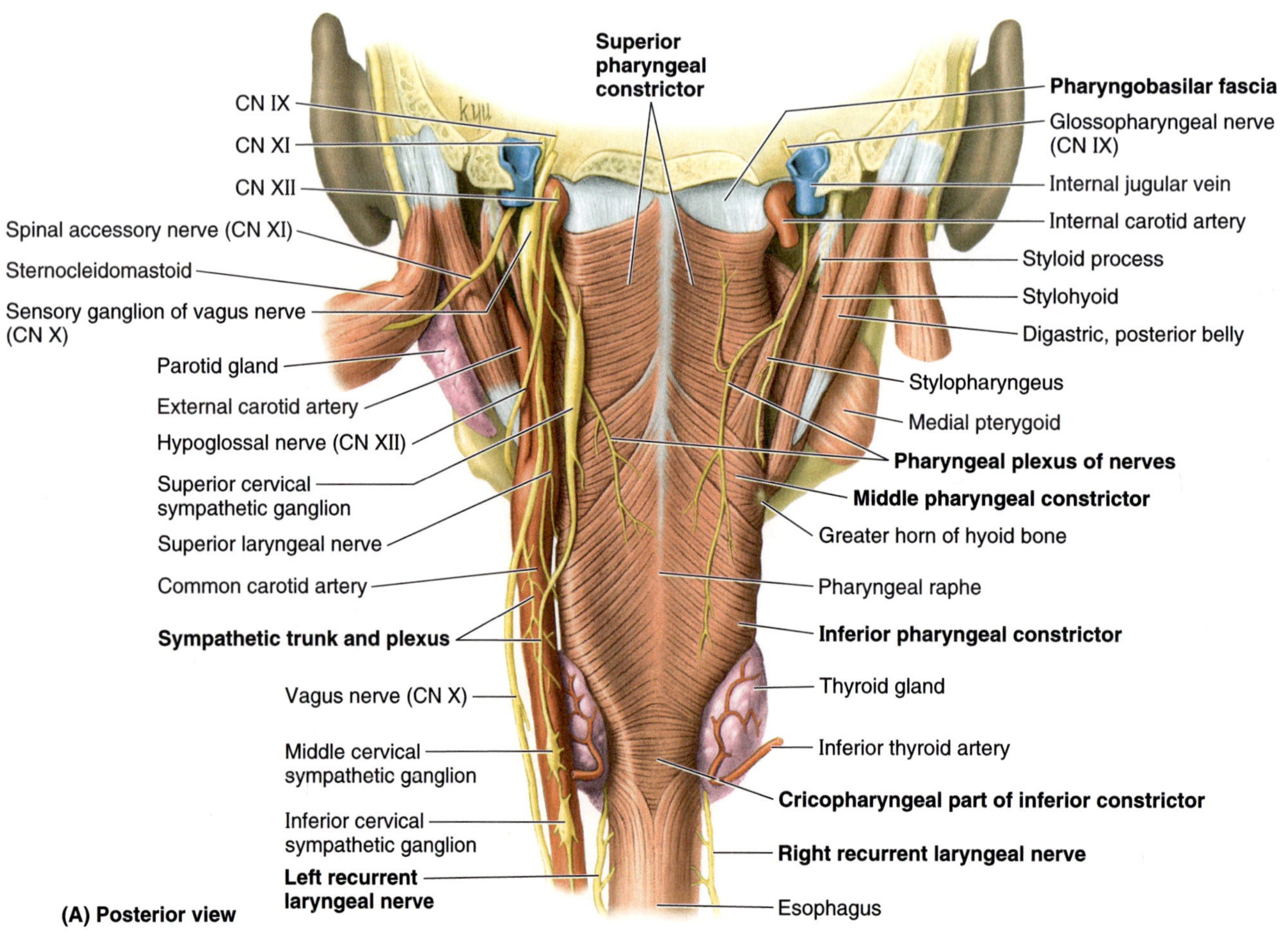

FIGURE 9.47. **Pharynx and cranial nerves. A.** This dissection shows the posterior aspect of the pharynx and associated structures. The buccopharyngeal fascia has been removed. Of the three pharyngeal constrictor muscles, the inferior muscle overlaps the middle one and the middle one overlaps the superior one. All three muscles form a common median pharyngeal raphe posteriorly.

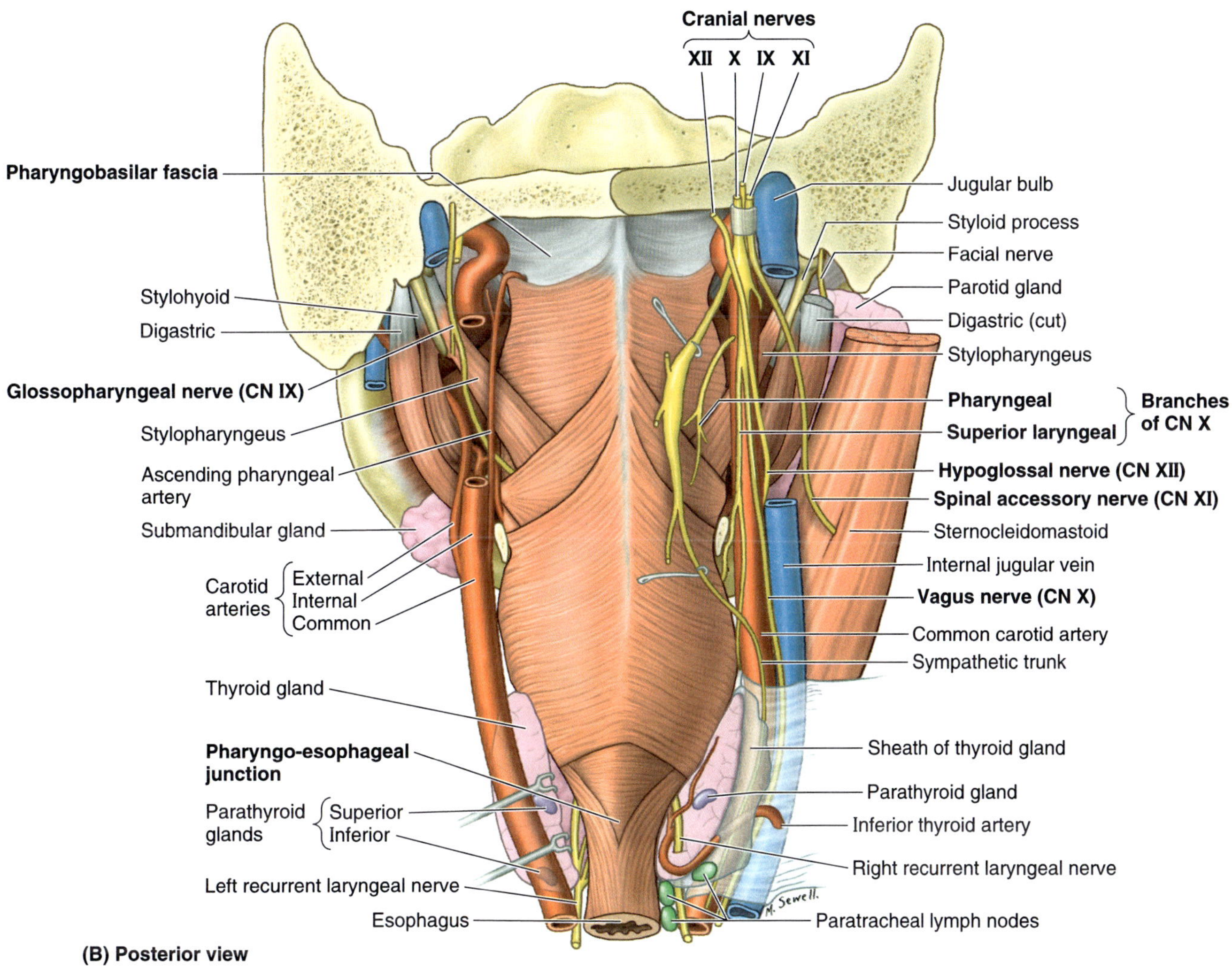

FIGURE 9.47. (Continued) B. The narrowest and least distensible part of the alimentary tract is the pharyngo-esophageal junction, where the laryngopharynx becomes the esophagus.

and *inferior pharyngeal constrictor muscles* (Fig. 9.47A, B). Internally, the wall is formed by the *palatopharyngeus and stylopharyngeus muscles*. The laryngopharynx communicates with the larynx through the **laryngeal inlet** on its anterior wall (Fig. 9.43).

AN36.3 The **piriform fossa** (recess) is a small depression of the laryngopharyngeal cavity on either side of the laryngeal inlet. This mucosa-lined fossa is separated from the laryngeal inlet by the **aryepiglottic fold**. Laterally, the piriform fossa is bounded by the medial surfaces of the thyroid cartilage and the *thyrohyoid membrane* (Fig. 9.40). Branches of the internal laryngeal and recurrent laryngeal nerves lie deep to the mucous membrane of the piriform fossa and are vulnerable to injury when a foreign body lodges in the fossa.

Pharyngeal Muscles. The wall of the pharynx is exceptional for the alimentary tract, having a muscular layer composed entirely of *voluntary muscle*, arranged with longitudinal muscles internal to a circular layer of muscles. Most of the alimentary tract is composed of smooth muscle, with a layer of longitudinal muscle external to a circular layer. The external circular layer of pharyngeal muscles consists of three **pharyngeal constrictors: superior, middle,** and **inferior** (Figs. 9.45B, 9.47A, B and 9.48). The internal longitudinal muscles consist of the **palatopharyngeus, stylopharyngeus**, and **salpingopharyngeus**. These muscles elevate the larynx and shorten the pharynx during swallowing and speaking. The pharyngeal muscles are illustrated in Figure 9.48, and their attachments, nerve supply, and actions of the pharyngeal muscles are described in Table 9.6.

The pharyngeal constrictors have a strong internal fascial lining, the *pharyngobasilar fascia* (Fig. 9.47B), and a thin external fascial lining, the *buccopharyngeal fascia* (Fig. 9.42A). Inferiorly, the buccopharyngeal fascia blends with the pretracheal layer of the *deep cervical fascia*. The pharyngeal constrictors contract involuntarily so that contraction takes place sequentially from the superior to the inferior end of the pharynx, propelling food into the esophagus. All three pharyngeal constrictors are supplied by the *pharyngeal plexus of nerves* that is formed by pharyngeal branches of the vagus and glossopharyngeal nerves and by sympathetic

(*continued on p.* 1103)

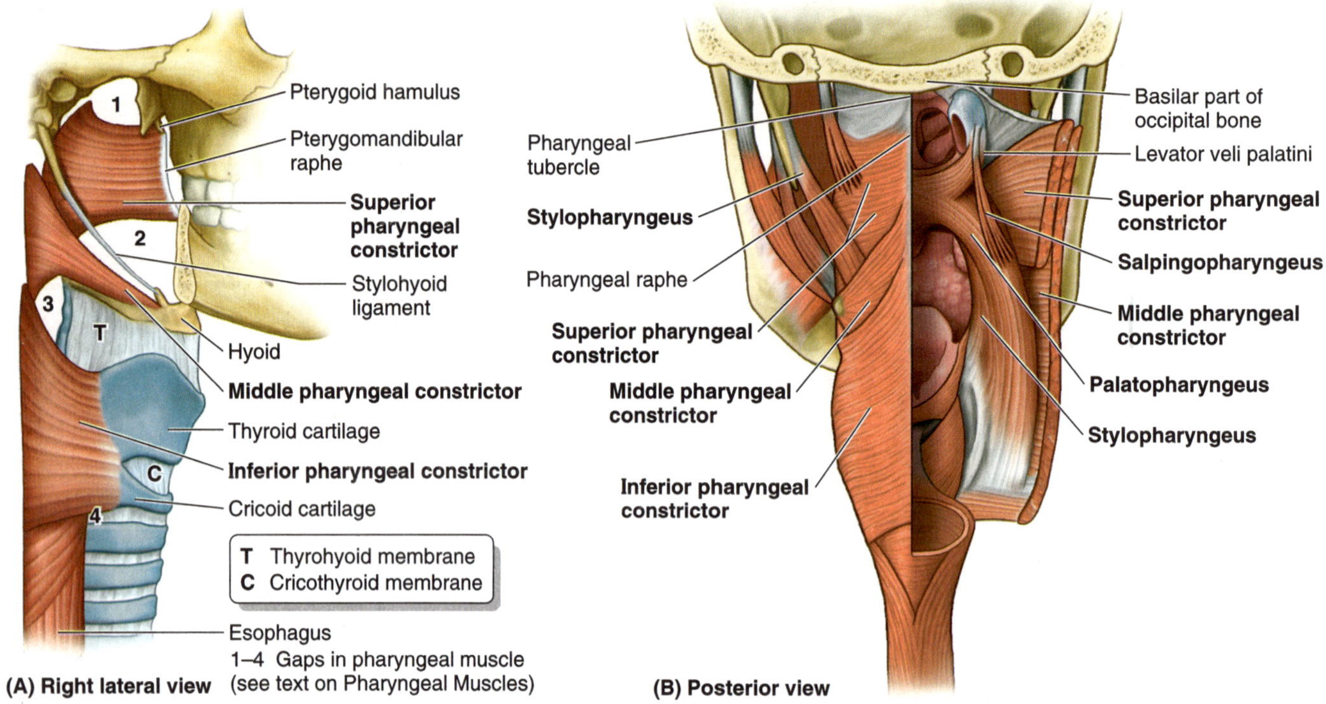

FIGURE 9.48. Muscles of pharynx.

TABLE 9.6. MUSCLES OF PHARYNX

Muscle	Origin	Insertion	Innervation	Main Action(s)
External layer				
Superior pharyngeal constrictor	Pterygoid hamulus, pterygomandibular raphe, posterior end of mylohyoid line of mandible, and side of tongue	Pharyngeal tubercle on basilar part of occipital bone	Pharyngeal branch of vagus (CN X) and pharyngeal plexus	Constrict walls of pharynx during swallowing
Middle pharyngeal constrictor	Stylohyoid ligament and greater and lesser horns of hyoid	Pharyngeal raphe	Pharyngeal branch of vagus (CN X) and pharyngeal plexus, plus branches of external and recurrent laryngeal nerves of vagus	
Inferior pharyngeal constrictor	Oblique line of thyroid cartilage and side of cricoid cartilage	Cricopharyngeal part encircles pharyngo-esophageal junction without forming a raphe		
Internal layer				
Palatopharyngeus	Hard palate and palatine aponeurosis	Posterior border of lamina of thyroid cartilage and side of pharynx and esophagus	Pharyngeal branch of vagus (CN X) and pharyngeal plexus	Elevate (shorten and widen) pharynx and larynx during swallowing and speaking
Salpingopharyngeus	Cartilaginous part of pharyngotympanic tube	Blends with palatopharyngeus		
Stylopharyngeus	Styloid process of temporal bone	Posterior and superior borders of thyroid cartilage with palatopharyngeus	Glossopharyngeal nerve (CN IX)	

branches from the superior cervical ganglion (Fig. 9.47A; Table 9.6). The pharyngeal plexus lies on the lateral wall of the pharynx, mainly on the middle pharyngeal constrictor.

The overlapping of the pharyngeal constrictor muscles leaves four gaps in the musculature for structures to enter or leave the pharynx (Fig. 9.48A):

1. Superior to the superior pharyngeal constrictor, the levator veli palatini, pharyngotympanic tube, and ascending palatine artery pass through a *gap between the superior pharyngeal constrictor and the cranium*. It is here that the pharyngobasilar fascia blends with the buccopharyngeal fascia to form, with the mucous membrane, the thin wall of the pharyngeal recess (Fig. 9.43).
2. A *gap between the superior and middle pharyngeal constrictors* forms a passageway that allows the stylopharyngeus, glossopharyngeal nerve, and stylohyoid ligament to pass to the internal aspect of the pharyngeal wall (Fig. 9.48).
3. A *gap between the middle and inferior pharyngeal constrictors* allows the internal laryngeal nerve and superior laryngeal artery and vein to pass to the larynx.
4. A *gap inferior to the inferior pharyngeal constrictor* allows the recurrent laryngeal nerve and inferior laryngeal artery to pass superiorly into the larynx.

Vessels of Pharynx. A branch of the facial artery, the **tonsillar branch** (Fig. 9.45B), passes through the superior pharyngeal constrictor muscle and enters the inferior pole of the palatine tonsil. The tonsil also receives arterial twigs from the ascending palatine, lingual, descending palatine, and ascending pharyngeal arteries. The large **external palatine vein** (paratonsillar vein) descends from the soft palate and passes close to the lateral surface of the tonsil before it enters the pharyngeal venous plexus.

AN36.2 The **tonsillar lymphatic vessels** pass laterally and inferiorly to the lymph nodes near the angle of the mandible and the **jugulodigastric node**, referred to as the *tonsillar node* because of its frequent enlargement when the tonsil is inflamed (*tonsillitis*) (see Fig. 9.51). The palatine, lingual, and pharyngeal tonsils form the **pharyngeal lymphatic** (tonsillar) **ring**, an incomplete circular band of lymphoid tissue around the superior part of the pharynx (Fig. 9.49). The antero-inferior part of the ring is formed by the *lingual tonsil* in the posterior part of the tongue. Lateral parts of the ring are formed by the palatine and tubal tonsils, and posterior and superior parts are formed by the pharyngeal tonsil.

Pharyngeal Nerves. The nerve supply to the pharynx (motor and most of sensory) derives from the **pharyngeal plexus of nerves** (Fig. 9.47A). Motor fibers in the plexus are derived from the vagus nerve (CN X) via its pharyngeal branch or branches. They supply all muscles of the pharynx and soft palate, except the stylopharyngeus (supplied by CN IX) and the tensor veli palatini (supplied by CN V_3). The inferior pharyngeal constrictor also receives some motor fibers from the external and recurrent laryngeal branches of the vagus. Sensory fibers in the pharyngeal plexus are derived from the glossopharyngeal nerve. They are distributed to all three

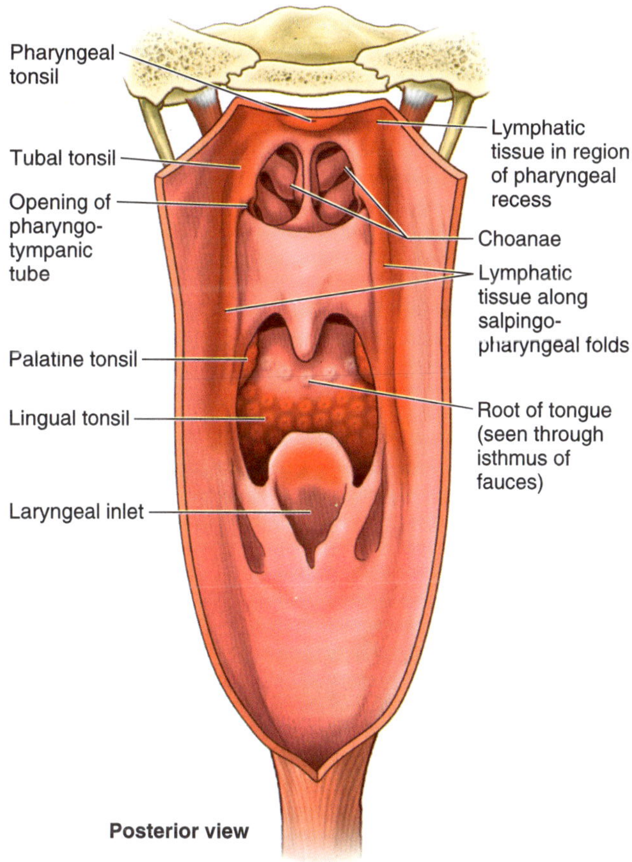

FIGURE 9.49. Lymphoid tissue in tongue and pharynx. The pharyngeal lymphatic (tonsillar) ring (*pink*) around the superior pharynx is formed of the pharyngeal, tubal, palatine, and lingual tonsils.

parts of the pharynx. In addition, the mucous membrane of the anterior and superior nasopharynx receives innervation from the maxillary nerve (CN V_2). The **tonsillar nerves** are derived from the *tonsillar plexus of nerves* formed by branches of the glossopharyngeal and vagus nerves.

ESOPHAGUS

The *esophagus* is a muscular tube that connects the pharynx to the stomach. It begins in the neck where it is continuous with the laryngopharynx at the **pharyngo-esophageal junction** (Figs. 9.43 and 9.47B). The esophagus consists of striated (voluntary) muscle in its upper third, smooth (involuntary) muscle in its lower third, and a mixture of striated and smooth muscle in between.

Its first part, the **cervical esophagus**, is part of the voluntary upper third. It begins immediately posterior to, and at the level of, the inferior border of the cricoid cartilage in the median plane. This is the level of the C6 vertebra.

Externally, the pharyngo-esophageal junction appears as a constriction produced by the **cricopharyngeal part of the inferior pharyngeal constrictor muscle** (the superior esophageal sphincter) and is the narrowest part of the esophagus. The cervical esophagus inclines slightly to the left as it descends and enters the superior mediastinum via the superior thoracic aperture, where it becomes the thoracic esophagus.

When the esophagus is empty, it is a slit-like lumen. When a food bolus descends in it, the lumen expands, eliciting reflex peristalsis in the inferior two thirds of the esophagus. The cervical esophagus lies between the trachea and the cervical vertebral column (Figs. 9.42 and 9.44A). It is attached to the trachea by loose connective tissue. The *recurrent laryngeal nerves* lie in or near the **tracheo-esophageal grooves** between the trachea and esophagus (Fig. 9.47). On the right of the esophagus is the right lobe of the *thyroid gland and* the right *carotid sheath* and its contents.

The esophagus is in contact with the cervical pleura at the root of the neck. On the left is the left lobe of the thyroid gland and the left carotid sheath. The thoracic duct adheres to the left side of the esophagus and lies between the pleura and the esophagus. For details concerning the thoracic and abdominal regions of the esophagus, see Chapter 4, Thorax, and Chapter 5, Abdomen.

Vessels of Cervical Esophagus. The arteries to the cervical esophagus are branches of the *inferior thyroid arteries*. Each artery gives off ascending and descending branches that anastomose with each other and across the midline. Veins from the cervical esophagus are tributaries of the *inferior thyroid veins*. Lymphatic vessels of the cervical part of the esophagus drain into the *paratracheal lymph nodes* and *inferior deep cervical lymph nodes* (see Fig. 9.51).

Nerves of Cervical Esophagus. The nerve supply to the cervical esophagus is somatic motor and sensory to the upper half and parasympathetic (vagal), sympathetic, and visceral sensory to the lower half. The cervical esophagus receives somatic fibers via branches from the *recurrent laryngeal nerves* and vasomotor fibers from the *cervical sympathetic trunks* through the plexus around the inferior thyroid artery (Fig. 9.47).

Surface Anatomy of Endocrine and Respiratory Layers of Cervical Viscera

AN43.5 The neck of an infant is short; therefore, the cervical viscera are located more superiorly in infants than in adults. The cervical viscera do not reach their final levels until after the 7th year. The elongation of the neck is accompanied by growth changes in the skin. Consequently, a midline incision in the inferior neck of an infant results in a scar that will lie over the superior part of the sternum as a child.

The U-shaped *hyoid bone* lies in the anterior part of the neck in the deep angle between the mandible and the thyroid cartilage at the level of the C3 vertebra (see Fig. 9.51). Swallow, and the hyoid will move under your fingers when they are placed at the angle between the chin and anterior neck. The greater horn of one side of the hyoid is palpable only when the greater horn on the opposite side is steadied.

The *laryngeal prominence* is produced by the meeting of the laminae of the thyroid cartilage at an acute angle in the anterior midline. This *thyroid angle*, most acute in postpubertal males, forms the laryngeal prominence ("Adam's apple"), which is palpable and frequently visible. During palpation of the prominence, it can be felt to recede on swallowing. The vocal folds are at the level of the middle of the laryngeal prominence.

The *cricoid cartilage* can be felt inferior to the laryngeal prominence at the level of the C6 vertebra. Extend your neck as far as possible and run your finger over the laryngeal prominence. As your finger passes inferiorly from the prominence, feel the *cricothyroid ligament*, the site for a needle *cricothyrotomy or coniotomy* (see the clinical box "Aspiration of Foreign Bodies and Heimlich Maneuver"). After your finger passes over the arch of the cricoid cartilage, note that your fingertip sinks in because the arch of the cartilage projects farther anteriorly than the rings of the trachea. The cricoid cartilage, a key landmark in the neck, indicates the

- level of the C6 vertebra.
- site where the carotid artery can be compressed against the transverse process of the C6 vertebra.
- junction of the larynx and trachea.
- joining of the pharynx and esophagus.
- point where the recurrent laryngeal nerve enters the larynx.
- site that is approximately 3 cm superior to the isthmus of the thyroid gland.

The **first tracheal cartilage** is broader than the others and is palpable (Fig. 9.33A). The second through fourth cartilages cannot be felt because the thyroid isthmus connecting the right and left lobes of the thyroid covers them.

The *thyroid gland* may be palpated by anterior or posterior approaches (i.e., standing in front of or behind the person). Place your fingertips anterior (for the isthmus) or immediately lateral (for the lobes) to the trachea and then direct the person to swallow (see Bickley, 2016, for details). Although both approaches to examining the thyroid are performed, the posterior approach usually allows better palpation, but the anterior approach allows observation. A perfectly normal thyroid gland may not be visible or distinctly palpable in some females, except during menstruation or pregnancy. The normal gland has the consistency of muscle tissue. AN43.6

The *isthmus of the thyroid gland* lies immediately inferior to the cricoid cartilage; it extends approximately 1.25 cm on either side of the midline. It can usually be felt by placing the fingertips of one hand on the midline below the cricoid arch and then asking the person to swallow. The isthmus will be felt moving up and then down. The apex of each *lobe of the thyroid gland* extends superiorly to the middle of the lamina of the thyroid cartilage (Fig. 9.50).

The surface anatomy of the posterior aspect of the neck is described in Chapter 2, Back. Key points are the following:

- The *spinous processes of the C6 and C7 vertebrae* are palpable and visible, especially when the neck is flexed.

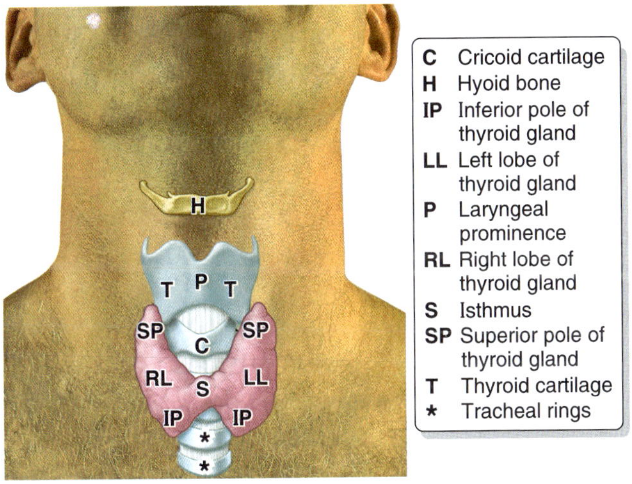

FIGURE 9.50. **Surface anatomy of endocrine and respiratory layers of neck.**

- The *transverse processes of the C1, C6, and C7 vertebrae* are palpable.
- The *tubercles of the C1 vertebra* can be palpated by deep pressure postero-inferior to the tips of the mastoid processes.

LYMPHATICS OF NECK

Most superficial tissues in the neck are drained by lymphatic vessels that enter the **superficial cervical lymph nodes**, which are located along the course of the EJV. Lymph from these nodes, like lymph from all of the head and neck, drains into **inferior deep cervical lymph nodes** (Figs. 9.51 and 9.52). The specific group of inferior deep cervical nodes involved here descends across the lateral cervical region with the spinal accessory nerve (CN XI). AN35.5

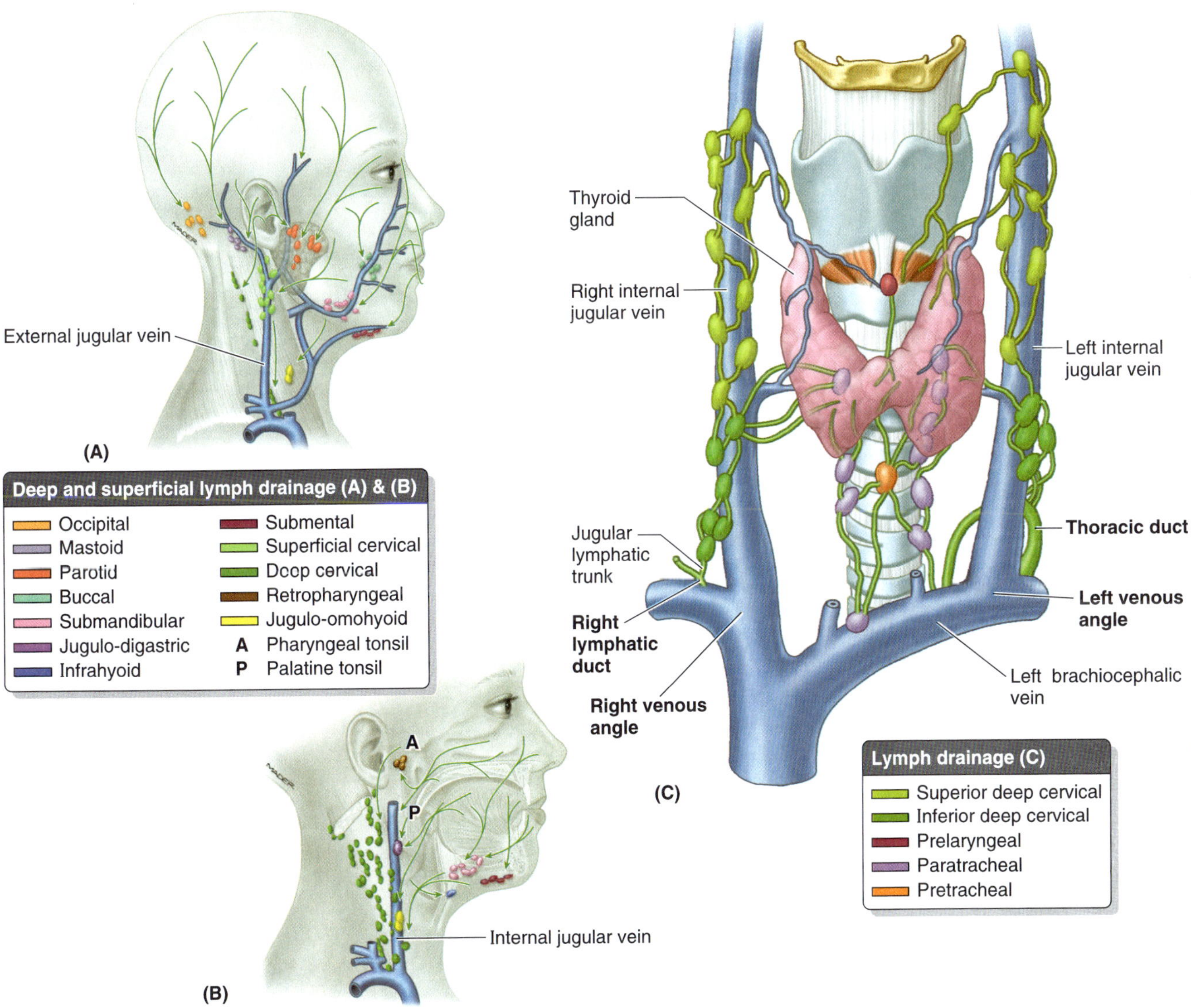

FIGURE 9.51. **Lymphatic drainage of head and neck. A, B.** The pathways of the superficial and deep lymphatic drainages are shown, respectively. **C.** The lymph nodes, lymphatic trunks, and thoracic duct are shown.

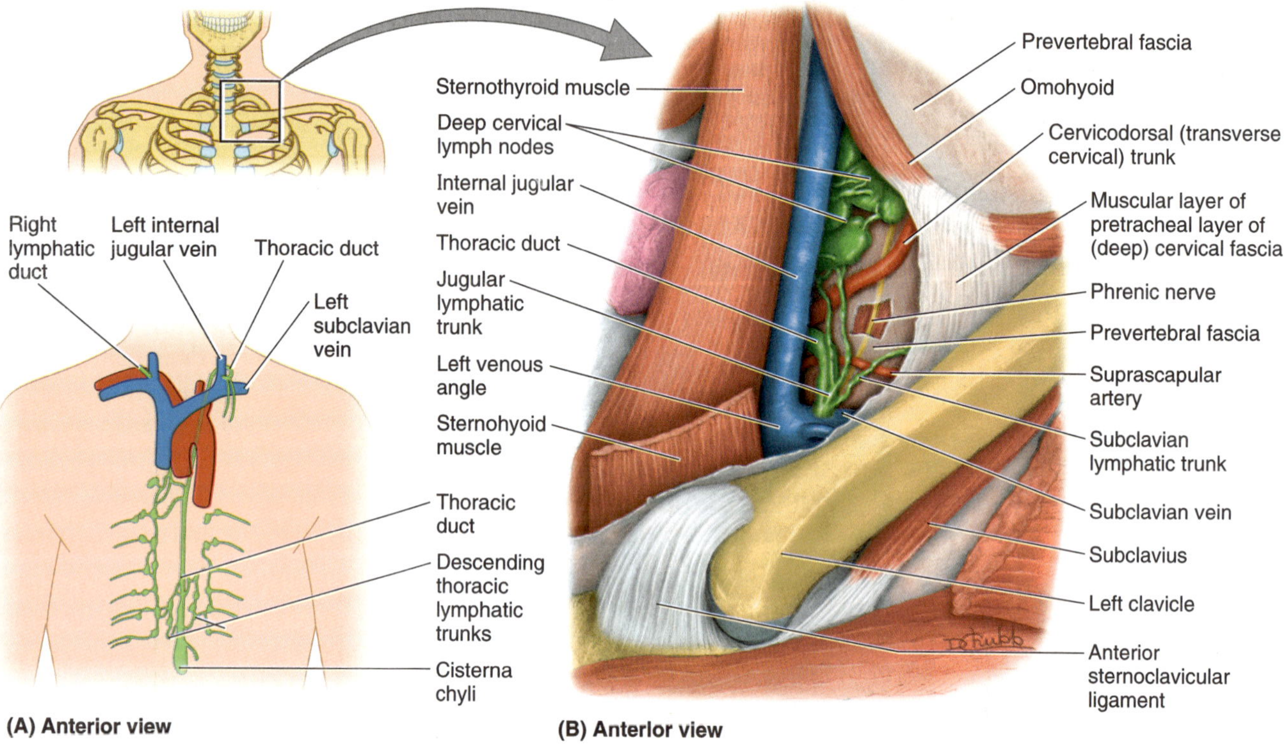

FIGURE 9.52. Lymphatic vessels in root of neck. A. This overview demonstrates the course of the thoracic duct and site of the termination of the thoracic and right lymphatic ducts. **B.** This dissection of the left side shows the deep cervical lymph nodes and the termination of the thoracic duct at the junction of the subclavian and internal jugular veins (left venous angle). The cervicodorsal trunk is often called the transverse cervical artery.

Most lymph from the six to eight lymph nodes then drains into the *supraclavicular group of nodes*, which accompany the cervicodorsal trunk. The main group of deep cervical lymph nodes forms a chain along the IJV, mostly under cover of the SCM. Other deep cervical nodes include the prelaryngeal, pretracheal, paratracheal, and retropharyngeal nodes. Efferent lymphatic vessels from the deep cervical nodes join to form the **jugular lymphatic trunks**, which usually join the thoracic duct on the left side and enter the junction of the internal jugular and subclavian veins (right venous angle) directly or via a short right lymphatic duct on the right.

The **thoracic duct** passes superiorly through the superior thoracic aperture along the left border of the esophagus. It arches laterally in the root of the neck, posterior to the carotid sheath and anterior to the sympathetic trunk and vertebral and subclavian arteries (Fig. 9.52B). The thoracic duct enters the left brachiocephalic vein at the junction of the subclavian and IJVs (*left venous angle*). When the right jugular, subclavian, and bronchomediastinal lymphatic trunks unite to form a right *lymphatic duct*, it enters the right venous angle as the thoracic duct does on the left (Fig. 9.52A). Often, however, these lymphatic trunks enter the venous system independently in the region of the right venous angle.

CLINICAL BOX

VISCERA AND LYMPHATICS OF NECK

Thyroid Ima Artery

In approximately 10% of people, a small, unpaired *thyroid ima artery* (L. *arteria thyroidea ima*) arises from the brachiocephalic trunk (Fig. B9.5); however, it may arise from the arch of the aorta or from the right common carotid, subclavian, or internal thoracic arteries. This small ima artery ascends on the anterior surface of the trachea to the isthmus of the thyroid gland, supplying branches to both structures. The possible presence of this artery must be considered when performing procedures in the midline of the neck inferior to the isthmus, because it is a potential source of bleeding (see the clinical box "Tracheostomy" in this chapter).

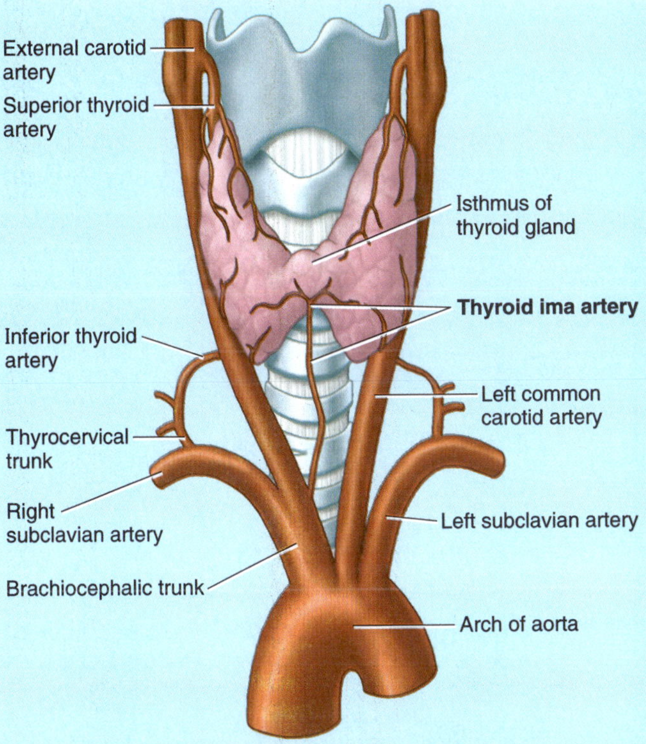

FIGURE B9.5. Thyroid ima artery.

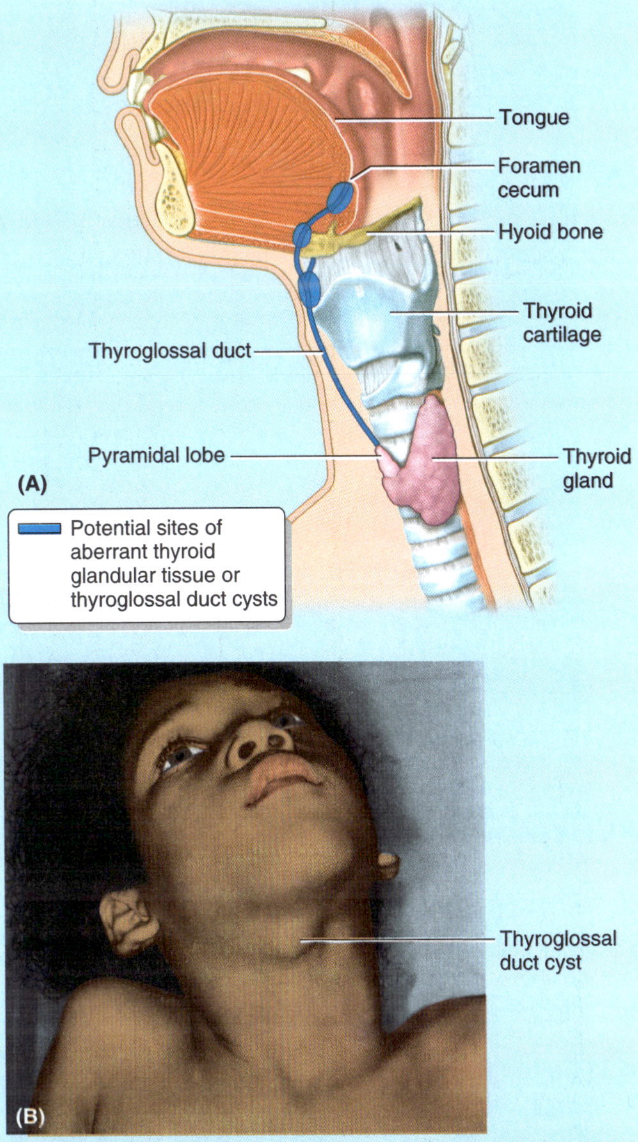

FIGURE B9.6. **A.** Thyroglossal duct vestiges. **B.** Child with thyroglossal duct cyst.

Thyroglossal Duct Cysts

AN43.4 Development of the thyroid gland begins in the floor of the embryonic pharynx at the site indicated by a small pit, the *foramen cecum*, in the dorsum of the postnatal tongue (Chapter 8, Head). Subsequently, the developing gland relocates from the tongue into the neck, passing anterior to the hyoid and thyroid cartilages to reach its final position anterolateral to the superior part of the trachea (Moore et al., 2016). During this relocation, the thyroid gland is attached to the foramen cecum by the **thyroglossal duct**. This duct normally disappears, but remnants of epithelium may remain and form a *thyroglossal duct cyst* at any point along the path of its descent (Fig. B9.6A). The cyst is usually in the neck, close or just inferior to the hyoid, and forms a swelling in the anterior part of the neck. Surgical excision of the cyst may be necessary. Most thyroglossal duct cysts are in the neck, close or just inferior to the body of the hyoid (Fig. B9.6B).

Aberrant Thyroid Gland

Aberrant thyroid glandular tissue may be found anywhere along the path of the embryonic thyroglossal duct. Although uncommon, the thyroglossal duct carrying thyroid-forming tissue at its distal end may fail to relocate to its definitive position in the neck. Aberrant thyroid tissue may be in the root of the tongue, just posterior to the foramen cecum, resulting in a **lingual thyroid gland**, or in the neck, at or just inferior to the hyoid (Fig. B9.7A). Cystic remnants of the thyroglossal duct may be differentiated from an undescended thyroid by radioisotope scanning (Fig. B9.7B). As a rule, an ectopic thyroid gland in the median plane of the neck is the only thyroid tissue present. Occasionally, thyroid glandular tissue is associated with a thyroglossal duct cyst. Therefore, it is important to differentiate between an ectopic thyroid gland and a thyroglossal duct cyst when excising a cyst. Failure to do so may result in a *total thyroidectomy*, leaving the person permanently dependent on thyroid medication (Leung et al., 1995).

Accessory Thyroid Glandular Tissue

Portions of the thyroglossal duct may persist to form thyroid tissue. *Accessory thyroid glandular tissue* may appear anywhere along the embryonic

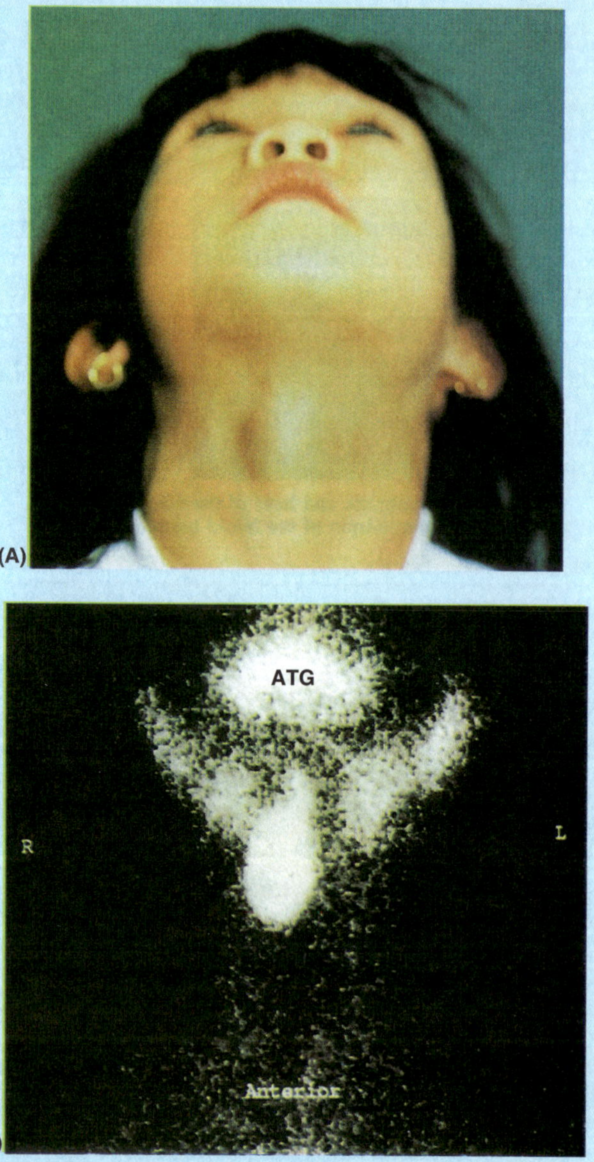

FIGURE B9.7. **Aberrant thyroid glandular tissue. A.** Aberrant tissue inferior to hyoid bone. **B.** Radioisotope scan demonstrating presence of aberrant thyroid glandular tissue (*ATG*). Glandular tissue in the typical position is present in irregularly shaped masses making up small tapering lobes and a large isthmus.

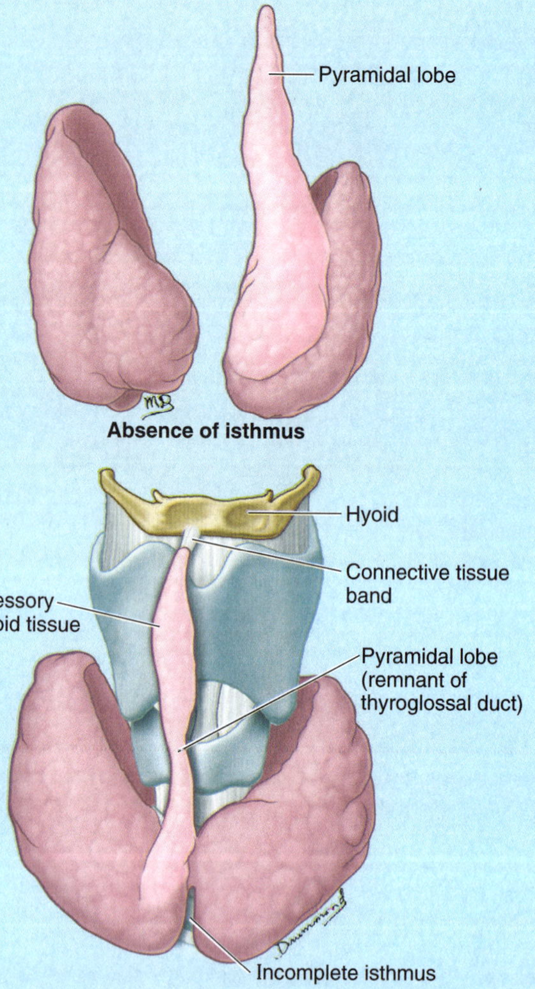

FIGURE B9.8. **Pyramidal lobe of thyroid gland.**

course of the thyroglossal duct (e.g., in the thymus inferior to the thyroid gland or in the thorax). An *accessory thyroid gland* may develop in the neck lateral to the thyroid cartilage; it usually lies on the thyrohyoid muscle (Fig. 9.29). Although the accessory gland may be functional, it is often of insufficient size to maintain normal function if the thyroid gland is removed.

Pyramidal Lobe of Thyroid Gland

Approximately 50% of thyroid glands have a *pyramidal lobe*. This lobe, which varies in size, extends superiorly from the isthmus of the thyroid gland, usually to the left of the median plane; the isthmus may be incomplete or absent (Fig. B9.8). A band of connective tissue, often containing accessory thyroid tissue, may continue from the apex of the pyramidal lobe to the hyoid. This narrow lobe and connective tissue band develop from remnants of the epithelium and connective tissue of the thyroglossal duct.

Enlargement of Thyroid Gland

AN35.8

A nonneoplastic, noninflammatory *enlargement of the thyroid gland*, other than the variable enlargement that may occur during menstruation and pregnancy, is called a *goiter*, which results from a lack of iodine. It is common in parts of the world where the soil and water are deficient in iodine. The enlarged gland causes a swelling in the neck that may compress the trachea, esophagus, and recurrent laryngeal nerves (Fig. B9.9). When the gland enlarges, it may do so anteriorly, posteriorly, inferiorly, or laterally. It cannot move superiorly because of the superior attachments of the overlying sternothyroid and sternohyoid muscles (Table 9.3). Substernal extension of a goiter is also common.

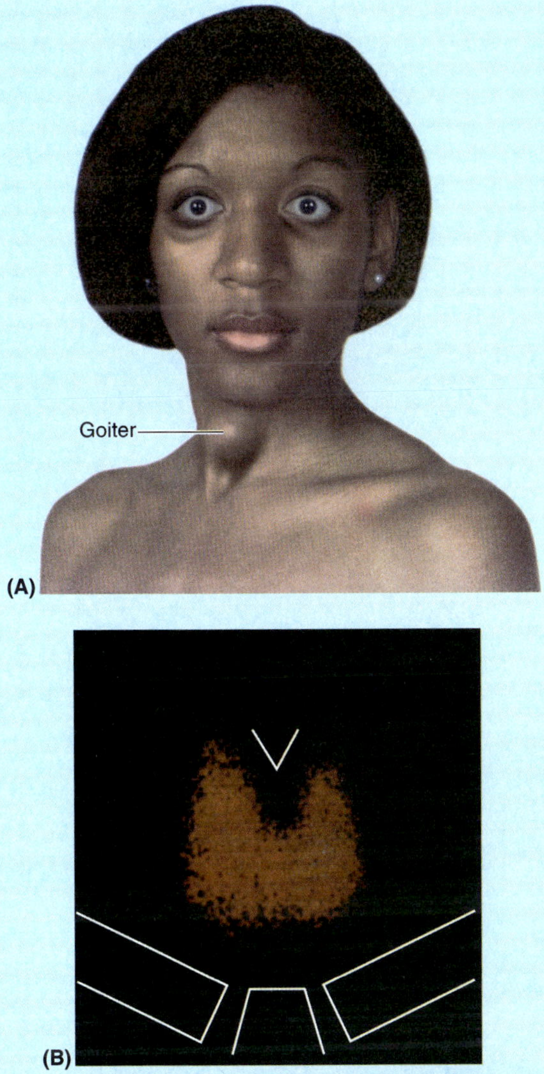

FIGURE B9.9. Enlarged thyroid. A. Individual with a goiter. **B.** Scintigram showing a diffuse, enlarged thyroid gland.

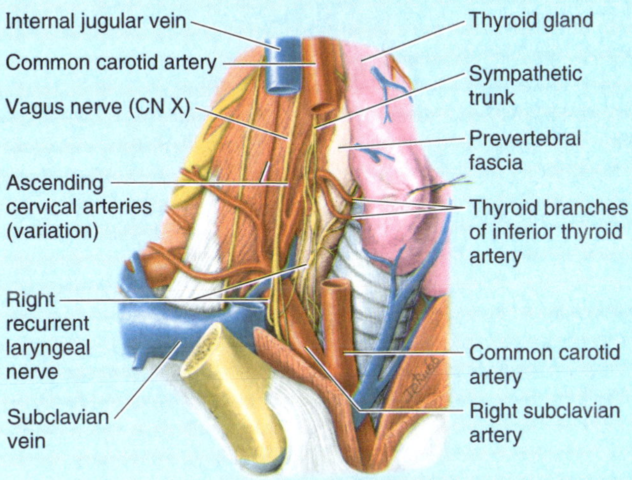

FIGURE B9.10. Injury to recurrent laryngeal nerves.

Thyroidectomy

Excision of a malignant tumor of the thyroid gland, or other surgical procedure, sometimes necessitates removal of part or all of the gland (*hemithyroidectomy* or *thyroidectomy*). In the surgical treatment of hyperthyroidism, the posterior part of each lobe of the enlarged thyroid is usually preserved, a procedure called *near-total thyroidectomy*, to protect the recurrent and superior laryngeal nerves and to spare the parathyroid glands. Postoperative hemorrhage after thyroid gland surgery may compress the trachea, making breathing difficult. The blood collects within the fibrous capsule of the gland.

AN38.3 Injury to Recurrent Laryngeal Nerves

The risk of *injury to the recurrent laryngeal nerves* is ever present during neck surgery. Near the inferior pole of the thyroid gland, the right recurrent laryngeal nerve is intimately related to the inferior thyroid artery and its branches (Fig. B9.10). This nerve may cross anterior or posterior to branches of the artery, or it may pass between them. Because of this close relationship, the inferior thyroid artery is ligated some distance lateral to the thyroid gland, where it is not close to the nerve. Although the danger of injuring the left recurrent laryngeal nerve during surgery is not as great, owing to its more vertical ascent from the superior mediastinum, the artery and nerve are also closely associated near the inferior pole of the thyroid gland (Fig. 9.28). Hoarseness is the usual sign of unilateral recurrent nerve injury; however, temporary *aphonia* or disturbance of phonation (voice production) and laryngeal spasm may occur. These signs usually result from bruising the recurrent laryngeal nerves during surgery or from the pressure of accumulated blood and serous exudate after the operation.

Inadvertent Removal of Parathyroid Glands

The variable position of the parathyroid glands, especially the inferior ones, puts them in danger of being damaged or removed during surgical procedures in the neck. The superior parathyroid glands may be as far superior as the thyroid cartilage, and the inferior glands may be as far inferior as the superior mediastinum (Fig. 9.31B). The aberrant sites of these glands are of concern when searching for abnormal parathyroid glands, as may be necessary in treating *parathyroid adenoma*, an ordinarily benign tumor of epithelial tissue associated with *hyperparathyroidism*.

Atrophy or inadvertent surgical removal of all the parathyroid glands results in tetany, a severe neurologic syndrome characterized by muscle twitches and cramps. The generalized spasms are caused by decreased serum calcium levels. Because laryngeal and respiratory muscles are involved, failure to respond immediately with appropriate therapy can result in death. To safeguard these glands during thyroidectomy, surgeons usually preserve the posterior part of the lobes of the thyroid gland.

In cases in which it is necessary to remove the whole thyroid gland (e.g., because of malignant disease), the parathyroid glands are carefully isolated with their blood vessels intact before removal of the thyroid gland. Parathyroid tissue may also be transplanted, usually to the arm, so it will not be damaged by subsequent surgery or radiation therapy.

Fractures of Laryngeal Skeleton

Laryngeal fractures may result from blows received in sports, such as kick boxing and hockey, or from compression by a shoulder strap during an automobile accident. Because of the frequency of this type of injury, most goalies in ice hockey and catchers in baseball have protective guards hanging from their masks that cover their larynges. Laryngeal fractures produce submucous hemorrhage and edema, respiratory obstruction, hoarseness, and sometimes a temporary inability to speak.

Laryngoscopy

Laryngoscopy is the procedure used to examine the interior of the larynx. The larynx may be examined visually by *indirect laryngoscopy* using a laryngeal mirror (Fig. B9.11A). The anterior part of the tongue is gently pulled from the oral cavity to minimize the extent to which the posterior part of the tongue covers the epiglottis and laryngeal inlet. Because the rima vestibuli is larger than the rima glottidis during normal respiration, the vestibular folds and vocal folds are visible during a laryngoscopic examination (Fig. B9.11B). The larynx can also be viewed by *direct laryngoscopy*, using a tubular endoscopic instrument, a laryngoscope. A *laryngoscope* is a tube or flexible fiber optic endoscope equipped with electrical lighting for examining or operating on the interior of the larynx through the mouth. The vestibular folds normally appear pink, whereas the vocal folds are usually pearly white.

Valsalva Maneuver

The sphincteric actions of the vestibular and vocal folds are important during the *Valsalva maneuver*, any forced expiratory effort against a closed airway, such as a cough, sneeze, or strain during a bowel movement or weight lifting. The vestibular and vocal folds abduct widely as the lungs inflate during deep inspiration. In the Valsalva maneuver, both the vestibular and vocal folds are tightly adducted at the end of deep inspiration. The anterolateral abdominal muscles then contract strongly to increase the intrathoracic and intra-abdominal pressures. The relaxed diaphragm passively transmits the increased abdominopelvic pressure to the thoracic cavity. Because high intrathoracic pressure impedes venous return to the right atrium, the Valsalva maneuver is used to study cardiovascular effects of raised peripheral venous pressure and decreased cardiac filling and cardiac output.

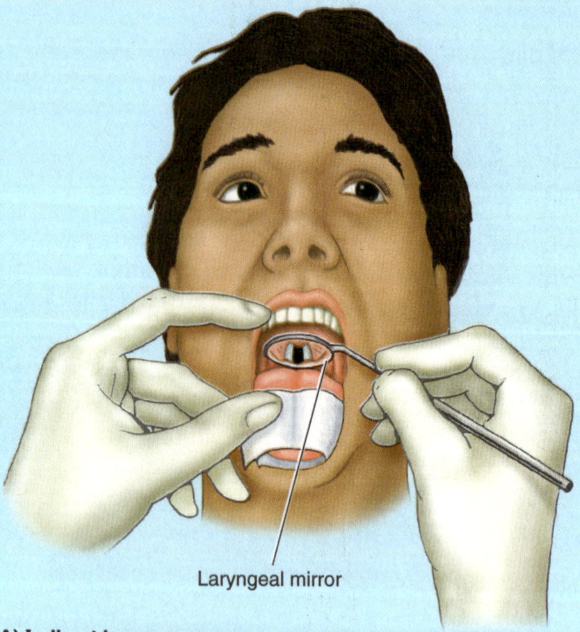

(A) Indirect laryngoscopy

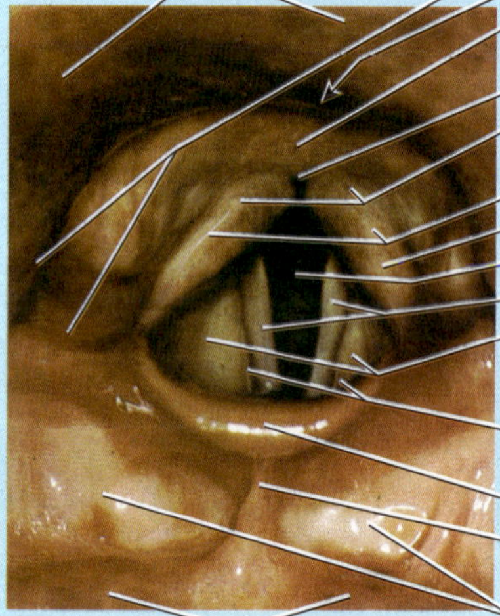

(B)

FIGURE B9.11. Laryngoscopy.

Aspiration of Foreign Bodies and Heimlich Maneuver

A foreign object, such as a piece of steak, may accidentally *aspirate* (be inhaled into the airways) through the laryngeal inlet into the vestibule of the larynx, where it becomes trapped superior to the vestibular folds. When a foreign object enters the vestibule of the larynx, the laryngeal muscles go into spasm, tensing the vocal folds. The rima glottidis closes, and no air enters the trachea. The resulting blockage may completely seal off the larynx (*laryngeal obstruction*) and choke the person, leaving the individual speechless because the larynx is blocked. *Asphyxiation* occurs, and the person will die in approximately 5 min from lack of oxygen if the obstruction is not removed.

A person who is choking will cough in an attempt to dislodge the object. The vestibular folds are part of the protective mechanism that closes the larynx. The mucosa of the vestibule is sensitive to foreign objects such as food. When an object passes through the laryngeal inlet and contacts the vestibular epithelium, violent coughing occurs. Emergency therapy must be given to open the airway. The procedure used depends on the condition of the person, the facilities available, and the experience of the person giving first aid.

Because the lungs still contain air, sudden compression of the abdomen (*Heimlich maneuver*) causes the diaphragm to elevate and compress the lungs, expelling air from the trachea into the larynx. This maneuver usually dislodges the food or other material from the larynx. To perform the Heimlich maneuver, the person giving first aid uses subdiaphragmatic abdominal thrusts to expel the foreign object from the larynx. First, the closed fist, with the base of the palm facing inward, is placed on the victim's abdomen between the umbilicus and the xiphoid process of the sternum (Fig. B9.12). The fist is grasped by the other hand and forcefully thrust inward and superiorly, forcing the diaphragm superiorly. This action forces air from the lungs and creates an artificial cough that usually expels the foreign object. Several abdominal thrusts may be necessary to remove the obstruction in the larynx.

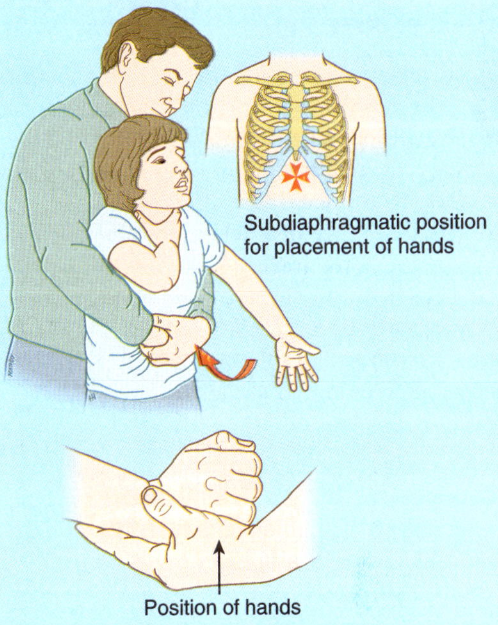

FIGURE B9.12. Heimlich maneuver.

Cricothyrotomy

In extreme emergency cases (e.g., severe airway obstruction, major facial or cervical trauma or angio-edema) where intubation isn't possible, experienced persons (e.g., physicians or EMT personnel) insert a large-bore needle through the cricothyroid membrane/ligament (Fig. 9.29) (*needle cricothyrotomy*, or "coniotomy") to permit fast entry of air. Later, a *surgical cricothyrotomy* (inferior laryngotomy) may be performed, which involves an incision through the skin and cricothyroid membrane and insertion of a *small tracheostomy tube* into the trachea (Fig. B9.13). Cricothyrotomy is a more expedient procedure than tracheostomy and manipulation of the cervical spine usually unnecessary.

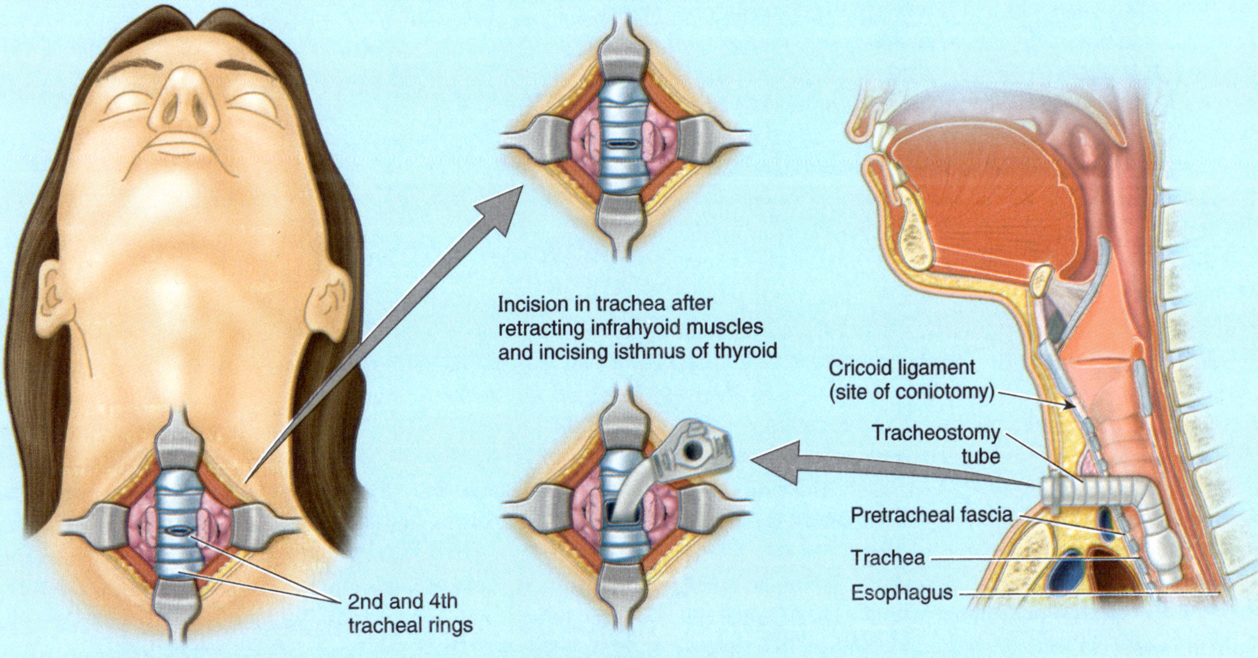

FIGURE B9.13. Tracheostomy.

Tracheostomy

A transverse incision through the skin of the neck and anterior wall of the trachea, *tracheostomy*, establishes an airway in patients with upper airway obstruction or respiratory failure (Fig. B9.13). The infrahyoid muscles are retracted laterally, and the isthmus of the thyroid gland is either divided or retracted superiorly. An opening is made in the trachea between the first and second tracheal rings or through the second through fourth rings. A *tracheostomy tube* is then inserted into the trachea and secured. To avoid complications during a tracheostomy, the following anatomical relationships are important:

- The *inferior thyroid veins* arise from a venous plexus on the thyroid gland and descend anterior to the trachea.
- A small *thyroid ima artery* is present in approximately 10% of people; it ascends from the brachiocephalic trunk or the arch of the aorta to the isthmus of the thyroid gland.
- The *left brachiocephalic vein*, jugular venous arch, and pleurae may be encountered, particularly in infants and children.
- The *thymus* covers the inferior part of the trachea in infants and children.
- The trachea is small, mobile, and soft in infants, making it easy to cut through its posterior wall and damage the esophagus.

Injury to Laryngeal Nerves

Because the inferior laryngeal nerve, the continuation of the recurrent laryngeal nerve, innervates the muscles moving the vocal fold, *paralysis of the vocal fold* results when *injury to laryngeal nerves occurs*. The voice is poor initially because the paralyzed vocal fold cannot adduct to meet the normal vocal fold. Within weeks, the contralateral fold crosses the midline when its muscles act to compensate. When bilateral paralysis of the vocal folds occurs, the voice is almost absent because the vocal folds are motionless in a position that is slightly narrower than the usually neutral respiratory position. They cannot be adducted for phonation, nor can they be abducted for increased respiration, resulting in *stridor* (high-pitched, noisy respiration) often accompanied by anxiety similar to that accompanying an asthmatic episode.

In progressive lesions of the recurrent laryngeal nerve, abduction of the vocal ligaments is lost before adduction; conversely, during recovery, adduction returns before abduction. Hoarseness is the common symptom of serious disorders of the larynx, such as carcinoma of the vocal folds.

Paralysis of the superior laryngeal nerve causes anesthesia of the superior laryngeal mucosa. As a result, the protective mechanism designed to keep foreign bodies out of the larynx is inactive, and foreign bodies can easily enter the larynx. Injury to the external branch of the superior laryngeal nerve results in a voice that is monotonous in character because the paralyzed cricothyroid muscle supplied by it is unable to vary the length and tension of the vocal fold (Table 9.5). Such an injury may be unnoticed in individuals who do not usually employ a wide range of tone in their speech, but it may be critical to singers or public speakers.

To avoid injury to the external branch of the superior laryngeal nerve (e.g., during thyroidectomy), the superior thyroid artery is ligated and sectioned more superior to the gland, where it is not as closely related to the nerve. Because an enlarged thyroid gland (goiter) may itself cause impaired innervation of the larynx by compressing the laryngeal nerves, the vocal folds are examined by laryngoscopy before an operation in this area. In this way, damage to the larynx or its nerves resulting from a surgical mishap may be distinguished from a pre-existing injury resulting from nerve compression.

Superior Laryngeal Nerve Block

A *superior laryngeal nerve block* is often administered with endotracheal intubation in the conscious patient. This technique is used for perioral endoscopy, transesophageal echocardiography, and laryngeal and esophageal instrumentation. The needle is inserted midway between the thyroid cartilage and the hyoid, 1–5 cm anterior to the greater horn of the hyoid. The needle passes through the thyrohyoid membrane and the anesthetic agent bathes the internal laryngeal nerve, the larger terminal branch of the superior laryngeal nerve. Anesthesia of the laryngeal mucosa occurs superior to the vocal folds and includes the superior surface of these folds.

Cancer of Larynx

The incidence of *cancer of the larynx* is high in individuals who smoke cigarettes or chew tobacco. Most persons present with persistent hoarseness, often associated with *otalgia* (earache) and *dysphagia* (difficulty in swallowing). Enlarged pretracheal or paratracheal lymph nodes may indicate the presence of laryngeal cancer. *Laryngectomy* (removal of the larynx) may be performed in severe cases of cancer. Vocal rehabilitation can be accomplished by an electrolarynx, a tracheo-esophageal prosthesis, or esophageal speech (regurgitation of ingested air).

Age Changes in Larynx

The larynx grows steadily until approximately 3 years of age, after which little growth occurs until approximately 12 years of age. Before puberty, no major laryngeal sex differences exist. Owing to the presence of testosterone at puberty in males, the walls of the larynx strengthen, and the laryngeal cavity enlarges. There is only a slight increase in the size of the larynx of most girls. In boys, all of the laryngeal cartilages enlarge and the laryngeal prominence becomes conspicuous in most males. The anteroposterior diameter of the rima glottidis almost doubles its prepubescent measurement in males, the vocal folds lengthening and thickening proportionately and abruptly. This growth accounts for the voice changes that occur in males: the pitch typically becomes an octave lower.

The pitch of the voice of *eunuchs*, males whose testes have not developed (*agonadal males*) or have been surgically removed (e.g., cancerous testes), does not become lower without administration of male hormones. The thyroid, cricoid, and most of the arytenoid cartilages often ossify as age advances, commencing at approximately 25 years of age in the thyroid cartilage. By 65 years of age, the cartilages are frequently visible in radiographs.

Foreign Bodies in Laryngopharynx

AN36.3 When food passes through the laryngopharynx during swallowing, some of it enters the piriform fossae. *Foreign bodies* (e.g., a chicken bone or fishbone) *entering the pharynx* may lodge in this recess. If the object is sharp, it may pierce the mucous membrane and injure the internal laryngeal nerve.

The superior laryngeal nerve and its internal laryngeal branch are also vulnerable to injury during removal of the object if the instrument used to remove the foreign body accidentally pierces the mucous membrane. Injury to these nerves may result in anesthesia of the laryngeal mucous membrane as far inferiorly as the vocal folds. Young children swallow a variety of objects, most of which reach the stomach and pass through the alimentary tract without difficulty. In some cases, the foreign body stops at the inferior end of the laryngopharynx, its narrowest part. A medical image such as a radiograph or a CT scan will reveal the presence of a radiopaque foreign body. Foreign bodies in the pharynx are often removed under direct vision through a pharyngoscope.

Tonsillectomy

AN36.4 *Tonsillectomy* (removal of the tonsils) is performed by dissecting the palatine tonsil from the tonsillar bed or by a guillotine or snare operation. Each procedure involves removal of the tonsil and surrounding connective tissue (Fig. B9.14). Because of the rich blood supply of the tonsil, bleeding commonly arises from the large *external palatine vein* (Fig. 9.45B) or, less commonly, from the tonsillar artery or other arterial twigs. The glossopharyngeal nerve (CN IX) accompanies the tonsillar artery on the lateral wall of the pharynx. Because this wall is thin, the nerve is vulnerable to injury. The internal carotid artery is especially vulnerable when it is tortuous and lies directly lateral to the tonsil (Fig. 9.47B).

Adenoiditis

Inflammation of the pharyngeal tonsils (adenoids—Fig. 9.44) is called *adenoiditis*, which can obstruct the passage of air from the nasal cavities through the choanae into the nasopharynx, making mouth breathing necessary. Infection from the enlarged pharyngeal tonsils may spread to the tubal tonsils, causing swelling and closure of the pharyngotympanic tubes. Impairment of hearing may result from nasal obstruction and blockage of the pharyngotympanic tubes. Infection spreading from the nasopharynx to the middle ear causes *otitis media* (middle ear infection), which may produce temporary or permanent hearing loss. Sometimes the palatine and pharyngeal tonsils are removed during the same operation (*tonsillectomy and adenoidectomy*; T&A).

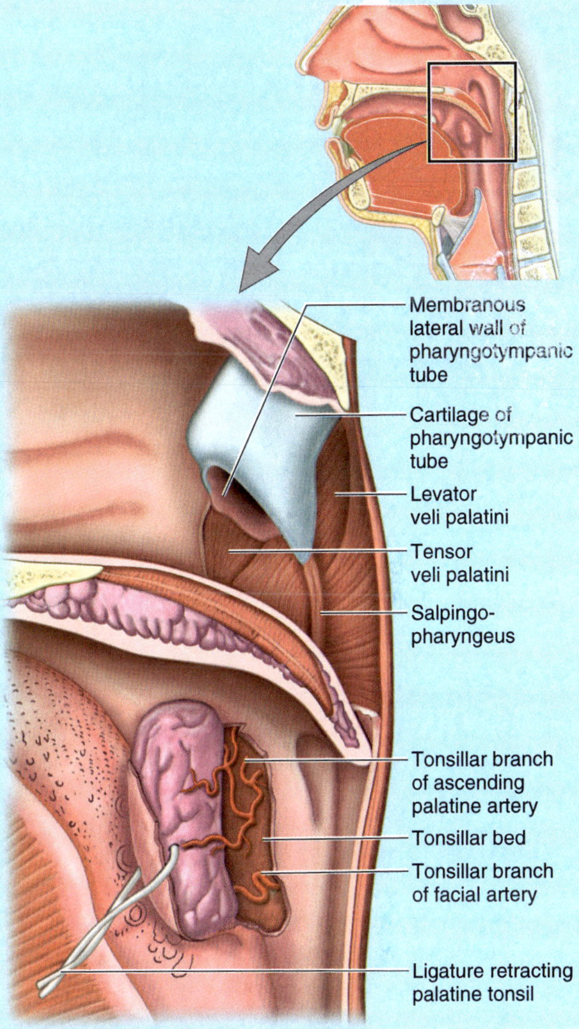

FIGURE B9.14. **Tonsillectomy.**

Branchial Fistula

A *branchial fistula* is an abnormal canal that opens internally into the tonsillar sinus (fossa) and externally on the side of the neck (Fig. B9.15A). Saliva may drip from the fistula, which may become infected. This uncommon cervical canal results from persistence of remnants of the 2nd pharyngeal pouch and 2nd pharyngeal groove (Moore et al., 2016). The fistula ascends from its cervical opening, usually along the anterior border of the SCM in the inferior third of the neck. It first passes through the subcutaneous tissue, platysma, and fascia of the neck to enter the carotid sheath. It then passes between the internal and the external carotid arteries on its way to its opening in the tonsillar sinus. Its course can be demonstrated by radiography (Fig. B9.15B). Refer *Langman's Medical Embryology*, South Asian Edition, Chapter 17, Head and Neck, p. 294 for **development of branchial apparatus** and pp. 300–301 for **congenital anomalies of branchial apparatus**. AN4

Branchial Sinuses and Cysts

When the embryonic cervical sinus fails to disappear, it may retain its connection with the lateral surface of the neck by a *branchial sinus*, a narrow canal. The

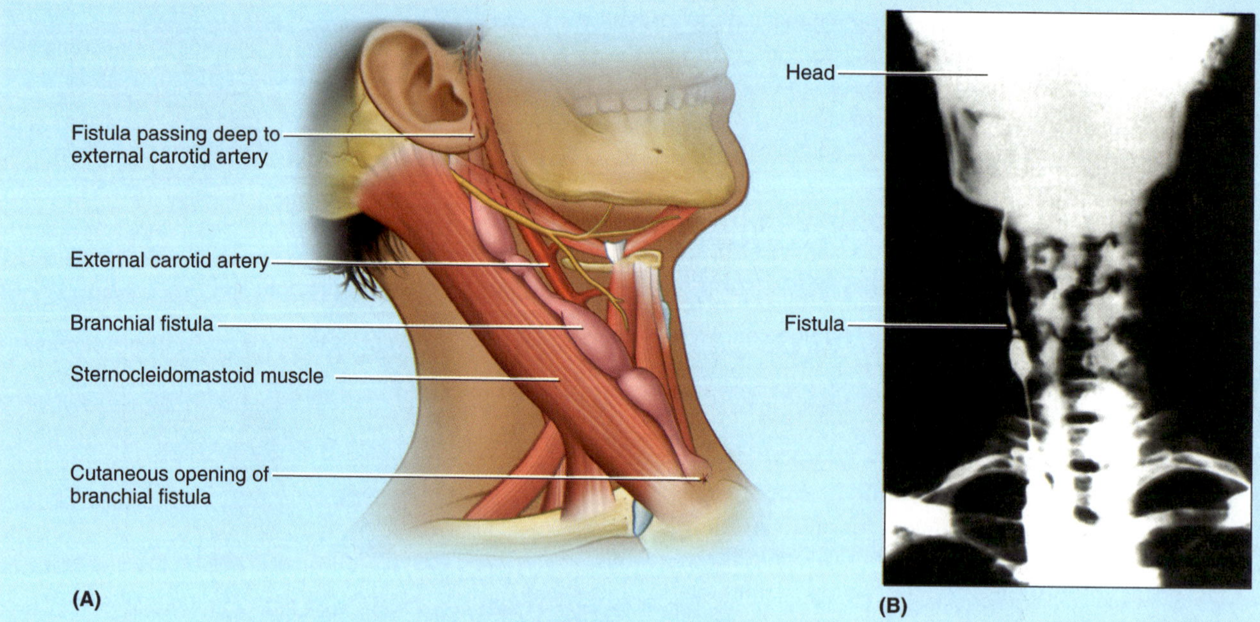

FIGURE B9.15. Branchial fistula.

opening of the sinus may be anywhere along the anterior border of the SCM (Fig. B9.16). If a remnant of the cervical sinus is not connected with the surface, it may form a *branchial cyst* (lateral cervical cyst), usually located just inferior to the angle of the mandible. Although branchial cysts may be present in infants and children, they may not enlarge and become visible until early adulthood. The sinus and cyst are usually excised. The cyst passes close to the hypoglossal, glossopharyngeal, and spinal accessory nerves (Fig. 9.47A). Therefore, care must be taken to avoid damage to these nerves during removal of the cyst.

Esophageal Injuries

Esophageal injuries are the rarest kinds of penetrating neck trauma; however, they are life threatening and cause the most complications after a surgical procedure or other treatment. Most esophageal injuries are iatrogenic (physician caused; 50–75%), occurring in conjunction with endoscopy, esophageal dilation, procedures involving strictures caused by radiation or tumor, and airway injuries. The latter occur because the airway lies anterior to the esophagus and provides some protection to it. Esophageal injuries are often occult (hidden), which makes the injury difficult to detect, especially if it is isolated. Unrecognized esophageal perforation is fatal in nearly all nonoperative cases (e.g., from vomiting—Boerhaave syndrome), in approximately 20% of iatrogenic occurrences, and in 7% of trauma perforations (Ezenkwele UA, 2016).

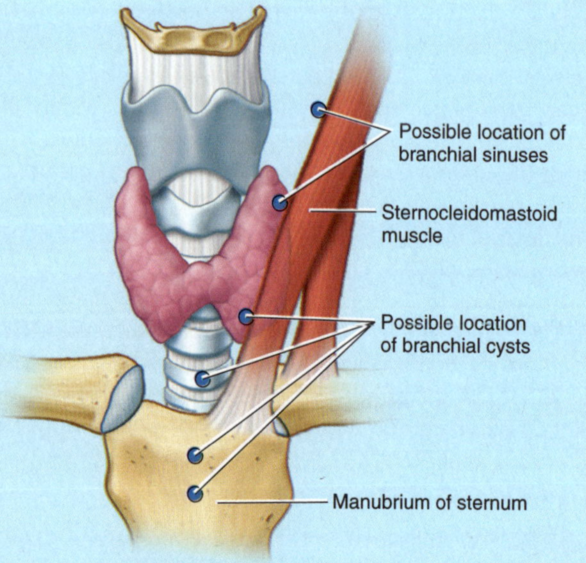

FIGURE B9.16. Branchial sinuses.

Tracheo-Esophageal Fistula

The most common birth defect of the esophagus is *tracheo-esophageal fistula (TEF)*. Usually, it is combined with some form of esophageal atresia. In the most common type of TEF (approximately 90% of cases), the superior part of the esophagus ends in a blind pouch and the inferior part communicates with the trachea (Fig. B9.17A). In these cases, the pouch fills with mucus, which the infant aspirates. In some cases, the superior esophagus communicates with the trachea and the inferior esophagus joins the stomach (Fig. B9.17C), but sometimes it does not, producing TEF with esophageal atresia (Fig. B9.17B). TEFs result from failures in partitioning of the esophagus and trachea (Moore et al., 2016). For embryological basis of tracheo-oesophageal AN25.4
fistula, refer *Langman's Medical Embryology*, South Asian Edition, Chapter 14, Respiratory System, p. 230.

Esophageal Cancer

The most common presenting complaint of *esophageal cancer* is *dysphagia* (difficulty in swallowing), which is not usually recognized until the lumen is reduced by 30–50%. *Esophagoscopy* is a common diagnostic

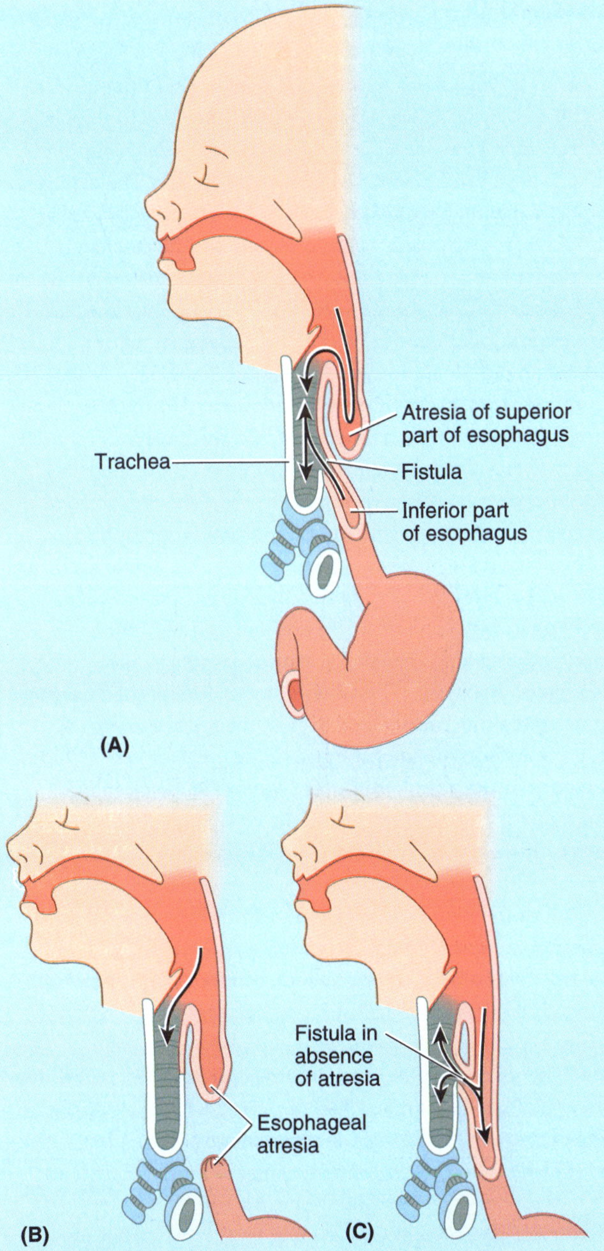

FIGURE B9.17. **Tracheo-esophageal fistulae (TEF).**

tool for observing these cancers. Painful swallowing in some patients suggests extension of the tumor to peri-esophageal tissues. Enlargement of the inferior deep cervical lymph nodes also suggests *esophageal cancer*. Compression of the recurrent laryngeal nerves by an esophageal tumor produces hoarseness.

Zones of Penetrating Neck Trauma

Three zones are common clinical guides to the seriousness of neck trauma (Fig. B9.18). The zones give physicians an understanding of the structures that are at risk with penetrating neck injuries:

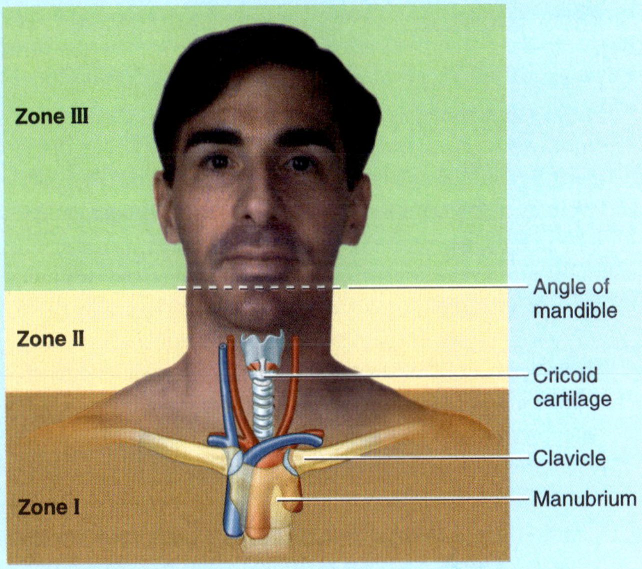

FIGURE B9.18. **Zones of penetrating neck trauma.**

- **Zone I**: includes the root of the neck and extends from the clavicles and the manubrium to the level of the inferior border of the cricoid cartilage. Structures at risk are the cervical pleurae, apices of lungs, thyroid and parathyroid glands, trachea, esophagus, common carotid arteries, jugular veins, and the cervical region of the vertebral column.
- **Zone II**: extends from the cricoid cartilage to the level of the angles of the mandible. Structures at risk are the superior poles of the thyroid gland, thyroid and cricoid cartilages, larynx, laryngopharynx, carotid arteries, jugular veins, esophagus, and cervical region of the vertebral column.
- **Zone III**: occurs at the angles of the mandibles superiorly. Structures at risk are the salivary glands, oral and nasal cavities, oropharynx, and nasopharynx.

Injuries in zones I and III obstruct the airway and have the greatest risk for **morbidity** (complications following surgical procedures and other treatments) and **mortality** (a fatal outcome) because the injured structures are difficult to visualize and repair and the vascular damage is difficult to control. Injuries in zone II are most common; however, morbidity and mortality are lower because physicians can control vascular damage by direct pressure and surgeons can visualize and treat injured structures more easily than they can in the other zones.

Radical Neck Dissections

Radical neck dissections are performed when cancer invades the cervical lymphatics. During the procedure, the deep cervical lymph nodes and tissues around them are removed as completely as possible. The major arteries, brachial plexus, CN X, and phrenic nerve are preserved; however, most cutaneous branches of the cervical plexus are removed. The aim of the dissection is to remove all tissue that bears lymph nodes in one piece. The deep cervical lymph nodes, particularly those located along the cervicodorsal trunk, may be involved in the spread of cancer from the thorax and abdomen. Because their enlargement may give the first clue to cancer in these regions, they are often referred to as the *cervical sentinel lymph nodes*.

The Bottom Line: Viscera of Neck

Endocrine layer of cervical viscera: Despite different developmental origins, the endocrine thyroid and parathyroid glands are intimately related. • Typically, the thyroid gland is roughly H-shaped, with right and left lobes linked by a thin central isthmus. • The thyroid gland wraps around the anterior and lateral aspects of the trachea at the level of the second to fourth tracheal rings; the isthmus lies anterior to the second and third rings. • Typically, there are four parathyroid glands (two superior and two inferior) within the capsule of the thyroid gland or in the gland itself. • An abundant blood supply, essential to the endocrine function, is provided to the thyroid gland by a four-way anastomosis between the right and left superior and inferior thyroid arteries, with the latter usually providing branches to the parathyroid glands. • Superior thyroid veins accompany the arteries of the same name, draining the area they supply. • Unaccompanied middle and inferior thyroid veins drain the inferior part of the thyroid gland: the superior and middle thyroid veins drain to the IJV, whereas the usually singular inferior thyroid vein enters the left brachiocephalic vein. • Vasomotor nerves course along the arteries, but the glands are regulated hormonally rather than by secretomotor nerve fibers. • Lymphatic vessels pass directly to the deep cervical lymph nodes or via nodes associated with the larynx and trachea.

Respiratory layer of cervical viscera: The larynx is the superior end of the lower respiratory tract, modified to regulate entry into or close off the lower respiratory tract. • The larynx also modifies the exit of air from the tract to produce tone for vocalization. • With the diaphragm, it regulates intra-abdominal pressure through air retention and the force and suddenness by which air exits the tract (e.g., exhaling verses coughing or sneezing). • The larynx consists of a cartilaginous articulating skeleton joined by ligaments, membranes, and muscles, lined with mucous membrane. • All the laryngeal muscles except one (posterior crico-arytenoid) participate in closure of the rima glottidis. • Active opening of the rima is required only during deep inspiration. • Otherwise, opening occurs passively by the tidal flow of air, with the other muscles controlling the amount and nature of resistance provided at the rima glottidis to produce tone and control its pitch. • In addition to intrinsically produced movements between its components, extrinsic musculature (hyoid muscles) can move the entire larynx for swallowing and to modify pitch further. • The internal laryngeal nerve, a branch of the superior laryngeal nerve, is the sensory nerve of the larynx. • The recurrent laryngeal nerve (via its terminal branch, the inferior laryngeal nerve) is the motor nerve, which supplies all muscles of the larynx, with one exception. • The external laryngeal nerve, a smaller branch of the superior laryngeal nerve, supplies the cricothyroid muscle. • The trachea is the median fibrocartilaginous tube extending between the cricoid cartilage at the C6 vertebral level and its bifurcation into main bronchi at the T4–T5 IV disc level (level of sternal angle).

Alimentary layer of cervical viscera: Although generally considered part of the alimentary tract, the pharynx is shared with the respiratory system. • The superior, noncollapsible nasopharynx is exclusively respiratory, and the air and food pathways cross within the oropharynx and laryngopharynx. • The contractile pharynx is unique within the alimentary tract in being constructed of voluntary muscle with the circular layer (pharyngeal constrictors) external to longitudinal muscle, the stylopharyngeus, palatopharyngeus, and salpingopharyngeus. • The flat posterior wall of the pharynx, abutting the musculoskeletal neck at the retropharyngeal space, is without openings; however, its anterior wall includes openings to the nose, mouth, and larynx. These openings determine the three segments of the pharynx. • The soft palate serves as a flap valve regulating access to or from the nasopharynx and oropharynx, whereas the larynx is the "valve" ultimately separating food and air before they enter the esophagus and trachea, respectively. • The superior two openings of the pharynx, which connect to the external environment, are encircled by a ring of lymphoid (tonsillar) tissue. • Gaps in the submucosal lateral wall, between attachments of the pharyngeal constrictor muscles, permit the passage of slip-like longitudinal muscles and neurovascular elements. • Innervation of the pharynx is from the pharyngeal nerve plexus, with the vagus providing the motor fibers and the glossopharyngeal providing sensory fibers. • At the level of the cricoid cartilage (C6 vertebral level), a relatively abrupt change is made to the muscular pattern more typical of the alimentary tract. • The cricopharyngeal part of the inferior pharyngeal constrictor, the most inferior part of the external circular layer, forms the superior esophageal sphincter. • Immediately inferior, as the outer muscular layer becomes longitudinal, the esophagus begins. • Also at approximately this point, sensory and motor innervation is transferred to the recurrent laryngeal nerves. • The cervical esophagus is composed of voluntary muscle.

Multiple-Choice Questions

1. **All of the following are branches of the external carotid artery EXCEPT:**
   a. Superior thyroid artery
   b. Ascending pharyngeal artery
   c. Transverse cervical artery
   d. Lingual artery
   (Ref: Page 1069)

2. **Venous drainage of cervical part of esophagus is into the:**
   a. Superior thyroid veins
   b. Inferior thyroid veins
   c. Common facial veins
   d. Anterior jugular veins
   (Ref: Page 1104)

3. **The clinical features of Horner's syndrome are all the following EXCEPT:**
   a. Ptosis
   b. Anhydrosis
   c. Enophthalmos
   d. Mydriasis
   (Ref: Page 1082)

4. **Which of the following nodes is called the tonsillar node?**
   a. Submandibular
   b. Jugulo-omohyoid
   c. Jugulodigastric
   d. Preauricular
   (Ref: Page 1103)

5. **The only abductor muscle of the vocal cords is:**
   a. Cricothyroid
   b. Lateral cricoarytenoid
   c. Posterior cricoarytenoid
   d. Thyroarytenoid
   (Ref: Page 1093)

6. **The ascending palatine artery is a branch of:**
   a. Facial artery
   b. Ascending pharyngeal artery
   c. Lingual artery
   d. Maxillary artery
   (Ref: Page 1069)

7. **The carotid sinus nerve is a branch of:**
   a. Trigeminal
   b. Glossopharyngeal
   c. Vagus
   d. Superior laryngeal
   (Ref: Page 1065)

8. **The carotid sheath encloses all the following EXCEPT:**
   a. Cervical sympathetic trunk
   b. Internal jugular vein
   c. Vagus nerve
   d. Internal carotid artery
   (Ref: Page 1053)

9. **The lingual artery runs deep to all the following EXCEPT:**
   a. Posterior belly of digastric
   b. Hypoglossal nerve
   c. Hyoglossus
   d. Middle pharyngeal constrictor
   (Ref: Page 1069)

10. **Which of the following nerves is in danger of injury during thyroid surgery?**
    a. Vagus
    b. Internal laryngeal
    c. Recurrent laryngeal
    d. Superior laryngeal
    (Ref: Page 1109)

11. Which one of the following is a typical cervical vertebra?

a. C1
b. C2
c. C6
d. C7

(Ref: Page 1049)

12. Which one of the following nerves passes deep to prevertebral fascia?

a. Phrenic nerve
b. Spinal accessory nerve
c. Supraclavicular nerve
d. Lesser occipital nerve

(Ref: Page 1061)

13. Which one of the following arteries is a branch of the second part of the subclavian artery?

a. Thyrocervical trunk
b. Costocervical trunk
c. Internal thoracic
d. Vertebral

(Ref: Page 1080)

14. The vertebral artery passes through foramen transversarium of all the following cervical vertebrae EXCEPT:

a. C3
b. C4
c. C6
d. C7

(Ref: Pages 1049, 1080)

15. Carotid tubercle is the anterior tubercle of the transverse process of which vertebra?

a. C4
b. C5
c. C6
d. C7

(Ref: Page 1079)

16. Post-mortem examination report of a case of strangulation mentions the fracture of a structure at vertebral level C3, which does not articulate with the rest of the skeleton. What structure is this?

a. Hard palate
b. Hyoid bone
c. Thyroid cartilage
d. Cricoid cartilage

(Ref: Page 1049)

17. During an ultrasound-guided supraclavicular brachial plexus block, the anesthetist observes an artery arising from the subclavian trunk, passing through the upper and middle trunks of the plexus and supplying levator scapulae and rhomboid muscles. Which artery is this?

a. Suprascapular artery
b. Subscapular artery
c. Dorsal scapular artery
d. Circumflex scapular artery

(Ref: Page 1059)

18. Which of the following arterial pulsations can be palpated in the greater supraclavicular fossa?

a. Superior thyroid artery
b. Subscapular artery
c. Superior laryngeal artery
d. Subclavian artery

(Ref: Page 1072)

19. Which of the following nerves is blocked when an anesthetic agent is instilled through a needle inserted midway between thyroid cartilage and hyoid, just anterior to its greater horn?

a. External laryngeal nerve
b. Recurrent laryngeal nerve
c. Superior laryngeal nerve
d. Inferior laryngeal nerve

(Ref: Page 1112)

20. An intern is asked to demonstrate inverted kite shape of rima glottidis during indirect laryngoscopy. What should he instruct the patient to do?

a. Deep inhalation
b. Normal respiration
c. Whisper
d. Valsalva maneuver

(Ref: Page 1092)

Answer Keys for MCQs

1. **c** 2. **b** 3. **d** 4. **c** 5. **c** 6. **a** 7. **b** 8. **a** 9. **d** 10. **c** 11. **c** 12. **a**
13. **b** 14. **d** 15. **c** 16. **b** 17. **c** 18. **d** 19. **c** 20. **a**

Refer to *Appendix A* at the end of the book for *Student Case Study Questions and Answers* of Volume 3.

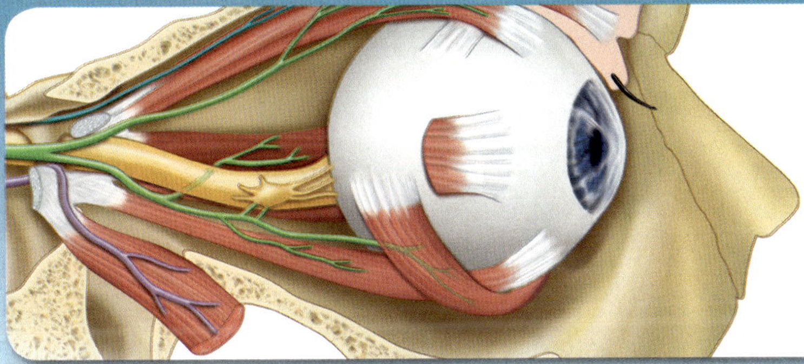

Summary of Cranial Nerves

10

OVERVIEW / 1120

TABLE 10.1. Cranial Nerves: Attachment to Central Nervous System, General Functions, and Distribution / 1121

TABLE 10.2. Summary of Cranial Nerves / 1124

TABLE 10.3. Cranial Parasympathetic Ganglia: Location; Sensory, Parasympathetic, and Sympathetic Roots and Main Distribution / 1127

OLFACTORY NERVE (CN I) / 1127

OPTIC NERVE (CN II) / 1128

OCULOMOTOR NERVE (CN III) / 1129

TROCHLEAR NERVE (CN IV) / 1132

TRIGEMINAL NERVE (CN V) / 1133

Ophthalmic Nerve (CN V_1) / 1135

Maxillary Nerve (CN V_2) / 1135

Mandibular Nerve (CN V_3) / 1135

ABDUCENT NERVE (CN VI) / 1135

TABLE 10.4. Summary of Divisions of Trigeminal Nerve (CN V) / 1136

FACIAL NERVE (CN VII) / 1138

Somatic (Branchial) Motor / 1140

Visceral (Parasympathetic) Motor / 1140

Somatic (General) Sensory / 1140

Special Sensory (Taste) / 1140

VESTIBULOCOCHLEAR NERVE (CN VIII) / 1140

GLOSSOPHARYNGEAL NERVE (CN IX) / 1142

Somatic (Branchial) Motor / 1142

Visceral (Parasympathetic) Motor / 1142

Somatic (General) Sensory / 1142

Special Sensory (Taste) / 1142

Visceral Sensory / 1142

VAGUS NERVE (CN X) / 1143

SPINAL ACCESSORY NERVE (CN XI) / 1146

TABLE 10.5. Summary of Vagus Nerve (CN X) / 1147

HYPOGLOSSAL NERVE (CN XII) / 1148

CLINICAL BOX: Cranial Nerves / **1151**

TABLE 10.6. Summary of Cranial Nerve Lesions / 1151

Multiple-Choice Questions / 1157

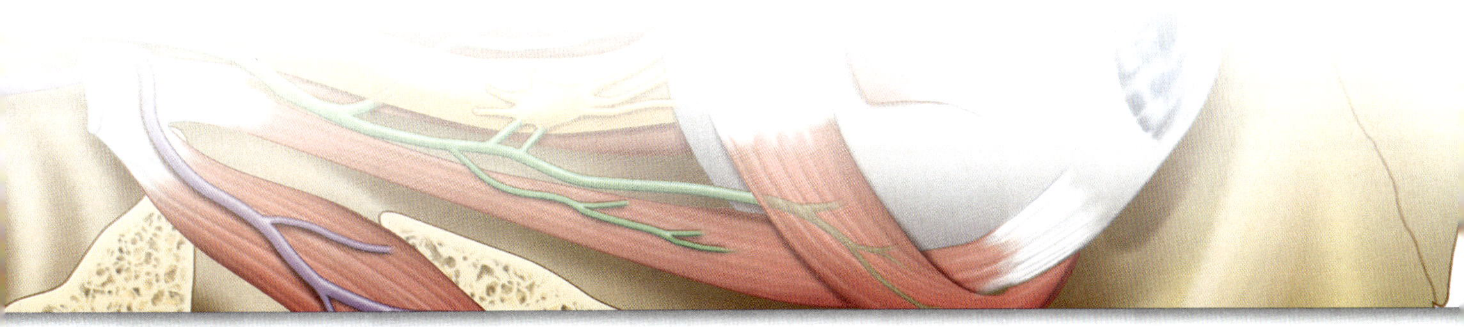

CLINICAL BOX KEY

Anatomical Variations | Diagnostic Procedures | Life Cycle | Surgical Procedures | Trauma | Pathology

Competencies Covered in the Chapter

AN28.4 Describe and demonstrate branches of facial nerve with distribution / 1138
AN28.7 Explain the anatomical basis of facial nerve palsy / 1154
AN30.5 Explain effect of pituitary tumors on visual pathway / 1152
AN31.2 Describe and demonstrate nerves in the orbit / 1129, 1132, 1135
AN31.5 Explain the anatomical basis of oculomotor nerve palsy / 972, 1152
AN31.5 Explain the anatomical basis of trochlear nerve palsy / 1153
AN31.5 Explain the anatomical basis of abducent nerve palsy along with strabismus / 972, 1154
AN34.1 Describe submandibular ganglion / 1127
AN35.7 Describe the course and branches of IX nerve in the neck / 1142
AN35.7 Describe the course and branches of X nerve in the neck / 1143
AN35.7 Describe the course and branches of XI nerve in the neck / 1146
AN35.7 Describe the course and branches of XII nerve in the neck / 1148
AN39.2 Explain the anatomical basis of hypoglossal nerve palsy / 1156
AN58.3 Enumerate cranial nerve nuclei in medulla oblongata with their functional group / 1121
AN59.3 Enumerate cranial nerve nuclei in pons with their functional group / 1121
AN62.1 Enumerate cranial nerve nuclei with its functional component / 1124

The regional aspects of the cranial nerves are described in the preceding chapters, especially those for the head and neck. This chapter summarizes all of the cranial nerves, largely in figures and tables. Figures 10.2 to 10.4 and Tables 10.1 and 10.2 summarize specific cranial nerves. Figure 10.5 and Table 10.3 summarize the cranial parasympathetic ganglia, their location, sympathetic and parasympathetic roots, and main distribution.

OVERVIEW

Like spinal nerves, **cranial nerves** are bundles of sensory or motor fibers that innervate muscles or glands, carry impulses from sensory receptors, or have a combination of motor and sensory fibers. They are called cranial nerves because they emerge from the cranial cavity via foramina or fissures in the cranium (Fig. 10.1) and are covered by tubular sheaths derived from the cranial meninges. There are 12 pairs of cranial nerves, which are numbered I–XII, from rostral to caudal (Figs. 10.1 to 10.4). Their names reflect their general distribution or function.

Cranial nerves carry one or more of the following five main functional components (Figs. 10.2 and 10.4; Tables 10.1 and 10.2).

- Motor (efferent) fibers
  1. *Motor fibers to voluntary* (striated) *muscle*. These include the somatic motor (general somatic efferent) axons. On the basis of the embryologic/phylogenetic derivation of certain muscles of the head and neck,[1] some motor fibers conveyed by cranial nerves to striated muscle have traditionally been classified as "special visceral." When appropriate, these fibers are designated somatic (branchial) motor, referring to the muscle tissue derived from the pharyngeal arches in the embryo (e.g., muscles of mastication).
  2. *Motor fibers involved in innervating involuntary* (smooth) *muscles or glands*. These include visceral motor (general visceral efferent) axons that constitute the cranial outflow of the parasympathetic division of the autonomic nervous system (ANS). The presynaptic (preganglionic)

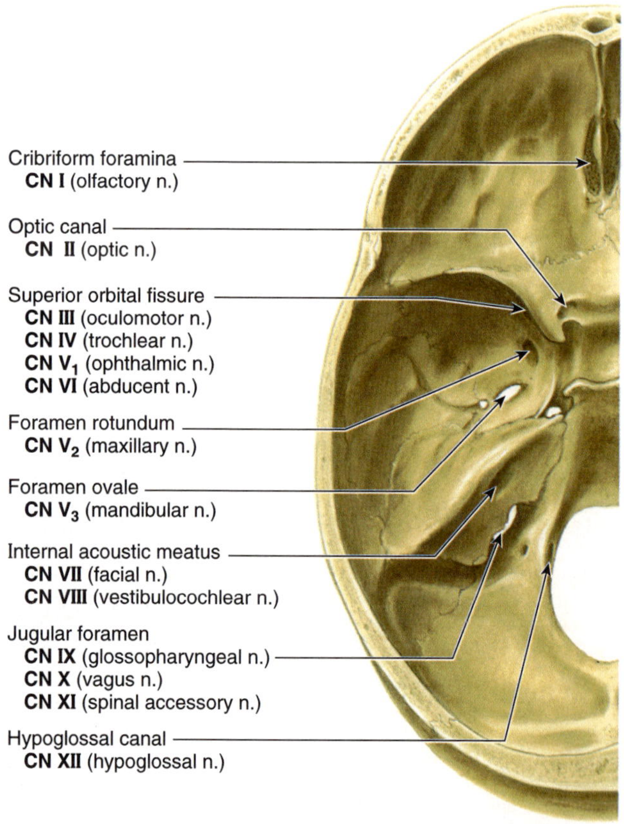

FIGURE 10.1. Cranial base and openings providing passage for cranial nerves.

[1]Historically, the sternocleidomastoid and trapezius have been classified as branchiomeric muscles. Students may see them classified as such in other references.

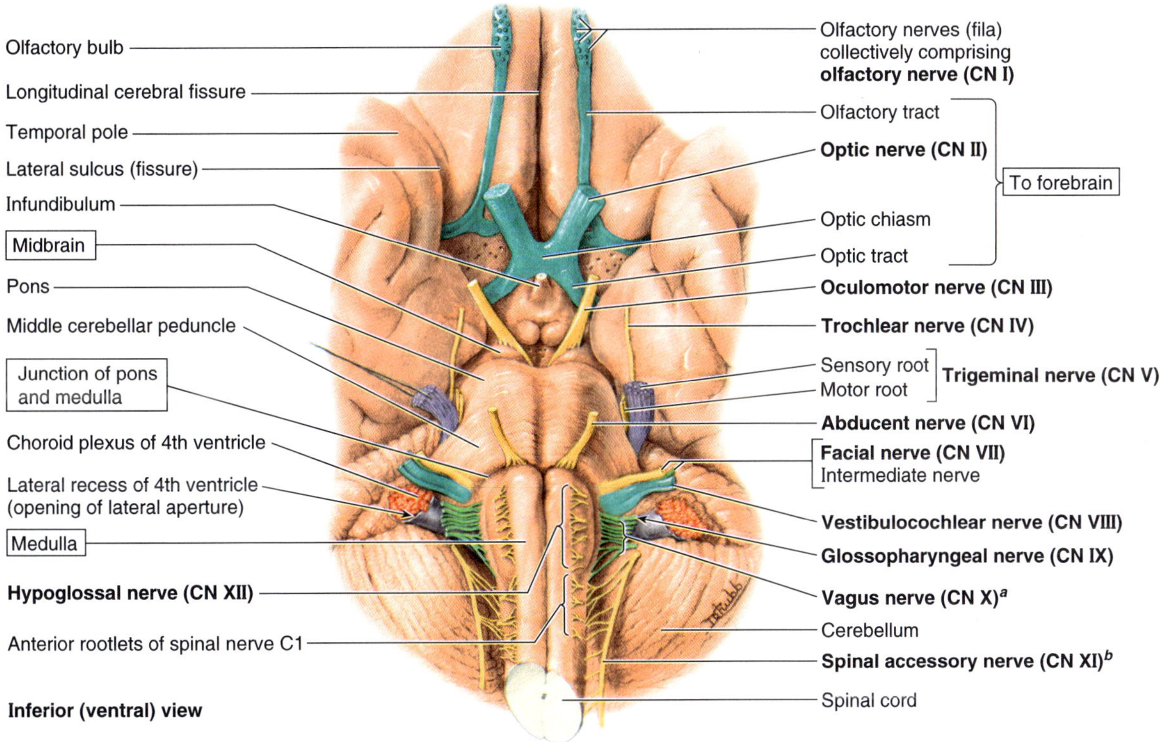

FIGURE 10.2. Superficial origins of cranial nerves from brain and spinal cord (except for CN IV, which arises from the posterior aspect of the midbrain). [a]The traditional "cranial root of the accessory nerve" is considered here as part of the vagus nerve. [b]The spinal accessory nerve as listed here refers to only the traditional "spinal root of the accessory nerve."

For cranial nerve nuclei in pons and medulla oblongata with their functional group, refer *Snell's Clinical Neuroanatomy*, South Asian Edition, Chapter 5,
AN58.3 Brainstem (Table 5-4), p. 216.

AN59.3 **TABLE 10.1. CRANIAL NERVES: ATTACHMENT TO CENTRAL NERVOUS SYSTEM, GENERAL FUNCTIONS, AND DISTRIBUTION**

Cranial Nerve Number	Cranial Nerve	Part of Central Nervous System from Which Nerve(s) Enter(s) or Emerge(s)		General Functional Types of Fibers[a]		General Distribution
I	**Olfactory**	Forebrain (pros-encephalon)	Cerebral hemispheres (telencephalon)	Special sensory		Olfactory mucosa of nose
II	**Optic**		Diencephalon			Retina of eye
III	**Oculomotor**	Midbrain (mesencephalon)		Motor[b]		Intra-ocular and four extra-ocular muscles
IV	**Trochlear**	Midbrain				One extra-ocular muscle (superior oblique)
V	**Trigeminal**	Brainstem	Pons (metencephalon)	Mixed	Motor root / Sensory root	Derivatives of frontonasal process and 1st pharyngeal arch
VI	**Abducent (abducens)**		Junction between pons and medulla	Motor[b]		One extra-ocular muscle (lateral rectus)
VII	**Facial**			Mixed	Primary root / Intermediate root	Derivatives of 2nd pharyngeal arch
VIII	**Vestibulocochlear**			Special Sensory[c]		Internal ear
IX	**Glossopharyngeal**		Medulla (myelencephalon)	Mixed		Derivatives of 3rd pharyngeal arch
X	**Vagus**					Derivatives of 4th pharyngeal arch
XI	**Spinal accessory**	Superior spinal cord		Motor[d]		Superficial layer of neck
XII	**Hypoglossal**	Brainstem	Medulla (myelencephalon)	Motor[e]		Muscles of tongue

[a]Note that the colors in this column match those of the nerves in Figure 10.2.
[b]The presence and function of proprioceptive afferent fibers to the extra-ocular muscles is controversial.
[c]The cochlear part of CN VIII, traditionally considered "purely sensory," actually conveys some efferent fibers that appear to modulate sensory sensitivity.
[d]Cranial nerve XI is purely motor as it leaves the CNS but gains pain and proprioceptive fibers from the cervical plexus in the lateral cervical region (posterior triangle) of the neck.
[e]Cranial nerve XII is purely motor as it leaves the CNS; pathways for proprioception associated with the tongue are unknown and may involve the lingual and glossopharyngeal nerves and cervical spinal nerves that communicate with CN XII.

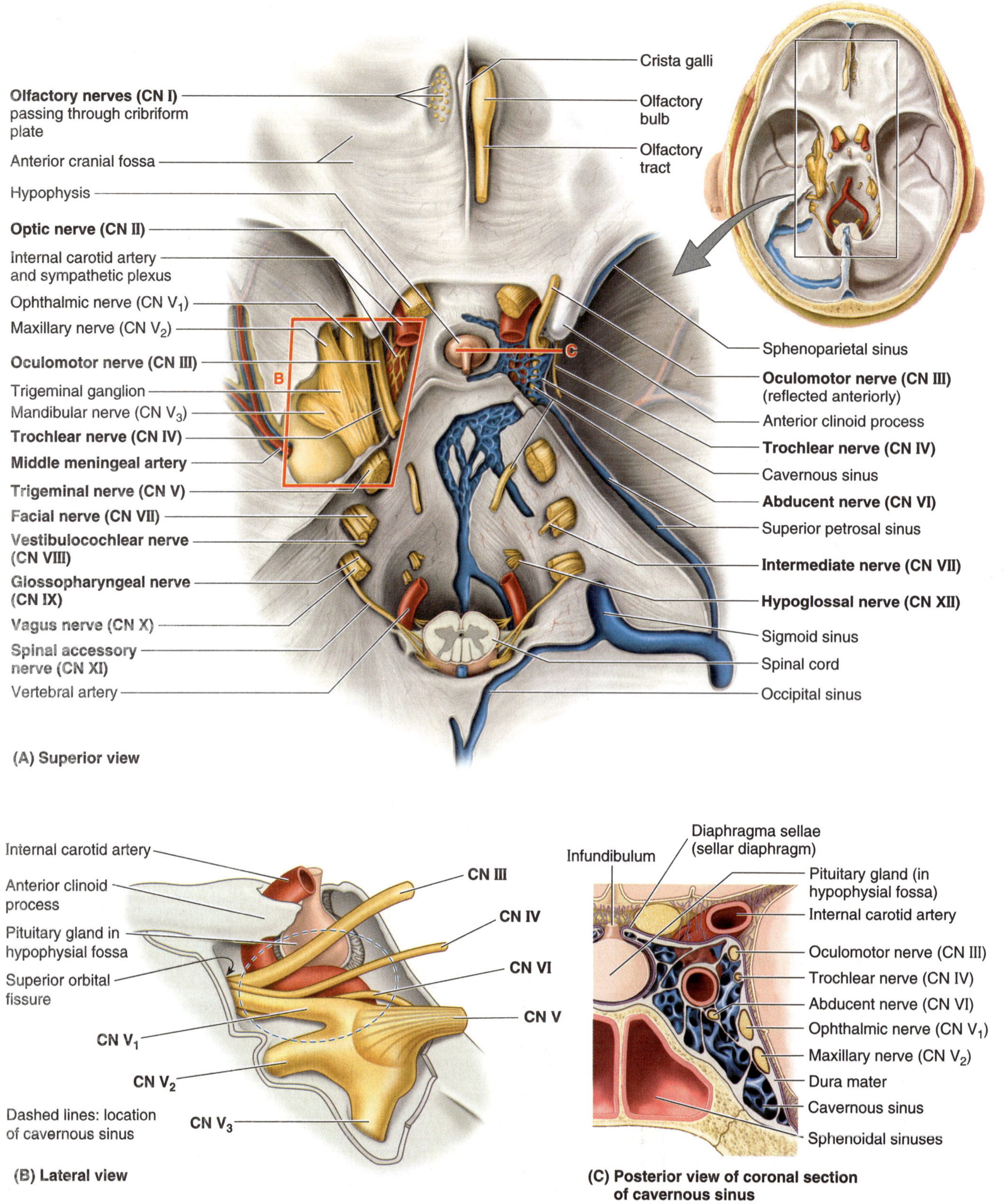

FIGURE 10.3. Cranial nerves in relation to internal aspect of cranial base and dural formations. A. The tentorium cerebelli has been removed, and the venous sinuses have been opened on the right side. The dural roof of the trigeminal cave has been removed on the left side, and CN V_1, CN III, and CN IV have been dissected from the lateral wall of the cavernous sinus. **B.** Lateral view of area outlined in red in **(A)**. Dura mater has been removed opening the trigeminal cave, cavernous sinus and hypophysial fossa, demonstrating contained cranial nerves, internal carotid artery, and hypophysis. **C.** Coronal section at plane indicated by line C in **(A)**. Structures and relationships within the cavernous sinus and its lateral wall.

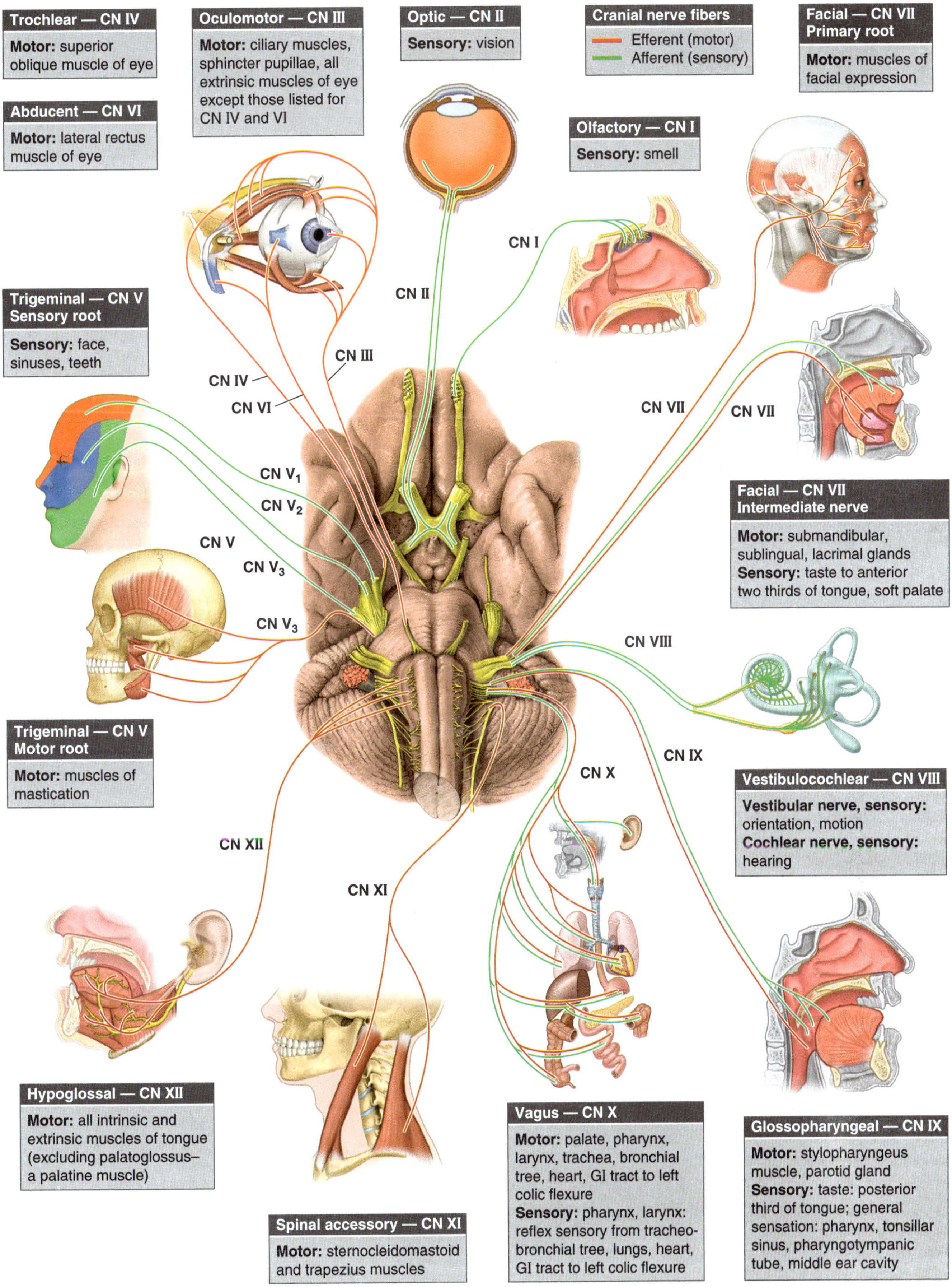

FIGURE 10.4. Summary of cranial nerves.

N62.1 **TABLE 10.2. SUMMARY OF CRANIAL NERVES**

Nerve	Components	Location of Nerve Cell Bodies (and Site of Synapse)	Cranial Exit	Function
Olfactory (CN I)	Special sensory (olfaction)	Olfactory epithelium (olfactory cells)	Foramina in cribriform plate of ethmoid bone	Smell from nasal mucosa of roof of each nasal cavity and superior sides of nasal septum and superior concha
Optic (CN II)	Special sensory (vision)	Retina (ganglion cells)	Optic canal	Vision from retina
Oculomotor (CN III)	Somatic motor	Midbrain (nucleus of oculomotor nerve)	Superior orbital fissure	Motor to superior rectus, inferior rectus, medial rectus, inferior oblique, and levator palpebrae superioris muscles; raises superior eyelid; rotates eyeball superiorly, inferiorly, and medially
	Visceral motor	*Presynaptic:* midbrain (Edinger-Westphal nucleus) *Postsynaptic:* ciliary ganglion		Parasympathetic innervation to sphincter pupillae and ciliary muscle; constricts pupil and accommodate lens of eye
Trochlear (CN IV)	Somatic motor	Midbrain (nucleus of trochlear nerve)		Motor to superior oblique to assist in turning eye inferolaterally (or inferiorly when adducted)
Trigeminal (CN V)				
Ophthalmic division ($CN\ V_1$)	Somatic (general) sensory	Trigeminal ganglion Synapse: sensory nucleus of trigeminal nerve		Sensation from cornea, skin of forehead, scalp, eyelids, nose, and mucosa of nasal cavity and paranasal sinuses
Maxillary division ($CN\ V_2$)			Foramen rotundum	Sensation from skin of face over maxilla including upper lip, maxillary teeth, mucosa of nose, maxillary sinuses, and palate
Mandibular division ($CN\ V_3$)			Foramen ovale	Sensation from the skin over mandible, including lower lip, side of head, mandibular teeth, temporomandibular joint, mucosa of mouth, and anterior two thirds of tongue
	Somatic (branchial) motor	Pons (motor nucleus of trigeminal nerve)		Motor to muscles of mastication, mylohyoid, anterior belly of digastric, tensor veli palatini, and tensor tympani
Abducent (CN VI)	Somatic motor	Pons (nucleus of abducent nerve)	Superior orbital fissure	Motor to lateral rectus to turn eye laterally
Facial (CN VII)	Somatic (branchial) motor	Pons (motor nucleus of facial nerve)	Internal acoustic meatus, facial canal, and stylomastoid foramen	Motor to muscles of facial expression and scalp; also supplies stapedius of middle ear, stylohyoid, and posterior belly of digastric
	Special sensory (taste)	Geniculate ganglion Synapse: nuclei of solitary tract		Taste from anterior two thirds of tongue and palate
	Somatic (general) sensory	Geniculate ganglion Synapse: sensory nucleus of trigeminal nerve		General sensation from skin of both aspects of auricle
	Visceral motor	*Presynaptic:* pons (superior salivatory nucleus) *Postsynaptic:* pterygopalatine ganglion and submandibular ganglion		Parasympathetic innervation to submandibular and sublingual salivary glands, lacrimal gland, and glands of nose and palate

TABLE 10.2. SUMMARY OF CRANIAL NERVES (Continued)

Nerve	Components	Location of Nerve Cell Bodies (and Site of Synapse)	Cranial Exit	Function
Vestibulocochlear (CN VIII)				
Vestibular	Special sensory (balance)	Vestibular ganglion Synapse: vestibular nuclei	Internal acoustic meatus	Vestibular sensation from semicircular ducts, utricle, and saccule related to position and movement of head
Cochlear	Special sensory (hearing)	Spiral ganglion Synapse: cochlear nuclei		Hearing from spiral organ
Glossopharyngeal (CN IX)	Somatic (branchial) motor	Medulla (nucleus ambiguus)	Jugular foramen	Motor to stylopharyngeus to assist with swallowing
	Visceral motor	*Presynaptic:* medulla (inferior salivatory nucleus) *Postsynaptic:* otic ganglion		Parasympathetic innervation to parotid gland
	Special sensory (taste)	Inferior sensory ganglion (nuclei of solitary tract)		Taste from posterior third of tongue and pharynx
	Somatic (general) sensory	Superior sensory ganglion (sensory nucleus of CN V)		Posterior auricle, tragus, posterior 1/3 of tongue, soft palate and pharynx
		Inferior sensory ganglion (sensory nucleus of CN V)		Tympanic cavity and membrane, pharyngo-tympanic tube, mastoid cells
	Visceral sensory	Inferior sensory ganglion (nuclei of solitary tract)		Carotid body (chemoreceptors) and sinus (baroreceptor)
Vagus (CN X)	Somatic (branchial) motor	Medulla (nucleus ambiguus)		Motor to constrictor muscles of pharynx, intrinsic muscles of larynx, muscles of palate (except tensor veli palatini), and striated muscle in superior two thirds of esophagus
	Visceral motor	*Presynaptic:* medulla *Postsynaptic:* intrinsic ganglia in, on, or near viscera		Parasympathetic innervation to smooth muscle of trachea, bronchi, digestive tract, and cardiac muscle
	Visceral sensory	Inferior ganglion Synapse: nuclei of solitary tract		Visceral sensation from base of tongue, pharynx, larynx, trachea, bronchi, heart, esophagus, stomach, and intestine
	Special sensory (taste)	Inferior ganglion Synapse: nuclei of solitary tract		Taste from epiglottis and palate
	Somatic (general) sensory	Superior ganglion Synapse: sensory nucleus of trigeminal nerve		Sensation from auricle, external acoustic meatus, and dura mater of posterior cranial fossa
Spinal accessory nerve (CN XI)	Somatic motor	Cervical spinal cord		Motor to sternocleidomastoid and trapezius
Hypoglossal (CN XII)	Somatic motor	Medulla	Hypoglossal canal	Motor to intrinsic and extrinsic muscles of the tongue (except palatoglossus)

fibers emerge from the brain and synapse outside the central nervous system (CNS) in parasympathetic ganglia (Fig. 10.5; Table 10.3). The postsynaptic (postganglionic) fibers continue to innervate smooth muscles and glands (e.g., the sphincter pupillae and lacrimal gland).

- Sensory (afferent) fibers
  3. *Fibers transmitting general sensation* (e.g., touch, pressure, heat, cold, etc.) *from the skin and mucous membranes*. These include somatic sensory (general somatic afferent) fibers, mainly carried by CN V but also by CN VII, CN IX, and CN X (Fig. 10.4; Tables 10.1 and 10.2).
  4. *Fibers conveying sensation from the viscera*. These fibers include visceral sensory (general visceral afferent) fibers conveying information from the carotid body and carotid sinus (see Fig. 9.18), pharynx, larynx, trachea, bronchi, lungs, heart, and gastrointestinal tract.
  5. *Fibers transmitting unique sensations*. These include special sensory fibers conveying taste and smell (special visceral afferent fibers) and those serving the special senses of vision, hearing, and balance (special somatic afferent fibers).

Some cranial nerves are purely sensory, others are considered purely motor, and several are mixed. CN III, CN IV, CN VI, CN XI, CN XII, and the motor root of CN V are considered to be "pure" motor nerves that appear to have evolved from primordial anterior roots. However, a small number of sensory fibers for proprioception (nonvisual perception of movement and position) are also present in these nerves, the cell bodies of which are probably located in the mesencephalic nucleus of CN V. The sensory root of CN V is purely a somatic (general) sensory nerve. Four cranial nerves (CN III, CN VII, CN IX, and CN X) contain presynaptic parasympathetic (visceral motor) axons as they emerge from the brainstem (Fig. 10.5; Table 10.3). CN V, CN VII, CN IX, and CN X are mixed nerves with both somatic (branchial) motor and somatic (general) sensory components. Each of these nerves supplies derivatives of a different pharyngeal arch (Fig. 10.4; Table 10.2).

The fibers of cranial nerves connect centrally to **cranial nerve nuclei**—groups of neurons in which sensory or afferent fibers terminate and from which motor or efferent fibers originate (Fig. 10.6). Except for CN I and CN II, which involve extensions of the forebrain, the nuclei of the cranial nerves are located in the brainstem. Nuclei of similar functional components (e.g., somatic or visceral motor, or somatic or visceral sensory) are generally aligned into functional columns in the brainstem.

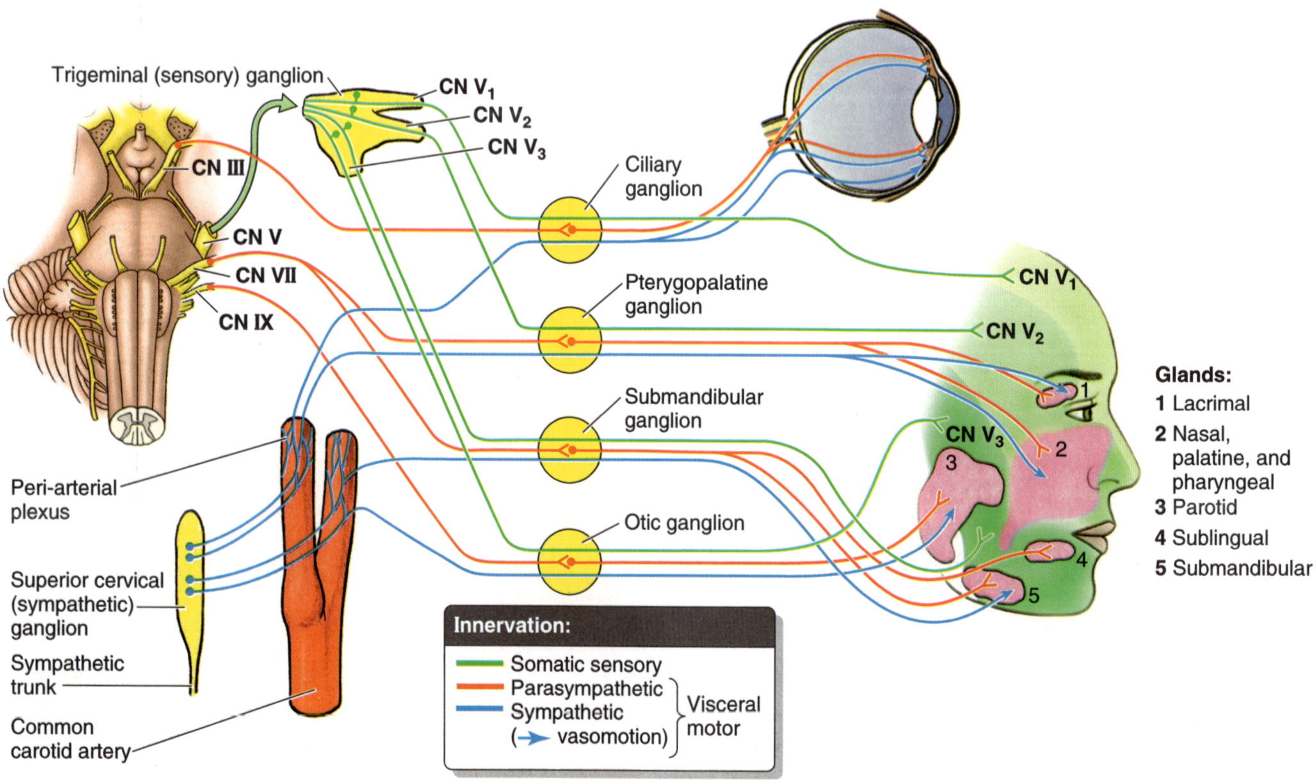

FIGURE 10.5. Summary of cranial parasympathetic ganglia and related visceral motor and sensory fiber distribution. CN III, VII, and IX are "parent nerves" bringing presynaptic parasympathetic fibers from the CNS. CN V conveys no ANS fibers from the CNS. However, the cranial parasympathetic ganglia are all associated with branches of CN V, and the postsynaptic parasympathetic fibers are distributed via branches of CN V.

AN34.1 **TABLE 10.3. CRANIAL PARASYMPATHETIC GANGLIA: LOCATION; SENSORY, PARASYMPATHETIC, AND SYMPATHETIC ROOTS AND MAIN DISTRIBUTION**

Ganglion	Location and Sensory Root	Parasympathetic Root	Sympathetic Root	Main Distribution
Ciliary	Between optic nerve and lateral rectus, tethered to nasociliary nerve (CN V) by sensory roots	Inferior branch of oculomotor nerve (CN III)	Branches from internal carotid plexus in cavernous sinus	Parasympathetic postsynaptic fibers from ciliary ganglion pass to ciliary muscle and sphincter pupillae of iris; sympathetic postsynaptic fibers from superior cervical ganglion pass to dilator pupillae and blood vessels of eye
Pterygopalatine	In pterygopalatine fossa, where it is suspended by ganglionic branches of maxillary nerve (CN V_2) by sensory roots; just anterior to opening of pterygoid canal and inferior to CN V_2	Greater petrosal nerve from facial nerve (CN VII) via nerve of pterygoid canal	Deep petrosal nerve, a branch of internal carotid plexus that is a continuation of postsynaptic fibers of cervical sympathetic trunk; fibers from superior cervical ganglion pass through pterygopalatine ganglion and enter branches of CN V_2.	Parasympathetic postganglionic (secretomotor) fibers from pterygopalatine ganglion innervate lacrimal gland via zygomatic branch of CN V_2; sympathetic postsynaptic fibers from superior cervical ganglion accompany branches of pterygopalatine nerve that are distributed to blood vessels of nasal cavity, palate, and superior parts of pharynx
Otic	On medial aspect of trunk of mandibular nerve (CN V_3), to which it tethered by a sensory root; between trunk and tensor veli palatine, and inferior to foramen ovale of sphenoid bone	Tympanic nerve from glossopharyngeal nerve (CN IX); continues from tympanic plexus as lesser petrosal nerve	Fibers from superior cervical ganglion come from plexus on middle meningeal artery	Parasympathetic postsynaptic fibers from otic ganglion are distributed to parotid gland via auriculotemporal nerve (branch of CN V_3); sympathetic postsynaptic fibers from superior cervical ganglion pass to parotid gland and supply its blood vessels
Submandibular	Suspended from lingual nerve by two ganglionic branches or sensory roots; lies on surface of hyoglossus muscle inferior to submandibular duct	Parasympathetic fibers join facial nerve (CN VII) and leave it in its chorda tympani branch, which unites with lingual nerve	Sympathetic fibers from superior cervical ganglion via plexus on facial artery	Parasympathetic postsynaptic (secretomotor) fibers from submandibular ganglion are distributed to sublingual and submandibular glands; sympathetic fibers from superior cervical ganglion supply sublingual and submandibular glands

OLFACTORY NERVE (CN I)

Function: Special sensory (special visceral afferent) for the special sense of smell. "*Olfaction* is the sensation of odors that results from the detection of odorous substances aerosolized in the environment" (Simpson, 2013).

The cell bodies of olfactory receptor neurons are located in the **olfactory organ** (the olfactory part of the nasal mucosa or olfactory area), which is located in the roof of the nasal cavity, and along the nasal septum and medial wall of the superior nasal concha (Fig. 10.7). **Olfactory receptor neurons** are both receptors and conductors. The apical surfaces of the neurons possess fine **olfactory cilia**, bathed by a film of watery mucus secreted by the **olfactory glands** of the epithelium. The olfactory cilia are stimulated by molecules of an odiferous gas dissolved in the fluid.

The basal surfaces of the bipolar olfactory receptor neurons of the nasal cavity of one side give rise to central processes that are collected into approximately 20 **olfactory nerves** (L. *fila olfactoria*), constituting the right or left **olfactory nerve** (**CN I**). They pass through tiny foramina in the *cribriform plate of the ethmoid bone*, surrounded by sleeves of dura mater and arachnoid mater, and enter the olfactory bulb in the anterior cranial fossa (Figs. 10.1 to 10.3). The **olfactory bulb** lies in contact with the inferior or orbital surface of the frontal lobe of the cerebral hemisphere. The olfactory nerve fibers synapse with **mitral cells** in the olfactory bulb. The axons of these secondary neurons form the **olfactory tract**. The olfactory bulbs and tracts are anterior extensions of the forebrain.

Each olfactory tract divides into lateral and medial **olfactory striae** (distinct fiber bands). The lateral olfactory stria terminates in the piriform cortex of the anterior part of the temporal lobe, and the medial olfactory stria projects through the anterior commissure to contralateral olfactory structures. The olfactory nerves are the only cranial nerves to enter the cerebrum directly.

The Bottom Line: Olfactory Nerve

- The olfactory nerves (CN I) have sensory fibers concerned with the special sense of smell. • The olfactory receptor neurons are in the olfactory epithelium (olfactory mucosa) in the roof of the nasal cavity. • The central processes of the olfactory receptor neurons ascend through foramina in the cribriform plate of the ethmoid bone to reach the olfactory bulbs in the anterior cranial fossa. These nerves synapse on neurons in the bulbs, and the processes of these neurons follow the olfactory tracts to the primary and associated areas of the cerebral cortex.

1

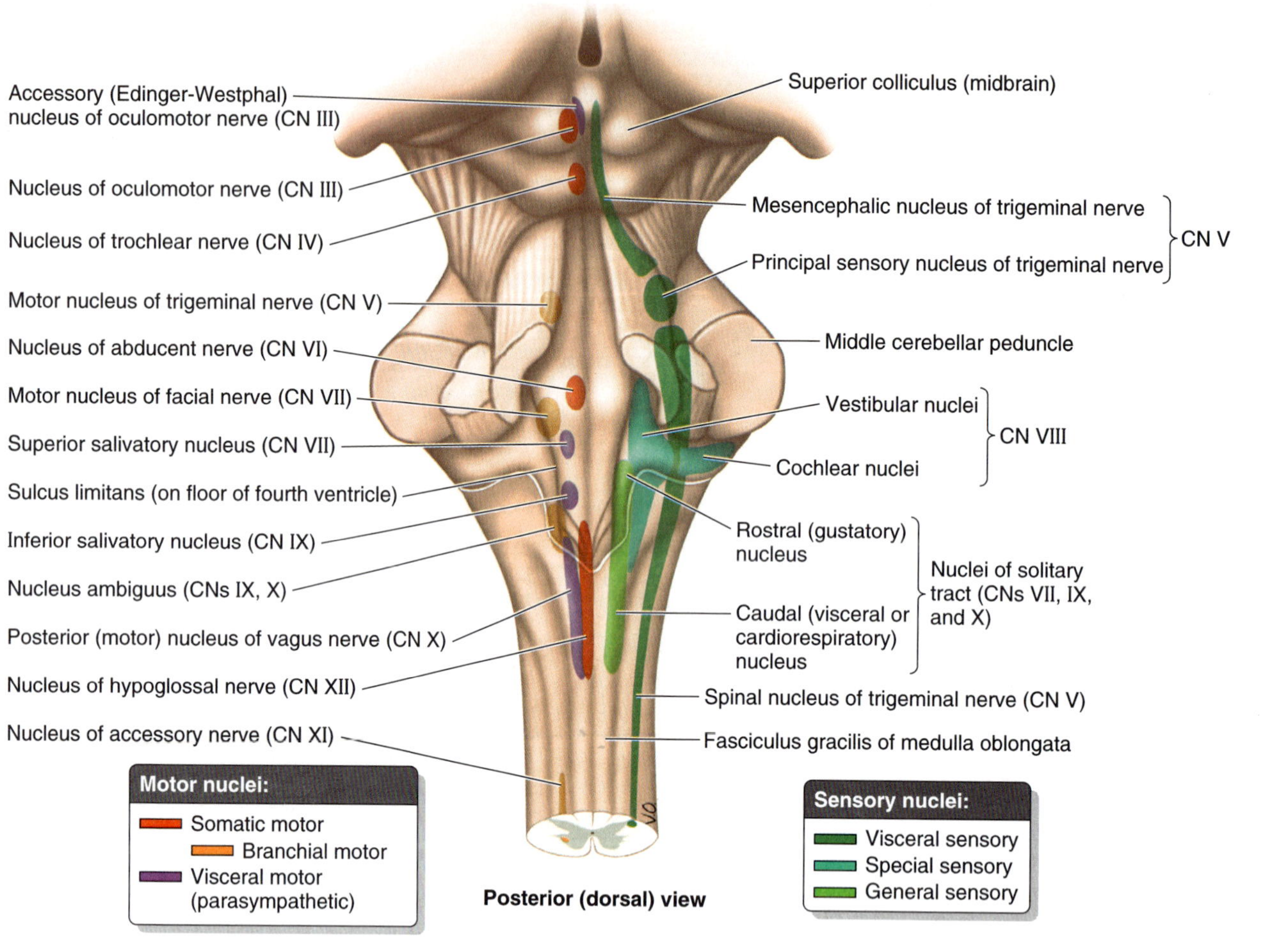

FIGURE 10.6. Cranial nerve nuclei. The motor nuclei are shown on the left side of the brainstem and the sensory nuclei on the right side. The sensory and motor nuclei are all bilaterally paired, that is, located on both the right and left sides of the brainstem.

OPTIC NERVE (CN II)

Function: Special sensory (special somatic afferent) for the special sense of vision.

Although officially nerves by convention, the **optic nerves** (CN II) develop in a completely different manner from the other cranial nerves. The structures involved in receiving and transmitting optical stimuli (the optical fibers and neural retina, together with the pigmented epithelium of the eyeball) develop as evaginations of the diencephalon. The optic nerves are paired, anterior extensions of the forebrain (diencephalon), and are therefore actually CNS fiber tracts formed by axons of **retinal ganglion cells** (Moore et al., 2016). In other words, they are third-order neurons, with their cell bodies located in the retina (Fig. 10.8B).

The optic nerves are surrounded by extensions of the cranial meninges and subarachnoid space, which is filled with cerebrospinal fluid (CSF). The meninges extend all the way to the eyeball. The central artery and vein of the retina traverse the meningeal layers and course in the anterior part of the optic nerve. Cranial nerve II begins where the unmyelinated axons of retinal ganglion cells pierce the sclera (the opaque part of the external fibrous coat of the eyeball) and become myelinated, deep to the *optic disc*.

The nerve passes posteromedially in the orbit, exiting through the *optic canal* to enter the middle cranial fossa, where it forms the **optic chiasm** (Figs. 10.2 and 10.8A). Here, fibers from the nasal (medial) half of each retina decussate in the chiasm and join uncrossed fibers from the temporal (lateral) half of the retina to form the **optic tract**.

The partial crossing of optic nerve fibers in the chiasm is a requirement for binocular vision, allowing depth-of-field perception (three-dimensional vision). Therefore, fibers from the right halves of both retinas form the right optic tract. The decussation of nerve fibers in the chiasm results in the right optic tract conveying impulses from the left visual field and vice versa. The **visual field** is what is seen by a person who has both eyes wide open and who is looking straight ahead. Most fibers in the optic tracts terminate in the **lateral geniculate bodies** of the thalamus. From these

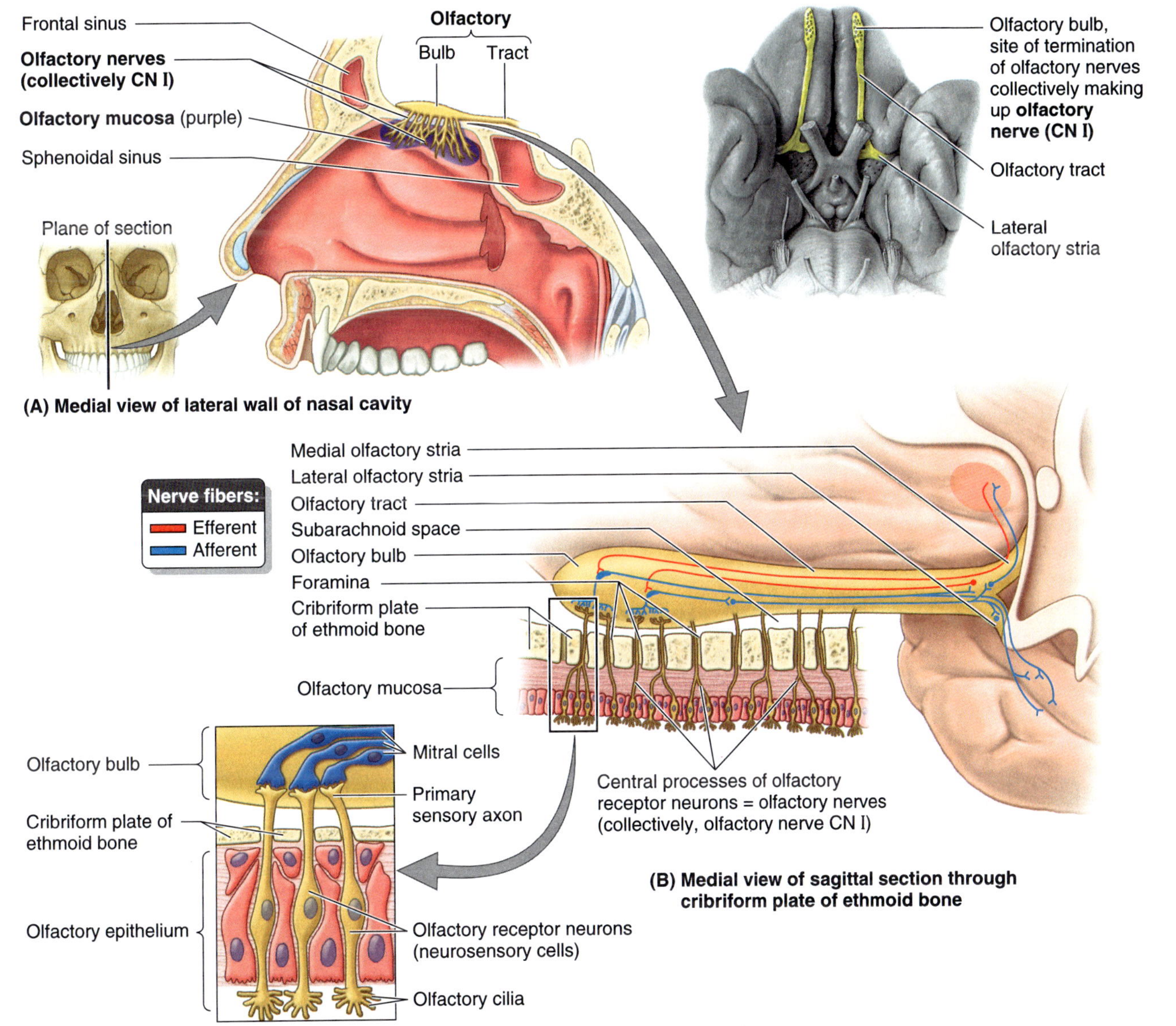

FIGURE 10.7. Olfactory system. A. This sagittal section through the nasal cavity shows the relationship of the olfactory mucosa to the olfactory bulb. **B.** The bodies of the olfactory receptor neurons are in the olfactory epithelium. These bundles of axons are collectively called the olfactory nerve (CN I).

nuclei, axons are relayed to the visual cortices of the occipital lobes of the brain.

The Bottom Line: Optic Nerve

- The optic nerves (CN II) have sensory fibers concerned with the special sense of vision. • The optic nerve fibers arise from ganglion cells in the retina. • The nerve fibers exit the orbit via the optic canals; fibers from the nasal half of the retina cross to the contralateral side at the optic chiasm. • The nerve fibers then pass via the optic tracts to the geniculate bodies of the thalamus, where they synapse on neurons whose processes form the optic radiations to the primary visual cortex of the occipital lobe.

OCULOMOTOR NERVE (CN III)

Functions: Somatic motor (general somatic efferent) and visceral motor (general visceral efferent–parasympathetic). AN31

Nuclei: There are two oculomotor nuclei, each serving one of the functional components of this nerve. The somatic motor **nucleus of the oculomotor nerve** is in the midbrain (Fig. 10.6). The visceral motor (parasympathetic) **accessory (Edinger-Westphal) nucleus of the oculomotor nerve** lies dorsal to the rostral two thirds of the somatic motor nucleus (Haines, 2013).

The oculomotor nerve (CN III) provides the following (Fig. 10.9):

- Motor innervation to the striated muscle of four of the six extra-ocular muscles (*superior*, *medial*, and *inferior*

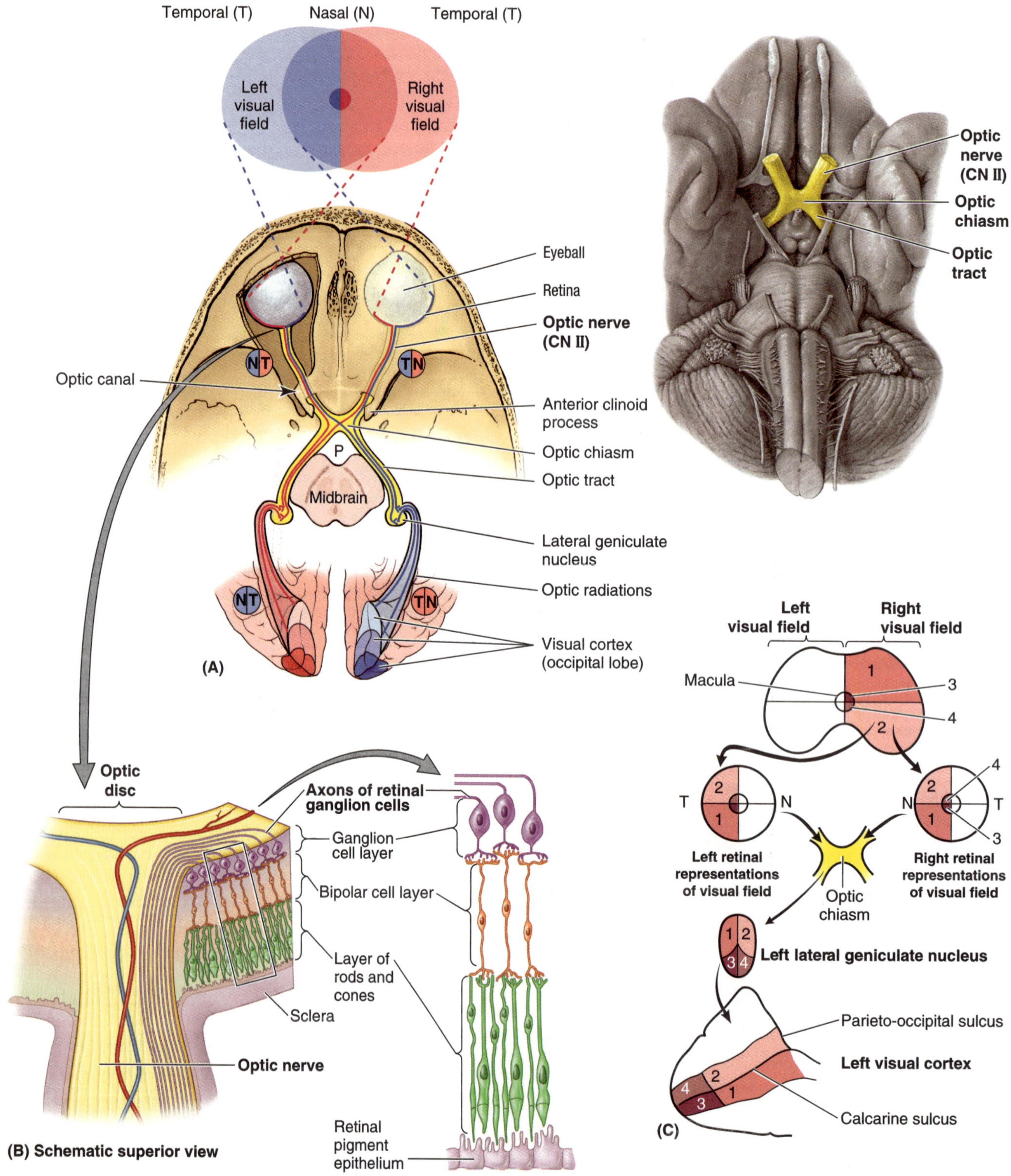

FIGURE 10.8. **Visual system. A.** The origin, course, and distribution of the visual pathway are shown. The axons of retinal ganglionic neurons convey visual information to the lateral geniculate body of the diencephalon (thalamus) through the optic nerve (CN II) and optic tract. Fibers from the lateral geniculate body project to the visual cortices of the occipital lobes. The axons of the ganglion cells of the nasal halves of the retinas cross in the optic chiasm; those from the temporal halves do not cross. **B.** The visual pathway begins with photoreceptor cells (rods and cones) in the retina. The responses of the photoreceptors are transmitted by bipolar cells (neurons with two processes) to ganglion cells in the ganglion cell layer of the retina. The central processes of this third-order neuron are the fibers conducted by the optic nerves. **C.** Right visual field represented on retinae, left lateral genicular nucleus, and left visual cortex.

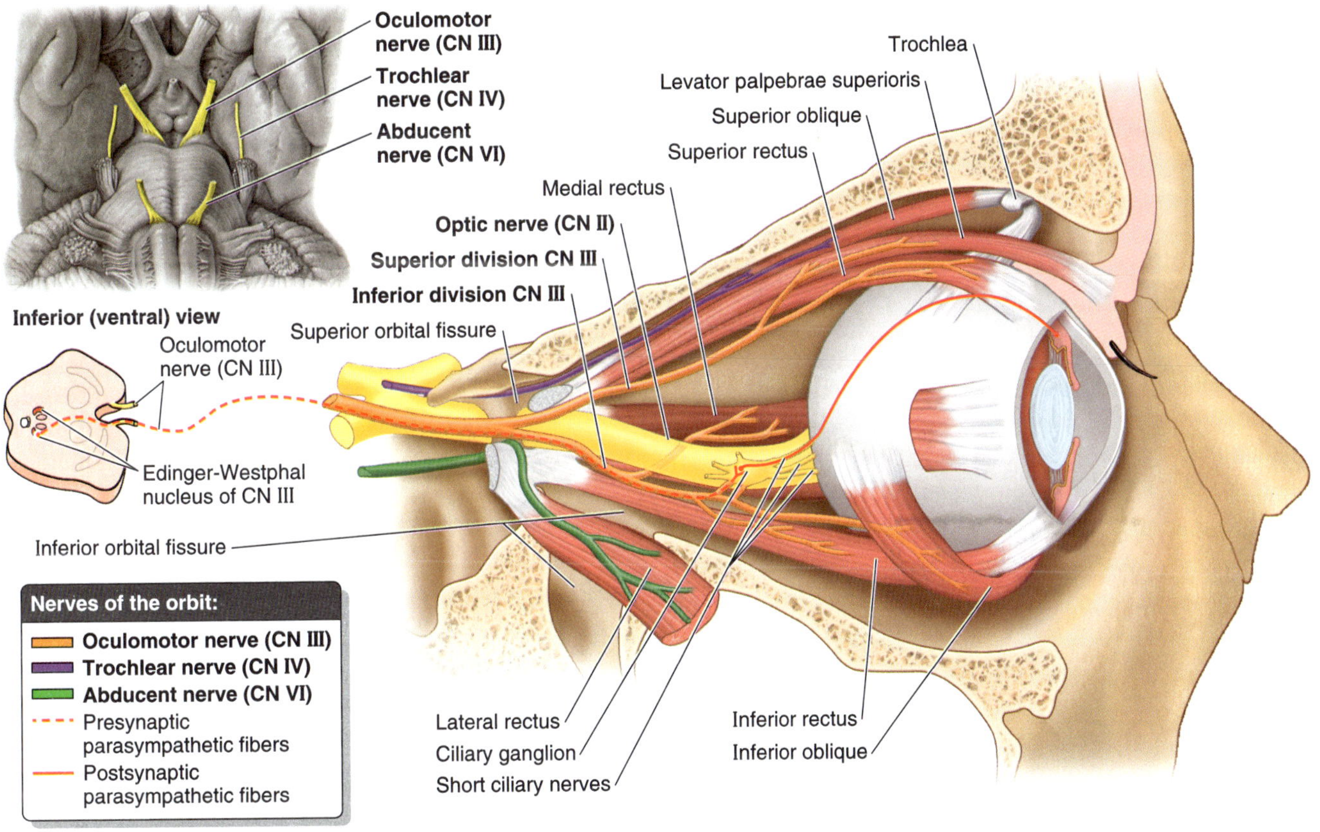

FIGURE 10.9. Distribution of oculomotor (CN III), trochlear (CN IV), and abducent (CN VI) nerves. CN IV supplies the superior oblique, CN VI supplies the lateral rectus, and CN III supplies five striated extra-ocular muscles (levator palpebrae superioris, superior rectus, medial rectus, inferior rectus, and inferior oblique) and two intra-ocular muscles (ciliary muscle and sphincter pupillae muscle—not shown; see Chapter 8, Head).

recti and *inferior oblique*) and superior eyelid (L. *levator palpebrae superioris*), hence the nerve's name.

- Parasympathetic innervation through the ciliary ganglion to the smooth muscle of the sphincter pupillae that causes constriction of the pupil and ciliary muscle, producing *accommodation* (allowing the lens to become more rounded) for near vision.

CN III is the chief motor nerve to the ocular and extra-ocular muscles. It emerges from the midbrain, pierces the dura mater lateral to the diaphragma sellae roofing over the hypophysis, and then runs through the roof and lateral wall of the *cavernous sinus*. CN III leaves the cranial cavity and enters the orbit through the *superior orbital fissure*. Within this fissure, CN III divides into a **superior division** (which supplies the superior rectus and levator palpebrae superioris) and an **inferior division** (which supplies the inferior and medial rectus and inferior oblique). The inferior division also carries presynaptic parasympathetic (visceral efferent) fibers to the *ciliary ganglion*, where they synapse (see Fig. 10.5; Table 10.3). Postsynaptic fibers from this ganglion pass to the eyeball in the *short ciliary nerves* to innervate the ciliary body and sphincter pupillae (see Fig. 8.51 in Chapter 8, Head).

Oculomotor nerve distribution and central connections are shown in Figure 10.10.

The Bottom Line: Oculomotor Nerve

● The oculomotor nerves (CN III) send somatic motor fibers to all extra-ocular muscles, except the superior oblique and lateral rectus. ● These nerves also send presynaptic parasympathetic fibers to the ciliary ganglion for innervation of the ciliary body and sphincter pupillae. ● These nerves originate from the brainstem, emerging medial to the cerebral peduncles, and run in the lateral wall of the cavernous sinus. ● These nerves enter the orbit through the superior orbital fissures and divide into superior and inferior branches.

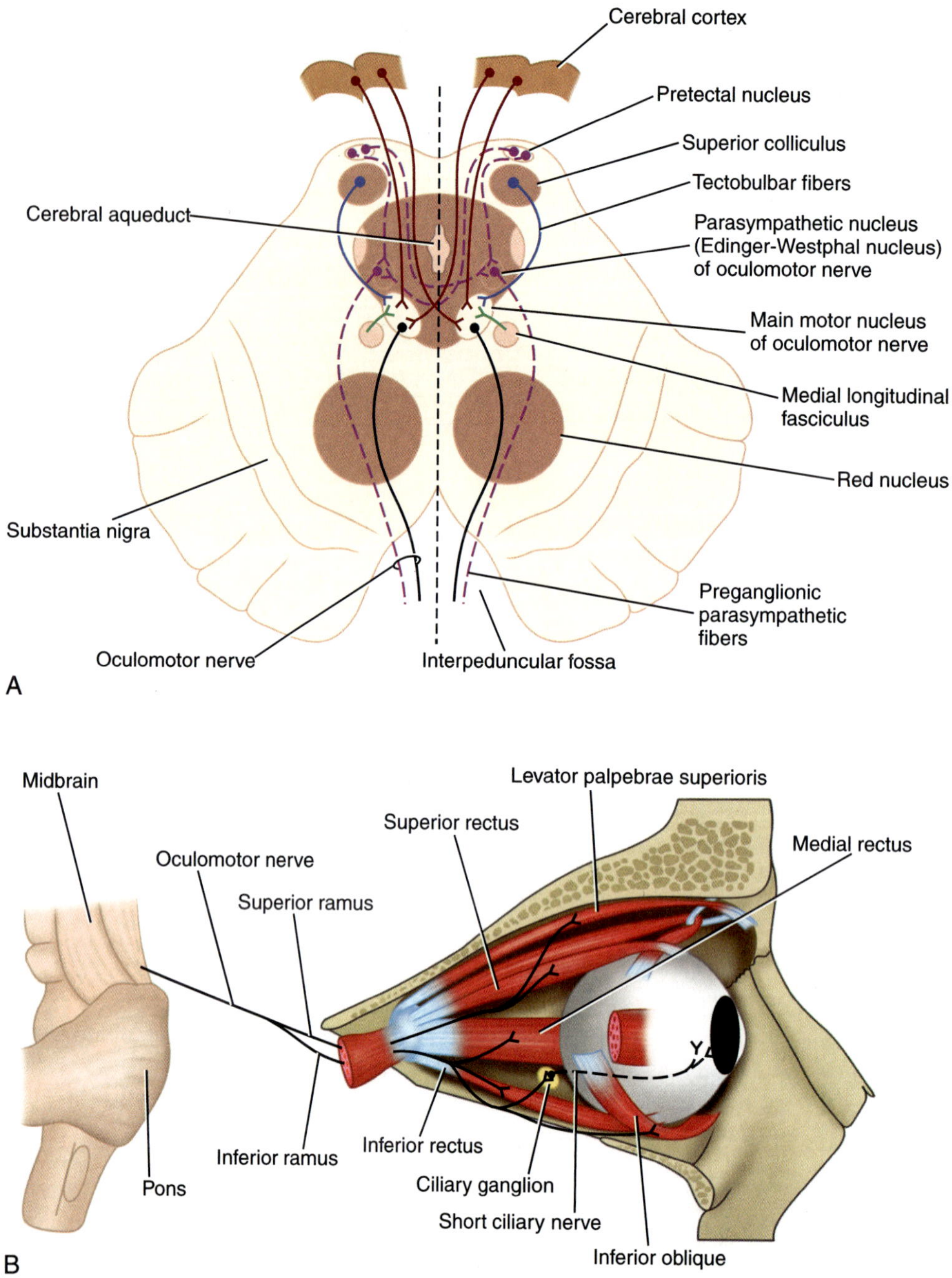

FIGURE 10.10. **A**. Oculomotor nerve nuclei and their central connections. **B**. The distribution of the oculomotor nerve.

TROCHLEAR NERVE (CN IV)

N31.2 **Functions:** Somatic motor (general somatic efferent) to one extra-ocular muscle (superior oblique).

Nucleus: The **nucleus of the trochlear nerve** is located in the midbrain, immediately caudal to the oculomotor nucleus (Fig. 10.6).

The **trochlear nerve** (CN IV) is the smallest cranial nerve. It emerges from the posterior (dorsal) surface of the midbrain (the only cranial nerve to do so), passing anteriorly around the brainstem. It has the longest *intracranial (subarachnoid) course* of the cranial nerves. The trochlear nerve pierces the dura mater at the margin of the tentorium cerebelli and passes anteriorly in the lateral wall of the cavernous sinus (Fig. 10.3A–C). CN IV then continues through the superior orbital fissure into the orbit, where it supplies the superior oblique—the only extra-ocular muscle that uses a pulley, or trochlea, to redirect its line of action (hence the nerve's name) (Fig. 10.9).

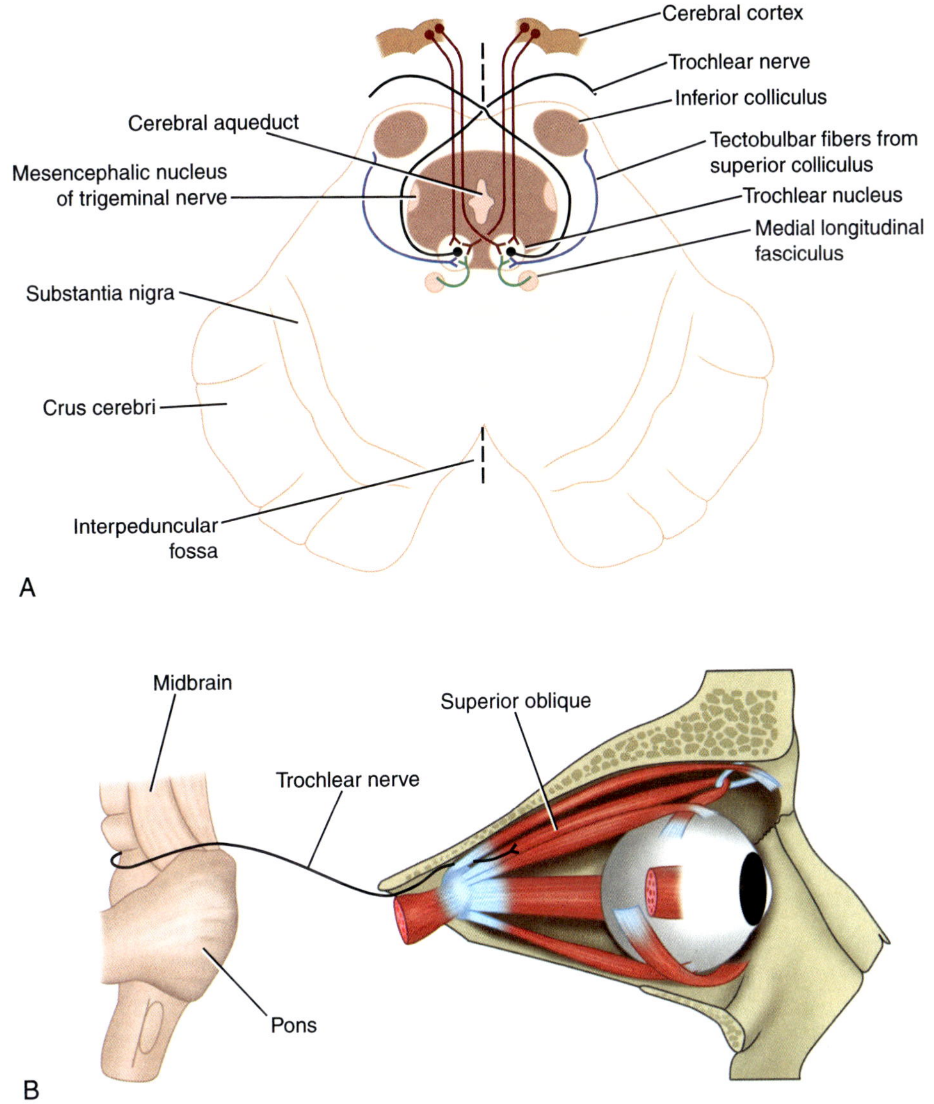

FIGURE 10.11. **A**. Trochlear nerve nucleus and its central connections. **B**. Distribution of the trochlear nerve.

Figure 10.11 shows trochlear nerve central connections and distribution.

The Bottom Line: Trochlear Nerve

- The trochlear nerves (CN IV) supply somatic motor fibers to the superior oblique muscles, which abduct, depress, and medially rotate the pupil. ● The trochlear nerves emerge from the posterior aspect of the brainstem. ● The nerves run a long intracranial course, passing around the brainstem to enter the dura mater in the free edge of the tentorium cerebelli close to the posterior clinoid process. ● The nerves then run in the lateral wall of the cavernous sinus, entering the orbit via the superior orbital fissures.

TRIGEMINAL NERVE (CN V)

Functions: Somatic (general) sensory and somatic (branchial) motor to derivatives of the 1st pharyngeal arch.

Nuclei: There are four trigeminal nuclei (Fig. 10.6)—one motor (**motor nucleus of trigeminal nerve**) and three sensory (**mesencephalic, principal sensory, and spinal nuclei of trigeminal nerve**).

The **trigeminal nerve** (CN V) is the largest cranial nerve (if the atypical optic nerve is excluded). It emerges from the lateral aspect of the pons of the brainstem by a large sensory root and a small motor root (Figs. 10.2 to 10.4). The roots of CN V are comparable to the posterior and anterior roots of spinal nerves. CN V is the principal somatic (general) sensory nerve for the head (face, teeth, mouth, nasal cavity, and dura mater of the cranial cavity). The large **sensory**

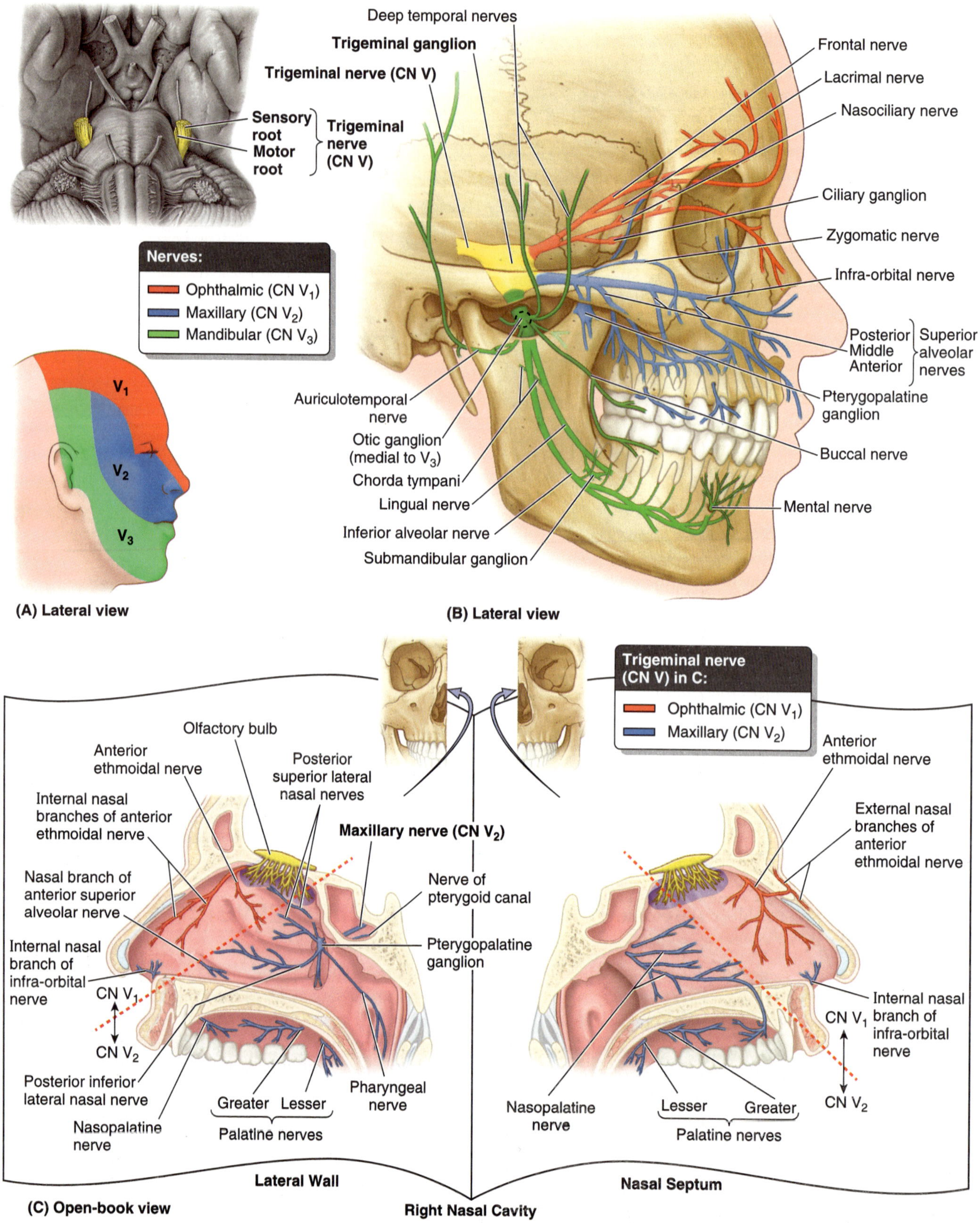

FIGURE 10.12. Distribution of trigeminal nerve (CN V). A. Cutaneous (sensory) zones are innervated by the three divisions of the trigeminal nerve. **B.** Each cranial nerve division supplies skin and mucous membranes and sends a branch to the dura of the anterior and middle cranial fossae. Each division is associated with one or two parasympathetic ganglia and delivers the postsynaptic parasympathetic fibers from that ganglion: CN V_1 for the ciliary ganglion, CN V_2 for the pterygopalatine ganglion, and CN V_3 for the submandibular and otic ganglia. **C.** This open-book view shows the innervation of the lateral wall and septum of the nasal cavity and palate. CN V_1 supplies the anterosuperior portions of the cavity, and CN V_2, the postero-inferior portions and the palate.

root of CN V is composed mainly of the central processes of the pseudounipolar neurons that make up the sensory **trigeminal ganglion** (Fig. 10.12). The ganglion is flattened and crescent shaped (hence its unofficial name, semilunar ganglion) and is housed within a dural recess (**trigeminal cave**) lateral to the cavernous sinus.

The peripheral processes of the ganglionic neurons form three nerves or divisions: *ophthalmic nerve* (CN V_1), *maxillary nerve* (CN V_2), and sensory component of the *mandibular nerve* (CN V_3). Maps of the zones of cutaneous innervation by the three divisions resemble the dermatome maps for cutaneous innervation by spinal nerves (Fig. 10.12A). Unlike spinal nerve dermatomes, however, there is little overlap in innervation by the divisions; lesions of a single nerve result in clearly demarcated areas of numbness.

The **motor root of CN V** passes adjacent to the trigeminal ganglion, bypassing the ganglion and merging with the mandibular division of CN V immediately distal to the ganglion. The motor fibers are distributed exclusively via the mandibular nerve (CN V_3), blending with its sensory fibers as the nerve traverses the foramen ovale to exit the cranium (Figs. 10.1, 10.3A–C and 10.4). This is similar to the way that anterior roots of spinal nerves bypass the spinal sensory (dorsal root) ganglia, also merging with the sensory fibers of the nerves immediately distal to the ganglion, as the nerves traverse the intervertebral foramina, exiting the spine (see Fig. 1.41 in Chapter 1, Overview and Basic Concepts). Motor fibers of the mandibular nerve are distributed to the muscles of mastication, mylohyoid, anterior belly of the digastric, tensor veli palatini, and tensor tympani (see Fig. 8.76 in Chapter 8, Head), which are derived from the 1st pharyngeal arch.

Although CN V conveys no presynaptic parasympathetic fibers from the CNS, all four parasympathetic ganglia are associated with the divisions of CN V. Postsynaptic parasympathetic fibers from the ganglia join branches of CN V and are carried to their destinations along with the CN V sensory and motor fibers (Fig. 10.5; Table 10.3).

Figure 10.13 illustrates trigeminal nerve nuclei seen in a coronal section of the pons and in the brainstem and their central connections.

Ophthalmic Nerve (CN V_1)

AN31.2 In contrast to the other two CN V divisions, CN V_1 is not a branchial nerve (i.e., it does not supply pharyngeal arch derivatives). It serves structures derived from the paraxial mesoderm of the embryonic frontonasal process. The ophthalmic nerve's association with the other CN V divisions is a secondary occurrence. The somatic (general) sensory fibers of CN V_1 are distributed to skin and mucous membranes and conjunctiva of the front of the head and nose (Fig. 10.12).

Testing CN V_1: The integrity of this division is tested by checking the corneal reflex—touching the cornea, which is also supplied by CN V_1, with a wisp of cotton will evoke a reflexive blink if the nerve is functional (Table 10.4; see also Fig. B8.14B).

Maxillary Nerve (CN V_2)

CN V_2 innervates derivatives of the maxillary prominence of the 1st pharyngeal arch. Exiting the cranial cavity via the foramen rotundum, its somatic (general) sensory fibers are mainly distributed to skin and mucous membranes associated with the upper jaw (Fig. 10.12; Table 10.4). The pterygopalatine (parasympathetic) ganglion is associated with this division of CN V, involved in innervating the lacrimal gland and glands of the nose and palate (Fig. 10.5; Table 10.3).

Mandibular Nerve (CN V_3)

CN V_3 innervates derivatives of the mandibular prominence of the 1st pharyngeal arch. CN V_3 is the only division of CN V to convey somatic (branchial) motor fibers, distributed to the striated muscle derived from mandibular prominence mesoderm, primarily the muscles of mastication. Two parasympathetic ganglia, the otic and submandibular, are associated with this division of CN V; both are concerned with the innervation of salivary glands.

Tables 10.1 to 10.3 provide a general summary of CN V. Table 10.4 summarizes the branches of the three divisions.

The Bottom Line: Trigeminal Nerve

- CN V is the chief nerve for general sensory innervation of the head. • Via its three divisions, it provides sensory innervation to dura of the anterior and middle cranial fossae, skin of the face, teeth, gingiva, mucous membrane of the nasal cavity, paranasal sinuses, and mouth. • The trigeminal nerve (CN V) supplies somatic motor fibers to the muscles of mastication, mylohyoid, anterior belly of the digastric, tensor tympani, and tensor veli palatini muscles. • It also distributes postsynaptic parasympathetic fibers of the head to their destinations. • CN V originates from the lateral surface of the pons by two roots: motor and sensory. • These roots cross the medial part of the crest of the petrous part of the temporal bone and enter the trigeminal cave of the dura mater lateral to the body of the sphenoid and cavernous sinus. • The sensory root leads to the trigeminal ganglion; the motor root runs parallel to the sensory root, bypasses the ganglion, and becomes part of the mandibular nerve (CN V_3).

ABDUCENT NERVE (CN VI)

Functions: Somatic motor (general somatic efferent) to one extra-ocular muscle, the *lateral rectus*.

Nucleus: The **abducent nucleus** is in the pons near the median plane (Fig. 10.6). AN31

TABLE 10.4. SUMMARY OF DIVISIONS OF TRIGEMINAL NERVE (CN V)

Divisions/Distributions	Branches
Ophthalmic nerve (CN V_1) Sensory only Passes through superior orbital fissure into orbit Supplies cornea; superior conjunctiva; mucosa of anterosuperior nasal cavity; frontal, ethmoidal, and sphenoidal sinuses; anterior and supratentorial dura mater; skin of dorsum of external nose; superior eyelid; forehead; and anterior scalp Somatic sensory CN V_1 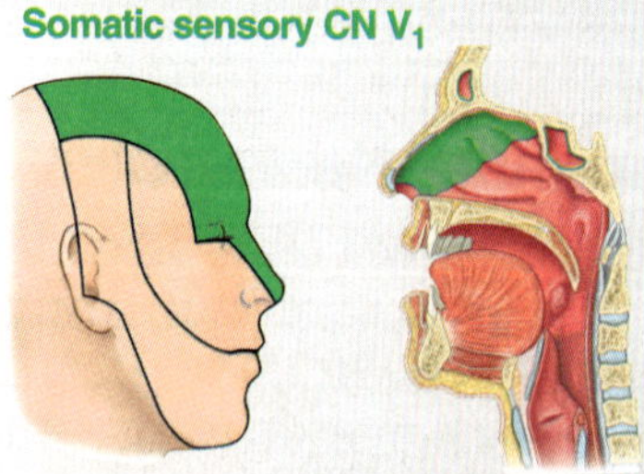	Tentorial nerve (a meningeal branch) Lacrimal nerve Communicating branch from zygomatic nerve Frontal nerve Supra-orbital nerve Supratrochlear nerve Nasociliary nerve Sensory root of ciliary ganglion Short ciliary nerves Long ciliary nerves Anterior and posterior ethmoidal nerves Infratrochlear nerves
Maxillary nerve (CN V_2) Sensory only Passes through foramen rotundum to enter pterygopalatine fossa Supplies dura mater of anterior part of middle cranial fossa; conjunctiva of inferior eyelid; mucosa of postero-inferior nasal cavity, maxillary sinus, palate, and anterior part of superior oral vestibule; maxillary teeth; and skin of lateral external nose, inferior eyelid, anterior cheek, and upper lip Somatic sensory CN V_2 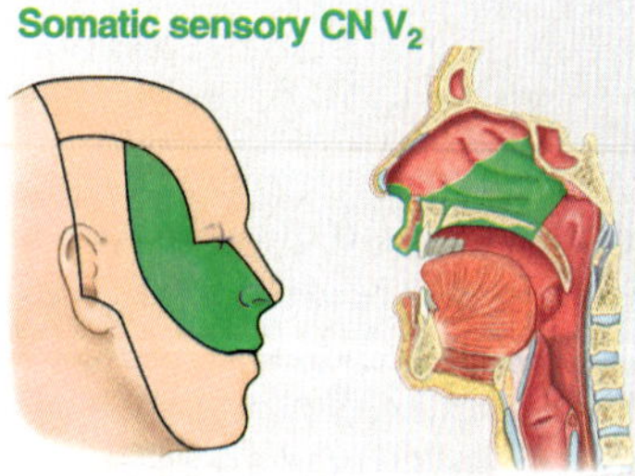	Meningeal branch Zygomatic nerve Zygomaticofacial branch Zygomaticotemporal branch Communicating branch to lacrimal nerve Ganglionic branches to (sensory root of) pterygopalatine ganglion Posterior superior alveolar branches Infra-orbital nerve Anterior and middle superior alveolar branches Superior labial branches Inferior palpebral branches External nasal branches Greater palatine nerves Posterior inferior lateral nasal nerves Lesser palatine nerves Posterior superior lateral nasal branches Nasopalatine nerve Pharyngeal nerve
Mandibular nerve (CN V_3) Sensory and motor Passes through foramen ovale into infratemporal fossa Supplies sensory innervation to mucosa of anterior two thirds of tongue, floor of mouth, and posterior and anterior inferior oral vestibule; mandibular teeth; and skin of lower lip, buccal, parotid, and temporal regions of face; and external ear (auricle, upper external acoustic meatus, and tympanic membrane) Supplies motor innervation to 4 muscles of mastication, mylohyoid, anterior belly of digastric, tensor veli palatini, and tensor tympani Somatic sensory CN V_3 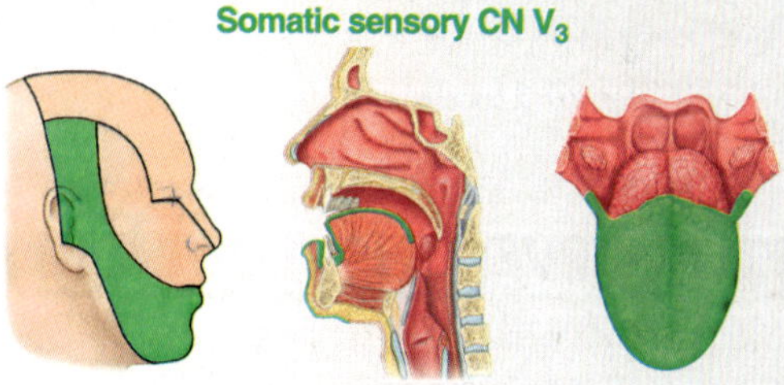 Somatic motor CN V_3 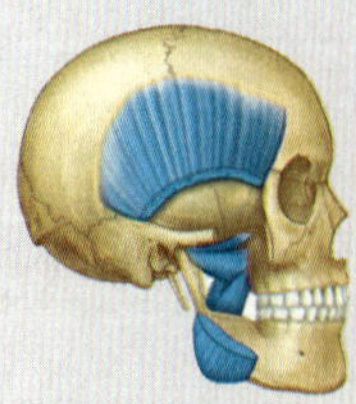	*Somatic (general) sensory branches* Meningeal branch (nervus spinosum) Buccal nerve Auriculotemporal nerve Lingual nerve Inferior alveolar nerve Inferior dental plexus Mental nerve *Somatic (branchial) motor branches* Masseteric nerve Deep temporal nerves Nerves to medial and lateral pterygoid Nerve to mylohyoid (and anterior belly of digastric) Nerve to tensor veli palatini Nerve to tensor tympani

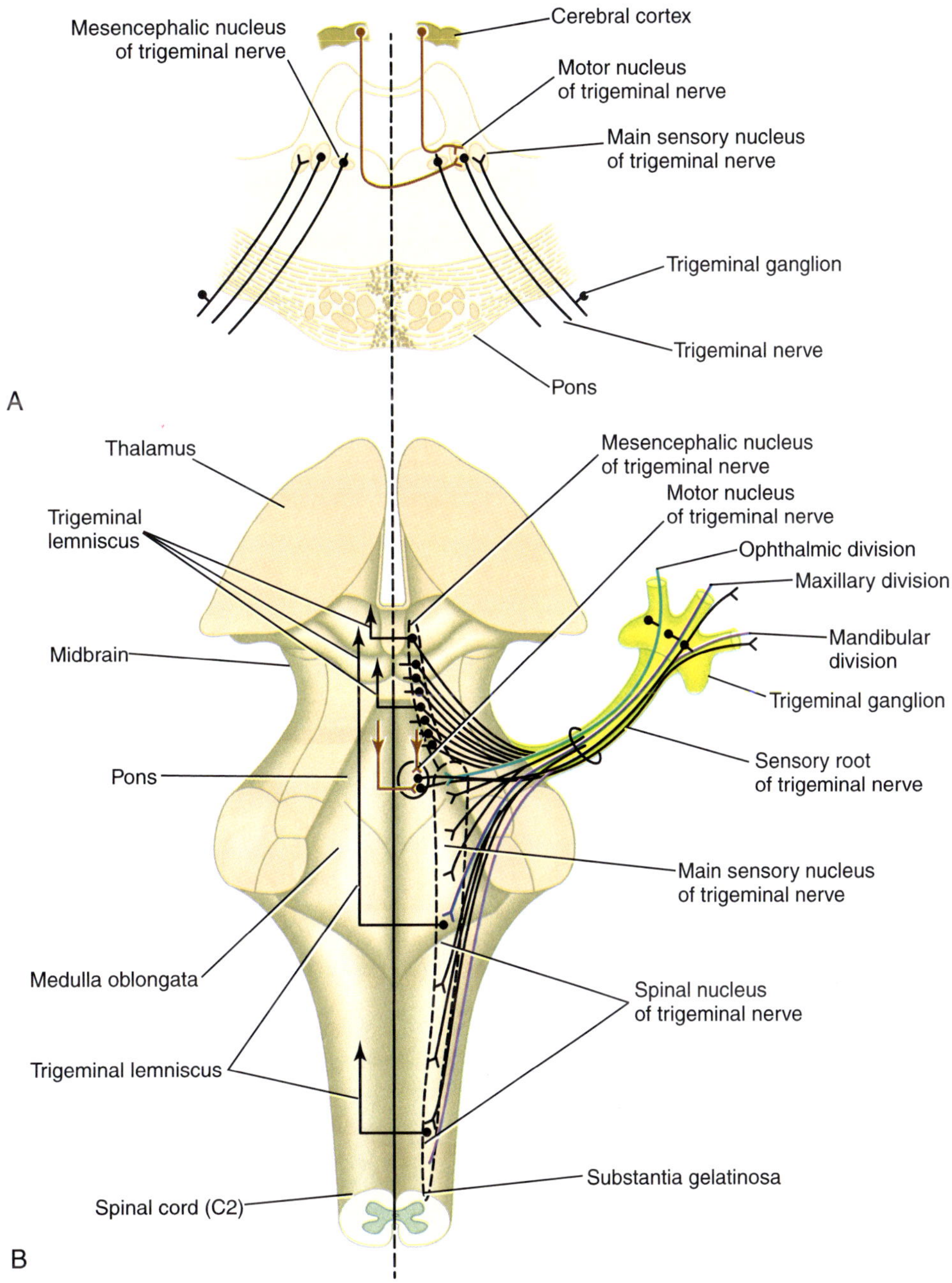

FIGURE 10.13. **A**. Trigeminal nerve nuclei seen in a coronal section of the pons. **B**. Trigeminal nerve nuclei in the brainstem and their central connections.

The **abducent nerve** (CN VI) emerges from the brainstem between the pons and the medulla and traverses the pontine cistern of the subarachnoid space, the right and left nerves straddling the basilar artery (Fig. 10.3A and inset; see also Fig. 8.42). Each abducent nerve then pierces the dura mater to run the *longest intradural course* within the cranial cavity of all the cranial nerves—that is, its point of entry into the dura mater covering the clivus is the most distant from its exit from the cranium via the superior orbital fissure. During its intradural course, it bends sharply over the crest of the petrous part of the temporal bone and then courses through the cavernous sinus, surrounded by the venous blood in the same manner as the internal carotid artery, which it parallels in the sinus (Fig. 10.3A–C). CN VI traverses the common tendinous ring (L. *anulus tendineus communis*) as it enters the orbit (see Fig. 8.55 in Chapter 8, Head), running on and penetrating the medial surface of the lateral rectus, which abducts the pupil (Fig. 10.9).

Abducent nerve nucleus and its central connections as well its distribution are shown in Figure 10.14.

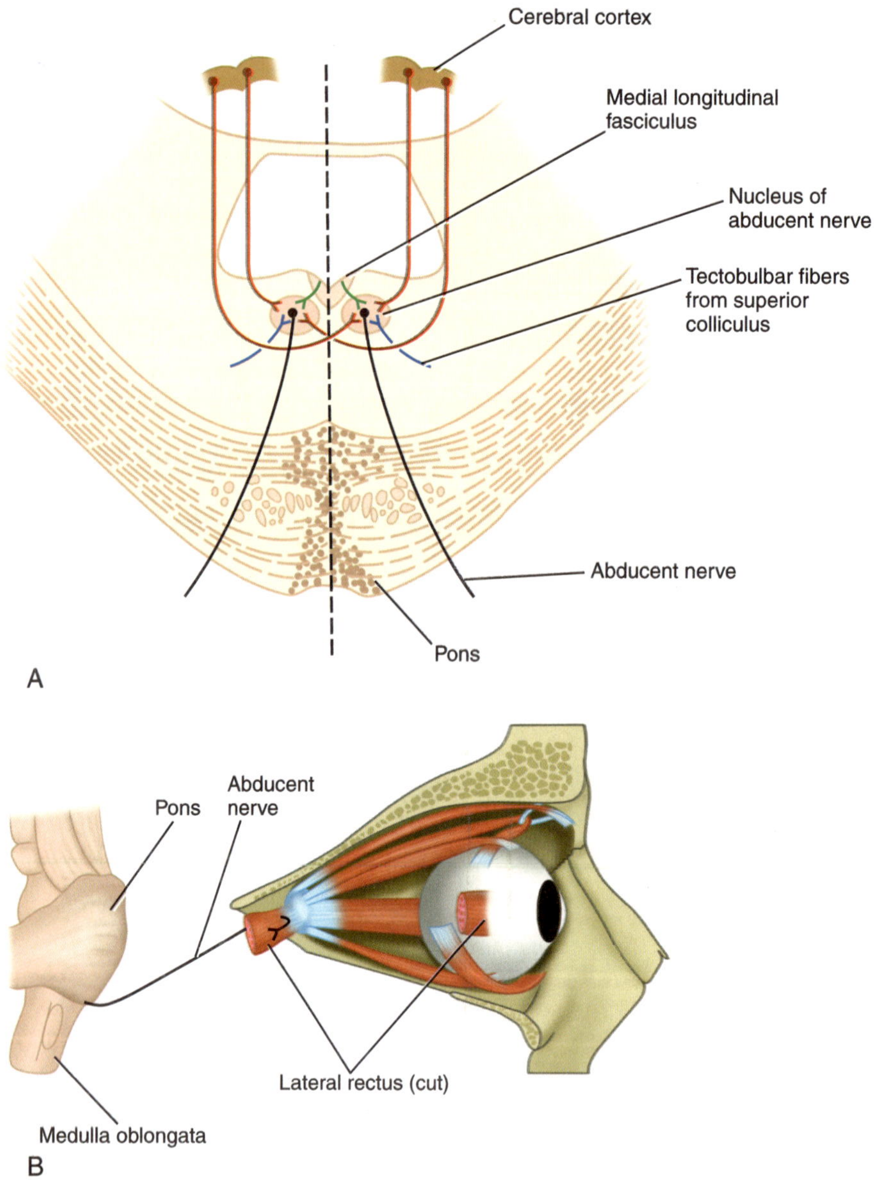

FIGURE 10.14. A. Abducens nerve nucleus and its central connections. B. Distribution of the abducens nerve.

The Bottom Line: Abducent Nerve

- The abducent nerves (CN VI) supply somatic motor fibers to the lateral rectus muscles of the eyeballs.
- The nerves originate from the pons, pierce the dura mater on the clivus, traverse the cavernous sinuses and superior orbital fissures, and enter the orbits.

FACIAL NERVE (CN VII)

AN28.4 **Functions:** *Sensory*—special sensory (taste) and somatic (general) sensory. *Motor*—somatic (branchial) motor and visceral (parasympathetic) motor. It also carries proprioceptive fibers from the muscles it innervates, although the muscles of facial expression include relatively few muscle spindles (mechanoreceptors for muscle stretch), so proprioceptive sensory fibers are fewer than in other motor nerves (Haines, 2013).

Nuclei: The **motor nucleus of the facial nerve** is a branchiomotor nucleus in the ventrolateral part of the pons of the brainstem (Fig. 10.6). The cell bodies of the primary sensory neurons are in the geniculate ganglion (Fig. 10.15). The central processes of those concerned with taste end in the nuclei of the solitary tract in the medulla. The processes of those concerned with general sensations (pain, touch, and thermal) from around the external ear end in the *spinal nucleus of the trigeminal nerve* (Fig. 10.5).

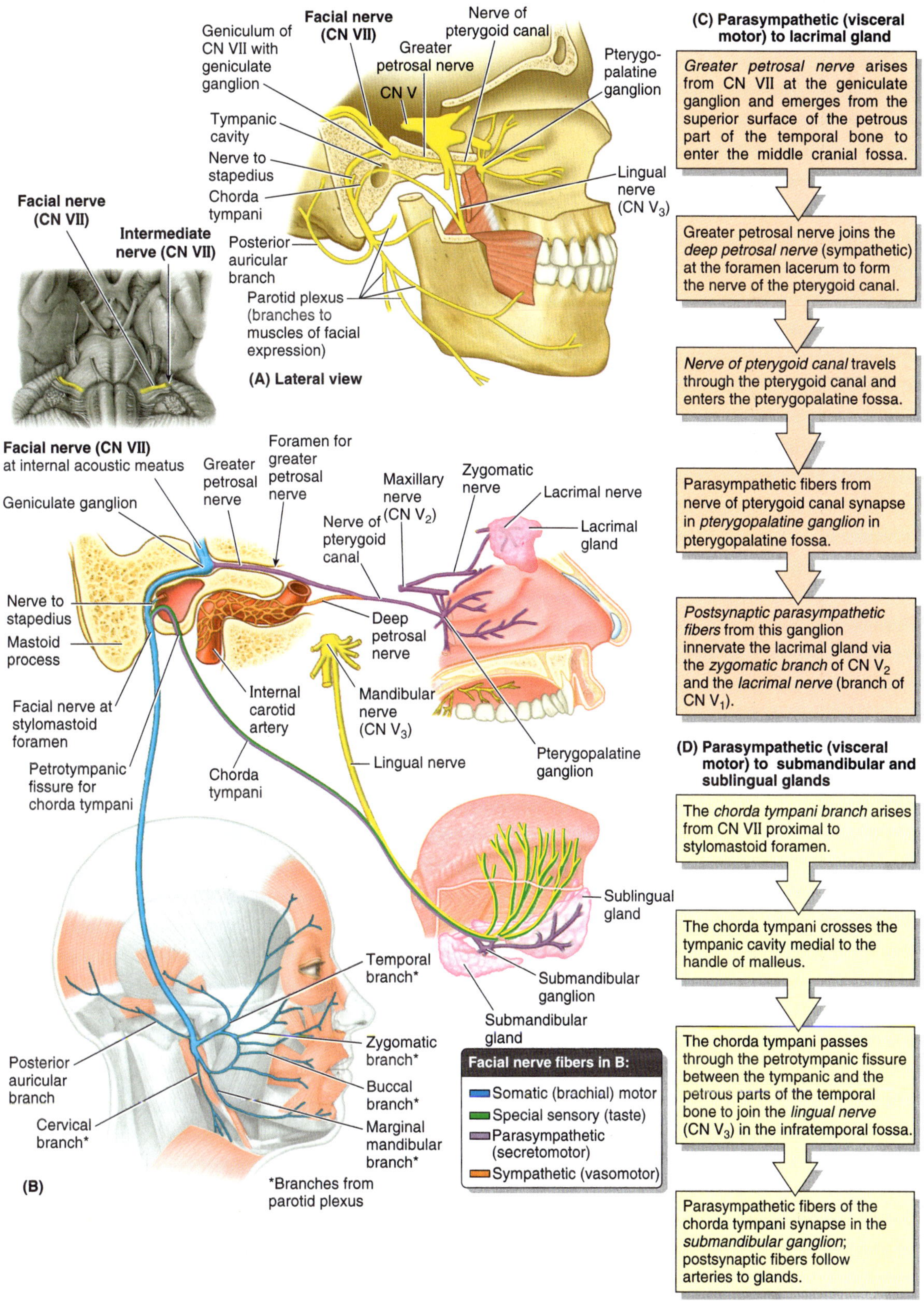

FIGURE 10.15. Distribution of facial nerve (CN VII). A. The facial nerve in situ demonstrates its intra-osseous course and branches. **B.** The distribution of the facial nerve fibers is shown. Observe that CN VII supplies (1) somatic (branchial) motor innervation (*blue*) to derivatives of the 2nd pharyngeal arch (muscles of facial expression, including the auricular and occipitofrontalis muscles plus the stapedius and posterior bellies of the digastric and stylohyoid); (2) special sensory (taste) and presynaptic parasympathetic (secretomotor) fibers (*green*) to the anterior tongue and submandibular ganglion via the chorda tympani; and (3) presynaptic parasympathetic (secretomotor) fibers (*purple*) to the pterygopalatine ganglion via the greater petrosal nerve. **C, D.** Parasympathetic innervation via CN VII. **C.** Innervation of the lacrimal gland. **D.** Innervation of the submandibular and sublingual glands.

The **facial nerve** (CN VII) emerges from the junction of the pons and medulla as two divisions: the primary root and the intermediate nerve (Fig. 10.2; Table 10.1). The larger **primary root** (facial nerve proper) innervates the muscles of facial expression, and the smaller **intermediate nerve** (L. *nervus intermedius*) carries taste, parasympathetic, and somatic sensory fibers. During its course, CN VII traverses the posterior cranial fossa, internal acoustic meatus, facial canal, stylomastoid foramen of the temporal bone, and parotid gland (Fig. 10.15A, B). After traversing the internal acoustic meatus, the nerve proceeds a short distance anteriorly within the temporal bone and then turns abruptly posteriorly to course along the medial wall of the tympanic cavity. The sharp bend, the **geniculum of the facial nerve** (L. *genu*, knee), is the site of the **geniculate ganglion**, the sensory ganglion of CN VII. While traversing the temporal bone within the facial canal (see Fig. 8.117B), CN VII gives rise to the:

- Greater petrosal nerve.
- Nerve to the stapedius.
- Chorda tympani nerve.

Then, after running the *longest intra-osseous course* of any cranial nerve, CN VII emerges from the cranium via the *stylomastoid foramen* (see Fig. 8.16B), gives off the posterior auricular branch, enters the *parotid gland*, and forms the parotid plexus, which gives rise to the following five terminal motor branches: temporal, zygomatic, buccal, marginal mandibular, and cervical (see Fig. 8.16).

Refer to *Snell's Clinical Neuroanatomy*, Chapter 11, Cranial Nerve Nuclei, Figure 11.11 for facial nerve nuclei and their central connections.

Somatic (Branchial) Motor

As the nerve of the embryonic 2nd pharyngeal arch, the facial nerve supplies striated muscles derived from its mesoderm, mainly the muscles of facial expression and auricular muscles. It also supplies the posterior bellies of the digastric, stylohyoid, and stapedius muscles.

Visceral (Parasympathetic) Motor

The visceral (parasympathetic) motor distribution of the facial nerve is presented in Figure 10.15C. CN VII provides presynaptic parasympathetic fibers to the *pterygopalatine ganglion* for innervation of the lacrimal, nasal, palatine, and pharyngeal glands and to the *submandibular ganglion* for innervation of the sublingual and submandibular salivary glands. The pterygopalatine ganglion is associated with the maxillary nerve (CN V_2), which distributes its postsynaptic fibers, whereas the submandibular ganglion is associated with the mandibular nerve (CN V_3). The distribution of visceral motor and sensory fibers to or through the parasympathetic ganglia supplied by the facial nerve and certain other cranial nerves is summarized in Figure 10.5 and Table 10.3. Parasympathetic fibers synapse in these ganglia, whereas sympathetic and sensory fibers pass through them.

Somatic (General) Sensory

Some fibers from the geniculate ganglion accompany the auricular branch of the vagus nerve to supply small areas of skin on both aspects of the auricle, in the region of the concha and at the opening of the external acoustic meatus.

Special Sensory (Taste)

Peripheral fibers of sensory neurons of the geniculate ganglion are carried by the chorda tympani. They join the *lingual nerve* of CN V_3 in the infratemporal fossa to supply taste buds of the anterior two thirds of the tongue and soft palate (Fig. 10.15B). Central fibers of the neurons pass to the brainstem via the intermediate nerve.

The Bottom Line: Facial Nerve

- The facial nerves (CN VII) supply motor fibers to the stapedius, posterior belly of the digastric, stylohyoid, facial, and scalp muscles. • They also supply presynaptic parasympathetic fibers via the intermediate nerve (smaller root of CN VII) destined for the pterygopalatine and submandibular ganglia via the greater petrosal nerve and chorda tympani, respectively. • CN VII is sensory to some skin of the external acoustic meatus and, via the intermediate nerve, is sensory to taste from the anterior two thirds of the tongue and the soft palate.
- CN VII originates from the posterior border of the pons and runs through the internal acoustic meatus and facial canal in the petrous part of the temporal bone.
- CN VII exits via the stylomastoid foramen; its main trunk forms the intraparotid nerve plexus.

VESTIBULOCOCHLEAR NERVE (CN VIII)

Functions: Special sensory (special somatic afferent), that is, special sensations of hearing, equilibrium, and motion (acceleration/deceleration).

Nuclei: Vestibular nuclei are located at the junction of the pons and medulla of the brainstem in the lateral part of the floor of the 4th ventricle; the **cochlear nuclei**, anterior and posterior, are in the medulla (Fig. 10.6).

The **vestibulocochlear nerve** (CN VIII) emerges from the junction of the pons and medulla and enters the *internal acoustic meatus* (Figs. 10.2, 10.3A, 10.4, and 10.16). Here, it separates into the vestibular and cochlear nerves.

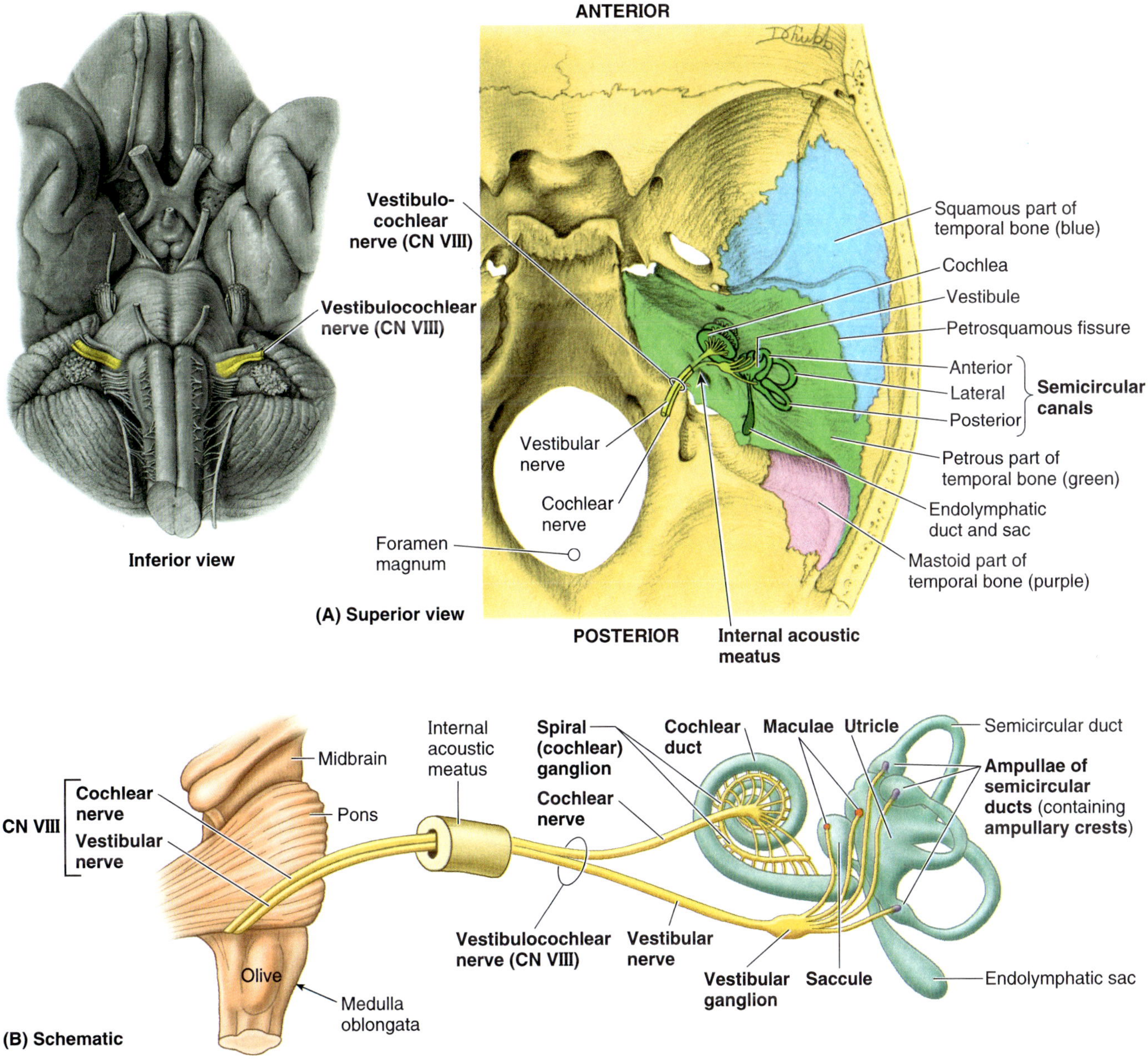

FIGURE 10.16. Vestibulocochlear nerve (CN VIII). A. Location of bony labyrinth of internal ear within temporal bone. **B.** Innervation of cochlea. The cochlear nerve of CN VIII provides innervation for the sense of hearing, and innervation of the vestibular apparatus is provided by the vestibular nerve of CN VIII, for equilibrium and motion.

- The **vestibular nerve** is composed of the central processes of bipolar neurons in the **vestibular ganglion**. The peripheral processes of the neurons extend to the *maculae of the utricle and saccule* (sensitive to linear acceleration and the pull of gravity relative to the position of the head) and to the cristae of the ampullae of the semicircular ducts (sensitive to rotational acceleration).
- The **cochlear nerve** is composed of the central processes of bipolar neurons in the **spiral ganglion**; the peripheral processes of the neurons extend to the spiral organ for the sense of hearing.

Within the internal acoustic meatus, the two divisions of CN VIII are accompanied by the primary root and intermediate nerve of CN VII and the labyrinthine artery (Fig. 10.3A; see also Figs. 8.42 and 8.43 in Chapter 8, Head).

Refer to *Snell's Clinical Neuroanatomy*, Chapter 11, Cranial Nerve Nuclei, Figures 11.13 and 11.14 for central connections of vestibular nerve nuclei and cochlear nerve nuclei.

The Bottom Line: Vestibulocochlear Nerve

• The vestibulocochlear nerves (CN VIII) carry fibers concerned with the special senses of hearing, equilibrium, and motion. • The nerves originate from the grooves between the pons and medulla. • They run through the internal acoustic meatus and divide into the cochlear and vestibular nerves. • The cochlear nerve is sensory to the spiral organ (for the sense of hearing). • The vestibular nerve is sensory to the cristae of the ampullae of the semicircular ducts and the maculae of the saccule and utricle (for the sense of equilibration and motion).

GLOSSOPHARYNGEAL NERVE (CN IX)

35.7 **Functions:** *Sensory*—somatic (general) sensory, special sensory (taste), and visceral sensory. *Motor*—somatic (branchial) motor and visceral (parasympathetic) motor for derivatives of the 3rd pharyngeal arch.

Nuclei: Four nuclei in the medulla send or receive fibers via CN IX: two motor (*nucleus ambiguus* and **inferior salivary nucleus**) and two sensory (*sensory nuclei of the trigeminal nerve* [CN V] and *nuclei of the solitary tract*). Three of these nuclei (in italics) are shared with CN X (Fig. 10.6).

The **glossopharyngeal nerve** (CN IX) emerges from the lateral aspect of the medulla and passes anterolaterally to leave the cranium through the anterior aspect of the *jugular foramen* (Figs. 10.17 and 10.18). At this foramen are the sensory **superior** and **inferior ganglia of CN IX**, which contain the pseudounipolar cell bodies for the afferent components of the nerve. CN IX follows the *stylopharyngeus*, the only muscle the nerve supplies, and passes between the superior and middle pharyngeal constrictor muscles to reach the oropharynx and tongue. It contributes sensory fibers to the *pharyngeal plexus of nerves*. CN IX is afferent from the tongue and pharynx (hence its name) and efferent to the stylopharyngeus and parotid gland.

Somatic (Branchial) Motor

Motor fibers pass to one muscle, the stylopharyngeus, derived from the 3rd pharyngeal arch.

Visceral (Parasympathetic) Motor

Following a circuitous route initially involving the tympanic nerve, presynaptic parasympathetic fibers are provided to the *otic ganglion* for innervation of the parotid gland (Fig. 10.19). The otic ganglion is associated with the mandibular nerve (CN V_3), branches of which convey the postsynaptic parasympathetic fibers to the parotid gland.

Somatic (General) Sensory

The general sensory branches of CN IX are as follows (Fig. 10.17):

- The *tympanic nerve* passes via the tympanic canaliculus between the carotid canal and jugular foramen to form the tympanic plexus within the tympanic cavity. The plexus provides sensory innervation for the mucosa of the tympanic cavity, antrum of mastoid air cells, and the posterolateral portion of the pharyngotympanic tube.
- The *pharyngeal, tonsillar*, and *lingual nerves* to the mucosa of the oropharynx and isthmus of the fauces (L., throat), including palatine tonsil, soft palate, and posterior third of the tongue. In addition to general sensation (touch, pain, temperature), tactile (actual or threatened) stimuli determined to be unusual or unpleasant here may evoke the **gag reflex** or even vomiting. The gag reflex is absent in about 37% of normal individuals (Davies et al., 1995). CN IX provides the afferent (sensory) limb of the reflex, while the efferent (motor) limb is via the vagus nerve (CN X).

Special Sensory (Taste)

Taste fibers are conveyed from the posterior third of the tongue to the sensory inferior ganglia of CN IX (Fig. 10.18). Details of the distribution of CN IX are outlined in Figure 10.17.

Visceral Sensory

The *carotid branch* of CN IX supplies the *carotid sinus*, a baroreceptor (pressoreceptor) sensitive to changes in blood pressure, and the *carotid body*, a chemoreceptor sensitive to blood gas (oxygen and carbon dioxide levels).

Glossopharyngeal nerve nuclei and their central connections are shown in Figure 10.20.

The Bottom Line: Glossopharyngeal Nerve

• The glossopharyngeal nerves (CN IX) send somatic motor fibers to the stylopharyngeus and visceral motor (presynaptic parasympathetic) fibers to the otic ganglion for innervation of the parotid gland. • They also send sensory fibers to the posterior third of the tongue (including taste), pharynx, tympanic cavity, pharyngotympanic cavity, carotid body, and carotid sinus. • The nerves originate from the rostral end of the medulla and exit from the cranium via the jugular foramina. • They pass between the superior and the middle pharyngeal constrictors to the tonsillar sinus and enter the posterior third of the tongue.

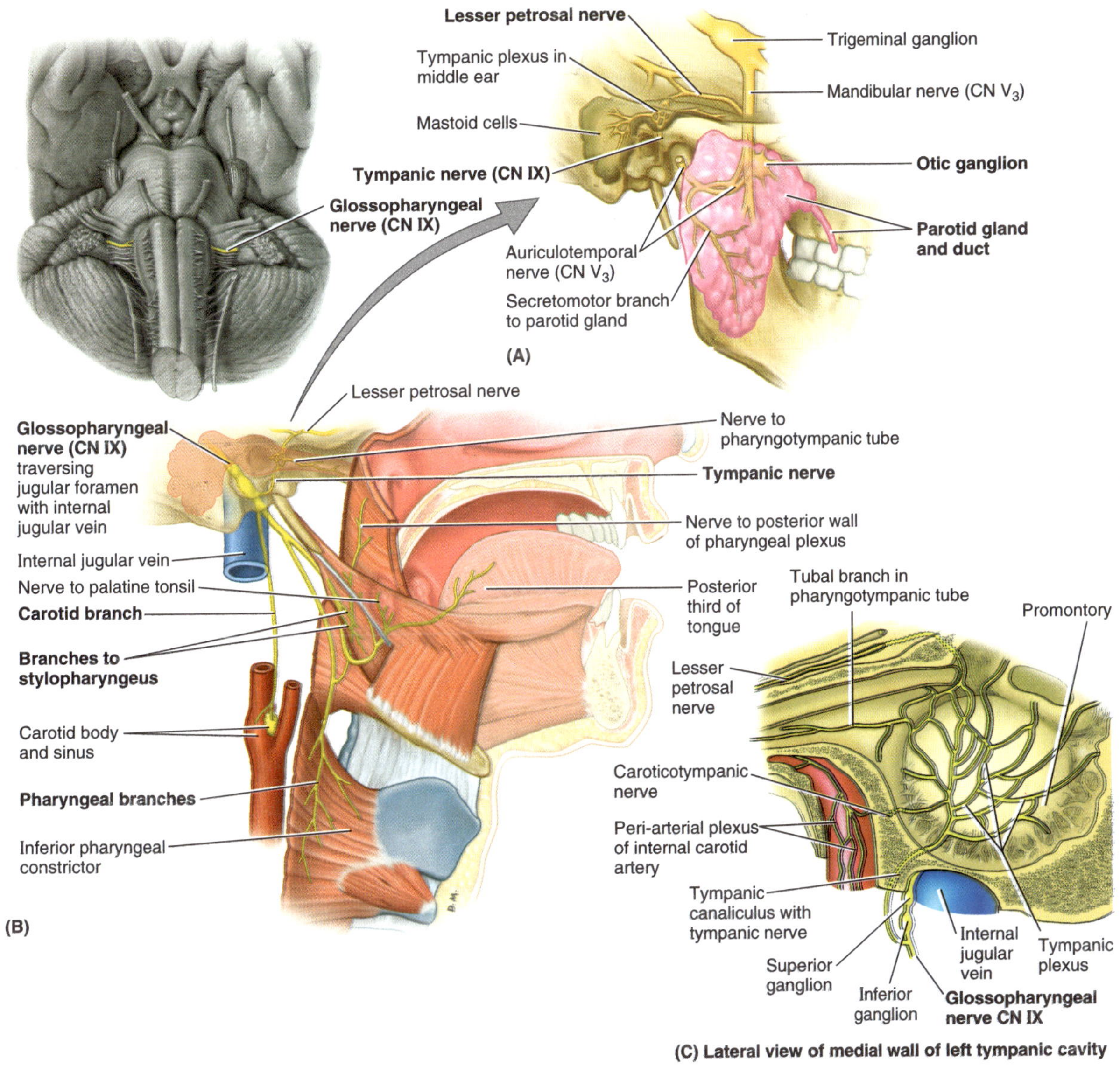

FIGURE 10.17. Distribution of glossopharyngeal nerve (CN IX). A. CN IX is motor to one striated pharyngeal muscle, the stylopharyngeus. It also carries sensory fibers from the carotid body and carotid sinus, conveying information about blood pressure and gas levels as well as somatic (general) sensation from the internal ear, pharynx, and fauces and taste from the posterior tongue. **B.** The parasympathetic component of CN IX supplies presynaptic secretory fibers to the otic ganglion; postsynaptic fibers pass to the parotid gland via the auriculotemporal nerve (CN V_3). **C.** Distribution of CN IX to middle ear (tympanic cavity and pharyngotympanic tube) and otic ganglion via tympanic nerve and plexus and lesser petrosal nerve.

VAGUS NERVE (CN X)

AN35.7 **Functions:** *Sensory*—somatic (general) sensory, special sensory (taste), visceral sensory. *Motor*—somatic (brachial) motor and visceral (parasympathetic) motor.

- Somatic (general) sensory from the inferior pharynx and larynx. The vagus provides the afferent (sensory) limb of the **cough reflex** stimulated by foreign irritants, preventing aspiration and infection.
- Visceral sensory from the thoracic and abdominal organs.
- Taste and somatic (general) sensation from the root of the tongue and taste buds on the epiglottis. Branches of the internal laryngeal nerve (a branch of CN X) supply a small area, mostly somatic (general) sensory but also some special sensation (taste).
- Somatic (branchial) motor to the soft palate, pharynx, intrinsic laryngeal muscles (phonation), and a nominal extrinsic tongue muscle, the palatoglossus, which is actually a palatine muscle based on its derivation and innervation.
- Proprioceptive to the muscles listed above.
- Visceral (parasympathetic) motor to thoracic and abdominal viscera.

Nuclei: *Sensory*—sensory nucleus of the trigeminal nerve (somatic sensory) and nuclei of the solitary tract (taste and visceral sensory). *Motor*—nucleus ambiguus (somatic

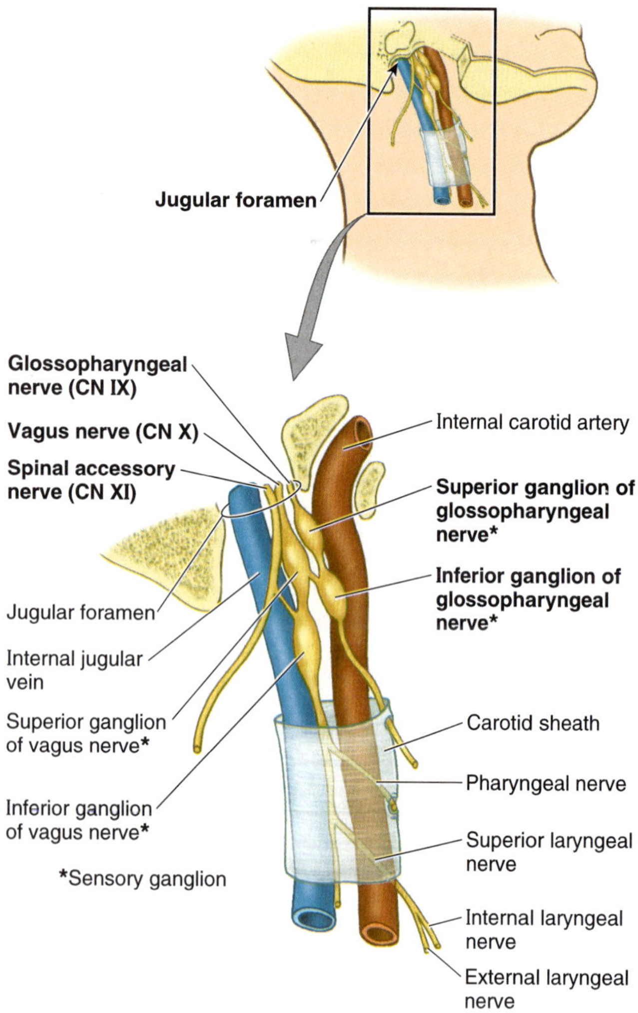

FIGURE 10.18. Relationship of structures traversing jugular foramen. CN IX, CN X, and CN XI are, in numerical order, anterior to the internal jugular vein as they traverse the foramen. They are immediately posterior to the internal carotid artery as they emerge from it. The superior and inferior sensory ganglia of CN IX and CN X are thickenings of those nerves immediately inferior to their exit from the cranium.

[branchial] motor) and **dorsal vagal nucleus** (visceral [parasympathetic] motor) (Fig. 10.6). Vagus nerve nuclei and their central connections are shown in Figure 10.21.

The **vagus nerve** (CN X) has the longest course and most extensive distribution of all the cranial nerves, most of which is outside of (inferior to) the head. The term *vagus* is derived from the Latin word *vagary*, meaning "wandering." CN X was called that because of its wide distribution extending far from the head (Table 10.5). It arises by a series of rootlets from the lateral aspect of the medulla that merge and leave the cranium through the *jugular foramen* positioned between CN IX and CN XI (Figs. 10.18 and 10.22).

What was formerly called the "cranial root of the accessory nerve" is actually a part of CN X (Fig. 10.23). CN X has a *superior ganglion* in the jugular foramen that is mainly concerned with the general sensory component of the nerve.

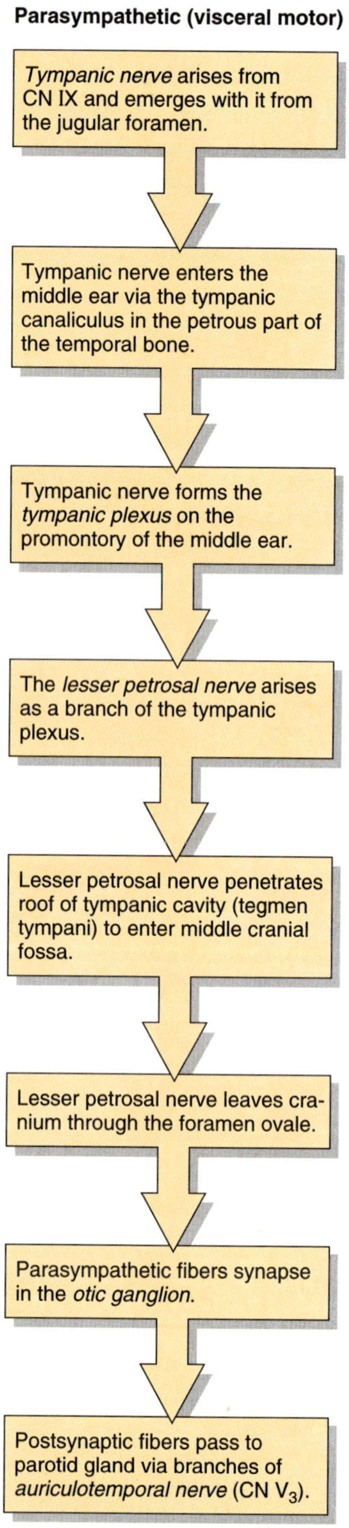

FIGURE 10.19. Parasympathetic innervation involving the glossopharyngeal nerve (CN IX). CN IX sends presynaptic parasympathetic (secretomotor) fibers to the otic ganglion via a convoluted route; postsynaptic fibers pass from the ganglion to the parotid gland via the auriculotemporal nerve (Fig. 10.17B).

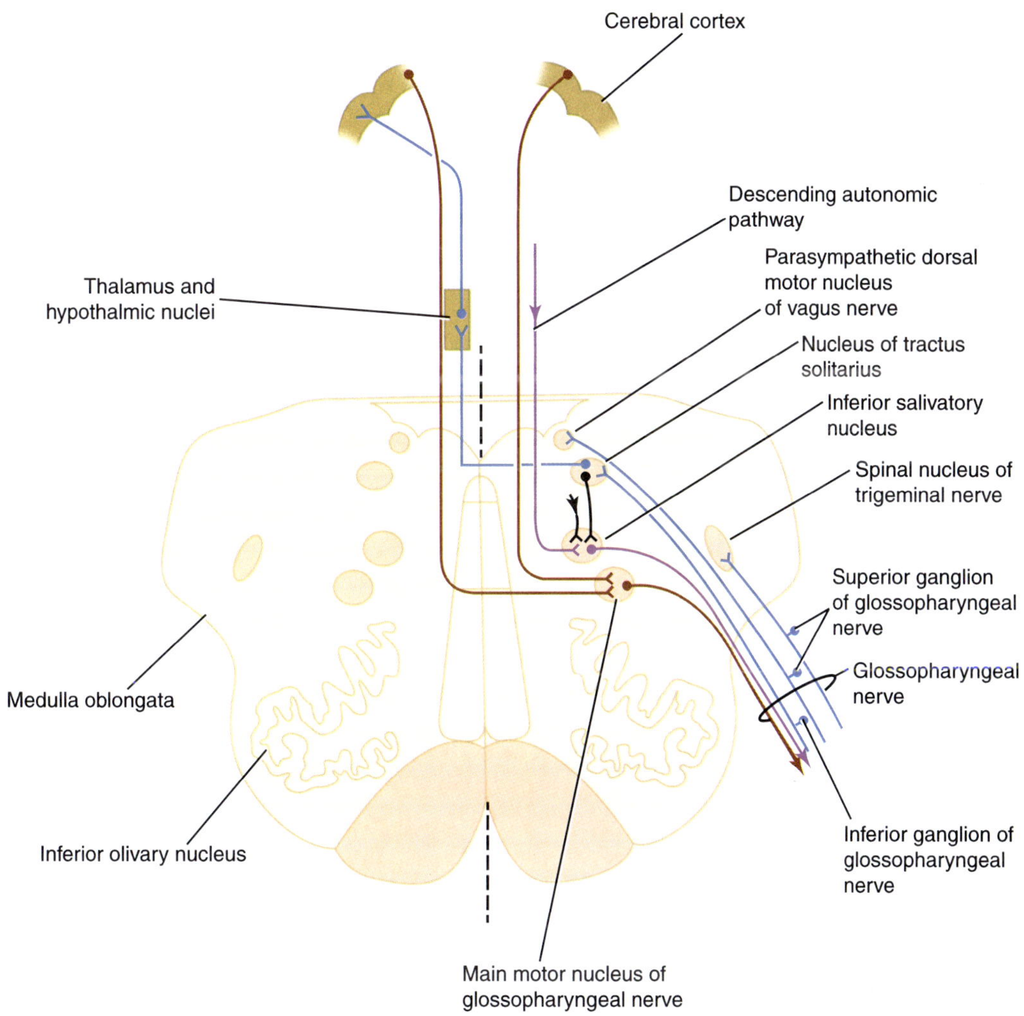

FIGURE 10.20. **Glossopharyngeal nerve nuclei and their central connections.**

Inferior to the foramen is an *inferior ganglion* (nodose ganglion) concerned with the visceral and special sensory components of the nerve (Fig. 10.18). In the region of the superior ganglion are connections to CN IX and the superior cervical (sympathetic) ganglion. CN X continues inferiorly in the *carotid sheath* to the root of the neck (see Chapter 9, Neck), supplying branches to the palate, pharynx, and larynx and cardiac branches to the cardiac and pulmonary plexuses (Fig. 10.22; Table 10.5).

The courses of the vagi (pl. of vagus) are asymmetrical in the thorax, a consequence of transitions of the great vessels and rotation of the midgut during development (see Chapter 4, Thorax and Chapter 5, Abdomen). CN X supplies branches to mixed motor and sensory plexuses that serve the heart, bronchi, lungs, and esophagus. **Anterior** and **posterior vagal trunks** form as continuations of the *esophageal plexus* surrounding the esophagus, which is also joined by branches of the sympathetic trunks. The trunks pass with the esophagus through the diaphragm into the abdomen, where the vagal trunks break up into branches that innervate the stomach and intestinal tract as far as the left colic flexure.

The Bottom Line: Vagus Nerve

- The vagus nerves (CN X) supply motor fibers to the voluntary muscles of the larynx and superior esophagus. • They also send visceral motor (presynaptic parasympathetic) fibers to the involuntary muscles and glands of (1) the tracheobronchial tree and esophagus via the pulmonary and esophageal plexuses, (2) to the heart via the cardiac plexus, and (3) to the alimentary tract as far as the left colic flexure via the vagal trunks. • The vagus nerves also send sensory fibers to the pharynx, larynx, and reflex afferents from these same areas (1–3 above). • They originate via 8–10 rootlets from the lateral sides of the medulla of the brainstem. They enter the superior mediastinum posterior to the sternoclavicular joints and brachiocephalic veins. • The nerves give rise to right and left recurrent nerves and then form the esophageal plexus, reform as anterior and posterior vagal trunks, and continue into the abdomen.

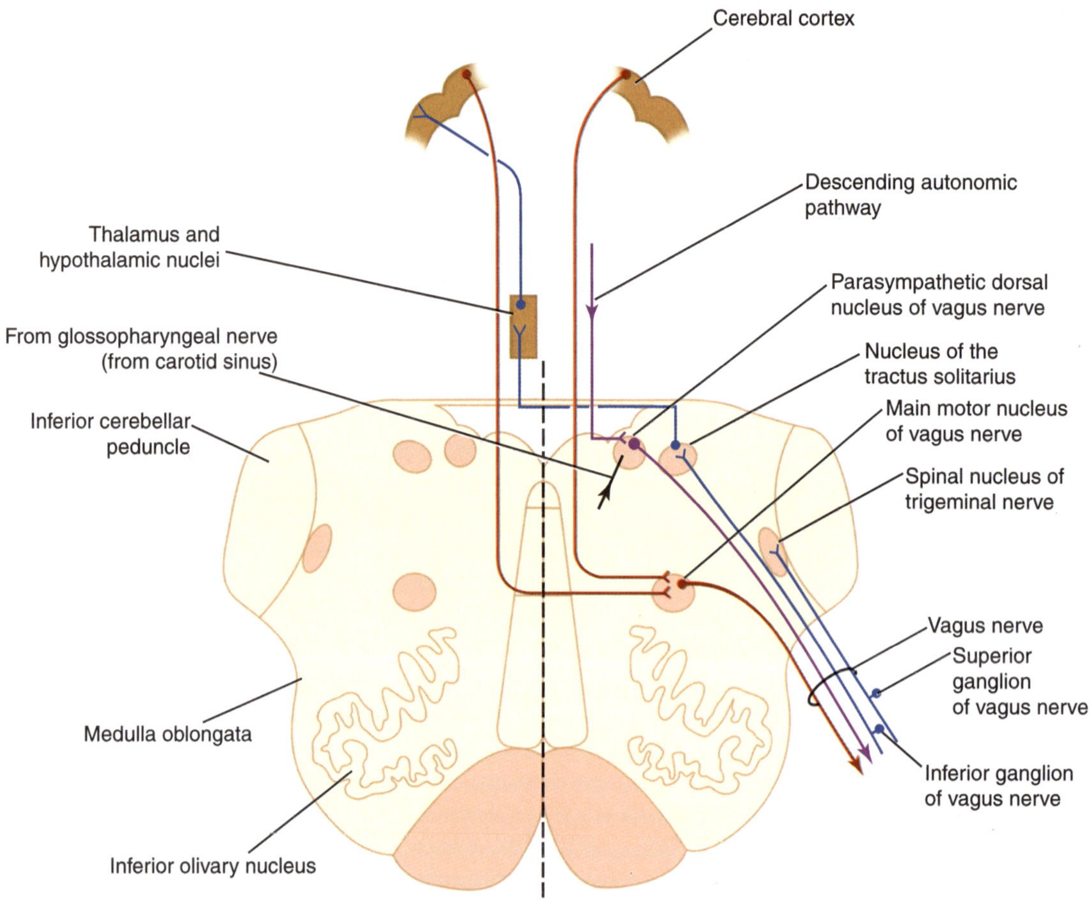

FIGURE 10.21. Vagus nerve nuclei and their central connections.

SPINAL ACCESSORY NERVE (CN XI)

N35.7 **Functions:** Somatic motor to the striated sternocleidomastoid and trapezius muscles.

Nuclei: The spinal accessory nerve arises from the **nucleus of the spinal accessory nerve**, a column of anterior horn motor neurons in the superior five or six cervical segments of the spinal cord (Fig. 10.6).

The traditional "cranial root" of CN XI is actually a part of CN X (Lachman et al., 2002). It may be united for a short distance with the **spinal accessory nerve** (CN XI) (Fig. 10.23). CN XI emerges as a series of rootlets from the first five or six cervical segments of the spinal cord. The spinal accessory nerve joins the CN X temporarily as they pass through the *jugular foramen*, separating again as they exit (Fig. 10.18). CN XI descends along the internal carotid artery, penetrates and innervates the sternocleidomastoid, and emerges from the muscle near the middle of its posterior border. Next, CN XI crosses the posterior cervical region and passes deep to the superior border of the trapezius to descend on its deep surface, providing multiple branches to the muscle. Branches of the cervical plexus conveying sensory fibers from spinal nerves C2–C4 join the spinal accessory nerve in the posterior cervical region, providing these muscles with pain and proprioceptive fibers.

Figure 10.24 shows cranial and spinal nuclei of the accessory nerve and their central connections.

The Bottom Line: Spinal Accessory Nerve

- The spinal accessory nerves (CN XI) supply somatic motor fibers to the sternocleidomastoid and trapezius muscles.
- The nerves arise as rootlets from the sides of the spinal cord in the superior five or six cervical segments.
- They ascend into the cranial cavity via the foramen magnum and exit through the jugular foramina, crossing the lateral cervical region, where pain and proprioceptive fibers from the cervical plexus join the nerves.

TABLE 10.5. SUMMARY OF VAGUS NERVE (CN X)

Divisions (Parts)	Branches
Cranial Vagi arise by a series of rootlets from medulla (includes traditional cranial root of CN XI)	Meningeal branch to dura mater (sensory; actually fibers of C2 spinal ganglion neurons that hitch a ride with vagus nerve) Auricular branch
Cervical Exit cranium/enter neck through jugular foramen; right and left vagus nerves enter carotid sheaths and continue to root of neck	Pharyngeal branches to pharyngeal plexus (motor) Cervical cardiac branches (parasympathetic, visceral afferent) Superior laryngeal nerve (mixed) internal (sensory) and external (motor) branches Right recurrent laryngeal nerve (mixed)
Thoracic Vagi enter thorax through superior thoracic aperture; left vagus contributes to anterior esophageal plexus; right vagus to posterior plexus; form anterior and posterior vagal trunks	Left recurrent laryngeal nerve (mixed; all distal branches convey parasympathetic and visceral afferent fibers for reflex stimuli) Thoracic cardiac branches Pulmonary branches Esophageal plexus
Abdominal Anterior and posterior vagal trunks enter abdomen through esophageal hiatus in diaphragm; distribute asymmetrically	Esophageal branches Gastric branches Hepatic branches Celiac branches (from posterior vagal trunk) Pyloric branch (from anterior vagal trunk) Renal branches Intestinal branches (to left colic flexure)

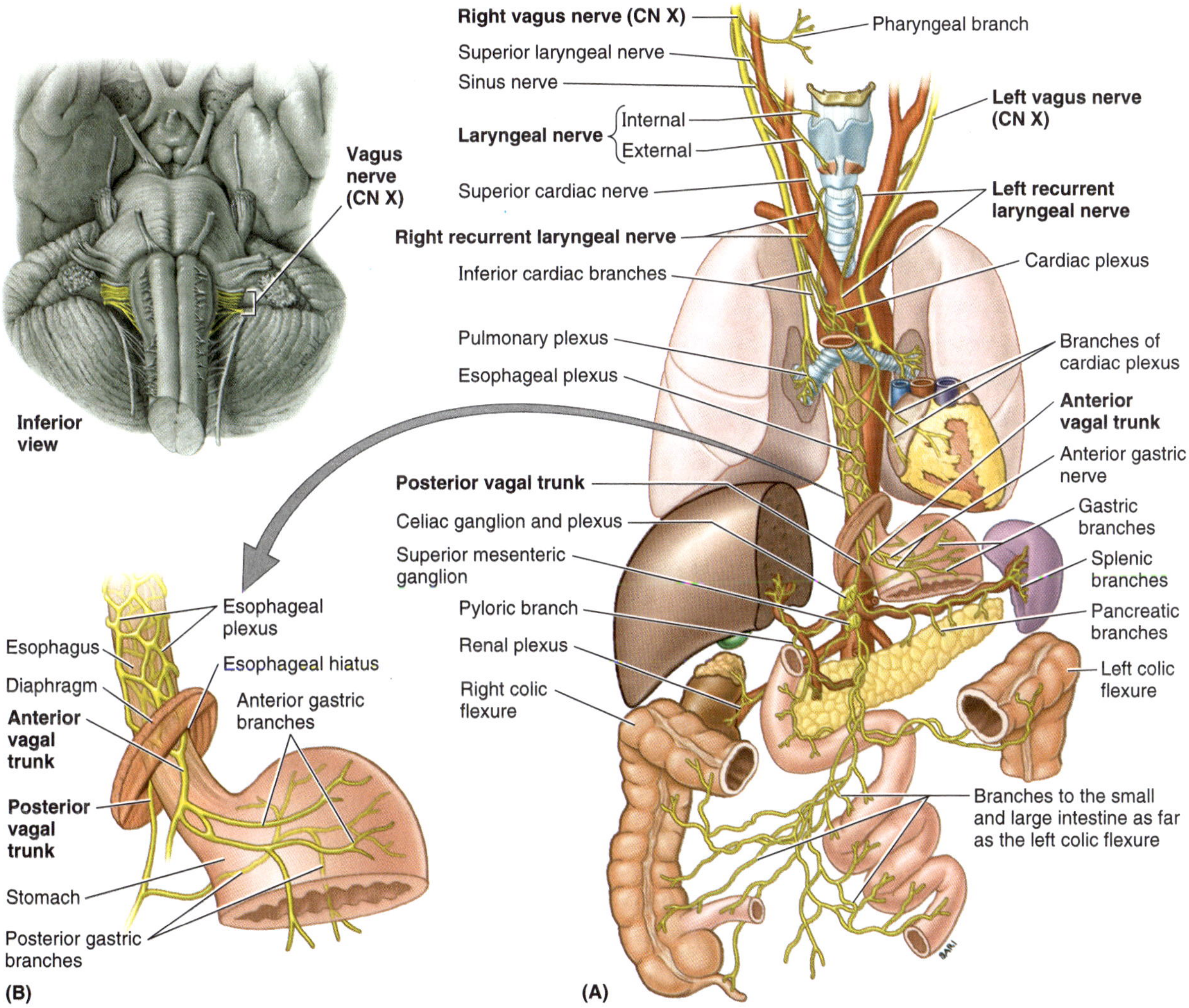

FIGURE 10.22. Distribution of vagus nerve (CN X). A. After supplying the palatine, pharyngeal, and laryngeal branches, CN X descends into the thorax. The recurrent laryngeal nerves ascend to the larynx, the left from a more inferior (thoracic) level. In the abdomen, the anterior and posterior vagal trunks demonstrate further asymmetry as they supply the terminal esophagus, stomach, and intestinal tract as far distally as the left colic flexure. **B.** Enlarged view of lower esophageal plexus transitioning to anterior and posterior vagal trunks.

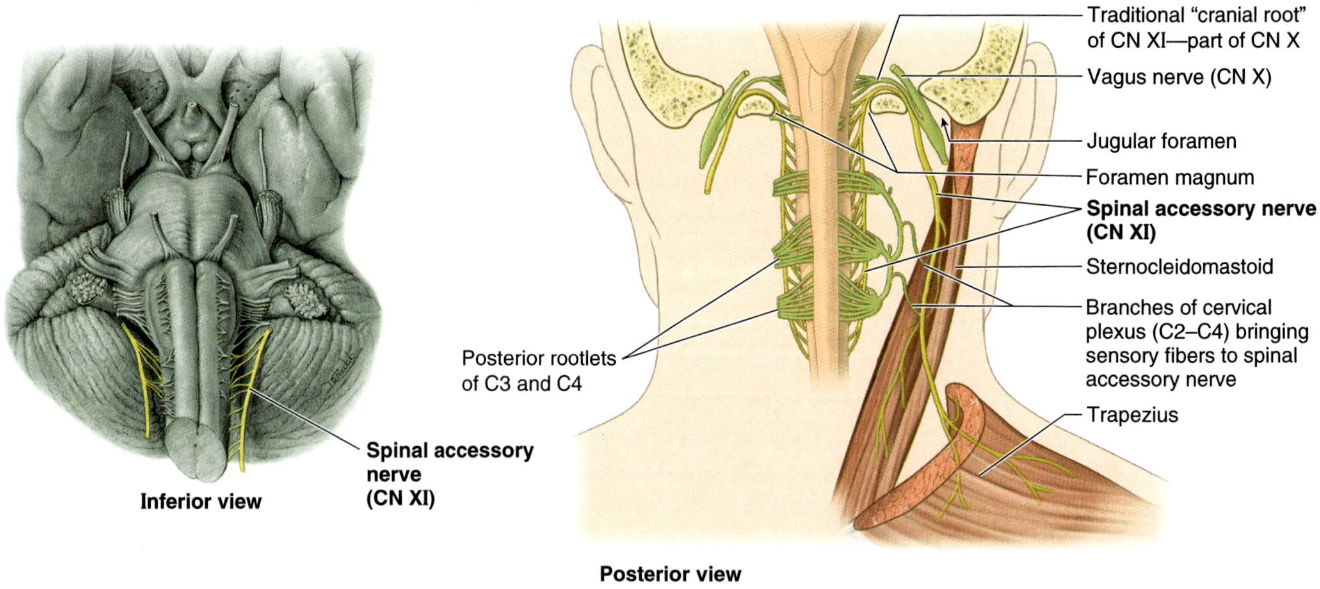

FIGURE 10.23. Distribution of spinal accessory nerve (CN XI).

HYPOGLOSSAL NERVE (CN XII)

AN35.7 **Functions:** Somatic motor to the intrinsic and extrinsic muscles of the tongue (G. *glossa*)—styloglossus, hyoglossus, and genioglossus.

The **hypoglossal nerve** (CN XII) arises as a purely motor nerve by several rootlets from the medulla and leaves the cranium through the *hypoglossal canal* (Figs. 10.2 and 10.3). After exiting the cranial cavity, CN XII is joined by a branch or branches of the cervical plexus conveying general somatic motor fibers from C1 and C2 spinal nerves and somatic (general) sensory fibers from the spinal ganglion of C2 (Fig. 10.25). These spinal nerve fibers "hitch a ride" with CN XII to reach the hyoid muscles, with some of the sensory fibers passing retrograde along it to reach the dura mater of the posterior cranial fossa (see Fig. 8.13B). CN XII passes inferiorly medial to the angle of the mandible and then curves anteriorly to enter the tongue (Fig. 10.25).

Hypoglossal nucleus and its central connections are shown in Figure 10.26.

CN XII ends in many branches that supply all the extrinsic muscles of the tongue, except the palatoglossus (a palatine muscle). CN XII has the following branches:

- A **meningeal branch** returns to the cranium through the hypoglossal canal and innervates the dura mater on the floor and posterior wall of the posterior cranial fossa. The nerve fibers conveyed are from the sensory spinal ganglion of spinal nerve C2 and are not hypoglossal fibers.
- The **superior root of the ansa cervicalis** branches from CN XII to supply the infrahyoid muscles (sternohyoid, sternothyroid, and omohyoid). This branch conveys only fibers from the cervical plexus (the loop between the anterior rami of C1 and C2) that joined the nerve outside the cranial cavity, not hypoglossal fibers (Fig. 10.25). Some fibers continue past the origin of the superior root to reach the thyrohyoid muscle.
- Terminal **lingual branches** supply the styloglossus, hyoglossus, genioglossus, and intrinsic muscles of the tongue.

The Bottom Line: Hypoglossal Nerve

- The hypoglossal nerves (CN XII) supply somatic motor fibers to the intrinsic and extrinsic muscles of the tongue, except the palatoglossus (a palatine muscle).
- They arise by several rootlets between the pyramids and the olives of the medulla.
- They pass through the hypoglossal canals and run inferiorly and anteriorly, passing medial to the angles of the mandible and between the mylohyoid and the hyoglossus to reach the muscles of the tongue.

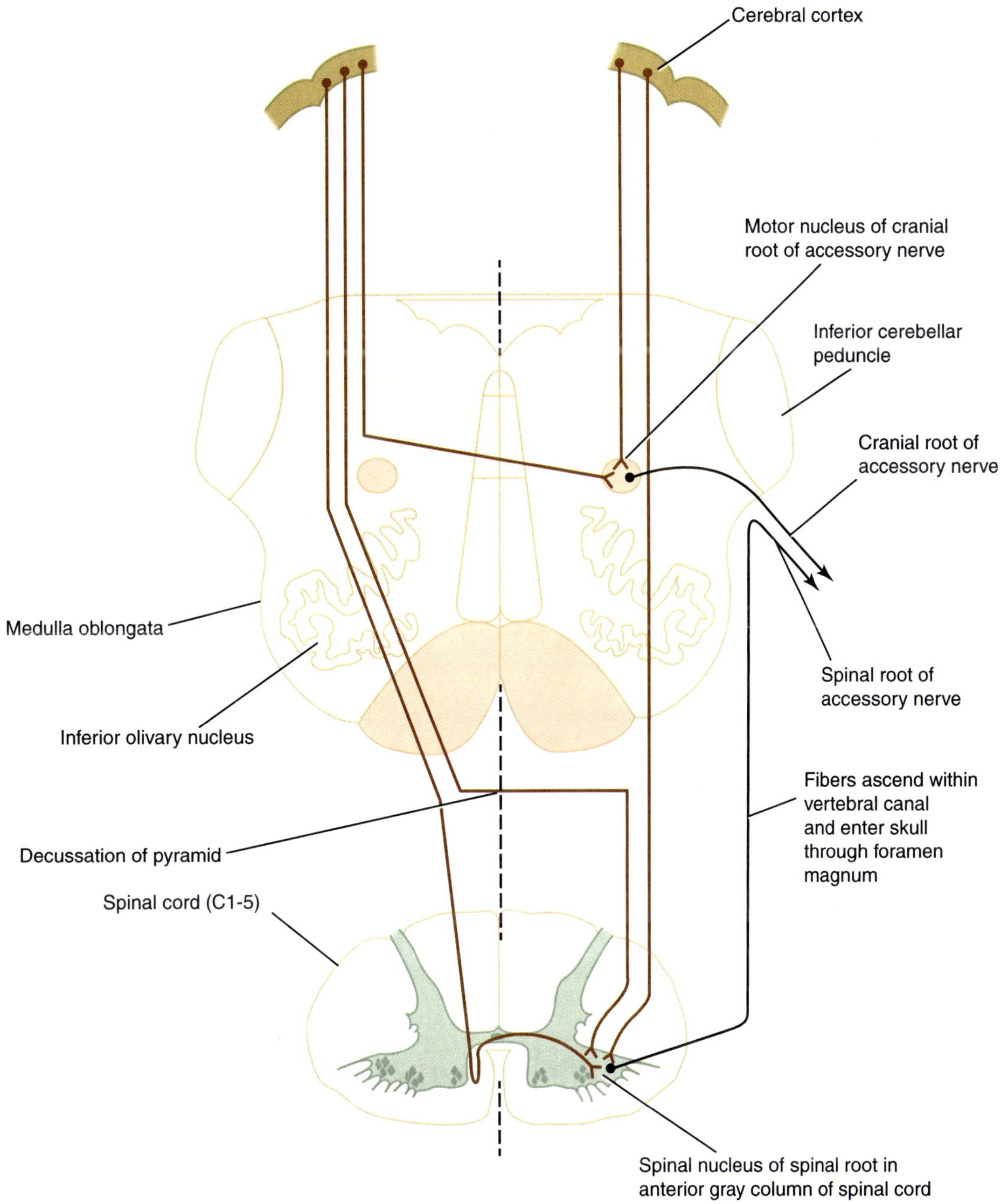

FIGURE 10.24. Cranial and spinal nuclei of the accessory nerve and their central connections.

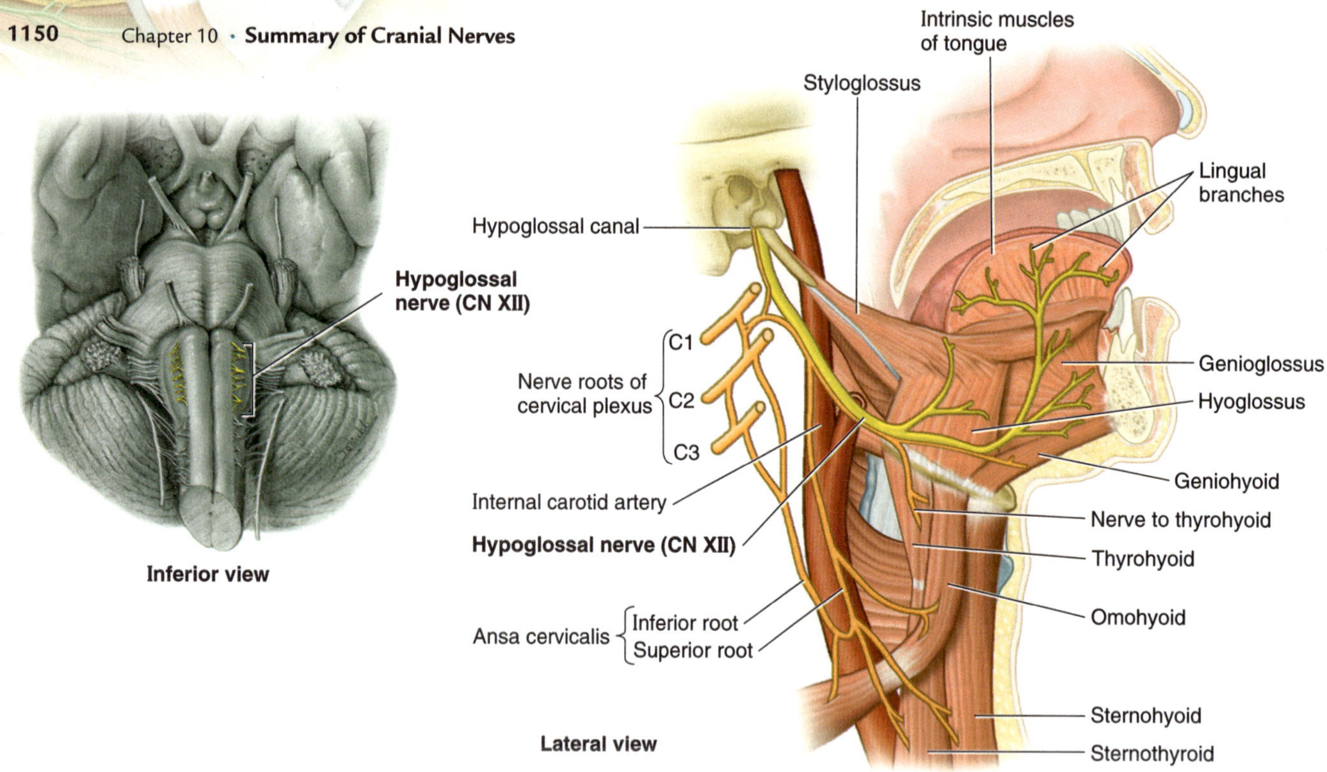

FIGURE 10.25. Distribution of hypoglossal nerve (CN XII). CN XII leaves the cranium through the hypoglossal canal and passes deep to the mandible to enter the tongue, where it supplies all intrinsic and extrinsic lingual muscles, except the palatoglossus. CN XII is joined immediately distal to the hypoglossal canal by a branch conveying fibers from the C1 and C2 loop of the cervical plexus. These fibers hitch a ride with CN XII, leaving it as the superior root of the ansa cervicalis and the nerve to the thyrohyoid muscle. Cervical spinal nerves, not CN XII, supply the infrahyoid muscles.

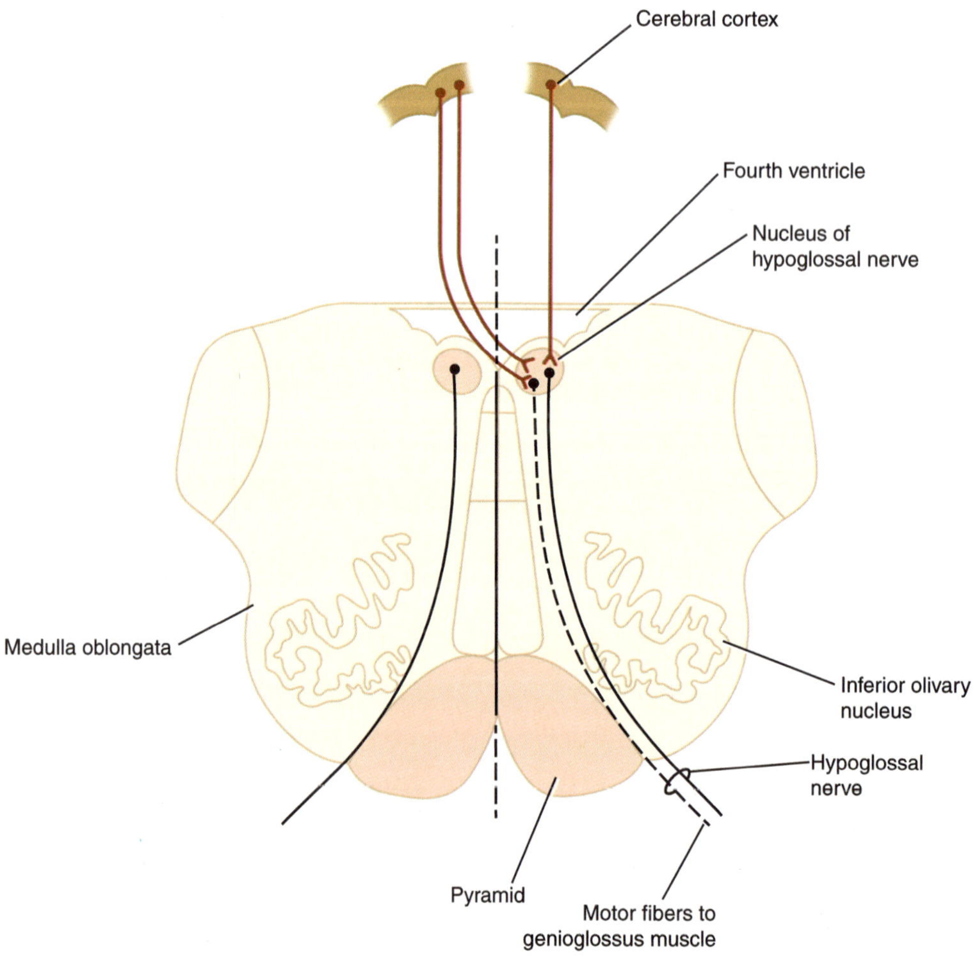

FIGURE 10.26. Hypoglossal nucleus and its central connections.

CLINICAL BOX

CRANIAL NERVES

Cranial Nerve Injuries

Table 10.6 summarizes some common cranial nerve injuries, indicating the type or site of lesions and abnormal findings that result. Injury to the cranial nerves is a frequent complication of a fracture in the base of the cranium. Furthermore, excessive movement of the brain within the cranium may tear or bruise cranial nerve fibers, especially those of CN I. Paralysis resulting from trauma may not be evident for several days. Further, cranial nerve injuries also commonly occur with traumatic injury to the brain, which can result in delayed diagnosis and intervention (Russo et al., 2016).

Because of their location within the confined cranial cavity, relatively fixed positions, and sometimes close relationships to bony or vascular formations, the intracranial portions of certain cranial nerves are also susceptible to compression owing to a tumor or aneurysm. In such cases, the onset of symptoms usually occurs gradually, and the effects depend on the extent of the pressure exerted. Because of their close relationship to the cavernous sinus, CN III, CN IV, CN V_1, and especially CN VI is susceptible to compression or injury related to pathologies (infections, thrombophlebitis) affecting the sinus.

OLFACTORY NERVE (CN I)

Anosmia: Loss of Smell

The loss of smell (anosmia) is frequently associated with upper respiratory infections, sinus disease, and head trauma. Loss of olfactory fibers occurs with aging. Consequently, elderly people often have reduced acuity of the sensation of smell, resulting from progressive reduction in the number of olfactory receptor neurons in the

TABLE 10.6. SUMMARY OF CRANIAL NERVE LESIONS

Nerve	Types(s) and/or Site(s) of Lesion	Abnormal Finding(s)
CN I	Fracture of cribriform plate	Anosmia (loss of smell); cerebrospinal fluid rhinorrhea
CN II	Direct trauma to orbit or eyeball; fracture involving optic canal	Loss of pupillary constriction
	Pressure on optic pathway; laceration or intracerebral clot in temporal, parietal, or occipital lobes of brain	Visual field defects. See Figure B10.1.
CN III	Pressure from herniating uncus on nerve; fracture involving cavernous sinus; aneurysms	Dilated pupil; ptosis; eye turns "down and out;" pupillary reflex on side of lesion will be lost. See Figure B8.32A.
CN IV	Stretching of nerve during its course around brainstem; fracture of orbit	Inability to look down when eye is adducted
CN V	Injury to terminal branches (particularly CN V_2) in roof of maxillary sinus; pathological processes affecting trigeminal ganglion	Loss of pain and touch sensations; paresthesia; masseter and temporalis muscles do not contract; deviation of mandible to side of lesion when mouth is opened
CN VI	Base of brain or fracture involving cavernous sinus or orbit	Eye fails to move laterally; diplopia on lateral gaze. See Fig. B8.32B.
CN VII	Laceration or contusion in parotid region	Paralysis of facial muscles; eye remains open; angle of mouth droops; forehead does not wrinkle
	Fracture of temporal bone	As above, plus associated involvement of cochlear nerve and chorda tympani; dry cornea; loss of taste on anterior two thirds of tongue
	Intracranial hematoma ("stroke")	Forehead wrinkles because of bilateral innervation of frontalis muscle, otherwise paralysis of contralateral facial muscles
CN VIII	Tumor of nerve (acoustic neuroma)	Progressive unilateral hearing loss; tinnitus (noises in ear)
CN IX	Brainstem lesion or deep laceration of neck	Loss of taste on posterior third of tongue; loss of sensation on affected side of soft palate
CN X	Brainstem lesion or deep laceration of neck	Sagging of soft palate; deviation of uvula to normal side; hoarseness owing to paralysis of vocal fold
CN XI	Laceration of neck	Paralysis of sternocleidomastoid and descending fibers of trapezius; drooping of shoulder
CN XII	Neck laceration; fractures of cranial base	Protruded tongue deviates toward affected side; moderate dysarthria (disturbance of articulation). See Figure B10.4.

olfactory epithelium. The chief complaint of most people with anosmia is the loss or alteration of taste; however, clinical studies reveal that in all but a few people, the dysfunction is in the olfactory system (Simpson, 2013). The reason is that most people confuse taste with flavor. Transitory olfactory impairment occurs as a result of viral or *allergic rhinitis*—inflammation of the nasal mucous membrane.

To test the sense of smell, the person is blindfolded and asked to identify common odors, such as freshly ground coffee placed near the external nares (nostrils). One naris is occluded and the eyes are closed. Because anosmia is usually unilateral, each naris is tested separately. If the loss of smell is unilateral, the person may not be aware of it without clinical testing.

Injury to the nasal mucosa, olfactory nerve fibers, olfactory bulbs, or olfactory tracts may also impair smell. In severe head injuries, the olfactory bulbs may be torn away from the olfactory nerves, or some olfactory nerve fibers may be torn as they pass through a *fractured cribriform plate*. If all the nerve bundles on one side are torn, a complete loss of smell will occur on that side; consequently, anosmia may be a clue to a fracture of the cranial base and cerebrospinal fluid *rhinorrhea* (leakage of the fluid through the nose).

A tumor and/or abscess in the frontal lobe of the brain or a tumor of the meninges (*meningioma*) in the anterior cranial fossa may also cause anosmia by compressing the olfactory bulb and/or tract (D'Amico et al., 2016).

Olfactory Hallucinations

Occasionally *olfactory hallucinations* (false perceptions of smell) may accompany lesions in the temporal lobe of the cerebral hemisphere. A lesion that irritates the lateral olfactory area (deep to the uncus) may cause *temporal lobe epilepsy* or "uncinate fits," which are characterized by imaginary disagreeable odors and involuntary movements of the lips and tongue.

OPTIC NERVE (CN II)

Demyelinating Diseases and Optic Nerves

Because the optic nerves are actually CNS tracts, the myelin sheath that surrounds the sensory fibers from the point at which the fibers penetrate the sclera is formed by oligodendrocytes (glial cells) rather than by neurolemma (Schwann) cells, as in other cranial or spinal nerves of the peripheral nervous system (PNS). Consequently, the optic nerves are susceptible to the effects of *demyelinating diseases* of the CNS, such as *multiple sclerosis* (MS), which usually do not affect other nerves of the PNS.

Optic Neuritis

Optic neuritis refers to lesions of the optic nerve that cause diminution of visual acuity, with or without changes in peripheral fields of vision (Odel et al., 2016). Optic neuritis may be caused by inflammatory, degenerative, demyelinating, or toxic disorders. The optic disc appears pale and smaller than usual on ophthalmoscopic examination. Many toxic substances (e.g., methyl and ethyl alcohol, tobacco, lead, and mercury) may also injure the optic nerve.

Visual Field Defects

Visual field defects result from lesions that affect AN30.5
different parts of the visual pathway. The type of defect depends on where the pathway is interrupted (Fig. B10.1):

- Complete section of an optic nerve results in blindness in the temporal (*T*) and nasal (*N*) visual fields of the ipsilateral eye (depicted in *black*).
- Complete section of the optic chiasm reduces peripheral vision and results in *bitemporal hemianopsia*, the loss of vision of one half of the visual field of both eyes.
- Complete section of the right optic tract at the midline eliminates vision from the left temporal and right nasal visual fields. A lesion of the right or left optic tract causes a contralateral homonymous hemianopsia, indicating that visual loss is in similar fields. This defect is the most common form of visual field loss and is often observed in patients with strokes (Swartz, 2014).

Defects of vision caused by compression of the optic pathway, as may result from tumors of the pituitary gland or berry aneurysms of the internal carotid arteries (see Chapter 8, Head), may produce only part of the visual losses described here. Patients may not be aware of changes in their visual fields until late in the course of disease, because lesions affecting the visual pathway often develop insidiously.

OCULOMOTOR NERVE (CN III) AN31.5

Injury to Oculomotor Nerve

A lesion of CN III results in *ipsilateral oculomotor palsy*, in which the eye is abducted and depressed, with the pupil dilated. This palsy is summarized in Table 10.6 and discussed and illustrated in the clinical box "Paralysis of Extra-ocular Muscles/Palsies of Orbital Nerves" in Chapter 8, Head.

Compression of Oculomotor Nerve

Rapidly increasing intracranial pressure (e.g., resulting from an extradural hematoma) often compresses CN III against the crest of the petrous part of the temporal bone. Because autonomic fibers in CN III are superficial, they are affected first. As a result, the pupil dilates progressively on the injured side. Consequently, the first sign of *CN III compression* is ipsilateral slowness of the pupillary response to light.

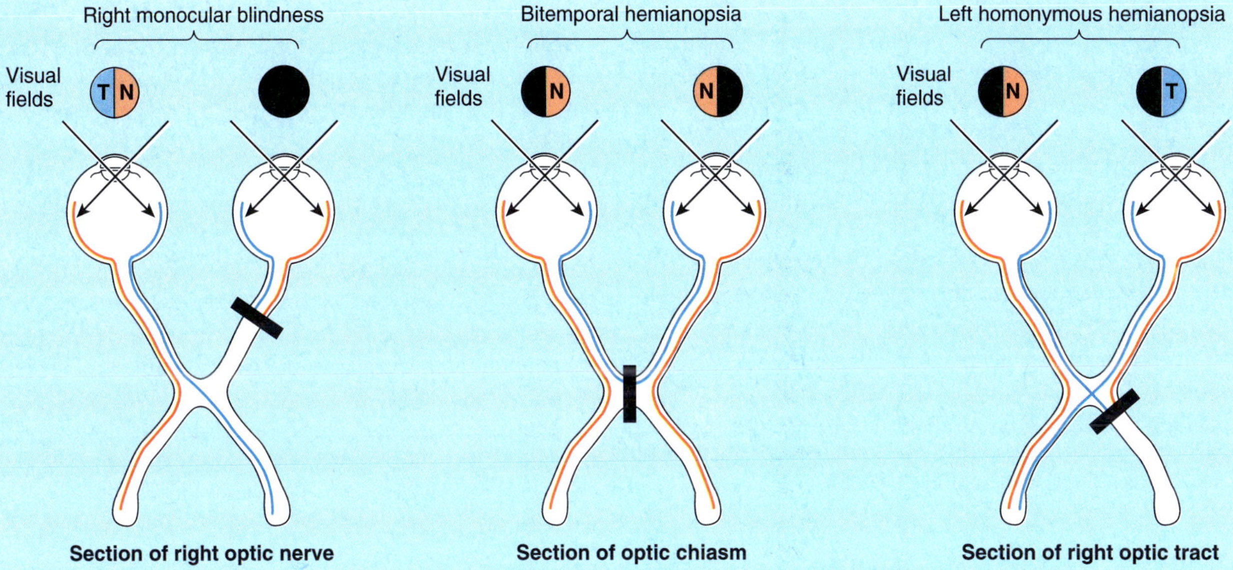

FIGURE B10.1. Visual field defects.

Aneurysm of Posterior Cerebral or Superior Cerebellar Artery

An aneurysm of a posterior cerebral or superior cerebellar artery may also exert pressure on CN III as it passes between these vessels. The effects of this pressure depend on its severity. Because CN III lies in the lateral wall of the cavernous sinus, injuries or infections of the sinus may also affect this nerve.

AN31.5 TROCHLEAR NERVE (CN IV)

CN IV is rarely paralyzed alone. *Lesions of the trochlear nerve* or its nucleus cause paralysis of the superior oblique and impair the ability to turn the affected eyeball inferomedially. CN IV may be torn when there are severe head injuries because of its long intracranial course. The characteristic sign of trochlear nerve injury is *diplopia* (double vision) when looking down. Diplopia occurs because the superior oblique normally assists the inferior rectus in depressing the pupil (directing the gaze downward) and is the only muscle to do so when the pupil is adducted. In addition, because the superior oblique is the primary muscle producing intorsion of the eyeball, the primary muscle producing extorsion (the inferior oblique) is unopposed when the superior oblique is paralyzed. Thus, the direction of gaze and rotation of the eyeball about its anteroposterior axis is different for the two eyes when an attempt is made to look downward and especially when looking downward and medially. The person can compensate for the diplopia by inclining the head anteriorly and laterally toward the side of the normal eye.

TRIGEMINAL NERVE (CN V)

Injury to Trigeminal Nerve

CN V may be injured by trauma, tumors, aneurysms, or meningeal infections (Cioroiu et al., 2016). It may be involved occasionally in poliomyelitis ("polio," a viral infantile disease) and generalized polyneuropathy, a disease affecting several peripheral nerves. The sensory and motor nuclei in the pons and medulla may be destroyed by intramedullary tumors or vascular lesions. An isolated lesion of the spinal trigeminal tract also may occur with multiple sclerosis (MS). *Injury to CN V* causes the following:

- Paralysis of the muscles of mastication with deviation of the mandible toward the side of the lesion (Table 10.6).
- Loss of the ability to appreciate soft tactile, thermal, or painful sensations in the face.
- Loss of corneal reflex (blinking in response to the cornea being touched) and the sneezing reflex (stimulated by irritants to clear the respiratory tract).

Common causes of facial numbness are dental trauma, *herpes zoster ophthalmicus* (infection caused by a herpes virus), cranial trauma, head and neck tumors, intracranial tumors, and idiopathic trigeminal neuropathy (a nerve disease of unknown cause).

Trigeminal neuralgia (tic douloureux), the principal disease affecting the sensory root of CN V, produces excruciating, episodic pain that is usually restricted to the areas supplied by the maxillary and/or mandibular divisions of this nerve. (See the clinical box "Trigeminal Neuralgia" in Chapter 8, Head, for a detailed discussion.)

10

Dental Anesthesia

Anesthetic agents are commonly administered by injection to block pain during dental procedures. CN V is of great importance in the practice of dentistry because it is the sensory nerve of the head, serving the teeth and mucosa of the oral cavity. Because the superior alveolar nerves (branches of CN V_2) are not accessible, the maxillary teeth are locally anesthetized by injecting the agent into the tissues surrounding the roots of the teeth and allowing the solution to infiltrate the tissue to reach the terminal (dental) nerve branches that enter the roots. By contrast, the inferior alveolar nerve (CN V_3) is readily accessible and is probably anesthetized more frequently than any other nerve. This procedure is described in the clinical box "Inferior Alveolar Nerve Block" in Chapter 8, Head.

N31.5 ABDUCENT NERVE (CN VI)

Because CN VI has a long intradural course, it is often stretched when intracranial pressure rises, partly because of the sharp bend it makes over the crest of the petrous part of the temporal bone after entering the dura mater. A space-occupying lesion, such as a brain tumor, may compress CN VI, causing paralysis of the lateral rectus. Complete *paralysis of CN VI* causes medial deviation of the affected eye, that is, it is adducted by the unopposed action of the medial rectus, leaving the person unable to abduct the eye lateral to the primary position. *Diplopia* (double vision) is present in all ranges of movement of the eyeball, except on gazing to the side opposite the lesion. Paralysis of CN VI may also result from:

- An aneurysm of the cerebral arterial circle (at the base of the brain). (See the clinical box "Strokes" in Chapter 8, Head for an illustrated discussion of berry aneurysm.)
- Pressure from an atherosclerotic (plaque-lined) internal carotid artery in the cavernous sinus, where CN VI is closely related to this artery. (See the clinical box "Brain Infarction" in Chapter 8, Head, for an illustration and explanation of atheromatous plaque.)
- Septic thrombosis of the cavernous sinus subsequent to infection in the nasal cavities and/or paranasal sinuses. (See the clinical box "Thrombophlebitis of Facial Vein" in Chapter 8, Head.)

N28.7 FACIAL NERVE (CN VII)

Among motor nerves, CN VII is the most frequently paralyzed of all the cranial nerves. Depending on the part of the nerve involved, injury to CN VII may cause paralysis of facial muscles without loss of taste on the anterior two thirds of the tongue or altered secretion of the lacrimal and salivary glands.

A *lesion of CN VII near its origin* or near the geniculate ganglion is accompanied by loss of motor, gustatory (taste), and autonomic functions. The motor paralysis of facial muscles involves superior and inferior parts of the face on the ipsilateral side.

A *central lesion of CN VII* (lesion of the CNS) results in paralysis of muscles in the inferior face on the contralateral side. Consequently, forehead wrinkling is not visibly impaired because it is innervated bilaterally. Lesions between the geniculate ganglion and the origin of the chorda tympani produce the same effects as that resulting from injury near the ganglion, except that lacrimal secretion is not affected. Because it passes through the facial canal in the temporal bone, CN VII is vulnerable to compression when a viral infection produces inflammation (viral neuritis) and swelling of the nerve just before it emerges from the stylomastoid foramen.

Because the branches of CN VII are superficial, they are subject to injury from knife and gunshot wounds, cuts, and birth injury. Damage to CN VII is common with fracture of the temporal bone and is usually detectable immediately after the injury. CN VII may also be affected by tumors of the brain and cranium, aneurysms, meningeal infections, and herpes viruses. Although injuries to CN VII cause paralysis of facial muscles, sensory loss in the small area of skin on the posteromedial surface of the auricle of the ear and around the opening of the external acoustic meatus is rare. Similarly, hearing is not usually impaired, but the ear may become more sensitive to low tones when the stapedius (supplied by CN VII) is paralyzed; this muscle dampens vibration of the stapes (see Chapter 8, Head).

Bell palsy is a unilateral facial paralysis of sudden onset resulting from a lesion of CN VII. See the clinical box, "Paralysis of Facial Muscles" in Chapter 8, Head, for an illustrated and detailed discussion of this syndrome.

VESTIBULOCOCHLEAR NERVE (CN VIII)

Injuries to Vestibulocochlear Nerve

Although the vestibular and cochlear nerves are essentially independent, peripheral lesions often produce concurrent clinical effects because of their close relationship. Hence, *lesions of CN VIII* may cause *tinnitus* (ringing or buzzing in ears), *vertigo* (dizziness, loss of balance), and impairment or loss of hearing. Central lesions may involve either the cochlear or vestibular divisions of CN VIII.

Deafness

There are two kinds of deafness (hearing loss): *conductive deafness*, involving the external or middle ear (e.g., otitis media, inflammation in the middle ear; see the clinical box, "Otitis Media" in Chapter 8, Head, for an illustrated and detailed discussion), and *sensorineural deafness* (damage to the hair cells in the inner ear), which results from disease in the cochlea or in the pathway from the cochlea to the brain.

Acoustic Neuroma

An *acoustic neuroma* (neurofibroma) is a slow-growing benign tumor of the neurolemma (Schwann) cells. The tumor begins in the vestibular nerve while it is in the internal acoustic meatus. The early symptom of an acoustic neuroma is usually loss of hearing. Dysequilibrium (derangement of the sense of motion and balance) and tinnitus occur in approximately 70% of patients (D'Amico et al., 2016).

Trauma and Vertigo

People with head trauma often experience headache, dizziness, vertigo, and other features of posttraumatic injury. *Vertigo* is a hallucination of movement involving the person or the environment (Roberts, 2016). It often involves a spinning sensation, but it may be felt as a swaying back and forth or falling. These symptoms, often accompanied by nausea and vomiting, are usually related to a peripheral vestibular nerve lesion.

GLOSSOPHARYNGEAL NERVE (CN IX)

Lesions of Glossopharyngeal Nerve

Isolated *lesions of CN IX* or its nuclei are uncommon and are not associated with perceptible disability (Russo et al., 2016). Most commonly, trauma to the nerve is *iatrogenic* (physician-caused, e.g., inadvertent injury during a tonsillectomy). Taste is absent on the posterior third of the tongue, and the gag reflex is absent on the side of the lesion. Ipsilateral weakness may produce a noticeable change in swallowing.

Injuries of CN IX resulting from infection or tumors are usually accompanied by signs of involvement of adjacent nerves. Because CN IX, CN X, and CN XI pass through the jugular foramen, tumors in this region produce multiple cranial nerve palsies, called the *jugular foramen (Vernet) syndrome*, in which *dysphagia* (difficulty in swallowing) and *dysarthria* (motor difficulty in speaking) are more apparent. The soft palate and posterior wall of the pharynx deviate to the contralateral side of the injury when the gag reflex is initiated ("curtain sign") (Fig. B10.2). Pain in the distribution of CN IX may be associated with involvement of the nerve in a tumor in the neck.

Glossopharyngeal Neuralgia

Glossopharyngeal neuralgia (glossopharyngeal tic) is uncommon and its cause is unknown. The sudden intensification of pain is of a burning or stabbing nature. These *paroxysms* (spasms or sudden attacks) of pain are often initiated by swallowing, protruding the tongue, talking, or touching the palatine tonsil (Yugrakh et al., 2016). Pain paroxysms occur during eating when trigger areas are stimulated.

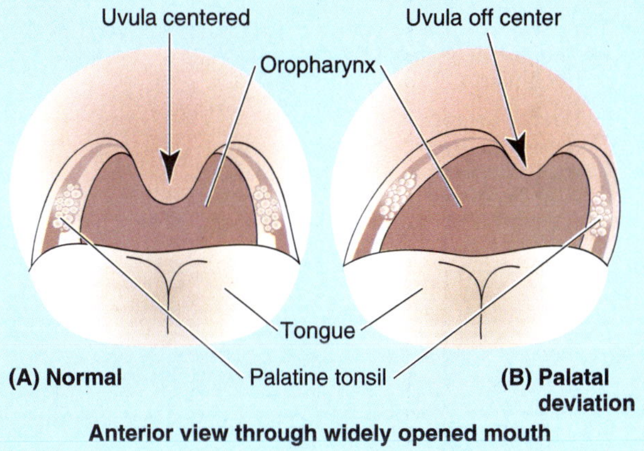

FIGURE B10.2. Gag reflex. A. Normal. **B.** Palatal deviation. Note that the palate and posterior wall of the pharynx deviate to the left side when the gag reflex is elicited. This "curtain sign" is due to a right CN IX/CN X lesion.

VAGUS NERVE (CN X)

Isolated *lesions of CN X* are uncommon. Injury to pharyngeal branches of CN X results in mild or severe *dysphagia* (difficulty in swallowing). Lesions of the superior laryngeal nerve produce anesthesia of the superior part of the larynx and paralysis of the cricothyroid muscle. (See the clinical box, "Injury to Laryngeal Nerves" in Chapter 9, Neck.) The voice is weak and tires easily. Injury of a recurrent laryngeal nerve may be caused by aneurysms of the arch of the aorta and may occur during neck operations. Injury of the recurrent laryngeal nerve causes *dysphonia* (hoarseness or weakness of voice) because of paralysis of the vocal folds (cords). Paralysis of both recurrent laryngeal nerves causes *aphonia* (loss of voice) and *inspiratory stridor* (a harsh, high-pitched respiratory sound). Paralysis of recurrent laryngeal nerves usually results from cancer of the larynx and thyroid gland and/or from injury during surgery on the thyroid gland, neck, esophagus, heart, and lungs. Because of its longer course, lesions of the left recurrent laryngeal nerve are more common than those of the right. Proximal lesions of CN X also affect the pharyngeal and superior laryngeal nerves, causing difficulty in swallowing and speaking.

SPINAL ACCESSORY NERVE (CN XI)

Because of its nearly subcutaneous passage through the lateral cervical region (posterior triangle of neck), *iatrogenic* (physician-caused) *injury of CN XI* may occur during surgical procedures such as *lymph node biopsy*, *cannulation of the internal jugular vein*, and *carotid endarterectomy* (Russo et al., 2016). Rare *high lesions of CN XI* result in paralysis of the ipsilateral sternocleidomastoid, manifest as impairment of rotation to the affected side (Fig. B10.3A) and of the trapezius, manifest as unilateral inability to shrug the

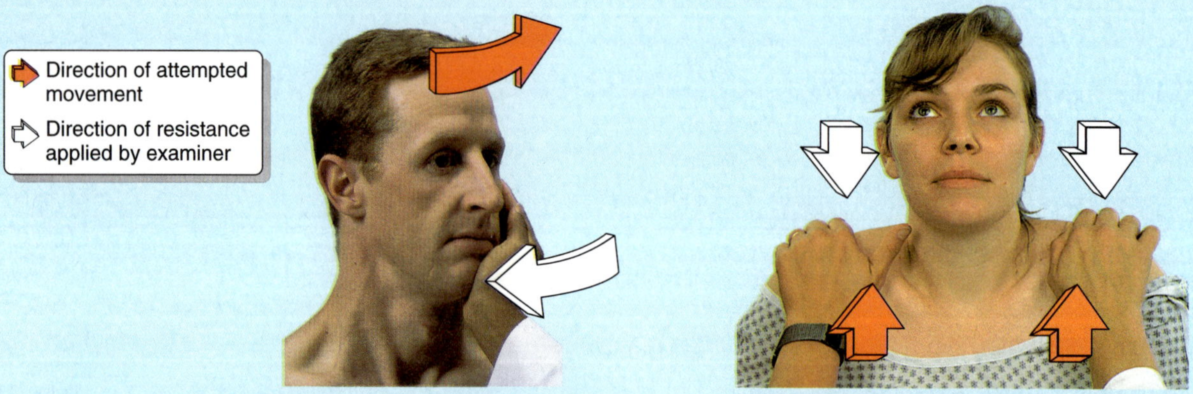

(A) Test for sternocleidomastoid function (B) Test for trapezius function

FIGURE B10.3. Testing function of sternocleidomastoid and trapezius and spinal accessory nerve.

shoulder (Fig. B10.3B), or winging of the scapula at rest. In the more common *lower lesion*, only the trapezius is affected. (See the clinical box, "Lesions of Spinal Accessory Nerve (CN XI)" in Chapter 9, Neck.)

HYPOGLOSSAL NERVE (CN XII)

39.2 Trauma to CN XII is also most often iatrogenic (e.g., injury during procedures including carotid endarterectomy, endotracheal intubation, or other airway device insertion and use). CN XII compression during head rotation results from a medially directed or elongated styloid process, sometimes associated with ossification of the stylohyoid ligament (Eagle syndrome). *Injury to CN XII* paralyzes the ipsilateral half of the tongue, resulting in *dysarthria*. After some time, the tongue atrophies, making it appear shrunken and wrinkled (Russo et al., 2016). When the tongue is protruded, its apex deviates toward the paralyzed side because of the unmatched action by the genioglossus and intrinsic muscles on the paralyzed side of the tongue, which remains unextended (Fig. B10.4).

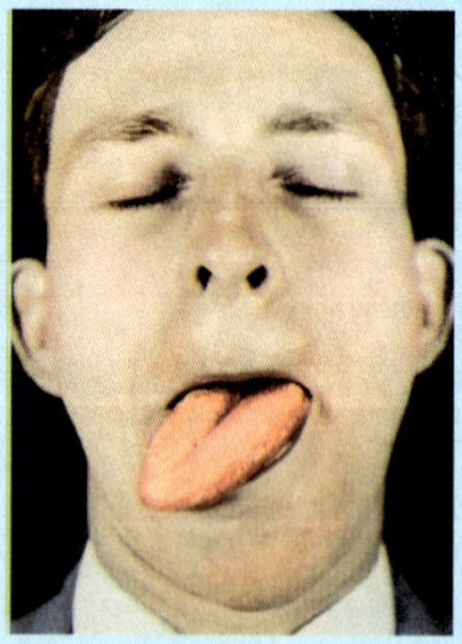

FIGURE B10.4. Hypoglossal nerve palsy.

Multiple-Choice Questions

1. **Preganglionic parasympathetic axons are contained in which of the following cranial nerves?**

   a. III, V, VII, IX
   b. III, V, VII, X
   c. III, VI, VII, IX
   d. III, VII, IX, X

   (Ref: Page 1126)

2. **Which of the following cranial nerve nucleus lies deep to facial colliculus of pons?**

   a. Facial nerve
   b. Glossopharyngeal nerve
   c. Abducent nerve
   d. Trigeminal nerve

   (Ref: Page 1128)

3. **The mandibular nerve supplies all the following muscles EXCEPT:**

   a. Mylohyoid
   b. Medial pterygoid
   c. Lateral pterygoid
   d. Stylohyoid

   (Ref: Page 1136)

4. **The facial nerve gives sercretomotor fibers to all the following EXCEPT:**

   a. Submandibular gland
   b. Parotid gland
   c. Lacrimal gland
   d. Nasal glands

   (Ref: Page 1140)

5. **Unilateral injury to the hypoglossal nerve causes the following signs EXCEPT:**

   a. Hemiatrophy of the involved side of the tongue
   b. On protrusion, the tongue deviates toward the paralyzed side
   c. Loss of taste sensation on the affected side of tongue
   d. Fasciculation of tongue

   (Ref: Page 1156)

6. **Motor fibers to muscles of pharynx and larynx arise from:**

   a. Dorsal nucleus of vagus
   b. Nucleus ambiguus
   c. Nuclei of solitary tract
   d. Mesencephalic nucleus of V nerve

   (Ref: Page 1125)

7. **The nucleus of origin of the facial nerve includes all of the following EXCEPT:**

   a. Motor nucleus
   b. Nuclei of solitary tract
   c. Superior salivatory
   d. Inferior salivatory

   (Ref: Page 1128)

8. **Following tonsillectomy, a patient had loss of general and taste sensation in the posterior third of tongue. Injury to which of the following nerves could cause this?**

   a. Chorda tympani
   b. Lingual
   c. Glossopharyngeal
   d. Facial

   (Ref: Page 1142)

9. **Branches of the trigeminal nerve exit the skull through all these foramina EXCEPT:**

   a. Foramen ovale
   b. Superior orbital fissure
   c. Foramen rotundum
   d. Foramen lacerum

   (Ref: Page 1136)

10. Injury to recurrent laryngeal nerves may cause all the following effects EXCEPT:

a. Paralysis of cricothyroid
b. Inspiratory stridor
c. Aphonia
d. Anesthesia of the lower part of larynx

(Ref: Page 1155)

11. A 42-year-old man with complete section of left optic tract will present with which of the following symptoms?

a. Right monocular blindness
b. Left monocular blindness
c. Right homonymous hemianopsia
d. Left homonymous hemianopsia

(Ref: Page 1152)

12. A 23-year-old male patient with history of aneurysms of the Circle of Willis presents to the ophthalmology clinic with his right eye abducted, depressed, and pupils dilated. Aneurysm in one of the following arteries can compress a cranial nerve resulting in this clinical presentation. Which artery is involved?

a. Anterior cerebral artery
b. Middle cerebral artery
c. Posterior cerebral artery
d. Anterior communicating artery

(Ref: Page 1153)

13. A 78-year-old male patient complains of paroxysms of pain in his tongue, throat, and ears whenever he eats or yawns. Which of the following cranial nerve is involved?

a. Maxillary nerve
b. Mandibular nerve
c. Facial nerve
d. Glossopharyngeal nerve

(Ref: Page 1155)

14. CT of temporal bone shows narrowing of vertical part of facial canal, distal to the geniculate ganglion. Which of the following branches of facial nerve will NOT be affected?

a. Posterior auricular nerve
b. Greater petrosal nerve
c. Nerve to stapedius
d. Chorda tympani nerve

(Ref: Pages 1014, 1140)

15. Which of the following conditions can result in paresis of IX, X, and XI cranial nerves?

a. Jugular foramen tumor
b. Cerebellopontine angle tumor
c. Acoustic neuroma
d. Cavernous sinus thrombosis

(Ref: Page 1155)

Answer Keys for MCQs

1. **d** 2. **c** 3. **d** 4. **b** 5. **c** 6. **b** 7. **d** 8. **c** 9. **d** 10. **a** 11. **c**
12. **c** 13. **d** 14. **b** 15. **a**

Refer to *Appendix A* at the end of the book for *Student Case Study Questions and Answers* of Volume 3.

APPENDIX A Student Case Study

Chapter 8 Head

Case Study 8-1

A young man was playing in a pickup hockey game when he was knocked down. He was not wearing a helmet and hit his head hard on the ice. He was momentarily stunned and said that he "saw stars." His vision was blurred for approximately 20 seconds. He skated to the bench and showed no other signs of injury except that he complained of a lingering headache.

Questions:

1. Do you think the person would have a fractured calvaria? Explain your answer.
2. What may the lingering headache indicate?
3. If you detected clear fluid dripping from the person's nose, what might be the source of the fluid?

Case Study 8-2

A hockey player was struck viciously on the lower face by an elbow during a scuffle in the corner of the rink. Profuse bleeding from the mouth was obvious, and he was unable to close his jaws normally.

Questions:

1. What bone may have been fractured?
2. A loss of integrity of the mandible results in a change of bite. What is this condition called? What results from this malformation?
3. What other structures may be fractured? Discuss these injuries.

Case Study 8-3

A batter was struck in the superolateral part of the right cheek by a baseball. His cheek appeared flat and depressed. There was soon swelling and ecchymosis around the eye. The player complained of dizziness, double vision in the right eyeball, and numbness of the cheek.

Questions:

1. What bone was most likely fractured?
2. What other bones may have been fractured?
3. What is the most common fracture of the upper cheek?
4. What symptom suggests that the eyeball and orbit may be injured?

Case Study 8-4

A shortstop fielding a ground ball was hit on the side of the nose when the ball bounced unexpectedly. Blood spurted from his, nose and his nasal airway was obstructed. His nose was deformed, and the nasal bones were displaced. Disruption of the nasal cartilages was also detected.

Questions:

1. What is epistaxis?
2. What causes spurting of blood from the nose? What specific structures are involved?
3. What causes obstruction to the nasal airway?
4. If the nasal fracture extends into the cranium, what may be the result?

Case Study 8-5

A 16-year-old youth was referred to a dermatologist for treatment of a severe case of acne (*acne vulgaris*). The physician observed a small abscess (boil) on the ala of the youth's nose that had developed a yellow "head" at its apex. She treated the youth with antibiotics but warned him not to pick or squeeze the boil because it might cause the infection to spread to the meninges (meningitis) and brain (*encephalitis*).

Questions:

1. Describe the danger triangle of the face.
2. Explain anatomically how an infection could spread from the nose to the meninges and brain.
3. Discuss the possible results of a meningeal infection.

Case Study 8-6

A figure skater fell on the ice, hitting the back of her head hard on the ice. She did not lose consciousness but was slightly confused and complained of temporary dizziness. Her pupils appeared normal. The fist-sized swelling on the back of her head was tense on palpation. The physician who examined her said that she probably had a hematoma of the scalp but would monitor her condition for several hours.

Questions:

1. In what layer of the scalp would the hematoma likely be located?
2. What limits the spread of a superficial hematoma of the scalp?
3. What initial treatment would likely be given?

Case Study 8-7

A young woman who was not wearing a seat belt hit her forehead on the dashboard of her 10-year-old car during a head-on collision. The frontal area of her scalp was lacerated and bleeding profusely. The wound was cleansed with a saline solution and covered with a sterile bandage. By the time the woman reached the hospital, she had two black eyes. Further examination revealed that there was no injury to her eyeballs.

Questions:

1. Why does the scalp bleed so profusely?
2. How could the scalp wound bleeding be controlled?
3. What is the anatomical basis for the circular dressing?
4. How could blood pass to both eyes when there was no injury to the orbital regions?
5. Does a deep wound of the scalp always require stitches? If yes, why?
6. Why are scalp wounds potentially dangerous?

Case Study 8-8

A 58-year-old man complained to his physician about a swelling on his cheek anterior to his ear lobule. He said that it had been growing rapidly for approximately 2 months and that this part of his face felt weak. He also experienced difficulty when he tried to whistle. The physical examination and subsequent pathological studies revealed a carcinoma of the parotid gland.

Questions:

1. How could this tumor cause weakness of the face and make it difficult for the man to whistle?
2. Where do tumor cells from this gland usually metastasize?
3. Is the facial paralysis likely to be permanent?

Case Study 8-9

A 72-year-old man was concerned about a pea-sized swelling posterior to his auricle. Physical examination of his external ear and scalp by a physician revealed an infected sebaceous cyst in the temporal region.

Questions:

1. How could an infection in the temporal region cause a swelling posterior to the auricle?
2. An infection of what other structures could produce a larger, more painful swelling posterior to the external ear?

Case Study 8-10

A young woman recovering from a severe cold with nasal congestion complained to her physician about pain in her upper jaw. She said that she had been to her dentist but he told her that her teeth were not infected.

Questions:

1. Infection of which structures in the woman's upper jaw could cause pain in this area of her cheek?
2. Infection of what dental structures could cause this type of facial pain?

Case Study 8-11

A 26-year-old man was examined in the emergency department after being hit in the eye with a pool cue during a brawl. Examination of the eyeball showed no serious injury except for bleeding into the anterior chamber. The physician was concerned about the appearance of the eyeball and referred the patient to an ophthalmologist.

Questions:

1. What type of orbital fracture may have occurred?
2. How do you think a nonpenetrating blow to the eye could result in serious problems?

Case Study 8-12

A young boy was taken to a pediatrician because of a severe earache. An otoscopic examination revealed a bulging, inflamed tympanic membrane. His mother told the physician that the boy was recovering from a severe cold and throat infection.

Questions:

1. Where do you think the ear infection was located? What is this type of inflammation called?
2. How could an infection in the throat cause inflammation and bulging of the tympanic membrane?

Case Study 8-13

A 27-year-old woman involved in a motorcycle accident was taken to the emergency department. She had facial lacerations but no obvious fractures. An eye examination revealed a medial strabismus of her right eyeball.

Questions:

1. What is the meaning of the term *strabismus*?
2. Injury to which cranial nerve would cause this eye abnormality?
3. Which muscle was paralyzed?

Case Study 8-14

The wife of a 45-year-old commercial traveler was awakened by the unusual nature of her husband's snoring and was puzzled when she noticed that he was sleeping with his left eye open. In the morning, she observed that the left side of his face was drooping. When he tried to examine his teeth, he found that his lips were also paralyzed on that side. He was unable to whistle or puff out his cheek because the air blew out through his lips on the left side. He also found that he was unable to raise his eyebrow or frown on that side. During breakfast, he had trouble chewing his food because it dribbled out of the left side of his mouth. Fearing that he may have had a mild stroke during the night, he made an appointment to see his physician.

Physical Examination: During the examination, the physician made the following observations: at rest, the left side of his face appeared flattened and expressionless. There were no lines on the left side of his forehead, and there was sagging in the left lower half of his face. Saliva drooled from the left corner of his mouth. He also had a loss of taste sensation on the anterior two thirds of the left side of his tongue and an absence of voluntary control of the left facial muscles. When he smiled, the lower portion of his face was pulled to the normal side and the right corner of his mouth was raised, but the left corner was not. During questioning, the patient related how he had driven home late the night before and, because of drowsiness, had rolled the window down part way. He also recalled that he had had a severe head cold and an ear infection a few days previously. He recalled that the physician who treated him said that his illness resulted from a viral infection.

Diagnosis: Bell palsy (facial paralysis). Paralysis of the facial muscles may occur without a known cause (idiopathic). Bell palsy (facial paralysis) may follow exposure to cold as occurs when riding in a car with the window open. Bell palsy occurs at all ages but is slightly more common in the third through fifth decades.

Questions:

1. Paralysis of what nerve would produce the signs exhibited by this person?
2. Why did the patient's left eye remain open even when he was sleeping? What other consequences involving the eye occur with this syndrome?
3. Explain the anatomical basis of the drooling and difficulty in chewing.
4. Why was there loss of taste sensation on the anterior two thirds of the left side of his tongue?
5. Where would the lesion of the nerve probably be located?
6. Is the paralysis permanent?

Case Study 8-15

A 62-year-old man complained to his dentist about sudden recurring attacks of excruciating, stabbing pain (*paroxysms*) on the left side of his face. They were of approximately 2-month duration and had been increasing in severity. Following examination, the dentist informed him that there was no dental cause for his pain. He recommended that he see a physician.

Physical Examination: The man told the physician that the stabbing pains, lasting 15–20 seconds, occurred several times a day and were so severe that he had once contemplated suicide. He said that the onset of pain seemed to be triggered by chewing and a cold wind blowing on his face. When the physician asked him to point to the area where the pains occurred, he pointed to his left upper lip and cheek. He said that the pain also radiated to his inferior eyelid, the lateral side of his nose, and the inside of his mouth. The physician applied firm, steady pressure over the person's left cheek and over his infra-orbital area. He detected no tenderness indicative of inflammation of the maxillary sinus. On further evaluation, the physician detected acute sensitivity to touch (*hyperesthesia*) on the left upper lip and over the entire left maxillary region but found no abnormality of sensation in the forehead or mandibular regions.

Diagnosis: Tic douloureux.

Questions:

1. Which branch of what major nerve supplies the area of skin and mucous membrane where the paroxysms were felt?
2. Where does the maxillary nerve leave the cranium?
3. What are the maxillary nerve's branches and how are they distributed?

Case Study 8-16

A 55-year-old farmer consulted his physician about a sore that had been on his lower lip for 6 months. He stated that he first thought it was a cold sore, but he became worried because it looked different and was getting larger.

Physical Examination: On examination, the physician observed an ulcerated lesion on the central part of the man's lower lip. Systematic palpation of the lymph nodes revealed enlarged, hard, submental lymph nodes. None of the submandibular or deep cervical lymph nodes was enlarged. A biopsy of the labial lesion was taken.

Diagnosis: Examination of the biopsy from the edge of the lesion revealed a *squamous cell carcinoma* (malignant tumor of epithelial origin).

Questions:

1. Into which lymph nodes does lymph from the central part of the lower lip drain?
2. Between the bellies of which muscles do these nodes lie?
3. What other structures, in addition to the central part of the lip, drain to these nodes?
4. To which lymph nodes do lymph vessels from the lateral part of the lip pass?

5. If the cancer had spread from the submental nodes, where would you expect to find metastases?

Case Study 8-17

A puck struck a 22-year-old medical student on the left temple during an interfaculty hockey game. He fell to the ice unconscious but regained consciousness in approximately 1 minute. A laceration approximately 3 cm superior to his left zygomatic arch was bleeding. As he was helped to the bench, he said that he felt weak and unsteady. Realizing that he may have sustained a cranial fracture, you asked a classmate to call a physician while you took him to the dressing room. Upon further examination, you found that the deep tendon reflexes in his limbs were equal. His pupils were equal in size and contracted to light. In approximately half an hour, your friend said that he was sleepy and wanted to lie down. His left pupil was now moderately dilated and reacted sluggishly to light. By the time the physician arrived, he was unconscious.

Physical Examination: The physician observed that the student's pupil on the left was widely dilated and did not respond to light, whereas the pupil on the right was slightly dilated but showed a normal reaction to light. The physician said, "We must get him to the hospital right away!"

Radiology Examination: In the hospital, several cranial radiographs and a CT scan of his head were taken. As the physician was almost certain of an intracranial hemorrhage, she called a neurosurgeon.

Diagnosis: Compressed fracture of the temporal squama, posterior to the pterion, and an extradural (epidural) hematoma (see Figure 8.1).

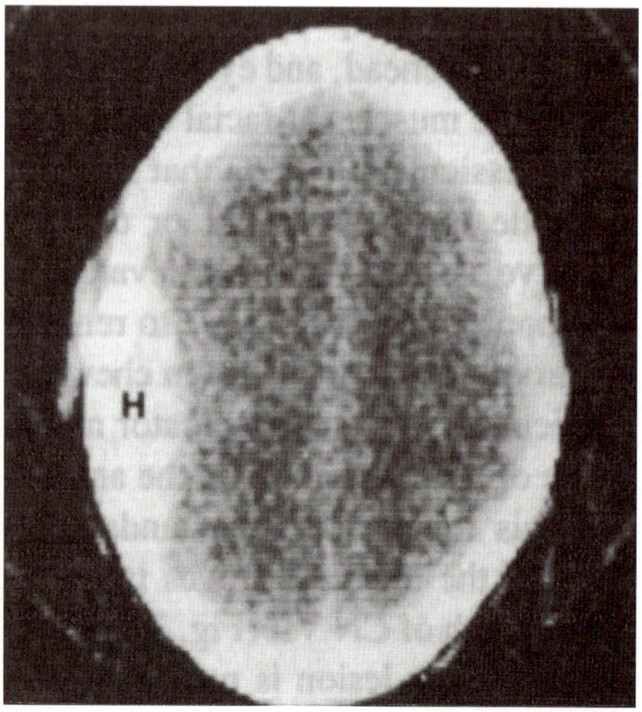

Questions:

1. Define the region known as the temple.
2. Delineate the cranial area known as the pterion.
3. In what part of the temporal fossa is the pterion located?
4. Why is the pterion clinically important?
5. What artery was most likely torn?
6. What other vessel may have been torn?
7. Where would the blood collect?
8. Differentiate between an extradural and a "subdural" hemorrhage.
9. What effect will an extradural hematoma likely have on the brain?

Case Study 8-18

A 49-year-old woman developed a throbbing headache that lasted for approximately 30 minutes and then slowly faded away. Similar headaches occurred occasionally for the next week. One day as she was lifting a heavy chair, she experienced a sudden, severe headache that was accompanied by nausea, vomiting, and a general feeling of weakness. A friend took her to a hospital immediately.

Physical Examination: The physician detected *nuchal rigidity* (neck stiffness) and an elevation of blood pressure. Visualization of the optic fundus through an ophthalmoscope showed *subhyaloid hemorrhages* (bleeding between the retina and vitreous body). Her deep tendon reflexes were symmetrical, and all modalities of sensation were normal. On the basis of these distinct signs and symptoms, the physician made a tentative diagnosis of subarachnoid hemorrhage. He requested radiographic studies and a lumbar puncture.

Radiology and Laboratory Reports: The arteriograms and CT scans showed a large, saccular aneurysm of the anterior communicating artery. The CSF was grossly bloody; after centrifugation, the supernatant fluid was xanthochromatic (yellow-colored).

Diagnosis: Ruptured aneurysm of the anterior communicating artery and a subarachnoid hemorrhage.

Questions:

1. Where would blood from the ruptured aneurysm most likely go?
2. How do you explain anatomically the formation of subarachnoid hemorrhages?
3. Why was the supernatant part of the CSF xanthochromatic?
4. Where do most single aneurysms occur?
5. If there had been markedly increased intracranial pressure due to the aneurysm or its rupture, would a lumbar puncture be performed? Why or why not?

Case Study 8-19

A 23-year-old man went to a dentist to have a badly decayed mandibular left third molar tooth extracted. The dentist explained he would likely experience considerable pain with removal of the tooth and informed the patient that he was going to inject a "local" anesthetic to desensitize the tooth and associated soft tissues. When agreeing to the extraction, the patient requested that plenty of anesthetic be given because he was extremely sensitive to pain. The dentist inserted the needle through the mucous membrane on the inside of the patient's mouth, where the needle came to rest near the lingula on the medial surface of the ramus of the mandible. In a few minutes, the patient stated that his gum, lip, chin, and tongue on the left side were numb (anesthetized). During the extraction procedure, the patient said he felt severe pain; the dentist injected more anesthetic. The tooth was removed without further incident.

As the patient was preparing to leave, he happened to look in the mirror. He was surprised to find that he was unable to close his eye on the affected side and that his mouth sagged on this side, particularly when he attempted to expose his teeth. He also noted that his ear lobule was numb. When he reported these unusual symptoms, the dentist explained that because of the large amount of anesthetic injected, other nerves in addition to those supplying the teeth had been anesthetized. He assured the patient that these effects would disappear in 3–4 hours.

Questions:

1. Name the nerve supplying the mandibular molar and premolar teeth.
2. Why were the patient's chin, lower lip, and tongue on the injected side also anesthetized?
3. When anesthetizing this nerve, what other nerves might be affected?
4. What probably caused the patient's facial paralysis and loss of sensation in his ear lobule?

Answers

Case Study 8-1

1. The young man probably does not have a fractured calvaria because he did not lose consciousness. The fall on his head resulted in the slight alterations in neurological function: "seeing stars" and blurred vision.
2. The lingering headache may indicate increasing intracranial pressure resulting from damage to the brain (e.g., contusion of the cerebral cortex).
3. A fracture of the cribriform plate of the ethmoid may tear the meninges and result in cerebral spinal fluid (CSF) rhinorrhea (loss of CSF through the nose).

Case Study 8-2

1. The player's lower jaw was probably fractured, which resulted in his teeth not fitting together (occluding) as they normally do. Fracture of the mandible is common in sports such as hockey, football, and rugby. Often two mandibular fractures, or a fracture–dislocation of the TMJ, occur in the jaw. The most common fracture site is near the angle of the mandible.
2. When the integrity of the jaw is lost, the teeth do not fit together normally (*malocclusion*). This leads to changes in speech patterns because the articulation of words is difficult (dental sounds, such as the "S" sound, may not be producible in the normal way or may be inadvertently produced, and the required movements of the jaw may be difficult and painful).
3. *Fractures of the teeth* may also occur when the jaws are hit by a hard blow. The fracture may occur through the enamel, pulp, or root of the tooth. Fractures exposing the pulp of the tooth cause severe pain and sensitivity to heat and cold. Root fractures cause mobility of the teeth.

Case Study 8-3

1. The zygomatic bone was most likely fractured.
2. The bones forming the orbit may also have fractured.
3. Fractures of the zygomatic bone are the most common fractures of the upper cheek, the most serious of which is the "tripod" fracture of the zygomatic bone involving three separate breaks of the cranial bones:
   a) Through the infra-orbital foramen and canal to the infra-orbital groove (a fracture of the maxilla).
   b) Through the zygomaticoparietal suture of the lateral margin of the orbit.
   c) Through the zygomatic arch, usually at its narrowest point, where the suture between the zygomatic process of the temporal bone and the temporal process of the zygomatic bone occurs.
4. The *diplopia* suggests that the eyeball and orbit may have been injured. Diplopia indicates malalignment of the visual axes. Temporary blurred vision may be a complication of zygomatic fractures.

Case Study 8-4

1. *Epistaxis* refers to nasal hemorrhage. The bleeding results from the richness of the blood supply to the nasal mucosa.
2. *Spurting of blood from the nose* results from ruptured arteries, particularly at the site of anastomosis of the sphenopalatine and greater palatine arteries on the nasal septum (Kiesselbach area).
3. The nasal airway is often obstructed when there is a nasal fracture because bone fragments may block the nose.
4. If the fracture extends into the floor of the anterior cranial fossa, the cribriform plate may fracture and the meninges may tear, resulting in *cerebral spinal fluid (CSF) rhinorrhea*, discharge of CSF through the nose.

Case Study 8-5

1. The *danger triangle of the face* has its base at the vermilion border of the upper lip and its apex at the bridge of the nose.

2. Inflammation of the facial vein associated with thrombus formation may result in the spread of infection from the facial vein through the superior and inferior ophthalmic veins to the meninges and the cavernous sinus.
3. *Cavernous sinus thrombosis* may result in meningitis, thrombophlebitis of cortical veins, and *cerebral edema*, an increase in brain volume resulting from an increase in water and sodium content. When severe, brain edema can cause various forms of herniation of the brain and pressure on the brainstem, which may result in failure of respiration and circulation.

Case Study 8-6

1. The hematoma was probably located in the thick, richly vascularized subcutaneous layer of connective tissue of the scalp (layer two).
2. A superficial hematoma of the scalp is limited by the fibrous tissue that binds the skin to the epicranial aponeurosis.
3. The initial treatment of the hematoma was probably the application of an ice pack to control the bleeding and swelling.

Case Study 8-7

1. The superficial arteries of the scalp, unlike most superficial arteries in subcutaneous tissue, course within the dermis superficial to the epicranial aponeurosis, with their walls firmly attached to the dense connective tissue. The severed arteries are thus unable to contract in response to the cut as other superficial arteries do, allowing clotting to occur sooner.
2. Bleeding from a deep scalp wound can be stopped by direct pressure with sterile gauze. Once the bleeding has stopped, a circular dressing can be applied for transportation to the hospital for further treatment (e.g., suturing the epicranial aponeurosis).
3. Because the arteries enter the scalp inferiorly and ascend toward to the vertex of the head, a horizontal headband type of bandage compresses the vertical arteries.
4. The skin of the scalp is continuous with that covering the forehead. Hence, bleeding in the loose connective layer can pass to the face, especially around the eyes, because this fourth layer of the scalp is somewhat like a sponge and may distend with blood from an injury. As the blood accumulates, it gravitates to the face and collects around the eyes.
5. A deep wound of the scalp involving the epicranius gapes widely because of the pull of the anterior and posterior parts of the occipitofrontalis and lateral pull of the temporoparietalis. Therefore, stitches must be used to close the gap in the epicranial aponeurosis.
6. A severe infection of the scalp may spread to the bones of the calvaria, meninges, and/or brain via diploic veins, possibly resulting in osteomyelitis (infection of the bone) or thrombosis of the dural sinuses or meningitis, which may be fatal.

Case Study 8-8

1. The facial nerve leaves the cranium through the stylomastoid foramen and almost immediately enters the parotid gland. Its branches spread out like the abducted fingers of the hand. Consequently, a malignant parotid tumor invades the facial nerve and interferes with its supply to the facial muscles, including those used to whistle.
2. Tumor cells from the carcinoma would metastasize to the deep cervical lymph nodes. These nodes form a chain along the course of the IJV from the cranium to the root of the neck.
3. The facial paralysis is likely permanent because severely injured cranial nerves do not regenerate.

Case Study 8-9

1. An infected sebaceous cyst in the temporal region could spread through the lymphatics to the mastoid lymph nodes located posterior to the auricle.
2. Inadequate treatment of a middle ear infection could spread through the mastoid antrum to the mastoid cells (*acute mastoiditis*) and produce a swelling posterior to the auricle.

Case Study 8-10

1. Infection of the maxillary sinuses—*maxillary sinusitis*—is a common complication of nasal infections. Infection of these sinuses is common because their ostia are near the roofs of the sinuses. Hence, the sinuses must be full before they will drain when the person is standing.
2. An infection from an abscess in a maxillary molar tooth could spread to the maxillary sinus because the apex of its root is in the thin floor of the maxillary sinus.

Case Study 8-11

1. A blowout fracture of the orbit may have occurred as a result of the sudden pressure increase in the orbit caused by the hard blow from the pool cue.
2. A nonpenetrating blow to the eye may produce herniation of the orbital contents inferiorly through a blowout fracture in the thin floor of the orbit into the maxillary sinus.

Case Study 8-12

1. An infection in the middle ear was most likely the cause of the inflamed tympanic membrane (*otitis media*).
2. If not adequately treated, a middle ear infection could spread through the mastoid antrum to the mastoid cells and produce *mastoiditis*.

Case Study 8-13

1. Strabismus is a deviation of an eye so that the visual axes of the eyes are not parallel, which the person cannot willfully overcome.

2. In this case, the right abducens nerve (CN VI) was injured, causing paralysis of the right lateral rectus muscle.
3. The patient cannot turn her right eyeball laterally because the lateral rectus is paralyzed. In the absence of opposition by the lateral rectus, the medial rectus pulls the eyeball medially (medial strabismus) (see Figure 8.2).

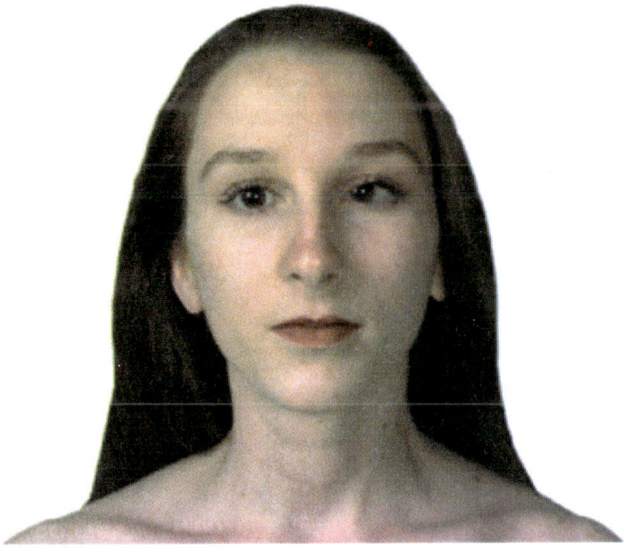

Abducent nerve injury

Case Study 8-14

1. The characteristic facial appearance results from a lesion of the facial nerve. In this patient, the motor supply to the muscles of the left face, forehead, and eyelids were most severely affected.
2. Paralysis of the muscles of facial expression on the left side explains the expressionless look on that side of the man's face and his inability to whistle, puff his cheek, or close his left eye. When the facial nerve is paralyzed, the levator palpebrae superioris (acting unopposed) causes the eye to remain open, even during sleep. Because of paralysis of the orbicularis oculi, the lacrimal puncta and often the entire inferior lid are no longer in contact with the cornea. As a result, tears tend to flow over the left inferior eyelid onto the cheek. The cornea may dry out during sleep (if an ointment is not used) because the eyelids on the affected side remain open. Drying of the cornea can also occur during the day owing to the inability to blink; this dryness could result in *corneal ulceration*.
3. The drooling and difficulty in chewing result from paralysis of the orbicularis oris and buccinator muscles.
4. Loss of taste sensation on the anterior two thirds of the left side of his tongue is understandable anatomically because this region of the tongue receives taste fibers through the chorda tympani branch of CN VII. This symptom also indicates that the nerve lesion must be proximal to the origin of the chorda tympani nerve in the facial canal.
5. The site of the lesion was most likely in the facial canal in the petrous part of the temporal bone, superior to the stylomastoid foramen.
6. The cause of the inflammation is generally thought to be due to a viral infection, which causes swelling (edema) of the facial nerve and compression of its fibers in the facial canal. Thus, in most cases, the nerve fibers are not permanently damaged and nerve degeneration is incomplete. As a result, recovery is slow but generally good. Some facial asymmetry may persist (e.g., slight sagging of the corner of the mouth).

Case Study 8-15

1. The area of the skin and mucosa where the stabbing pain was felt is supplied by the maxillary nerve, the second division of the trigeminal nerve.
2. This wholly sensory nerve leaves the cranium through the foramen rotundum.
3. At its termination as the infra-orbital nerve, it gives rise to branches that supply the ala of the nose, the inferior eyelid, and the skin and mucous membrane of the cheek and upper lip. Branches of the maxillary nerve also innervate the maxillary teeth and the mucous membranes of the nasal cavities, palate, mouth, and tongue.

Case Study 8-16

1. The central part of the lower lip drains to the submental lymph nodes.
2. The submental lymph nodes lie on the fascia covering the mylohyoid muscle between the anterior bellies of the right and left digastric muscles.
3. The floor of the mouth and the apex of the tongue also drain to the submental nodes.
4. The lateral part of the lower lip drains to the submandibular nodes.
5. If cancer cells had spread further, metastases would have developed in the submandibular nodes because efferents from the submental lymph nodes pass to them. Because all parts of the head and neck ultimately drain into the deep cervical nodes, they might also be sites of metastases. Specifically, the jugulo-omohyoid node receives drainage from the submental and submandibular nodes and could be involved. It is located where the omohyoid muscle crosses the IJV.

Case Study 8-17

1. The temple is the area of the temporal fossa between the temporal lines and the zygomatic arch, where the cranium is thin and covered by the temporal muscle and fascia.
2. The pterion is a somewhat variable H-shaped area that lies deep to the temporal muscle. Here, four bones (frontal, parietal, temporal, and sphenoid) approach each other or meet.

3. The center of the pterion is approximately 4 cm superior to the zygomatic arch and 3.5 cm posterior to the frontozygomatic suture. It lies in the anterior part of the temporal fossa.
4. The pterion is an important bony landmark because it indicates the location of the frontal branch of the middle meningeal artery.
5. The thin squamous part of the temporal bone is grooved on its internal aspect by the middle meningeal artery and its branches. The thin bones forming the temporal squama are easily fractured, and the broken pieces may tear this artery and its branches as they pass superiorly on the external surface of the dura mater, especially when the artery is coursing in a bony groove.
6. The middle meningeal artery is usually accompanied by a meningeal vein that also may have been torn.
7. This situation results in a slow accumulation of blood in the extradural space, forming an *extradural (epidural) hematoma*.
8. An *extradural hematoma* is a hemorrhage into the potential space between the inner table of bone of the calvaria and the periosteal layer of dural matter. A *"subdural" hematoma* is a hemorrhage into the interface between dura and arachnoid mater, forming a localized mass of extravasated blood close to the surface of the brain. Although these lesions are commonly called "subdural," there is no natural occurring space. They are more correctly called "dural border hematomas."
9. Because the dura is firmly attached to the bones by fibers that provide some resistance, "extradural" hematomas form relatively slowly, often allowing a lucid interval following recovery of the loss of consciousness, if any, resulting from the trauma and the onset of cerebral symptoms. In addition, this kind of a space-occupying intracranial lesion can be tolerated for a short time because some blood and CSF are squeezed out of the calvaria through the veins. However, because the cranium is nonexpansible, the intracranial pressure soon rises, producing drowsiness and then coma (G. *koma*, deep sleep). The increased intracranial pressure forces the supratentorial part of the brain, usually the uncus, through the tentorial notch (incisure), squeezing the oculomotor nerve between the brain and the sharp, free edge of the tentorium. Compression of CN III causes *third nerve palsy*, which results in a dilated, nonreacting pupil on the side of the lesion. An extradural hemorrhage in the characteristic position, illustrated by the present case, primarily causes compression of the temporal lobe underlying the pterion. Immediate surgical intervention is necessary to relieve the intracranial pressure and avoid further compression of the brain, which could cause death by interfering with the cardiac and respiratory centers in the medulla.

Case Study 8-18

1. Blood from the ruptured aneurysm would enter the subarachnoid space.
2. *Subarachnoid hemorrhages* occur as a result of rupture of any artery or aneurysm, the most common type of the latter being a *berry aneurysm* occurring in the vessels of or near the cerebral arterial circle and the medium-sized arteries at the base of the brain. Blood escaping from the ruptured artery or aneurysm would enter the subarachnoid spaces around the brain and spinal cord.
3. After centrifugation of the CSF, the supernatant fluid was xanthochromatic because it contained serum bilirubin and products of hemolyzed red blood cells.
4. Most single aneurysms occur in relationship to the anterior portion of the cerebral circulation, usually on the internal carotid artery. The most common site is its junction with the posterior communicating artery. Aneurysms of the anterior cerebral artery are usually on the anterior communicating artery, as in this case, or close to it.
5. A lumbar puncture would be performed to see if there was blood in the CSF. However, some authorities recommend against a lumbar puncture in an obvious case of subarachnoid hemorrhage, as in this instance. The lowering of CSF pressure in the spinal subarachnoid space by removing CSF might cause inferior movement of the brain, resulting in herniation (e.g., of part of the cerebellum).

Case Study 8-19

1. The inferior alveolar nerve supplies the mandibular molar and premolar teeth, and its branches supply the canine and incisor teeth. Hence, the inferior alveolar nerve supplies all teeth in one half of the mandible.
2. Anesthetizing the inferior alveolar nerve also anesthetizes the chin and lower lip because the mental nerve supplying these structures is a terminal branch of the inferior alveolar nerve. Because the lingual nerve descends just anterior to the inferior alveolar nerve near the mandibular foramen, the tongue was also anesthetized. This is often advantageous because the lingual nerve supplies sensory fibers to the mandibular gingiva as well as the tongue.
3. Because a relatively large amount of anesthetic was injected, it may have spread into the parotid gland anesthetizing branches of the facial nerve, or it could reach branches of the great auricular nerve.
4. Paralysis of the muscles of facial expression resulted from anesthetizing branches of the facial nerve. The patient's ear lobule was numb because intermediate branches of the great auricular nerve were also anesthetized. The anterior branches of this nerve supply skin on the postero-inferior part of the face, and its intermediate branches supply the inferior part of the auricle on both surfaces.

Chapter 9 Neck

Case Study 9-1

A 4-year-old girl's grandmother noticed that she was holding her head to one side. The child's mother took the girl to the pediatrician, who confirmed the grandmother's observation. On examination, he observed that the child's head was tilted to the right, her occiput was rotated toward her shoulder, and her chin was rotated to the left and elevated. The pediatrician also detected a palpable mass in the inferior part of the child's sternocleidomastoid (SCM). The remainder of the muscle was prominent throughout its course in the neck. He diagnosed the condition as *congenital muscular torticollis*.

Questions:

1. What is the common name for this anomaly?
2. What is the common cause of this abnormality?
3. When does it usually occur?
4. Why does it take so long for the torticollis to develop?
5. Can the injury be diagnosed during infancy and treated before torticollis develops?
6. If the torticollis is not treated, what further developmental abnormalities may develop?

Case Study 9-2

Following removal of a malignant tumor from the right posterosuperior region of the neck of a 52-year-old man, the surgeon decided to do a radical neck dissection of the region to remove the enlarged lymph nodes. One enlarged lymph node was in the submandibular triangle, deep to the superior end of the SCM. After the operation, the man informed the surgeon that he had difficulty shrugging his right shoulder and turning his face to the left side against resistance.

Questions:

1. What nerve was probably injured during the surgical removal of the enlarged lymph nodes?
2. What is the relationship of this nerve to the superior end of the SCM? Describe the course and function of this nerve.
3. Which lymph nodes do you think the surgeon removed?
4. From what areas do these nodes receive lymph?
5. If malignant cells from these nodes had metastasized, to which lymph nodes would they most likely go?

Case Study 9-3

A 42-year-old woman told her family physician that she recently observed a swelling in the anterior part of her neck. She also said that her breathing seemed to be abnormal. Physical examination revealed a firm swelling on the left side of her thyroid gland, which moved up and down during swallowing. An ultrasound scan revealed a solid nodule in the left lobe of her thyroid gland. A needle biopsy indicated that malignant changes had occurred in the cells.

Questions:

1. Why did this nodular swelling move up and down when the woman swallowed?
2. Why was her breathing affected?
3. Based on your knowledge of the lymphatic vessels of the thyroid gland, to which lymph nodes do you think the cancerous cells would most likely metastasize?

Case Study 9-4

A 62-year-old man consulted his physician about his difficulty in swallowing and breathing. He said that his wife was also concerned about the swelling in the anterior part of his neck, which she thought was a *goiter*. Physical examination, an ultrasound scan, and a needle biopsy revealed that the man had *thyroid cancer*. It was decided to perform a thyroidectomy and a neck dissection to search for and remove enlarged lymph nodes.

Questions:

1. What is a goiter?
2. Why was the man having difficulty breathing and swallowing?
3. Why is a total thyroidectomy usually not performed?
4. How can one avoid damaging the nerves during a thyroidectomy?

Case Study 9-5

A 65-year-old woman consulted her physician about muscle weakness, anorexia, nausea, constipation, and polyuria (passage of large volumes of urine). After taking a thorough history and performing an extensive physical examination, the physician ordered laboratory studies of her blood and urine. The laboratory reports revealed an elevated serum calcium concentration, an elevated serum level of parathormone, and an elevated urinary calcium excretion. A diagnosis of *parathyroid adenoma* was made. It was decided that resection of the enlarged gland(s) should be performed. The surgeon located the superior parathyroid glands without difficulty and found them to be normal in size. She could locate only one inferior parathyroid gland. Because it was enlarged and a frozen section suggested parathyroid hyperplasia and *parathyroid adenoma*, the gland was removed. She systematically searched the anterior part of the neck for the fourth parathyroid gland but was unable to find it. Continued searching resulted in detection of the gland.

Questions:

1. How many parathyroid glands are usually present?
2. Where would you expect to find a displaced or ectopic parathyroid gland?
3. If the ectopic parathyroid gland was not detected in the neck, where do you think the surgeon would search for it?

4. How would you explain displacement of these glands?
5. Which parathyroid gland(s) is/are most likely to be found in an ectopic position?

Case Study 9-6

An infant was referred by a family physician to a pediatrician because of respiratory distress and excessive salivation. The infant was coughing and choking during feeding. During the physical examination, the pediatrician observed an excessive amount of mucous secretion and saliva in the infant's mouth. She also observed that the infant experienced some difficulty in breathing and that gastric distension was present. As she was unable to pass a nasogastric tube very far along the esophagus, she told the mother that the infant had an esophageal anomaly.

Questions:

1. What congenital anomaly of the esophagus do you think was present?
2. What other anomaly is usually associated with this type of esophageal anomaly? Describe this condition.
3. What do you think might cause the gastric distension associated with the infant's esophageal and tracheal anomalies?

Case Study 9-7

A 6-year-old child was taken to a family physician for treatment of a persistent sore throat. During physical examination, the physician observed infection and hypertrophy of the tonsils and adenoids. He also detected an *enlarged tonsillar lymph node*. Although the boy's tonsils were the site of chronic infection, he was reluctant to recommend a tonsillectomy and adenoidectomy (T & A).

Questions:

1. Which lymph node is commonly referred to as the tonsillar lymph node?
2. Where is this node located?
3. Because of the vascularity of the palatine tonsils, tonsillectomy can be dangerous. Which vessels may bleed after tonsillectomy?

Case Study 9-8

A young man was deeply slashed with a knife in the middle of the right lateral cervical region. The cut ended anterior to the middle of the SCM. The bleeding was arrested, and the wound was sutured. The patient, who was right-handed, later complained that he had difficulty combing his hair and tilting his head to the right.

Questions:

1. Which blood vessel was likely severed?
2. What large nerves would likely be injured? Describe the course of these nerves.
3. Explain why the patient had difficulty combing his hair and laterally flexing his head.

Case Study 9-9

During an automobile accident, the neck of an 82-year-old man was injured by the safety belt as the vehicle stopped suddenly. He complained of difficult breathing and a sore "Adam's apple." The physician who examined him realized that it was necessary to perform an emergency *cricothyroidotomy* to secure an adequate airway.

Questions:

1. What structures in the anterior part of the neck were most likely injured by the safety belt during the automobile accident? How could this cause difficult breathing?
2. Why is the laryngeal skeleton more easily fractured in elderly people?
3. What structure is incised to enter the trachea during a cricothyroidotomy?
4. What surgical procedure do you think would be performed to support an airway over an extended period of time?
5. Based on your knowledge of the relations of the trachea, what structures may be injured during this procedure?

Case Study 9-10

A 58-year-old man consulted his physician about difficulty in swallowing. He said that he first had difficulty swallowing solid foods, but recently, he has had difficulty swallowing soft foods and liquids. He also said that he has lost considerable weight in the last 2 months. Physical examination of the man's neck revealed a large, firm lump deep to the anterior border of the SCM. A biopsy of the tumor and surrounding tissues revealed a malignant tumor of the cervical esophagus that had begun to infiltrate the periesophageal tissues.

Questions:

1. What caused the man's dysphagia?
2. What do you think caused the large lump deep to the SCM?
3. Describe the path of lymphatic drainage from the cervical esophagus.
4. Into which periesophageal tissues do you think the cancer would infiltrate?

Case Study 9-11

A 20-year-old man with moderate fever and a sore throat noticed a swelling on the side of his face anterior to his ear. He was also concerned when another swelling appeared below his jaw. He quickly arranged an appointment with his family physician. During the physical examination, the physician observed enlargement of the right parotid and submandibular glands. Palpation of the parotid gland was painful. Examination of the oral cavity revealed redness of the openings of the ducts of these glands. The pain of the swollen parotid gland increased when he was asked to sip lemon juice. The physician diagnosed the man with mumps.

Questions:

1. In which triangle of what region of the neck is the submandibular gland located?
2. Where do the ducts of the submandibular glands open?
3. Why is swelling of the parotid gland painful, especially during chewing? What nerve conveys this pain?

Case Study 9-12

A 3-year-old boy was playing with some coins that he found on the floor. He put a nickel into his mouth and accidentally swallowed it. He suddenly began to cough, drool, and choke. The boy was rushed to the hospital. A lateral radiograph of his neck revealed that the coin was lodged in his esophagus.

Questions:

1. Where would the coin probably lodge in the cervical esophagus?
2. If the coin passed further down the esophagus into the thorax, where might it lodge?
3. What would make the child choke?
4. How do you think the coin might be removed?

Case Study 9-13

A 30-year-old man was eating a fish dinner when he suddenly started to choke. He told his wife that he believed a fishbone was stuck in his throat. She drove him to the emergency department of a hospital. The attending physician examined the man's larynx with a laryngeal mirror; however, he was unable to see a fishbone. He then inserted an endoscope into the patient's laryngopharynx and was able to locate and remove the bone.

Questions:

1. Where do you think the fishbone was lodged?
2. What structure might be injured if the bone pierced the mucous membrane?
3. What would be the result of injury to this structure?

Case Study 9-14

The mother of an 11-year-old child consulted her physician about a swelling in the anterior aspect of her daughter's neck. Although the swelling was painless, the mother was concerned because the lump was slowly getting larger. The physician explained that this type of neck swelling is common in children. He told the mother that these swellings often represent developmental anomalies that do not become apparent until childhood, adolescence, or early adulthood. He also stated that these midline masses tend to be benign (nonmalignant).

Physical Examination: Physical examination revealed that none of the cervical lymph nodes was enlarged or tender. The physician noted that the swelling was located just inferior to the hyoid and that it was cystic and freely movable (see Figure 9.1). The physician held the swelling gently between his first and second fingers and asked the patient to swallow. The swelling moved superiorly during swallowing. He then asked the patient to stick her tongue out as far as possible and then retract it. The physician noted a definite superior tug on the mass as the patient's tongue protruded. The physician aspirated fluid from the swelling for laboratory investigation.

Laboratory Report: The fluid consists of a thin, watery substance containing gelatinous material.

Diagnosis: Thyroglossal duct cyst.

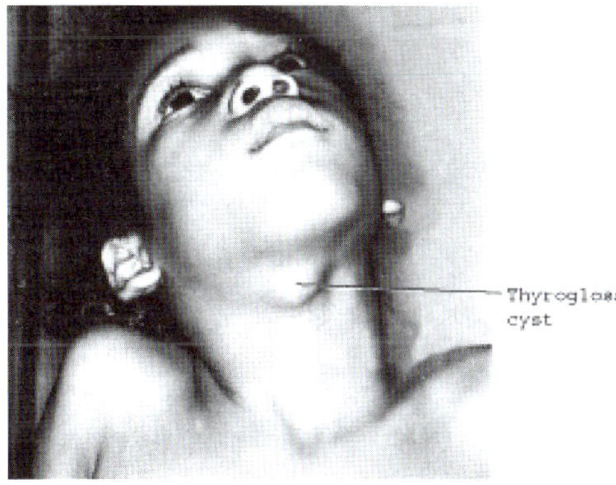

Questions:

1. Explain the embryological basis of this cyst.
2. Where are these cysts usually found?
3. What is the anatomical basis for the cyst's superior movement when the child protruded her tongue and swallowed?
4. What glandular tissue may be associated with this type of cyst?
5. What would this condition be called if a midline cervical opening into the cyst had been present?

Case Study 9-15

A 27-year-old medical student consulted her clinical instructor about a painless, plum-shaped swelling in the anterior cervical region, inferior to the angle of her mandible (see Figure 9.2). As her mandibular third molar teeth had not erupted, she thought the swelling might be caused by a dental abscess in the submandibular triangle because her third molar on that side was producing some pain. She also feared that the swelling might be caused by a tumor of her submandibular gland or be the result of an enlarged jugulodigastric lymph node.

History: The physician asked the student several questions.

When did you first notice the lump? I first saw it approximately 3 months ago.

Does it hurt? No, but the swelling has been slowly getting larger.

Have you had any ear or throat infections recently? No, but I had a cold approximately 2 weeks ago.

Have you detected any hoarseness since this swelling appeared? No.

Physical Examination: The physician palpated the neck lump and told the student that it was a cystic swelling just anterior to the upper third of her left SCM. He aspirated fluid from the cyst for laboratory investigation. The physician examined her left third molar tooth and said that it was impacted and that the gingiva was slightly inflamed; however, he assured her that the infection in her tooth was not related to the neck swelling.

Laboratory Report: The cyst contains cloudy, cholesterol crystal–laden fluid.

Diagnosis: Branchial cyst.

Surgical Treatment: The physician arranged to have the cyst surgically removed (*cystectomy*).

During excision of the cyst, a sinus tract was observed to pass superiorly from it. The sinus tract was carefully dissected and removed.

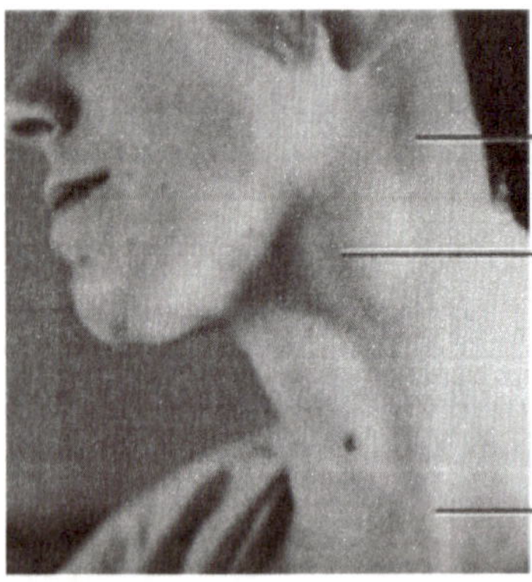

Questions:

1. Explain the embryological basis of a branchial cyst.
2. Where did the sinus tract probably terminate?
3. What nerve could be damaged during the cystectomy?
4. What signs would be present if this nerve was injured?
5. If the sinus tract had passed inferiorly, where would it probably open?
6. If the cystic swelling was painful during palpation, do you think it could still be a branchial cyst?

Case Study 9-16

After completing your first anatomy examination, your father decided to celebrate and take you out for a steak dinner. After a few drinks, you noted that he was eating his steak rapidly and that his speech was slurred. Later, you noticed your father's face change suddenly. He had a terrified look and then collapsed on the floor. At first, you suspected that he had passed out, but as you examined him more closely, you thought that perhaps he was having a stroke, a heart attack, or a seizure. Your examination also revealed that his pulse was strong, but his face began to turn blue. You then realized that your father was suffering from *asphyxia*. You opened his mouth widely and observed a large piece of steak caught in the posterior part of his throat. First you reached into his mouth with your index finger and tried to pull it out. On being unsuccessful, you rolled him into the prone position and performed the *Heimlich maneuver*. This increased his intra-abdominal pressure and moved his diaphragm superiorly, forcing the air out of his lungs and expelling the piece of steak.

Questions:

1. Where was the piece of steak most likely lodged?
2. Discuss the common causes of laryngeal obstruction.
3. If the Heimlich maneuver had not been successful and a physician had come to help you, what lifesaving measures do you think he or she might have taken?

Case Study 9-17

A 30-year-old woman was concerned about a swelling in the anterior part of her neck, nervousness, and loss of weight. She told her physician that her family complains that she is irritable, excitable, and cries easily.

Physical Examination: The physician detected a swelling on each side of her neck, inferior to the larynx. During palpation of the patient's neck from a posterior position, the physician felt an enlarged thyroid gland and noted that it moved up and down during swallowing. The following signs were also detected: protrusion of the eyeballs, rapid pulse, tremor of the digits, moist palms, and loss of weight.

Diagnosis: Hyperthyroidism (exophthalmic goiter, Graves disease). When the patient did not respond to medical treatment, a subtotal thyroidectomy was performed. After the operation, the patient complained of hoarseness.

Questions:

1. What is the rationale for removal of thyroid tissue from this patient?
2. What is the anatomical basis for the enlarged thyroid gland moving up and down during deglutition?
3. Because the patient's thyroid gland was enlarged, what nerves might have been compressed?
4. What deficits could result from injury of these nerves?
5. What are other possible causes of the patient's hoarseness?
6. If a total thyroidectomy had been done, what other important structures might inadvertently have been removed?
7. What would result from this surgical error?

Case Study 9-18

A 10-year-old boy was admitted to the hospital with a sore throat and earache. He had a high fever (temperature, 40.5°C), rapid pulse rate, and rapid respirations.

Physical Examination: Examination of the boy's throat by the attending physician revealed diffuse redness and swelling of the pharynx, especially of the palatine tonsils. His left tympanic membrane was also bulging. The boy's medical history revealed that he had had chronic symptoms of inflammation of the nasal mucous membrane (*rhinitis*), including the pharyngeal tonsils (*adenoiditis*), resulting in persistent mouth breathing.

Diagnosis: Tonsillitis–inflammation of the tonsils, especially the palatine tonsils.

Treatment: Following antibiotic treatment, the infection resolved. In view of the boy's history, it was decided to readmit him 3 or 4 months later for a tonsillectomy and adenoidectomy.

Questions:

1. What is meant by the term "tonsils"? What is their function?
2. Explain the anatomical basis of the boy's earache.
3. Which lymph node would likely be swollen and tender in this case?
4. What is the probable source of hemorrhage during a tonsillectomy?
5. Compression of what vessel would control severe arterial bleeding in the tonsillar bed?

Answers

Case Study 9-1

1. This relatively common abnormality of the neck is usually called a "wry neck" by lay persons.
2. Lesions of the SCM may result from fixed positioning of the head and neck in the uterus that causes tearing of the muscle fibers and *fibrosis* (formation of fibrous tissue as a reparative or reactive process). Excessive stretching of the neck during a difficult delivery may also cause tearing of fibers and bleeding within the SCM. The resulting *hematoma* is contained within its own fascial compartment, which results in increased pressure on the muscle fibers. This damages the muscle and results in an area of *ischemia*. The damaged muscle fibers gradually undergo fibrosis.
3. Congenital muscular torticollis usually occurs at birth.
4. The torticollis develops slowly as fibrosis, and contraction of the SCM occurs. It may not be noticed until the child is 4–6 years old.
5. A thorough examination may reveal a hematoma in the inferior third of the SCM. If this swelling is massaged and daily passive neck stretching exercises are carried out, the hematoma may disappear and no fibrosis and shortening of the SCM may develop.
6. Failure to correct muscular torticollis results in asymmetrical development of the facial bones. Wedge-shaped deformities of the cervical vertebrae may also develop.

Case Study 9-2

1. Most likely the spinal accessory nerve (CN XI) was injured.
2. This nerve pierces the deep surface of the superior part of the SCM and supplies it. CN XI then crosses the lateral cervical region and supplies the trapezius. The SCM tilts the head laterally and rotates the neck, explaining why the patient had difficulty turning his head. The trapezius elevates, retracts, and rotates the scapula, explaining why he had difficulty shrugging his shoulder.
3. The enlarged lymph nodes the surgeon removed would be *submandibular lymph nodes*, located beneath the investing layer of deep cervical fascia.
4. The submandibular nodes receive lymph from a wide area, including lymph vessels from the submental, buccal, and lingual groups of lymph nodes.
5. Efferent lymphatic vessels from the submandibular nodes pass to the superior and inferior deep cervical lymph nodes. Consequently, these nodes would also enlarge because of the spread of malignant cells from the primary tumor.

Case Study 9-3

1. The thyroid gland and the nodular swelling in it are invested by the visceral layer of pretracheal deep cervical fascia, which attaches the gland's capsule to the cricoid cartilage and tracheal rings. Consequently, when the woman swallows, her thyroid gland and the nodule within it move up and down as the larynx (and upper trachea) are elevated and then depressed by the suprahyoid and infrahyoid muscles, respectively.
2. Her breathing was affected because each lobe of the thyroid gland is closely related to the trachea. Consequently, an enlarged lobe resulting from a large tumor is likely to compress the trachea and partially occlude its lumen, causing *dyspnea*.
3. Because malignant cells were in the thyroid nodule, the cells would likely metastasize to the prelaryngeal, pretracheal, and paratracheal lymph nodes. From these nodes, the malignant cells would likely pass to the inferior deep cervical lymph nodes.

Case Study 9-4

1. The term *goiter* refers to enlargement of the thyroid gland that produces a swelling in the anterior part of the neck.
2. The man had dyspnea and dysphagia because the enlarged thyroid gland was compressing the trachea and esophagus and partially occluding their lumina, causing difficulty in breathing and swallowing.
3. Total thyroidectomy is usually not performed because of the danger of injuring the recurrent laryngeal nerves and inadvertently removing all the parathyroid glands. Medially, the recurrent laryngeal nerves are closely related to the posterior part of the capsule of the thyroid gland. The parathyroid glands, when in their usual

position, lie in close relationship to the posterior aspect of the thyroid gland, outside its fibrous capsule but inside its fascial sheath.

4. Surgeons avoid injury to the recurrent laryngeal nerves during thyroidectomy by not cutting through the posterior aspect of the fibrous capsule of the thyroid, especially medially where these nerves lie in the tracheoesophageal grooves.

Case Study 9-5

1. Typically, a person has four parathyroid glands; however, more than four glands are present in approximately 5% of the population.
2. An ectopic parathyroid gland is commonly found in association with the thymus or embedded in the inferior part of the thyroid gland.
3. If the gland is not in the neck, the surgeon might explore the superior mediastinum.
4. The superior parathyroid glands are derived from the fourth pair of pharyngeal pouches and the inferior ones from the third pair, as does the thymus. As the embryo develops, the thymus descends and usually separates from the inferior parathyroid glands. Usually the separation occurs when they lie posterior to the inferior lobe of the thyroid gland.
5. This migration is extremely variable, and as a result, the inferior glands are more likely to be in an ectopic position.

Case Study 9-6

1. Inability to pass a catheter through the esophagus of a newborn infant into the stomach indicates *esophageal atresia*.
2. Esophageal atresia in an infant is commonly associated with a tracheoesophageal fistula (TEF). Most often the esophagus forms a blind pouch, and the distal esophagus is connected to the tracheobronchial tree just superior to the carina, the ridge separating the openings of the right and left main bronchi at their junction with the trachea.
3. A TEF forces air through the fistula into the gastrointestinal tract, causing gastric distension, which precipitates passage of gastric contents into the trachea and bronchi.

Case Study 9-7

1. Lymph from the palatine tonsil drains to the superior deep cervical lymph nodes, especially the *jugulodigastric node*, often referred to as the tonsillar node.
2. The jugulodigastric lymph node lies on the IJV where the posterior belly of the digastric muscle crosses the IJV.
3. Sometimes the large *tonsillar artery*, a branch of the facial artery, may have to be ligated when bleeding occurs after a tonsillectomy. Bleeding often results from incising veins from the pharyngeal venous plexus, especially the large external palatine vein.

Case Study 9-8

1. The EJV was most likely severed. This large vessel passes inferolaterally across the SCM and pierces the investing layer of deep cervical fascia just superior to the clavicle.
2. The *transverse cervical nerve* was likely cut because it turns around the middle of the posterior border of the SCM and crosses the muscle deep to the platysma. It then divides into branches that supply the skin on the side and anterior part of the neck. Superior to the middle of the posterior border of the SCM, the spinal accessory nerve (CN XI) crosses the lateral cervical region obliquely. It supplies the SCM and trapezius.
3. The patient had difficulty combing his hair because the knife had cut his CN XI, paralyzing his trapezius. To raise his hand to his head, the trapezius, assisted by the serratus anterior, must rotate the scapula so the glenoid cavity faces superolaterally. He experienced some difficulty tilting his head to the right side because of paralysis of the SCM, which is also supplied by the spinal accessory nerve.

Case Study 9-9

1. The laryngeal cartilages, particularly the protruding thyroid cartilage, were likely fractured. The displaced laminae of the thyroid cartilage probably blocked the airway. In addition, edema of the submucosa of the larynx may have obstructed the passage of air.
2. The laryngeal skeleton, particularly the thyroid cartilage, is more easily fractured in elderly people because of ossification of the cartilages.
3. To facilitate breathing, the *cricothyroid membrane* was likely incised and a small tracheostomy tube was inserted into the trachea.
4. When an extended period of airway support is required and rapid entry into the trachea is not necessary, a *tracheostomy* is usually performed. This procedure may be performed either superior or inferior to the isthmus of the thyroid. Division of the isthmus allows exposure of the upper trachea (i.e., between the first and second tracheal rings). Some surgeons prefer to make a vertical incision through rings two to four.
5. In a tracheal incision that extends too far posteriorly, the posterior tracheal wall and esophagus may be damaged, especially in children. In some cases, injury to the recurrent laryngeal nerves may occur during a tracheostomy

Case Study 9-10

1. Dysphagia, present in approximately 80% of patients with malignant tumors of the esophagus, is caused by gradual pressure from the tumor and closure of the esophageal lumen.
2. The dysphagia is usually progressive. The hard lump deep to the SCM was likely a cancerous deep cervical lymph node located near the IJV. The malignancy had metastasized through the lymphatics to this node.

3. The lymphatic drainage of the cervical esophagus is to the paratracheal and inferior deep cervical lymph nodes.
4. Invasion of the trachea or main bronchi is likely to occur with advanced esophageal cancer.

Case Study 9-11

1. The submandibular gland is in the posterior part of the *submandibular triangle*, one of the four subdivisions of the anterior cervical region.
2. The submandibular duct opens by one to three orifices on the small sublingual papilla beside the lingual frenulum.
3. Inflammation of the parotid gland (*parotiditis*) is painful because the gland is enclosed within a strong capsule that is continuous with the investing layer of deep cervical fascia and the capsule resists enlargement of the gland. The overlying skin may also be tightly stretched. The greater auricular nerve innervates the parotid sheath and overlying skin. Usually the pain is greater during chewing because the parotid gland is wrapped around the posterior border of the ramus of the mandible and compressed against the mastoid process when the mouth is open.

Case Study 9-12

1. The coin would most likely lodge where the laryngopharynx joins the superior end of the esophagus, which is located at the level of the inferior border of the cricoid cartilage.
2. If the coin passed into the thoracic esophagus, it would likely lodge in the second constriction at the level of the arch of the aorta.
3. Choking of the infant would result from compression of the larynx or trachea by the localized enlargement of the esophagus.
4. Removal of the coin would likely be performed under direct vision with an *esophagoscope*.

Case Study 9-13

1. The fishbone was likely lodged in the *piriform fossa* between the aryepiglottic fold and the lateral wall of the laryngopharynx. Foreign bodies such as fishbones and chicken bones often pass into these pear-shaped recesses because when food passes through the laryngopharynx during swallowing, it is forced to flow through these recesses. Sharp objects may lodge in them and pierce the floors of the recesses.
2. The internal laryngeal nerve may be injured because both nerves run immediately deep to the mucous membrane lining the recess.
3. This nerve supplies sensory fibers to the laryngeal mucosa superior to the vocal folds, including the superior surface of these folds. The mucous membrane of the superior part of the larynx is sensitive, and contact by a foreign object causes immediate explosive coughing to expel it. Lack of sensation in this mucosa resulting from a nerve injury could allow food to enter the larynx and cause choking.

Case Study 9-14

1. A thyroglossal duct cyst develops from a remnant of the embryonic *thyroglossal duct*, which connects the thyroid gland with the base of the tongue in the embryo. Normally the thyroglossal duct atrophies and degenerates as the thyroid gland descends to its final site in the neck.
2. Remnants of this duct may persist anywhere along the anterior midline of the neck between the foramen cecum of the tongue and the thyroid gland. These remnants may give rise to cysts in the tongue or neck, but they usually lie just inferior to the hyoid.
3. Often the cyst is in intimate contact with the anterior part of the hyoid. It may be connected superiorly by a duct with the foramen cecum, inferiorly with a pyramidal lobe, or the isthmus of the thyroid gland, or both. Thus, thyroglossal cysts may move up and down during deglutition and when the tongue is protruded.
4. Sometimes thyroid tissue is associated with a thyroglossal duct cyst and, in unusual cases, the entire thyroid gland is attached to the cyst because it failed to descend to its normal position during the embryonic period.
5. A thyroglossal duct cyst may develop an opening onto the surface of the neck (*thyroglossal sinus*). This results from erosion of cervical tissues following infection and rupture of the cyst.

Case Study 9-15

1. All of the conditions that came to the student's mind could have caused the swelling in the side of her neck. Branchial cysts are usually derived from remnants of the cervical sinus, the second pharyngeal groove, or the second pharyngeal pouch. Although they may be associated with branchial sinuses, as in the present case, and may drain through them, these cysts often lie in the neck just inferior to the angle of the mandible. They usually develop along the anterior border of the SCM. The cyst may extend deep to this muscle and involve other structures.
2. In the present case, the cyst was probably derived from a remnant of the embryonic cervical sinus. The sinus tract running superiorly from it was likely derived from the second pharyngeal pouch. It probably passed between the internal and external carotid arteries. It likely terminated in or close to the tonsillar cleft of the palatine fossa, the adult derivative of the cavity of the second pharyngeal pouch.
3. The surgical excision of ascending sinuses associated with branchial cysts may bruise or injure the hypoglossal nerve, causing temporary or prolonged unilateral lingual paralysis.
4. Unilateral lingual paralysis resulting from hypoglossal nerve injury would be indicated by hemiatrophy of the tongue and deviation of the tongue to the paralyzed side when it was protruded, a result of the unopposed action of the tongue muscles on the other side.

5. If the sinus tract had passed inferiorly, it probably would have opened in the inferior third of the neck, along the anterior border of the SCM.
6. A branchial sinus that opens externally is likely derived from remnants of the second pharyngeal groove. If the cystic swelling had been painful during the physical examination, the cyst could be one that was secondarily infected (e.g., resulting from leakage of fluid from it into the surrounding tissues).

Case Study 9-16

1. The piece of steak was probably lodged in the *laryngeal inlet*.
2. Choking on food is a common cause of laryngeal obstruction, particularly in children, in persons who have consumed too much alcohol, and in persons with neurological impairment. Many so-called restaurant deaths thought to be caused by heart attacks have been shown to result from choking. Persons with dentures and/or who are impaired by excessive alcohol intake are less able to chew their food properly and to detect a bite that is too large. The mucous membrane of the superior part of the larynx is sensitive, and contact by a foreign body such as a piece of steak causes immediate explosive coughing to expel it. However, neurological or alcohol impairment may reduce or eliminate this response.

   Sometimes a foreign body enters the piriform fossa or passes through the larynx and becomes lodged in the trachea or a main bronchus. Usually, as in the present case, the piece of steak is only partly in the larynx, but entry of air into the trachea and lungs is largely prevented. The patient would likely have died within 5 minutes, almost certainly before there was time to get him to a hospital, if the piece of steak had not been dislodged using the Heimlich maneuver, which re-established adequate respiration.
3. Had your emergency procedure not been successful, the physician would likely have first tried to get the piece of steak out of the patient's larynx with a long spoon or a slender fork. If these procedures had failed, he would likely have performed a lifesaving *emergency inferior laryngotomy* (surgical incision of the larynx). If he happened to have a large bore needle with him, he would have inserted it through the *cricothyroid ligament*. If not, he probably would have used a penknife or a steak knife to make an incision through the midline of the neck into the cricothyroid ligament (*cricothyrotomy*).

Case Study 9-17

1. The surgical treatment of hyperthyroidism is to remove part of each lobe of the thyroid (*subtotal thyroidectomy*), thereby leaving less glandular tissue to secrete hormones.
2. The enlarged thyroid gland producing the swelling in the neck moves up and down during swallowing because the gland attaches to the respiratory layer by the pretracheal layer of deep cervical fascia. The respiratory layer (larynx and trachea) and pharynx are both elevated during swallowing by the suprahyoid muscles and then are depressed (to their original positions) by gravity afterward.
3. Thyroidectomy may cause injury to the recurrent laryngeal nerves because they are closely related to the thyroid gland and trachea and, near the inferior poles of the thyroid gland, they are intimately related to the inferior thyroid arteries. The nerves may cross anterior or posterior to this artery or between its branches before ascending in or near the groove between the trachea and esophagus. The left recurrent laryngeal nerve is more vulnerable to trauma and disease than the right nerve because of its longer course around the arch of the aorta.
4. The recurrent laryngeal nerves supply all muscles of the larynx except the cricothyroids. Damage to or severance of one of the nerves could seriously affect speech (e.g., causing hoarseness, as in the present case, or a change in the quality of the voice to a brassy sound). Some people also have difficulty clearing their throats. Injury to both recurrent laryngeal nerves—an unusual occurrence—may completely paralyze the intrinsic muscles, severely impairing breathing and speech because the vocal folds remain partly adducted. In this case, the rima glottidis is not fully open.
5. Temporary malfunction of the recurrent laryngeal nerves may also result from postoperative edema. A common cause of temporary hoarseness after surgery is trauma to the mucous membrane of the larynx by the endotracheal tube that the anesthetists insert as an airway. If the nerves are compressed as a result of inflammation or the accumulation of fluid, the breathing and speech defects normally disappear following healing and drainage of the operative site.
6. The parathyroid glands could be removed. Typically, the parathyroids lie on the posterior surface of the thyroid gland; thus, posterior parts of the lobes are left to prevent inadvertent removal of these glands. At least one of them is essential for secretion of parathormone, which maintains the normal level of calcium in the blood and body fluids.
7. Removal of the parathyroid glands causes a convulsive disorder known as *tetany*. The signs are nervousness, twitching, and spasms in the facial and limb muscles.

Case Study 9-18

1. There are numerous aggregates of lymphoid tissue in the pharyngeal walls. Major aggregates of this tissue are called tonsils. Unless otherwise stated, reference to the tonsils refers to the *palatine tonsils*. The other tonsils are the lingual, pharyngeal, and tubal tonsils. Collectively, all the tonsils form a *tonsillar ring* around the pharyngeal isthmus, where the oropharynx communicates with the nasopharynx. Although it is often stated that the tonsillar ring acts as a barrier to infection, its function is not clearly

understood. However, it is certain that this lymphoid tissue is important in the immune reaction to infection.

2. In the present case, the infection had spread along the pharyngotympanic tube into the middle ear, producing *otitis media* and bulging of the tympanic membrane. This bulging would likely be the chief cause of the boy's earache. Twigs from the glossopharyngeal nerve innervate the tonsils and, because the tympanic branch of this nerve supplies the mucous membrane of the tympanic cavity, some of the pain related to the tonsillitis may have also been referred to the ear. When the opening of the pharyngotympanic tube is closed, as it probably was in the present case, pressure changes in the middle ear can also cause earache.
3. The numerous lymphatic vessels of the tonsils penetrate the pharyngeal wall and terminate principally in the *jugulodigastric node* in the deep chain of cervical lymph nodes. Enlargement of this tonsillar node is commonly associated with tonsillitis.
4. The external palatine vein is usually the chief source of hemorrhage following tonsillectomy. This important and sometimes large vein descends from the soft palate and is immediately related to the lateral surface of the tonsil before it pierces the superior constrictor muscle of the pharynx.
5. In cases of severe and uncontrolled bleeding (e.g., from the tonsillar branch of the facial artery), hemorrhage may be controlled by compressing or clamping the external carotid artery at its origin. This artery supplies blood to the tonsillar arteries.

APPENDIX B References and Suggested Reading

CHAPTER 8 Head

Bickley LS: *Bates' Guide to Physical Examination and History Taking*, 12th ed. Baltimore, Wolters Kluwer Health, 2016.

Chou DE, Headache and pain syndromes. *In* Louis ED, Mayer SA, Rowland LP (eds): *Merritt's Neurology*, 13th ed. Philadelphia, Wolters Kluwer Health, 2016.

Corbett JJ, Haines DE, Ard MD, Lancon JA: The ventricles, choroid plexus, and cerebrospinal fluid. *In* Haines DE (ed): *Fundamental Neuroscience for Basic and Clinical Applications*, 4th ed. Philadelphia, Elsevier/Saunders, 2013.

Esenwa CC, Czeisler BM, Mayer SA: Acute ischemic attack. *In* Louis ED, Mayer SA, Rowland LP (eds): *Merritt's Neurology*, 13th ed. Philadelphia, Wolters Kluwer Health, 2016.

Fernandez-Valencia R, Gomez Pellico L: Functional anatomy of the human saccus lacrimalis. *Acta Anat (Basel)* 139:54–59, 1990.

Haines DE (ed): *Fundamental Neuroscience for Basic and Clinical Applications*, 4th ed. Philadelphia, Elsevier/Saunders, 2013.

Haines DE: *Neuroanatomy in a Clinical Context: An Atlas of Structures, Sections, and Systems*, 9th ed. Baltimore, Lippincott Williams & Wilkins, 2015.

Haines DE, Harkey HL, Al-Mefty O: The "subdural" space: A new look at an outdated concept. *Neurosurgery* 32:111, 1993.

Jubelt B, Nathan BR: Acute bacterial meningitis and infective endocarditis. *In* Louis ED, Mayer SA, Rowland LP (eds): *Merritt's Neurology*, 13th ed. Philadelphia, Wolters Kluwer, 2016.

Kiernan JA, Rajakumar N: *Barr's The Human Nervous System: An Anatomical Viewpoint*, 10th ed. Baltimore, Wolters Kluwer Health, 2013.

Kliegman RM, Stanton BMD, St. Geme J, Schor NF (eds): *Nelson Textbook of Pediatrics*, 20th ed. Philadelphia, Elsevier/Saunders, 2016.

Louis ED, Mayer SA, Rowland LP: *Merritt's Neurology*, 13th ed. Philadelphia, Wolters Kluwer Health, 2016.

Marshall RS: Transient ischemic attack. *In* Louis ED, Mayer SA, Rowland LP (eds): *Merritt's Neurology*, 13th ed. Philadelphia, Wolters Kluwer Health, 2016.

Mayer SA: Brain edema and disorders of intracranial pressure. *In* Louis ED, Mayer SA, Rowland LP (eds): *Merritt's Neurology*, 13th ed. Philadelphia, Wolters Kluwer Health, 2016.

Moore KL, Persaud TVN, Torchia MG: *The Developing Human: Clinically Oriented Embryology*, 10th ed. Philadelphia, Elsevier/Saunders, 2016.

Murkerji SS, Lyons JL: Viral infections. *In* Louis ED, Mayer SA, Rowland LP (eds): *Merritt's Neurology*, 13th ed. Philadelphia, Wolters Kluwer Health, 2016.

Olson TR, Ger R, Abrahams P: *Ger's Essentials of Clinical Anatomy*, 3rd ed. New York, Cambridge University Press, 2009.

Organek N, Frontera JA: Cerebral venous and sinus thrombosis. *In* Louis ED, Mayer SA, Rowland LP (eds): *Merritt's Neurology*, 13th ed. Philadelphia, Wolters Kluwer Health, 2016.

Russo JF, Mikell CB, Winfree CJ: Traumatic cranial and peripheral nerve injuries. *In* Louis ED, Mayer SA, Rowland LP (eds): *Merritt's Textbook of Neurology*, 13th ed. Philadelphia, Wolters Kluwer, 2016.

Sevusch-Garcy J, Elkind MSV: Global burden of neurologic disease. *In* Louis ED, Mayer SA, Rowland LP (eds): *Merritt's Neurology*, 13th ed. Philadelphia, Wolters Kluwer Health, 2016.

Standring S (ed): *Gray's Anatomy: The Anatomical Basis of Medicine and Surgery*, 41st British ed. London, Churchill Livingstone/Elsevier, 2016.

Storper IS: Ménière syndrome, benign paroxysmal positional vertigo, and vestibular neuritis. *In* Louis ED, Mayer SA, Rowland LP (eds): *Merritt's Neurology*, 13th ed. Philadelphia, Wolters Kluwer Health, 2016.

CHAPTER 9 Neck

Agur AMR, Dalley AF: *Grant's Atlas of Anatomy*, 14th ed. Philadelphia: Wolters Kluwer Health, 2017.

Bickley LS: *Bates' Guide to Physical Examination and History Taking*, 12th ed. Baltimore, Wolters Kluwer Health, 2016.

Cioroiu CM: Pain, numbness, and paresthesias. *In* Louis ED, Mayer SA, Rowland LP (eds): *Merritt's Neurology*, 13th ed. Philadelphia, Wolters Kluwer, 2016.

Ezenkwele UA, Long CM: Esophageal rupture and tears in emergency medicine. *Medscape*, 2016. Available at http://emedicine.medscape.com/article/775165-overview

Fahn S: Dystonia. *In* Louis ED, Mayer SA, Rowland LP (eds): *Merritt's Neurology*, 13th ed. Philadelphia, Wolters Kluwer, 2016.

Kliegman RM, Stanton BMD, St. Geme J, Schor NF (eds): *Nelson Textbook of Pediatrics*, 20th ed. Philadelphia, Elsevier/Saunders, 2016.

Lachman N, Acland RD, Rosse C: Anatomical evidence for the absence of a morphologically distinct cranial root of the accessory nerve in man. *Clin Anat* 15:4–10, 2002.

Leung AKC, Wong AL, Robson WLLM: Ectopic thyroid gland simulating a thyroglossal duct cyst: A case report. *Can J Surg* 38:87, 1995.

Louis ED, Mayer SA, Rowland LP. *Merritt's Neurology*, 13th ed. Philadelphia, Wolters Kluwer Health, 2016.

Moore KL, Persaud TVN, Torchia MG: *The Developing Human: Clinically Oriented Embryology*, 10th ed. Philadelphia, Elsevier/Saunders, 2016.

Olson TR, Ger R, Abrahams P: *Ger's Essentials of Clinical Anatomy*, 3rd ed. New York, Cambridge University Press, 2009.

Quinn CE, Udelsman R: The parathyroid glands. *In* Townsend CM, Beauchamp RD, Evers BM, Mattox KL (eds): *Sabiston Textbook of Surgery*, 20th ed. Philadelphia, Elsevier, 2017.

Sevush-Garcy J, Elkind MSV: Global burden of neurologic disease. *In* Louis ED, Mayer SA, Rowland LP (eds): *Merritt's Neurology*, 13th ed. Philadelphia, Wolters Kluwer, 2016.

Shih T: Syncope and spells. *In* Louis ED, Mayer SA, Rowland LP (eds): *Merritt's Neurology*, 13th ed. Philadelphia, Wolters Kluwer, 2016.

Skandalakis JE, Skandalakis PN, Skandalakis LJ: *Surgical Anatomy and Technique. A Pocket Manual*, 4th ed. New York, Springer-Verlag, 2014.

Smith PW, Hanks LR, Salomone LJ, Hanks JB: Chapter 36. Thyroid. *In* Townsend CM, Beauchamp RD, Evers BM, Mattox KL (eds): *Sabiston Textbook of Surgery*, 20th ed. Philadelphia, Elsevier, 2017.

Standring S (ed): *Gray's Anatomy: The Anatomical Basis of Medicine and Surgery*, 41st British ed. London, Churchill Livingstone/Elsevier, 2016.

Townsend CM, Beauchamp RD, Evers BM, Mattox KL: *Sabiston Textbook of Surgery*, 20th ed. Philadelphia, Elsevier, 2017.

Weiglein AH, Morrigl B, Schalk C, et al.: Arteries in the posterior cervical triangle in man. *Clin Anat* 18:533–557, 2005.

CHAPTER 10 Summary of Cranial Nerves

Agur, AMR, Dalley AF: *Grant's Atlas of Anatomy*, 14th ed. Philadelphia, Wolters Kluwer, 2017.

Brannigan TH, Tanji K: Acquired peripheral neuropathies. *In* Louis ED, Mayer SA, Rowland LP (eds): *Merritt's Textbook of Neurology*, 13th ed. Philadelphia, Wolters Kluwer, 2016.

Cioroiu CM, Brannagan TH: Bell's palsy and cranial nerve lesions. *In* Louis ED, Mayer SA, Rowland LP (eds): *Merritt's Textbook of Neurology*, 13th ed. Philadelphia, Wolters Kluwer, 2016.

D'Amico RS, Sisti MB: Acoustic neuromas and other skull base tumors. *In* Louis ED, Mayer SA, Rowland LP (eds): *Merritt's Textbook of Neurology*, 13th ed. Philadelphia, Wolters Kluwer, 2016.

Davies AE, Kidd D, Stone SP, MacMahon J: Pharyngeal sensation and gag reflex in healthy subjects. *Lancet* 345(8948):487–488, 1995.

Haines DE: *Fundamental Neuroscience for Basic and Clinical Applications*, 4th ed. New York, Elsevier/Saunders, 2013.

Haines DE: *Neuroanatomy in a Clinical Context: An Atlas of Structures, Sections, and Systems*, 9th ed. Baltimore, Lippincott Williams & Wilkins, 2015.

Haines DE, Mihailoff GA: An overview of the brainstem. *In* Haines DE (ed): *Fundamental Neuroscience for Basic and Clinical Applications*, 4th ed. New York, Elsevier/Saunders, 2013.

Kiernan JA, Rajakumar N: *Barr's the Human Nervous System: An Anatomical Viewpoint*, 10th ed. Baltimore, Lippincott Williams & Wilkins, 2014.

Lachman N, Acland RD, Rosse C: Anatomical evidence for the absence of a morphologically distinct cranial root of the accessory nerve in man. *Clin Anat* 15:4, 2002.

Louis ED, Mayer SA, Rowland LP (eds): *Merritt's Textbook of Neurology*, 13th ed. Philadelphia, Wolters Kluwer, 2016.

Lynch JC, Corbett JJ: The visual system. *In* Haines DE (ed): *Fundamental Neuroscience for Basic and Clinical Applications*, 4th ed. New York, Elsevier/Saunders, 2013.

Moore KL, Persaud TVN, Torchia MG: *The Developing Human: Clinically Oriented Embryology*, 10th ed. Philadelphia, Elsevier/Saunders, 2016.

Odel JG, Mallory J: Visual disturbances. *In* Louis ED, Mayer SA, Rowland LP (eds): *Merritt's Textbook of Neurology*, 13th ed. Philadelphia, Wolters Kluwer, 2016.

Roberts JK: Dizziness, vertigo, and hearing loss. *In* Louis ED, Mayer SA, Rowland LP (eds): *Merritt's Textbook of Neurology*, 13th ed. Philadelphia, Wolters Kluwer, 2016.

Russo JF, Mikell CB, Winfree CJ: Traumatic cranial and peripheral nerve injuries. *In* Louis ED, Mayer SA, Rowland LP (eds): *Merritt's Textbook of Neurology*, 13th ed. Philadelphia, Wolters Kluwer, 2016.

Sevush-Garcy J, Elkind MSV: Global burden of neurologic disease. *In* Louis ED, Mayer SA, Rowland LP (eds): *Merritt's Textbook of Neurology*, 13th ed. Philadelphia, Wolters Kluwer, 2016.

Simpson KL, Sweazey RD: Olfaction and taste. *In* Haines DE (ed): *Fundamental Neuroscience for Basic and Clinical Applications*, 4th ed. New York, Elsevier/Saunders, 2013.

Swartz MH: *Textbook of Physical Diagnosis: History and Diagnosis*, 7th ed. Philadelphia, Elsevier/Saunders, 2014.

Wilson-Pauwels L, Stewart PA, Akesson EJ, Spacey SD: *Cranial Nerves: Function and Dysfunction*, 3rd ed. Shelton, CT, People's Medical Publishing House-USA, 2010.

Yugrakh MS, Chou DE: Cranial neuralgias and facial pain disorders. *In* Louis ED, Mayer SA, Rowland LP (eds): *Merritt's Textbook of Neurology*, 13th ed. Philadelphia, Wolters Kluwer, 2016.

Index
Volumes 1–3

Volume 1: Pages 1–427; **Volume 2:** 428–875; **Volume 3:** Pages 876–1158.
Note: Page numbers in **boldface** indicate the primary entry for the term, which appears in boldface or as a heading on the page indicated and is followed by a definition or explanation; page numbers in *italics* denote figures; those followed by "t" denote tables.

A

Abbreviations, **5**
Abdomen, **431**–578
acute, 446, 509
fat accumulation on, 445
functions of, 431–432
hernias of, 445
medical imaging of, 575, *575–578*
paracentesis of, **472**
protuberance of, **445**
regions of, **432–434**, *433*
ultrasound of, **575**, *575*
viscera of, *431*, **474**–558
innervation of, **553**–558
overview of, **474**–476
physiology of, 475
sympathetic innervation of, **553**, *554*
walls of (*see* Abdominal wall)
Abdominal wall, **432**
anterolateral, **432**, **434**–464
blood vessels of, **443**
elements of, 432, *435*
fascia of, **434**–435
incisions of
gridiron (muscle-splitting), 447
longitudinal, **446**–447
median, 446
midline, 446
oblique, **447**
paramedian, 446–447
Pfannenstiel, *447*
suprapubic, 447
transverse, **447**
internal surface of, **449**–450
lymphatic system for, 443
muscles of, **435**–441
nerves of, **441**–443, 442t
palpation of, **446**
physical examination of, 434
structure of, *437*
surface anatomy of, **458**–459
inferior, *439*
posterior, **563**–570
arteries of, **567**–570
autonomic nerves of, *554*
blood vessels of, **567**–570
fascia of, **563**, *557*
lymphatic system of, *569*, **569**–570
muscles of, **565**–566, 565t, *566*
nerves of, *566*, **566**–567
subdivisions of, *434*
Abdominopelvic splanchnic nerves, **61**
Abduction, *9*, *10–11*, **956**
Abductor muscles
digiti minimi, 256, *258–259*, **259,** 260t, **261**
pollicis brevis, 256–257, *258–259*, **259**, 260t
pollicis longus, *229*, *234*, 234t–235t, *235*, *236–237*, *240*, **240**
Abscess
ischio-anal, **675**–676
parotid gland, **985**
pelvirectal, 675, *675*
peri-anal, **675**–677, *675*
perinephric, **549**
peritoneal, **473**
popliteal, **806**
psoas, **571**
retro-auricular, 1039, *1039*
retropharyngeal, 1054
seminal gland, **639**
subphrenic, **533**
tooth, **1007**
Accessory obturator artery, **763**, *763*
Accessory saphenous vein, **731**
Accessory soleus, **810**
AC joint—*See* Acromioclavicular joint
Acetabular labrum, **829**
Acetabular notch, **711**
Acetabular rim, **829**
Acetabulum, *27*, *449*, *587*, *707–710*, **711**, *753*, 828–829
fracture of, *594*
lunate surface of, **711**
Acetylcholine, 58
ACL. *See* Anterior cruciate ligament
Acoustic neuroma, **1155**
Acromioclavicular (AC) joint, *149*, *151*, 276, *276*, *278*, **279**
Acromion of scapula, *27*, *149*, *156*, *180*, 1056
Acute abdomen, 446, 509
Acute arterial occlusion, 827
Acute respiratory distress, 363
Adduction, **9**, *10–11*, 12, **956**
Adductor brevis, **749**, *750*, 750t, 751
Adductor canal, **752**, *757*, **757**
Adductor hiatus, **751**
Adductor longus, **749**, *750*, 750t
injury to, **760**–761
Adductor magnus, 749, *750*, 750t, **751**
Adductor tubercle, **713**
Adenocarcinoma, ductular, 533
Adenoid. *See* Tonsil, pharyngeal
Adenoiditis, **1113**
Adenoma, parathyroid, 1109–1110
Adhesions, **472**
diaphragmatic, *483*
peritoneal, **472**
pleural, **364**
splenic, *483*
Adhesiotomy, **472**
Adhesive capsulitis, **298**
Adrenal gland. *See* Gland, suprarenal
Adrenaline. *See* Epinephrine
Afferent fibers, 50
Aging
of costal cartilage, **320**
of vertebrae, **95–96**
Ala, of ilium, *768*
Alar folds, **838**
Alimentary system, **4**
Alveolus/alveoli, *352*
dental, *990*
pulmonary, **353**
Amastia, **342**
Ampulla
bony (of semicircular canals), **1035**, *1141*
of ductus deferens, 603, *604*, *634*, **635**
duodenum, **489**
hepatopancreatic, **489**, *515*, **515**, *525*, 527
rectal, *623*, **628**, *628*, *669*
of semicircular canals, *1141*
of semicircular ducts (labyrinthine), *1034*, **1036**, *1036*
of uterine tube, **642**
Anastomosis/Anastomoses **41–42**
of arteries
bronchial-pulmonary, 364
cerebral, **944**
colic, 498, 500
coronary, 385, *386*, 387t, 388, 398
epigastric, 443
facial, 920
of foot, 804, *818–819*, *821*, 822, 827

Anastomosis/Anastomoses (*Continued*)
gastric, 481, 505
gastro-omental, *471*, *481*, 505
gluteal, 776, 778t,
intercostal, *208*
internal iliac, 619
ovarian-uterine, 611, *612*
palatine, 996
pelvic, 607, *608*, 609t–610t
popliteal, *786*, 844, *846*
rectal, 629, 672
of scalp, 921
testicular, 457
ureteric, 631
arteriolovenular, **42**
arteriovenous (AVAs), 672, 676, 682, 1006
cruciate, of thigh, 776
cubital, **217**, *217*, 225–226, 242t, 243, 272
of face, 912
genicular *789*, **844**, *846*
peri-articular arterial, 28
of elbow (cubital), **217**, *217*, 225–226, 242t, 243, 272
of knee (genicular), *789*, **844**, *846*
of shoulder (scapular), *196*, 197t, **197**, **207**, *208*
of wrist and hand, 242t, 295
scapular, *196*, **197**, **207**, *208*
splenorenal, 539, *539*
surgical
peritoneum and, 471
of veins
axillary, 198
azygos system, 413
epigastric, 443
of face, 912, 915
portocaval, 539, *614*, 629, 676
portal-systemic, **529–**530, 538, 540
rectal, 629, 672
saphenous, 731
vena cava, 447
Anatomical
planes, **6**–7, *7*
position, **6**
snuff box, 158, *236*, **240**, *240*, 269
variations, **12**
Anatomy, **2–5**
clinical, **5**
history of, 2
radiographic, **3**
regional, **2**–4, *3*
study approaches for, **2**–5
surface, **3** (*see also under* Surface anatomy)
systemic, **4**–5
Andrology, 4
Anesthesia
blocks
brachial plexus, **211**
buccal nerve, **919**
caudal epidural, **93**, *93*, 657, *657*
cervical plexus, 1074
cervicothoracic ganglion, **1082**
epidural, **140**
fibular nerve, **827**
greater palatine nerve, **1009**
inferior alveolar nerve, **986**
infra-orbital nerve, **918**–919
intercostal nerve, **333**
lateral cervical region, **1074**
mandibular nerve, **986**
mental nerve, **919**
nasopalatine nerve, **1008**–1009
phrenic nerve, **1074**
pudendal nerve, 657, *657*
sciatic nerve, **784**
spinal, **140**, 656–657
superficial fibular nerve, **827**
superior laryngeal nerve, 1112
trigeminal nerve, **1153**
for childbirth, **656–657**
dental, **1154**
epidural
caudal, **93–**94
transsacral, 94
general, 656
regional
for childbirth, 656
of lower limbs, **742**
spinal, **140**
Aneurysm
abdominal aorta, **572**–573
aortic arch, **418**
ascending aorta, **418**
berry, 945
of cerebellar artery, 1154
popliteal, **806**–807
rupture of, 944
saccular, 944
Angina pectoris, **398**, 1010
Angiography. *See also* Arteriograms
aortic, **419**, *419*
cardiac, 762
coronary, **396–**397
magnetic resonance, *424*
Angioplasty, percutaneous transluminal, coronary, 399, *399*
Angle(s)
acromial, *149*, **157**, 187, *187*
costal, **310**
of declination, **713**
of eye, **949**, *967*
of flexion (of uterus), 643, *645*
of inclination, **711**
infrasternal, *309*, *314*, **314**, 338, *338*
iridocorneal, *952*
of Louis 5, **314** (*see* Angle, sternal)
lumbosacral, 74, **86**
of mandible, *976*, *978*, 1070, *1071*, *1115*
of mouth, **916**
Q-angle, *836*, **863**
of rib, *121*
of scapula, *149–150*, **151**, *187*, 188, *309*
inferior, *183*
lateral, *182*
superior, *183*
sternal, 5, *309*, **314**, 336, *338*, *368*, *1096*
subcostal, *309*, *314*
subpubic, **586**, *588*, 588t, 591
of torsion, **713**
venous, 355, **1080**
left, 335, 337, 412, *1105–1106*, 1106
right, 335, *1105*, 1106
of Wiberg, 861
Ankle joint, 811, **849**, *849*
articular surfaces, **849**
blood supply, **851**
capsule, **849**–850
dorsiflexion of, 850
injuries, **868**, *868*
ligaments, **850**
movements, **850**
nerve supply of, **851**
plantarflexion of, 850
Pott fracture-dislocation of, 868
radiographs of, *849*
retinacula of, *811*
surface anatomy of, **824–**826, **859**, *860*
Anosmia, **1151**–1152
Anoxia, 945
Ansa cervicalis, **1061**, *1063*, 1066, **1148**, *1150*
ANS. *See* Autonomic nervous system
Ansa subclavia, *1079*
Antagonist, **35**
Antebrachial fascia, **165**, *166*, *224*, *230*
Anteflexion (of uterus), 650, *651*, 652
Anterior, **7**, 9
Anterograde degeneration, 58
Anterolateral tibial (Gerdy) tubercle, **716**
Antihelix, 1026, *1027*
Antitragus, *1027*
Antrum
mastoid, 1027, **1030**, *1031*
pyloric, **480**, *480–481*
Anulus fibrosus, 98, *98*, 109, *109*
degeneration of, 109
Anus, *662*, 663, *664–665*, **670**, *694*
Aorta, *40*
abdominal, *455*, *493*, *530*, **567**–568, *578*, *628*
aneurysm of, **572–**573,
branches of, **568**, 568t
relations of, **568**
angiograms of, **419**
arch of, 350, *378*, *386*, 404, *404*, *406*, *410*, *1094*
aneurysm of, **418**
anomalies of, **417**–418
branches of, **417**
computed tomography of, *421–422*
double, *417*, **418**

lymph nodes of, *355*
right, **418**
ascending, *329*, *373*, *378*, *384*, *386*, **403**, *407*
aneurysm of, **418**
branches of, 412t
computed tomography of, *422*
bifurcation of, *577*
branches of, 412t
coarctation of, **418**
computed tomography of, *576*
descending, **403**, *404*, *406–408*
branches of, **410**
computed tomography of, *422*
descending thoracic, *569*
magnetic resonance imaging of, *577*
pulsations of, **572**, *573*
thoracic, *329*, 330t, *336*, *356*, *405*, **409–**410, *410*
branches of, *411*, 412t
ultrasound of, **575**, *575*
Aperture
diaphragmatic, **561**–562
median, *936*, **936**, *937*
thoracic
inferior, *314*, **315**
superior, *314*, **314–315**, *368*, 1079
Apex, **715**
of axilla, **193**, *194*
beat, **377**, **415**
of coccyx, *85*, **87**
of heart, *346*, **377**, *378*, *386*, *431*
of lung, *346*, **348**, *368*, *431*
of maxillary sinus, **1023**
of nose, *916*, **1015**
of sacrum, **86**
of tongue, **997**, *1010*
of urinary bladder, *623*, **624**
Aphonia, 1155
Aponeurosis, aponeuroses, **31**, 434
of abdominal wall, *564*
bicipital, *166*, **212**, *218*, 219, 221, *230*, *250*
epicranial, *129*, 129t, **900**, *901*, *902*, *911*, *1022*
oblique abdominal
external, **435**, 436t, 437, *437–439*, 441, *442*, 447, *450*, *452*, 452t, *454*
internal, 435, 436t, *437*, **439**, *440*, 441, *442*, 447, *452*, 452t, *454*
of transversus abdominis, *437*
palatine, **994**, 995
palmar, *161*, *229*, **254**, 256, *256*
plantar, **812**
of scalp, **900**, *902*
transverse (of transverse abdominis), *118*, **439**
triceps, **216**
Apophyses, **721**
Appendectomy, **509**–510
Appendicitis, **509**
Appendix, 432, *474–475*, *487*, *491*, *493*, 494, **494**, *496–498*, 506
of abdomen (*see* Appendix, vermiform)
of epididymis, 463, *463*
epiploic, *628*
lymphatic system of, 497, *501*
nerves of, *501*
omental, **494**
retrocecal, 498, 509
rupture of, 509
of testis, 463, *463*
vermiform, 497
Aqueduct
cerebral, *936*, **936**, *1029*
cochlear, **1035**
vestibular, *1029–1030*, *1034*, **1035**
Arachnoid mater
cranial, *901*, *923*, **929**
spinal, **134**, *135–136*
Arcades, arterial, *493*
Arch
alveolar, of maxillae, **887**
anterior, of cervical vertebrae, 80
of aorta, 350, *378*, *386*, 404, *404*, *406*, *410*, *1094*
aneurysm of, **418**
anomalies of, **417**–418
branches of, **417**
computed tomography of, *421–422*
double, *417*, **418**
lymph nodes of, *355*
right, **418**
of azygos vein, **404**, *408–409*, *413*
carpal
dorsal, *236*, *242*, 242t, *264*
palmar, *242*, 242t, *261*, *264*
coraco-acromial, **281**
costal (*see* Margins, costal)
dental, **987**
of foot
longitudinal, 718, **857**, *858*, *860*
transverse, **857**, *856*
iliopectineal, *565*
lateral longitudinal, **857**
medial longitudinal, **857**
neural, **87**
palatoglossal, *994*, **994**, *996*, *999*, *1010*, *1098–1099*
palatopharyngeal, *994*, **994**, *996*, *999*, *1010*, *1098–1099*, 1099
palmar arterial
deep, *40*, *242–243*, *264*, 264, 264t 270
laceration of, **272**
superficial, *242*, *258*, *264*, **264**, 264t, 270
wounds to, 275
plantar arterial, *730*, *804*, *818–819*, **822**
posterior of C1, *127*, 127t
pubic, **586**, *587*, 588t
superciliary, *915*, *1021*
superficial palmar, *40*
tendinous
of levator ani, **599**, *604*
of pelvic fascia, **603**, *604*
of soleus, **802**, *802*, *837*
venous
deep palmar, *243*, **244**
dorsal, *693*, 731, **822**
jugular, *1065*, **1070**, **1080**
plantar, *823*
superficial palmar, *243*
vertebral
of cervical vertebrae, 75, **76**, 77–78
fractures of, 92
joints of, **100**
lamina of, *99*
zygomatic, *976*, *1012*, *1022*
Arcuate artery, **822**
Arcuate popliteal ligament, **838**
Area
diaphragmatic, *518*
esophageal, *349*
Kiesselbach, 1019
olfactory, **1016**
respiratory, **1016**
Areola, **332**, *334*, 334–335, *340*
Arm, **212**–227
arteries of, *217*
cutaneous nerves of, *169*
muscles of, 212–216, 215t–216t
nerves of, 218–220
surface anatomy of, 221
veins of, 217–218
Arterial circle of Willis. *See* Circle, cerebral arterial
Arterial pulses, 3
Arteries (in general), **39**
conducting, 39
distributing, 40
function of, 39
small, **40**
submucosal, 478
types of, 39
veins and, comparisons between, 41
Arteries (named)
alveolar
inferior, *981*, **993**, *1022*
superior, *981*, **993**
angular, **912**, 913t
anterior tibial, **792**
recurrent, **789**
appendicular, *496*, **497**, *498–499*, 500t
arcuate, *819*, **822**, *846*
auricular
deep, *981*
posterior, 913t, *1068*, **1069**

Arteries (named) (*Continued*)
axillary, *178*, **195**, *195*, *208*, *325*, *329*, 331, 337, 1060
aneurysm of, **209**
branches of, 195
compression of, 209
occlusion of, 208
right, *1073*
basilar, *138*, **939**, *941*, 942t, *1083*
brachial, *196*, *208*, **217**, *218*, *336*
compression of, 225
deep artery of arm (*see* Arteries, profunda brachii)
division of, **250**, *250*
humeral nutrient artery, **217**
brachiocephalic, *407*
right, **337**
bronchial, *329*, *352*, **354**, 371, *390*, 412t
left, **354**
right, **354**
buccal, *981*
cardiovascular system, 39–41
carotid
common, *346*, 406, *406*, *410*, *1047*, *1064*, 1065, *1081*, *1086*, *1091*, *1100–1101*
left, *329*, *378*, **406**, *406–407*, *417*, *421–422*, **1066**, *1068*, *1078*
right, *329*, *407*, *417*, *419*, **1066**, *1068*, *1078*
external, **912**, *984*, *1002*, *1032*, *1064*, 1066, *1081*, *1084*, *1086*, *1100–1101*, *1114*
ligation of, 1074
internal, **926**, *930*, **939**, *940*, 942t, *978*, *1013*, *1031*, 1066, *1081*, *1084*, *1100–1101*, *1083*, *1139*, *1144*, *1150*
pulse taking, 1072, 1075
stenosis of, **920**
stenosis of, 945
celiac, *516*, *575*
central, of retina, *952*, 954, **965**, *964*, 965t, **972**
cerebellar
aneurysm of, **1153**
anterior inferior, *941*, 942t
posterior inferior, *138*, *941*
superior, *941*
cerebral
anastomoses of, **944**
anterior, **939**, *941–942*, 942t
middle, **939**, *941–942*, 942t
posterior, *138*, **939**, *941–942*, 942t
superior, *138*
cervical
ascending, *138*, *1078–1079*
deep, *138*
transverse, *194*, *205*, 1060, *1078–1079*
ciliary
anterior, *952*, *964*, 965t
long posterior, *952*, **965**, *964*, 965t
short posterior, **965**, *964*, 965t
circumflex
femoral, *608*, *756*, **755**, 756t
humeral, **197**, 197t
iliac, 444, 444t
scapular, *189*, **197**, 197t
colic
left, **498**, *498–499*, 500t, *501*, 502
middle, **498**, *498–499*, 500t, *501*, 502
right, **498**, *498–499*, 500t, *501*
collateral
middle (medial), **217**, *217*, *242*
radial, **217**, *217*, *242*
ulnar, inferior, **217**, *217*, *242*
superior, **217**, *217*, *242*
communicating
anterior, **939,** *941–942*, 942t
posterior, **939**, *941–942*, 942t
coronary, 371
left, *384*, **385**, *386*
right, *384–385*, **385**
variations of, **388**
cremasteric, 455, *455*, *628*
cricothyroid, **1094**
cystic, *484*, 484t, *515*, 527, *527–528*
deep
of arm (*see* Arteries (named), profunda brachii)
of clitoris, 671t
of penis, 671t, **681**
plantar, **821**
of thigh (*see* Arteries (named), profunda femoris)
digital
dorsal, *261*, *819*, **822**, *846*
plantar, *258*, *261*, 264, *819*, *821*
proper palmar, *264*, **264**, 264t
dorsal
of clitoris, **670**, 671t
digital, **822**
of foot (*see* Arteries (named), dorsalis pedis; Arteries (named), profunda brachii)
of penis, 612, **670**, 671t, *679*, *681*, **681**
dorsal digital, **822**
dorsalis indicis, *236*, *264*
dorsalis pedis, *40*, 796t, *818*, *821*, **821**–822
pulse, **827**
dorsalis pollicis, *236*, *264*
of ductus deferens, 457
epigastric
inferior, **443**, *444*, 444t, *449*, *598*, *611*, *669*
superficial, *438*, **443**, *444*, 444t
superior, *329*, 331, *440*, **443**, 444t
epiphysial, *22–23*, 23
esophageal, 371, 412t
ethmoidal
anterior, *963–964*, 965t, 1019
posterior, *963–964*, 965t, 1019
facial, *911*, 912, 913, 913t, *1064*, *1068*
compression of, **920**
pulse taking, **920**
tonsillar branch of, *1099*
transverse, *913*, 913t, 978
femoral, *438*, *444*, *455*, *697*, **755**, *756*, 756t
cannulation of, 761
circumflex
lateral, *608*
medial, *608*
compression of, **761**
deep (*see* Arteries (named), profunda brachii)
laceration, 761
palpation of, **761**
fibular, 725, *797*, *802*, **804**, *823*, *846*
circumflex, *804–805*
perforating branch(es), *794*, *797*, **798**, 827, *846*, 847, 849
of foot, *821*, 821–822
gastric
left, 478, **482**, *483*, *484*, 484t, *488*, *526*, *535*, *544*, *575*
posterior, *476*, **482**, *483–484*, 484t
right, **482**, *484*, 485t
short, **482**, *483–484*, 484t
gastroduodenal, *484*, 485t, *488*, **490**, *493*, *515–516*, 517, 527, *527*, *529*, *535*, *575*
gastro-omental (gastro-epiploic)
left, **482**, *483–484*, 484t
right, **482**, *484*, 485t, *488*, *493*, *516*
genicular
descending, *789*, *846*
inferior lateral, *788–789*, *796*, 796t
inferior medial, *788–789*, 796 796t, 846
middle, *789*, *846*
superior lateral, *788–789*, *796*, 796t, 846
superior medial, *788*, **789**, *789*, *796*, 796t, 840, 846
gluteal, **776**–777, *777*, 778t
inferior, *608*, 610t, *611*, **612**, *612*, 669
superior, 609t, *611*, **612**
hepatic, *484*, 484t, *488*, 524, 526, *575*
aberrant, **534**
common, *488*, *493*, *516*, 519, *520*, **524**
left, *535*
proper, *488*, **524**
relationships of, **534**
right, 527, *527*, *535*
humeral, circumflex, 188
ileal, *493*, *498–499*
ileocolic, *493*, *496*, **496**

iliac
  circumflex, *608*
    deep, *444*, 444t
    superficial, *444*, 444t
  common, *567*, 607 *608*, *611*, *634*
    left, *541*
    right, *455*, *541*, *547*
  external, 440, 449, 455, 555, 567, 598, 605, 608, 611, 621, 628, 634
  internal, 331, *455*, *555*, *605*, **607**, 609t–610t, 610, *611*, *615*, *634*, *643*
    ligation of, **619**
    posterior division of, **612**
iliolumbar, *608*, 610t, *611*, **612**, *615*
infra-orbital, **965**, *966*, 965t, *981*, *984*, 1013, 1022
intercostal, **331**, *409*
  anterior, *326*, *329*, 330t, **331**, *336*
  lumbar, *138*
  posterior, *106*, *138*, *326*, *329*, 330, 330t, **331**, 412t, *444*, 444t
  superior, **331**
  supreme, *410*
interosseous
  anterior, *242*, 242t, *264*, *288*
  common, *242*, 242t, *288*
  posterior, *236*, *242*, 242t, *264*, *288*
  recurrent, *242*, 242t
intestinal, *498*, 500t
jejunal, *488*, *493*, *498*, *499*
juxtacolic, 498
labial
  inferior, *913*, 913t, **988**
  superior, *913*, 913t, **988**, 1019
labyrinthine, *941*, *942*
lacrimal, *967*, 965t
large elastic, 39–40
laryngeal, *1068*, 1094
lateral circumflex femoral, **755**
lateral plantar, **822**
lateral tarsal, **821**
lingual, **1069**
  deep, **1000**, *1064*
  dorsal, **1000**
lobar
  middle, 353
  superior, 353
lumbar, 568
mammary, internal (*see* Arteries (named), thoracic, internal)
marginal, **498**, *499* 500
  left, **385**, *386*
  right, **385**, *386*
masseteric, *981*
maxillary, 980, **1023**, 1066
  branches of, *981*, *1032*
medial circumflex femoral, **755**
medial plantar, **822**
mediastinal, **410**
medium muscular, 40
medullary
  anterior segmental, *137*, *139*
  posterior segmental, **137**, *138*
meningeal
  accessory, *981*
  middle, **928**, 932, *964*, *984*, *1122*
    branches of, **928**
mental, *913*, 913t
mesenteric
  inferior, *476*, *493*, *498*, *499*, 500t, *508*, *515*, *541*, *546–547*, *555*, *567*, *608*
  superior, 476, 488, 489, *490*, 491, 493, 498, 499, 500t, 508, *515–516*, *526*, *541*, *546*, 567, 575–576
metacarpal, palmar, *261*, **264**
metaphysial, *23*
metatarsal
  dorsal, *819*, 821
    1st, **821**
    2nd, **822**
    3rd, **822**
    4th, **822**
  plantar, *818*
musculophrenic, *329*, **331**, *370*, 371, *444*, 444t, 560
nasal
  dorsal, *964*, 965t
  lateral, *913*, 913t
  posterior, *1013*
nodal
  atrioventricular, **389**
  sino-atrial, **385**
nutrient, **23**, 106
  of fibula, *804*, **804**
  humeral, **217**
  of tibia, *804*, **805**
obturator, **610–611**, *611*, *669*
  accessory, **611**
  replacement of, **763**
occipital, *913*, 913t, *1032*, 1018, *1019*, 1068, 1069, 1070
ophthalmic, *952*, **963**, *964*, 965t
  muscular branches of, *964*, 965t
ovarian, 605 609t, *612*, *614*, 642, *643*
  ligation of, **619**
palatine
  ascending, **996**, 1069
  descending, *981*, *1013*
  greater, **996**, 1019
  lesser, **996**
pancreatic, **517**
  dorsal, *516*
  greater, *488*, *516*
pancreaticoduodenal
  anterior, *488*, *516*, 517
  inferior, *484*, 485t, *488*, **490**, *516*, 517
  posterior, *488*, 527, *527*
  superior, *484*, 485t, *490*, *516*, 517
perforating, *236*, *756*, *768*, *777*, **778**, 778t, 818
pericardiacophrenic, *370*, *409*, 560
perineal, *670*
  posterior scrotal branches of, **457**
peroneal (*see* Arteries (named), fibular)
pharyngeal, *1013*, 1031, *1032*
  ascending, *1068*, **1069**
phrenic
  inferior, *476*, 478, *541*, *546*, **560**
  superior, 371, 410, 412t, **560**
plantar
  deep,
  lateral, *801*, 804, *804*, *817*, *821*, **822**, 846
  medial, *801*, 804, *804*, *821*, **822**
  perforating branches of, **822**
plantar digital, **822**
popliteal, *756*, *788–789*, *796*, 796t, *804*, 846
posterior retinacular, **755**
princeps pollicis, *264*, 264t, 265, *265*
profunda brachii, *191*, *196*, 197t, *208*, 213, 216, 217, 217,
profunda femoris, *608*
of pterygoid canal, *981*
pudendal
  external, *438*, 457, **678**, 689
  internal, *455*, 610t, *611*, *612*, 616, 629, 643, 647, 671t, 681, 689
pulmonary, *349*, *352*
  left, *353*, **353**, *378*, *386*, *406*, *410*, 421–422
  left inferior, *378*
  left superior, *378*
  right, *353*, **353**, *378*, *406*, *421–422*
  right inferior, *378*
  right superior, *378*
radial, *40*, *229*, 242t, **243**, *258*, **264**, 264, 399
  aberrant, *266*
  dorsal carpal branch of, 242t, 243
  muscular branches of, 243
  palmar carpal branch of, 242t, 243
  palpation of, 253
  pulse measurements, **250–251**
  superficial branch of, *266*
  variations in origin of, **251**
radialis indicis, *258*, *261*, *264*, 264t
radicular
  anterior, **137**, *138*
  posterior, *137*, *138–139*
rectal
  inferior, 500t, **629**, *629*, *669*, **670**, 671t, 672, 680
  median, *608*
  middle, 500t, *605*, *608*, *611*, **612**, 629, 629, 672
  superior, *498–499*, 500t, 609t, **613**, 616, 629, 629, 669, 672

Arteries (named) (*Continued*)
recurrent
anterior tibial, **789**, *789*, *796*
anterior ulnar, *242*, 242t, 243
interosseous, *242*, 242t
posterior ulnar, 242 242t, 243
radial, *242*, 242t, 243
renal, *544*
accessory, *547*, *550*
left, 455, 526, 546, 546–547, 576
right, *455*, **546**, *546–547*, *576*
ureteric branch of, *546*
retinacular, **832**
posterior, **755**
sacral
latera, *138*
lateral, 609t–610t, *611*, **612**, *615*
median, **568**, 609t, **613**, *615*
scapular
circumflex, *196*
dorsal, *196*, **1060**, 1080
scrotal
anterior, *455*, **678**
posterior, 671t, **678**
segmental
of kidney (renal), 546
of liver (tertiary branches), *522*
of lungs (pulmonary), **353**
sigmoid, 498, *498*, *499*, 500t
sphenopalatine, *981*, *984*, *998*, *1013*, 1019, 1019
spinal
anterior, **137**, *138*, *941*
posterior, *137*, *139*
splenic, *476*, 483, *484*, 484t, 488, 513, 513, 514, 526, 575
sternocleidomastoid, *1064*
of stomach, 482, *484*
subclavian, *325*, 331, *336*, *346*, *370*, 390, 409–410, 1057, 1068, 1072, 1079, 1086
branches of, *1060*, *1068*
groove for, *349*
left, *329*, *378*, **406**, *406–407*, *1068*, 1078
right, *407*, *417*, *1068*, *1073*, *1078*
retro-esophageal, *417*
subcostal, *329*, 330t, *444*, 444t, 567
submental, **1004**, 1005, *1064–1065*
subscapular, *191*, 197t, *208*
sulcal, *137*, *139*
superior gluteal, **776**
supraduodenal, *488*
supra-orbital, *913*, 913t, *964*, 965t, 1018
suprarenal
inferior, **548**, *546–547*
middle, **548**, *546–547*
superior, **547**, *546–547*
suprascapula, *1060*, **1060**, *1078–1079*
supratrochlear, *913*, 913t, *964*, 965t
tarsal
lateral, **821**, *821*, *846*
medial, *821*, *846*
temporal, *913*, 913t, *976*, *981*, 1026, *1028*
superficial, 1066, *1068*, 1069
testicular, *452*, *455*, 456t, **457**, *541*, 609t, 634–635, 681
left, *455*, *546*, *547*
right, *455*, *546–547*
thoracic
internal, *325–326*, *329*, 330t, 331, 370, 405–407, 409, 1078–1079, **1080**
lateral, *178*, *191*, 197, 197t, *336*
superior, 195, *196*, 197t, *208*
thoraco-abdominal, *195*
thoraco-acromial, *196*, *197*, 197t
thoracodorsal, *196*, *197*, 197t
thyrocervical, *197*
thyroid
inferior, 196, 197t, 208, 1068, 1078–1079, 1080, 1084, 1085, 1094, 1100–1101, 1104
superior, *1064*, *1068*, **1069**, *1070*, 1083, 1084
thyroid ima, *417*, **1106–1107**
tibial
anterior, *40*, *789*, *791*, **792**, *796*, 796t, 804, 819, 821 846
anterior recurrent, **789**, *789*, *796*
posterior, 789 *796*, 796t, *804*, **804**, 818–819, 821, 846
tonsillar, *1068*
tympanic, anterior, *981*
ulnar, *218*, 230, 241, *241*, *242*, 242t, 243, 258, 264, 264
dorsal branch of, *266*
superficial, 250
ulnar collateral, *188*, 189t
inferior, *217* **217**, *242*
superior, *217*, **217**, *242*
umbilical, 609, **610**, *669*
obliterated, 456t, *628*
uterine, *605*, *608*, 609t, **611**, *611*, *612*, 643, 647
ligation-related injury to, **619**
vaginal, *608*, 609t, *611*, **611–612**, *612*, 647
vertebral, **929**, **939**, *941*, *942*, 942t, 1078–1079, 1081, 1091, 1083
cervical part of, 1080
cranial part of, **1080**
suboccipital part of, **1080**
vertebral part of, **1080**
vertebral, *81*, *103*, *127*, 127t, *138*
vesical
inferior, 609t, **611**, *611*, *612*, *634*, *669*
superior, *605*, 609t, *611*, *612*, *669*
vitelline, *508*
zygomaticofacial, *964*, 965t
zygomaticotemporal, *964*, 965t
Arteries (of organs or regions)
of abdominal wall
anterolateral, 443
posterior, **567**–570
of alimentary tract, 475, *476*
of anal canal, **672**
of arm, *217*
of bile duct, 524
of brain, **939**–940
of breasts, 335, *336*
of cecum, 497, 500t
of cervical region
anterior, **1066–1069**
lateral, 1057, **1060–1062**
of diaphragm, 560, *561*
to ductus deferens, 609t, *634*, 635, *669*
of duodenum, 489
of dura mater, *929*
of ejaculatory ducts, **635**
of face, **912**, *913*, 913t
of foot, *819*, *821*, **821–822**
sole of, **822**
of forearm, *217*, **241–434**
functional terminal, 41
of gluteal region, 776, *777*, 778t
gonadal, 609t
of hand, **262–264**, *264*, 264t
of hip joint, 834
of kidneys, 546, *546*
of large intestine, *493*
of larynx, 1094
of leg
anterior compartment, **505**
posterior compartment, **804–805**
of liver, 524
of lungs, **353**
to muscles, **35**
of nose, *1019*, **1019**–1020
of pancreas, *516*
of penis, 679–681
of pericardium, 371
of perineum, *671*
of pharynx, 1103
of pleurae, **353**
of popliteal fascia, *789*
of prostate gland, 638
of rectum, **629**
of root of neck, 1079–1080
of scalp, **920**
to sciatic nerve, **775**
of scrotum, **678**
of seminal glands, **635**
of small intestine, *493*
of sole of foot, **822**
of spinal cord, 137, *138*
of spinal nerve roots, 137
of stomach, 484t
of suprarenal glands, *546*, 547
of teeth, 993
of thigh
anterior, *756*, 756t

medial, *756*, 756t
posterior, 776, *777*, 778t
of thoracic wall, **330–331**
of thyroid gland, 1083
of tongue, 1000
of ureters, **621**
of urethra
female, **626**
male, **626**, **677**
of urinary bladder, **624–625**
of uterus, *643*, **646**
of vagina, **647**
of vertebral column, 105–106
of vulva, **689**
of wrist, *242*, 242t
Arteriograms
aortic, *419*
axillary, *196*
carotid, *941*
coronary, 395
popliteal, *797*
superior mesenteric, *499*
of wrist and hand, *265*
Arterioles, 29–40
Arteriolovenular anastomoses (AVAs), **42**
Arteriosclerosis, 130
Arteriosus
conus, *380*, **380**, 422
truncus, **395**
Arthritis
osteoarthritis, 111
temporomandibular joint, **986**
Arthrology, 4
Arthroplasty. *See* Total Knee Replacement Arthroplasty
Arthroscopy, **29**
of knee joint, *866*, **866–867**
Arthrosis, 863
Articularis genu, **749**
Articular ligaments, 848
Articular surfaces, 848
Articular system, **4**
Articulation(s)
of elbow joint, **284**
humeroradial, 284, 302
humero-ulnar, 284, 302
of knee joint, **836**
femorotibial, 836
femoropatellar, 836
talocrural (*see* Ankle joint)
Ascites, **471**–472
Aspiration
of foreign bodies, **360**, 1111–1112
of knee joint, **867**
pneumonia, 1050
Asterion, 885t
Astrocytes, 47
Atelectasis, 358, 359, **361–362**
Atheroma, 42
Atheromatous plaque, 945
Atherosclerosis, *377*, **396**
Atlas (vertebra C1), *75*, *79*, **80**, *88*, *1017*, 1049, 1096
dislocation of, 92
fracture of, 92
Atrial fibrillation, 401
Atrial septal defects, 391–392
Atrium/atria, of heart
left, 375, *375*, *378*, *384*, 391, *420*
thrombi on, 393
right, 375, *375*, *378–379*, **379**, *420*, 421–422
embryology of, 391
physiology of, 383
Atrophy, 24
Auditory ossicles, *1026*, 1027, **1029**, *1029*, *1030*, 1031–1033
Auricle, **1026**–1027
left, *364*, *378*, 391
right, *378*, **379**, 391
Auscultation
of heart, 415
of lungs, 359, **360**
triangle of, *179*, **190**
Autonomic nervous system (ANS), **58**
enteric nervous system (ENS), 30t, 63–65, 64, 66, 494, 495, 553, 554, 556–558, 557
functions, 65–66, 65t
parasympathetic division, *63*, *64*
sympathetic division, *58*–61, *59–63*, 63
visceral sensation, 66
Avascular epidermis, 13
Avascular necrosis, **25**
of femoral head, 862
of lunate, 301
Avulsion fractures, 759
Axial line, **734**
Axilla, **193**–210
floor of, *164*
walls of, *164*, 193, *194*, *198*, *214*
Axillary fascia, **163**, *164*, *194*
Axillary fat, 193, *194*
Axis (pelvic), *586*, **596**, *597*
Axis (vertebra (C2)), *75*, *88*, *1017*, 1049
characteristics of, 80, 80t
dens of, *81*, *102*, *1087*
fracture of, 92
Axon, 46

B

Babinski sign, 827
Back, **73–139**
muscles of, **118–130**
extrinsic, *118*, **118–119**
intrinsic, **119**
deep layer of, **120–122**, *122*
intermediate layer of, **120**, *121*
superficial layer of, *120*, **120**
spasm of, **129–130**
surface anatomy of, *126*
overview of, 74
sprain of, *129*, 129–130, 129t
strain of, 129–130
vertebrae (*see* Vertebrae)
vertebral column (*see* Vertebral column)
Back pain, **108**
localized, 108
low, 108
Band
longitudinal, *102*, 103
myocardial, ventricular, **377**
navicular, *851*
Bar, costotransverse, **89**, *1048*
Bare areas, **468**
Bartholinitis, 691
Base
of axilla, **185**, *186*
of brain, *941*
cranial (basicranium), *81*, **879**, 887, 926, 1083
external surface of, **887**–890
internal surface of, **890**–893
fractures of, **933**
of heart, **377**, *378*
of lung, **350**
of maxillary sinus, **1023**
of metacarpals, 154
of patella, *758*, *841*
of sacrum, **86**
Baseball finger, **249**
Basicranium, **879**
Basilic veins, 164, *165*, **165**, *199*, 217, *218*, 221
Basi-occiput, *888*
Bed
bladder, **624**
breast, **334**
capillary, 42
parotid, **974**
of stomach, **481**, *483*
tonsillar, *1099*, **1100**
Biceps femoris, **773**
long head of, **773**
short head of, **773**
Bicipital aponeurosis, *166*, **212**, *218*, 219, 222, 223, 250
Bicornate uterus, **650**, *651*
Bilateral, **9**
Bile, **516**
Bile canaliculi, **527**
Biopsy
of liver, **536**
mediastinal, 372
splenic, **532**
sternal, **321**
Bipedalism, **861**
Birth defect, **12**
Bitemporal hemianopsia, 1152, *1152*
Bladder, urinary, **622**, *694*, *696*
apex of, **624**
arteries of, **624–625**

Bladder, urinary (*Continued*)
- body of, **624**
- in children, 622
- cystocele, **631–632**, *632*
- cystoscopy of, *632*, **632**
- fundus of, *623*, **624**
- in infants, 622
- innervation of, *625*, **625–626**
- interior of, *627*
- ligaments of
  - lateral, **603**, *605*
  - pubovesical, **603**
- lymphatic system of, *659*
- micturition, 624
- neck of, **24**
- rupture of, **632**
- surfaces of, 624, *624*
- trigone of, **624**
- uvula of, **624**
- walls of, 624

Block (anesthetic)
- brachial plexus, **211**
- buccal nerve, **919**
- caudal epidural, **657**, *657*
- cervical plexus, **1074**
- cervicothoracic ganglion, **1082**
- epidural, **140**
- fibular nerve, **827**
- greater palatine nerve, **1008**
- inferior alveolar nerve, **986**
- infra-orbital nerve, **917**–918
- intercostal nerve, **333**
- lateral cervical region, **1074**
- mandibular nerve, **986**
- mental nerve, **919**
- nasopalatine nerve, **1008**
- phrenic nerve, 1074
- pudendal nerve, 657, *657*
- sciatic nerve, **784**
- spinal, **140**, 656–657
- superficial fibular nerve, **827**
- superior laryngeal nerve, 1113
- trigeminal nerve, 1153

Block (pathological)
- bundle branch, 400
- heart, 400

Blood vessels. *See also* Arteries; vein(s)
- of abdominal wall
  - anterolateral, 443
  - posterior, **567**–570
- of ankle joint, 851
- arteries, 39–41
- capillaries, 42
- of elbow joint, **286**
- of femoral neck, 834
- of hip joints, 834
- of knee joints, 844
- of liver, **524**
- of posterior mediastinum, 413–414
- of stomach, 480
- structure, 39, *39*
- veins, 41–42
- of wrist, 291

Body
- anococcygeal, *598*, **598**
- of bone, *21*
- carotid, *1065*, **1065–1066**, 1066
- ciliary, **953**
- of clitoris, *689*
- of corpus callosum, *937*
- of epididymis, 456, *463*
- fat, of ischio-anal fossa, 669
- of gallbladder, **529**
- geniculate, lateral, *1132*, **1133**
- of hyoid, **1049**
- of ilium, 586, *587*
- of ischium, 586, **709**
- layer-based organization of, 3
- of lumbar vertebra, *542*
- of mandible, **886**
- of pancreas, *483*, **514**–515
- parts of, *3*, 7, 9
- of penis, 678, **679**
- perineal, *600*, *647*, 673, *680*, 683t, *687*
- pineal, *936*, *937*
- of pubis, 586
- of ribs, *306*, *307*
- of scapula, **147**
- of sphenoid, *927*, *1097*
- of sternum, *177*, *305*, *313*, **314**, 338, *368*
- of stomach, **479**, *481*
- talar, 718
- of talus, **718**
- of tongue, **997**
- of urinary bladder, **624**
- of uterus, *641*, **643**, *696*
- vertebral, *99–100*, *99–100*, 117, *1091*
  - cervical vertebrae, *79*, *81*
  - computed tomography of, *576*
  - joints of, 97–100
  - lumbar vertebrae, **83–85**
  - magnetic resonance imaging of, *577*
  - thoracic vertebrae, 82t, 422
- vitreous, 952, **955**

Bone(s) (in general)
- accessory, 23–24
- age-related changes in, 20
- atrophy of, 24
- classification of, 20–21
- compact, *20*, *21*
- development of, 22–23
- flat, 19
- function of, 20–21
- grafts, 724–725, *725*
- growth of, 25
- heterotopic, 24
- hip, **708**–709, *709*
- hypertrophy of, 24
- innervation, 23
- irregular, 24
- long, *21*, 22, 23
- markings, 21, 21–22
- osteoporotic, *24*
- pneumatized, **882**
- remodeling of, 24
- rider's, 24
- sesamoid, 21, 262, *719*, *720*, *803*, *817*, 857, 860
  - fracture of, **726**
- short, 21
- spongy, 21, *21*, *76*
- supernumerary, 23–24
- sutural, 24
- trauma to, 24
- vasculature of, 23, *23*

Bone(s) (named). *See also* specific bones
- carpal, *149*, *229*
- ethmoid, **948**
- femur, **711**, *712*, 713–715, *714*, 722
- fibula, *716*, **717**, 724
- foot, **718**, *719–720*, 720–721
- frontal, **884**
- general images of, *20*
- hip, **708**–709, *709*
  - in children, 586
  - in infants, 586
  - left, 585
  - pubertal fusion of, 586
  - right, 585
- hyoid, *20*, *907*, *999*, *1001*, *1004*, *1047*, 1048, 1063, 1070, 1089, 1098, 1104
  - fracture of, 1050
- ilium, **709**, *710*, 711
- lacrimal, *946*
- occipital, *127*, 127t, *129*, 129t, *926*, *1051*, 1097
- palatine, *995*, 1011, *1012*, *1098*
- parietal, *926*
- patella, *715*, **715**
- pubic, *696*
- sesamoid, 21, 262, *719*, *720*, *803*, *817*, 857
  - fracture of, **726**
- sphenoid, *880–881*, **889**
- tarsal, 21
- temporal
  - fracture of, **920**
  - petrous part of, *926*, *1029*, *1142*
  - squamous part of, *926*, *1029*, *1142*
- tibia, 21, **715**–717, *716*, 722, *723*
  - border of, *716*, **716**, 806
  - fractures of, **722–724**
  - functions of, 715–716
  - general images of, *18*
  - right, *716*
  - shaft of, *716*, **716**, 806
  - surface anatomy of, **717–718**
- zygomatic, *976*

Bone(s) (of regions)
- of foot, **718–720**
- of forearm, 152–153
- of hand, 153–155, 254, *290*
- of knee joint, *836*

of lower limb, *705*, 705–721, 707
arrangement, *707*, **707**, *708*
surface anatomy of, **713–714**
of neck, **1047–1049**
of pelvic girdle, **585–586**
of upper limb, 152–162
of wrist, 153–155, *290*
Bone marrow, *311*
Border
axillary, 152
of heart, 377, *378*
interosseous, 154, 716
of lungs
anterior, *349*, **350**
inferior, *349*, **350**
left, 350
posterior, **350**
right, 350
of mandible, *880-881*
of scapula, **152**
of spleen, *513*, **514**
superior, of manubrium, *314*
of tibia, 806
of ulna, *149*, 159
vermilion, *916*
vertebral, 152
Bow stringing, 18
Brachial fascia, 163, *218*, *230*
Brain, 935–945
arteries of, **939**–940
base of, *941*
cephalic brain, *557*
enteric brain, *557*
infarction of, 945
parts of, **935**
ventricles of
1st, 935
2nd, 935
3rd, *923*, *936*, **936**, *937*, *943*
4th, *923*, *936*, *937*, *943*, *1087*, *1122*
lateral, *937*, *943*
Brainstem, **130**, *936*
Branches
of abdominal cutaneous nerves
anterior, *438*
lateral, *438*
of aorta, 412t
of aortic arch, 417
atrioventricular nodal, **385**, *386*, 387t
of axillary artery, *195*
of bronchial artery, 412t
circumflex
of left coronary artery, 385, *386*
of subscapular artery, *191*
of coronary arteries
left, 385, *386*, 387t
right, 385, *386*, 387t
cutaneous
of cervical plexus, **1061**
lateral, 442t
of median nerve, *245*, 245t
of obturator nerve, *734*
of posterior rami, *118*
of subcostal nerve, *734*
of sural nerve, *823*
of thoraco-abdominal nerves, **441**
of ulnar nerve, *258*
of cutaneous nerve, lateral (of arm)
anterior branches, *327*
posterior branches, *327*
of descending aorta, 409
of esophageal artery, 412t
of facial artery, *1099*
of facial nerve, *911*, **912**
gastric
anterior, *479*
posterior, *479*
of genitofemoral nerve, 455, 457, 678
of hypoglossal nerve, 1149, *1150*
of ileocolic artery, *496*, **497**
of intercostal nerve, 330, *349*
of internal thoracic arteries, **403**
interventricular
anterior, 385, *386*
posterior, *386*, 387t
intraventricular, of left coronary artery, 385, *386*
malleolar, of fibular artery, *804*
mammary, *336*
of mandibular nerve, 1136t
marginal, right, 385, *386*, 387t
of maxillary artery, *981*
of maxillary nerve1136t
of median nerve, 244, *266*, *267*, 789
mediastinal, anterior, **403**
meningeal, of spinal nerves, **106**
of musculophrenic artery, *370*
of ophthalmic nerve, 1136t
pericardial, **410**
of perineal nerve, 670
of phrenic artery, 412t
of posterior intercostal arteries, *336*
of posterior rami, *118*
pubic, of obturator artery, 610
sacral, **568**
sinu-atrial nodal, 385, *386*, 387t
spinal, 106
of spinal nerve, **106**
of sural nerve, *64*
calcaneal, *64*
of thoracic aorta, *411*
of thoracic spinal arteries, 441–442
of thoraco-abdominal nerve, *442*
of tibial nerve, *64*
calcaneal, *64*
of ulnar nerve, *258*, 268t
of uterine artery, *643*
of vaginal artery, 612
of vagus nerve(s) (named), *1148*
Breast(s), **332**, *334*, 334–335, *336–340*
alveoli of, 335
amastia, **342**
areola of, **332**, *334*, 334–335, 340, *340*
arteries of, 335, *336*
axillary tail of, 334, *334*, *340*
carcinoma (cancer) of, **340–342**, *341*
in men, **342–343**
changes in, **340**
computed tomography, *399*
female, **334–335**
gynecomastia of, **343**
lymphatic drainage of, 335, *337*
mammary glands in, **334**, *334*
nerves of, **335**
nipple of, *334*, **335**, *340*
polymastia, **342**
polythelia, **342**
pregnancy-related changes in, 335
pubertal development of, 334
quadrants of, *340*, **340**
supernumerary, 342
surface anatomy of, 340, 343
surgical incisions in, **342**
vasculature of, **335**, *336*
veins of, 335, *336*
Breast-conserving surgery, 342
Bregma, *880*, 885t, **887**
Brim, pelvic, **586**, *586*
Bronchioles, *353*
conducting, *353*, **353**
respiratory, *353*, **353**
terminal, *352*, **353**
Bronchodilators, 355
Bronchoscopy, *361*, **361**
Bronchus/bronchi
carina of, 361, *361*
foreign body aspiration in, 360
lobar, **352**
inferior, *349*
middle, *349*
superior, *349*, *351*
main, **351**
left, **351**, *351–352*, 421
right, *351*, **351**, *361*, 421
right lower lobe, *351*
segmental, *351–352*, 352
Bud
periosteal, 22, *22*
taste, *999*
tooth, **989**, *991*
Bulb
jugular, *1101*
olfactory, *907*, *941*, *1020*, **1020**, *1121*–1122, 1127, 1128
of penis, *627*, *634*, 671t
of vestibule, **689**
Bulla, ethmoidal, *1017*, **1019**, *1020*
Bull rider's thumb, **301**
Bundle
atrioventricular, *377*, *386*, *389*, **389**
right branch of, 382
left, **390**
right, **390**

Bunion, 869
Burns, 16–17
Bursa(e), **18**
  of anconeus, *287*
  anserine, *848*, 848t
  bicipitoradial, **287**
  calcaneal, 799t, 800
  gastrocnemius, *842*, *848*, 848t
  glenohumeral joint, 284
  gluteal, **806**
  gluteofemoral, **767**, *768*
  infrapatellar, **844**, *848*, 848t
  ischial, **767**
  knee joint, **844**, *848*, 848t
  obturator, **770**
  olecranon, *285*, **287**
  omental, 465, 469–470, *469–470*, 508
  popliteal, **803**, *842*, 847, *848*, 848t
  prepatellar, *749*, *839*, 844, *848*, 848t
  retromammary, **334**
  semimembranosus, *842*, *848*, 848t
  subacromial, **284**
  subcutaneous, 18
  subdeltoid, *281*, 284
  subfascial, 18
  subscapular, *281*, 284
  subtendinous, 18
  suprapatellar, *749*, *837*, **844**, *848*, 848t
  trochanteric, **767**
Bursitis
  calcaneal, **809**
  elbow joint, **298–299**, *299*
  friction, 783
  infrapatellar, 867
  ischial, **783**
  prepatellar, 867
  subacromial, 297
  suprapatellar, 867
  trochanteric, **783**
Buttocks, **704**
Buttresses, of cranium, *893*, **893**
  frontonasal, **893**
  lateral orbital margin, **893**

C

Cage, thoracic, **308**, *309*, *435*
  flexibility of, 310
  functions of, 310
  shape of, 310
Calcaneal bursitis, *809*
Calcaneal fractures, 725, *726*
Calcaneal spur, 826
Calcaneal tendon, **799**
  reflex, 809
  rupture of, 809
Calcaneal tuberosity, **718**
Calcaneocuboid joint, **853**
Calcaneofibular ligament, **850**
Calcaneus, *708*, 718, **718**, *719*
  bursa of, 799t, 800
  fractures of, **725**, *726*
  tendinitis of, **808–809**
  tendons of, *32*, *794*, 799, 799t, *803*, 806, 851, 858
    reflex, **809**
    ruptured, **809**
  tuberosity of, **718**, *719*, 799
Calcitonin, 1083
Calculi
  renal, **551**–552
  ureteric, **551**–552, **631**
Calculus, **1010**
Callus, 869
Calvaria, *21*, **879**
  molding of, *898*
Calyces
  major, **543**, *544*
  minor, **543**, *544*
Canal(s)
  adductor, **752**, *757*, **757**, 758
  Alcock (*see* Canal(s), pudendal)
  anal, *487*, *623*, *629*, **670**, 672, *695*, *697*
    anorectal flexure of, **628**
    arteries of, **672**
    innervation of, **673**
    veins of, **672–673**
  auditory, external, *1012*
  birth, **643**, 646
  carotid, *888*, 890
  central, *937*
  cervical, *641*, **643**, 646, *696*
  cervico-axillary, 193, *198*
  condylar, *886*, 891t
  femoral, 755
  gastric, **480**
  Guyon (ulnar), 244, *246*, 274–275
  hypoglossal, 1148
  incisive, 1019, *1020*
  inguinal, *439–440*, **451**–454, *452*
    boundaries of, 452t
    development of, 453, *453–454*
      in females, 454
      in males, 453
    intra-abdominal pressure effects on, 454
  of Nuck, 460
  obturator, *599*, 615
  optic, *946*, **948**, *1120*, 1128
  palatine, *1021*
  pelvic, **593**
  pericardioperitoneal, **344**
  pterygoid, *907*, 950, *981*, **1012**, *1013*, *1021*, 1031, 1139
  pudendal, (Alcock), *661*, *665*, *669*, **670**, 680
  pulp, 991
  pyloric, **480**
  root, 991, *993*
  sacral, **85**, *86*, *95*, 657
  of Schlemm, *953*, 955
  semicircular, *1026*, *1029*, *1030*, *1031*, *1034*, 1035, 1141
  spiral, of cochlea, **1035**, *1141*
  vertebral, *75*, *109*, *131*, *577*
    contents of, 130–141
Canaliculi, lacrimal, *949*, **950**
Cancer. *See also* Carcinoma
  cervical, **652–653**
  esophageal, 1114–1115
  lung, **364**
  pancreatic, 533, 571–572
  scrotal, 462
  spread of, 45–46
  testicular, 461
  uterine, 459–460
Capillary
  arrangement of, 42
  beds, 42
  blood, 42
  characteristics of, 42
  lymphatic, **43**
  periosteal, 22
  walls of, 42
Capitate, *154*, **155**, *274*, *290*
Capitulum, 21, *151*, **152**
  of humerus, 21
Capsule
  of acromioclavicular joint, *278*, **279**
  of ankle joint, 849–850
  articular, **25**
  of atlanto-occipital joint, *101*, *103*
  of cricothyroid joint, *1089*
  of elbow joint, **284–285**
  of glenohumeral joint, *911*
  Glisson (hepatic), 524
  of hip joints, 832
  of intercarpal joints, **293**
  joint, **25**, *98*, 315
  of knee joint, *788*, **836**, *837*, *839*
  of lens, **954**
  of liver, *521*, 524, **524**, 529
  otic, *1034*, **1035**, *1036*
  pararenal fat, *542*
  perinephric fat, *542*
  of prostate, **636**
  of spleen, 513
  of sternoclavicular joint, 276, 277
  of temporomandibular joint, *977*
  of thyroid gland, 1083, *1084*
  of wrist, 291
Caput medusae, 538, *538*
Carcinoma. *See also* Cancer
  breast, **340–342**, *341*
  bronchogenic, **364–365**
  lingual, **1010**
  lymphogenous spread of, 45
  squamous cell, of lip, **921**
  stomach, 505
Cardiac arrest, 401
Cardiac catheterization, 391
Cardiac cycle, *375*, **376**, 389
Cardiac striated muscle, 30t, **31**, **37**
Cardiac tamponade, **373**

Cardiology, 4
Cardiopulmonary resuscitation, 401
Cardiopulmonary splanchnic nerves, 60
Cardiovascular system, **4**, **38**, *40*
  arteries (*see* Arteries; Arteries (named))
  arteriosclerosis, 42–43, *43*
  blood vessels
    arteries, 39–41
    capillaries, 42
    structure, 39, *39*
    veins, 41–42
  capillaries (*see* Capillary)
  varicose veins, 43, *43*
  vascular circuits, 38, 38–39
  veins (*see* Vein(s))
Caries, dental, *1007*, **1007**
Carotid endarterectomy, 1075
Cartilage (in general), **20**, *22*
  age-related changes in, *22*
  articular, **20**, *23*
  fibrocartilage, *1049*
  functions of, *21*
  hyaline, 350
Cartilage (named)
  alar, **1015**
  arytenoid, **1088**, *1089–1090*, *1092*
  corniculate, **1088**, *1089–1090*, *1110*
  costal, *438*, *471*, *560*, *577*, *1067*, 1067t
  costal, *88*, *309*, **310**, *314*, *323*, *405*, 421
  cricoid, *477*, *1085*, **1088**, *1091*, *1096–*1098, 1104, 1115
  cuneiform, **1088**, *1089–1090*
  epiglottic, **1088**, *1089–1090*
  nasal, lateral, *1021*
  septal, **1016**
  sesamoid, *1021*
  thyroid, 1047, *1049*, *1068*, **1088**, *1089–*1091, 1107
  tracheal, *1089*, **1095**
  triradiate, 586, *587*
  triticeal, *1089*
Caruncle
  hymenal, *687*, **690**
  lacrimal, *949*, 968
  sublingual, **999**, *1000*, *1010*
Catabolic, 64
Cataracts, **970**
Catheterization
  right cardiac, 1073
  urethral, in males, **684–685**
Cauda equina, *75*, *85*, 86, *109*, *131*, *133*, 138
Caudal, **8**, **9**
Caudal epidural anesthesia, **93–94**
Cave, trigeminal, *1122*, **1135**
Cavity
  abdominal, **434**, *586*, *597*
    regions of, *433*, 434
  abdominopelvic, **432**, *432*, *597*
  articular. (*see* Cavity, joint)
  cranial, 50, **890**, 893
    division(s) of, 922, 924
    entrances/exits (*see under* Fissures and Foramen/Foramina)
    floor of, 885, 887, *892*, 938 (*see also* cranial base)
    meninges and, **931–934**
    Monro-Kellie doctrine and, 938
    surgical access to (craniotomy), **896**, 917
    walls of, **893**
  of epididymis, 457
  glenoid, *151*, *281*
  infraglottic, **1088**, *1090–1091*
  joint, *25*, *26*, 29
  laryngeal, **1088**
  medullary, of bone, *21*
  nasal, 994, *994*, **1016**, 1018–1019, 1019, *1020*
  oral, *996*, *1098–1099* (*see also specific anatomy*)
    parts of, 987
    proper, 987, 994, *994*
  pelvic, 432, **596**–607, *597*
    floor of, 597–601
    walls of, 596–597, *598*, 599t
  pericardial, *370*, **369**, *1096*
  peritoneal, **465**–473, **601–603**, *623*
    abscess formation in, **473**
    embryology of, **466**–467
    shape of, 466
    subdivisions of, **469**–471
  pleural, **344**, *345*, *1096*
    left, *577*
    pneumothorax, 358–359
    primordial, 369
    right, *577*
    thoracotomy into, *319*, **319–320**
  pulmonary, **343**
    base of, *347*
    lining of, 344, *345*
  pulp, **991**, *993*
  thoracic, **308**, *597*
    changes in dimension with respiration, 317
    compartments of, 343–344, *345*
    viscera of, 343–424
  tympanic, *1026*, **1027**, *1029*, 1030, *1030*, *1031*
  uterine, *696*
Cecum, *431*, *474*, 487, **494**–497
  arteries of, 497, 500t
  lymphatic system of, 497
  nerves of, 497, *501*
  subhepatic, 509
Cell(s)
  acinar, 514
  astrocytes, 47
  body, 46
  chromaffin, 545
  ethmoidal, **1024**
    anterior, **1020**, *1021*
    middle, *1017*, 1019, **1020**, *1021*
    posterior, *1017*, 1019, **1020**, *1021*
  ganglion
    parasympathetic, 355
    sympathetic, 355
  hair, in maculae, **1035**
  of Hensen, *1036*
  mastoid, *1143*
  mitral, **1127**, *1129*
  neural crest, 545
  neurons, *46*, *47*, *57*
  satellite, 36, 47
  Schwann, *47*, *49*
Cement, 991, *993*
Central nervous system (CNS), **4**, 46–47
Cephalic arterial ramus, **60**
Cephalohematoma, **918**
Cerebellum, *923*, **935**, *1087*
Cerebral cortex, 46
Cerebral embolism, **944**
Cerebrospinal fluid (CSF), 47, 132–137
  circulation of, 938
  functions of, **938**
  hydrocephalus, 943, *943*, 944
  leakage of, **944**
  otorrhea, 944
  rhinorrhea, 944
  secretion of, **938**
Cerebrovascular accidents, **393**
Cerebrum, **935**
  concussion, 942
  contusions, 943
  lacerations to, 943
Cerumen, 1027
Cervical dystonia, 1073
Cervix, of uterus, *641*, **643**, *645*
  cancer of, **652–653**
  examination of, 652–653, *654*
  ligaments of, *604*, *605*
  ultrasound image of, *646*
Chalazia, 969
Chambers
  of eyeball, anterior, **971**
  of heart, 375–376
Cheeks, 987–988
  muscles of, **903**–905
Chemosis, 933
Chest, 308. *See also* Thorax
  pain, **319**
  tube, **359–360**
  wall of (*see* Thorax, wall of)
Chiasm
  optic, *937*, *1130*, **1128**
  tendinous, **262**
Childbirth, anesthesia for, **656–657**
Choanae, *997*, *1097*
Cholecystectomy, 473, 538
Cholecystokinin, 529
Chondroblasts, 22
Chondromalacia patellae, 759
Chordae tendineae, 380
Chorda tympani, *984*, *1139*

Choroid, **951**, *952*
Chronic traumatic encephalopathy, 943. *See also* Punchdrunk syndrome
Chyle cistern. *See* Cisterna chyli
Chylothorax, 419
Chyme, 479
Cilia, olfactory, **1127**, *1129*
Cineradiography, 391
Circle, cerebral arterial (of Willis), **940**, 941
  variations of, **944**
Circulation
  of cerebrospinal fluid, **938**
  collateral, **41**
  coronary collateral, **388**
  pulmonary, **38**, **39**, *353*
  systemic, **38**, **39**
Circulatory system, **4**
  functions of, 38
Circumcision
  female (*see* Female genital cutting)
  male, **685–686**
Circumduction, **11**, **12**
Circumflex femoral arteries, 755
Circumflex fibular artery, 804–805
Cirrhosis of liver, 502, **535**–536, 676
Cistern
  ambient, **938**
  cerebellomedullary, *937*, **937**–938, *1017*
  chiasmatic, *937*, **938**
  chyle (*see* Cisterna chyli)
  interpeduncular, *937*, **938**
  lumbar, *109*, *131*, 132, 137
  pontocerebellar, *937*, **938**
  quadrigeminal, *937*, **938**
  subarachnoid, *937*
Cisterna ambiens, **938**
Cisterna chyli, 45, *455*, 568, *569*, 570, 1106
Cisterna magna. *See* Cistern, cerebellomedullary
Cisternal puncture, 943
Clavicle, 147, 149, *151*, *309*, *356*, *431*, 1070, 1072, 1073, 1115
  fracture of, 158–159
  ossification of, 159
  radiographic appearance of, *67*
  surface anatomy of, 186, 335, *338*
Clavipectoral fascia, **164**, *164*, *198*
Claw hand, 211
Claw toes, 870, *870*
Cleavage lines. *See* Tension lines of skin
Cleft
  gluteal, *697*
  intergluteal, *87*, **87**, 126, *662*, *697*
  intermammary, *337*, **338**, *340*
  lip, *1006*, **1006**
  natal (*see* Cleft, intergluteal)
  palate, *1009*, **1009**
  pudendal, **688**
  of sternum, 321, 338
Clitoris, *645*, *662*, *664*, **689**
Clivus, 939, *939*
Clubfoot, **870**, *871*
Clunial nerves, **773**, 775
Coccyx, **85–86**, 586, 589, 590, 662, *694*, *696*
  injury of, **94–95**
  surface anatomy of, 86–87, *87*
  tip of, *598*
Cochlea, *1029*, **1035**, *1036*, *1141*
Coelom, intraembryonic, 466
Colectomy, **510**
Colic
  biliary, 537, 538
  ureteric, **551**–552
Coli, teniae, **494**, 500
Colitis, **510**
Collar of callus, 24, *24*
Collateral circulation, **41**
Colon, **497**–498, 500, 502. *See also* Intestine(s); Rectum
  ascending, *431*, *474*, *480*, *487*, *496*, **497**
  descending, *431*, 469, *474*, *487*, *496*, 544, 554
  sigmoid, *431*, *474*, *487*, *496*, 498, **511**, 623, 628, 669
  transverse, *431*, 467, *468*, *469*, 481, 487, 498, 520, 536
Colonoscopy, **510**, *511*
Colorectal cancer, **510**, *511*
Colostomy, **510**
Colostrum, 340
Column
  anal, **672**
  intermediolateral cell, **58**
  vertebral (*see* Vertebral column)
Commissures
  anterior, *936*
  labial, 903t, **916**
    anterior, *687*, 688
  posterior, *687*, 688
  palpebral
    lateral, *949*, **949**
    medial, *949*, **949**
Common tendinous ring, **955**
Compartment(s)
  of arm, **164**
  central
    of sole of foot, *813*
    of palm of hand, 256, *257*
  of cranial cavity,
    infratentorial, 924
    supratentorial, 924, 935
  fascial, *17*, *17*
  of femoral sheath, 755
  of foot, *813*
  of forearm, 228, *229*, *230*, *236*
    anterior compartment muscles, 228, *231*, 231t–232t, 232–233
    posterior compartment muscles, 233, *234*, 234t–235t, 235, *236*, 237, 239–240
  of hand, 256, 257
  hypothenar, **256**, *257*
  infracolic, **469**
  infratentorial, 924
  of leg, *790*
    anterior (dorsiflexor), *729*, *772*, 790, 790, 792
      artery in, 792
      muscles of, **790**, 792, 794
      nerve of, **792**, *795*, 795t
    infections, 807
    lateral (evertor), *790*, 793t, 794–798, 797–798
      blood vessels in, **798**
      muscles in, **794**, 797–798
      nerve of, **798**
    medial, *729*, *772*
    posterior (plantarflexor), 798–805, 799, 799t, 800, 800t, 801, 802, 803, 804, 805
      arteries in, **804–805**
      muscles of, 798–804, 799t–800t
      nerves in, **804**
  of palm of hand, 256, *257*
    central, 256, *257*
    hypothenar, **256**, 257
    interosseous, 256, 257
    thenar, **256**, 257,
  of sole of foot
    central, 812
    dorsal, 812
    interosseous, 812
    lateral, 812
    medial, 812
  supracolic, **469**
  supratentorial, 924, 935
  thenar, **256**, *257*
  of thigh, 728, *729*, 745
    anterior, **746**
      muscles of, *746–747*, 746–749, 746t–747t
    medial (adductor), 749
    muscles of, 749–751, *750*, 750t
    posterior, 770–779
      muscles of, 770–773, *771*, 771t
Compartment syndromes, 741
Compression
  of axillary artery, **209**
  of brachial artery, 225
  of facial artery, **920**
  of femoral artery, **761**
  of oculomotor nerve, **1152**
  of ulnar nerve, 252, 274
  of veins, 42
Computed tomography (CT), **68–69**, *70*
  of abdomen, *576*
  of breasts, *420*
  of thorax, *420–424*
Conchae
  of auricle, **1026**, *1027*

nasal
inferior, 997, *998*, 1018, *1021–1022*, 1087, 1098
middle, *994*, *998*, 1018, *1021–1022*, 1087, 1098
superior, *994*, *998*, 1018, *1022*, *1098*
Concussion, cerebral, 942
Condyle(s), 21
femoral
lateral, *21*, *708*, **713**, 715
medial, *708*, **713**, 715
humeral, *151*, **151**
of mandible, *978*
occipital, **80**, *1012*
tibial
anterolateral, *781*, *805*
lateral, *708*, 716, *720*, *765*, 765t
medial, *708*, 716, *720*
Cone, medullary, *75*, *131*, *133*, *140*
Confluence, portal, *577*
Congestive heart failure, 372
Congenital anomaly, **12**
Conjunctiva
bulbar, *947*, **948**, *952*, 964
hyperemia of, **969**
palpebral, *907*, *947*, **948**, 967, *967*
plica semilunaris of, *949*
Constriction
cervical, *477*, **477**
diaphragmatic, *477*, **477**
thoracic, *477*, **477**
Contraction of muscles, **33**
phasic, *33*, **33**
isometric, *33*, **33**
isotonic, *33*, **33**
concentric, **33**, **34**
eccentric, **33**, **34**
reflexive, **33**
tonic, **33**
Contralateral, **9**
Contusions
cerebral, 943
extensor digitorum brevis, **826**
hip, **759**
thigh, **759**
Conus elasticus, **1088**, *1089–1092*
Conventional radiography, *68*, 68–69, *69*
Convergent muscles, 33
Cord(s)
spermatic, *438*, 451, *452*, **454**–456, 457, 634, 695
hydrocele of, **460**, *462*
torsion of, 461–462
spinal, *75*, **130**, **132**, 136, *136*, *923*, 1087, 1096
arteries of, 137, *138*
injuries to, 136, **141**
ischemia of, **140–141**
motor neuron of, 34
nerve roots, **130**, **132**
shock, 141
transection of, 141
vasculature of, **137–139**
veins of, *137*, *139*
tendinous, *380*, **380**, *382*, *384*
umbilical, *508*
Cornea, **951**, *952*, 954, *964*, *967*
abrasions of, **971**
lacerations of, **971**
transplantation of, **971**
ulcers of, **971**
Cornua, coccygeal, **86**
Coronary angiography, **395–396**
Coronary artery bypass grafting, 373, *397*, 397
Coronary artery disease, **396–397**
Coronary ligaments, **844**
Cor pulmonale, 364
Corpus callosum, *936*, *937*
Corpus cavernosum, *634*, *678*, *680*, 694–695
Corpus spongiosum, *634*, *678*, **678**, *679*, 694–695
Cortex
cerebral, *901*
suprarenal, **545**
Cough reflex, 361
Coxa valga, **722**
Coxa vara, **722**
Cranial, **8**, **9**
Cranial parasympathetic outflow, 63
Craniosynostosis, **899**
Craniotomy, 917
Cranium, **879**–900
age-related changes in, **899**
base of (basicranium), **879**, *880*, *926*
fractures of, **933**
buttresses of, *893*, **893**
calvaria of, *21*, 879, 896
craniometric points of, 885t
development of, **896**–898
facial aspect of, **884**–886
frontal bone of, *880–881*
general images of, *20*
lacrimal bone of, *880*
lateral aspect of, **886**
malformations of, **899**
nasal bone of, *880*
neurocranium, **879**, *880*
newborn, joints of, **28**
occipital aspect of, **886**–887
occiput of, *886*, **886**
ossification of, 896–897
parts of, 879
sphenoid bone of, *880–881*
superior aspect of, **887**
surfaces of
external, **887**–890
internal, **890**–893
sutures of (*see* Suture(s))
viscerocranium, *880*, 881
Creases
cutaneous, inferior, 342
digital, **271**
flexion, 270
palmar, **270**
wrist, **270**
Crest, 22
ampullary, *1036*, **1036**
of bone, 21, 22
ethmoidal, *1017*
frontal, 924, *926*
iliac, *21*, 434, *458*, *565*, 586, *587*
infratemporal, *976*, *1012*
intertrochanteric, *708*, *712*, **713**, 832
of lacrimal bone, *946*
occipital
external, *929*
internal, *926*
pubic, 434, *435*, 459, *541*, 586, *587*
sacral
intermediate, **86**, *85*
lateral, **86**, *85*
median, *85*, **86**
sphenoidal, **890**, *892*
of spine of scapula, *150*, 156
supinator, **152**
supramastoid, *976*
supraventricular, *380*, **380**
urethral, **626**, *627*
Cribriform fascia, **728**
Cricothyrotomy, 1104, 1111
Crista galli, *1022*
Crohn disease, 510
Crown, of teeth, **991**
Cruciate ligaments, **841**
Crura
of clitoris, *689*
of diaphragm, **559**
of penis, **678**, **679**
Crus
lateral, *450*, **451**
of external oblique aponeurosis, *439*
medial, *450*, **451**
of external oblique aponeurosis, *439*
Cryptitis, 675
CSF. *See* Cerebrospinal fluid
Cubital tunnel syndrome, **252–253**
Cuboid, tuberosity of, **718**
Culdocentesis, **655**
Cuneiforms, *811*
intermediate, **718**, *719*
lateral, **718**, *719*
medial, *708*, **718**, *719*, *720*
1st, *852*
Cup, optic, 954, **969**
Cupula, pleura, **344**, *346*
Curvature (in general)
cervical, 104
lumbar, 104
primary, 104
sacral, 104–105

Curvature (in general) (*Continued*)
secondary, 105
of vertebral column, **104–105**
Curvature (named)
greater, **480**, *480–481*
lesser, **480**, *480–481*
Cusps
anterior, *380*
of aortic valve, 384, **393–394**
of mitral valve, 383
of pulmonary valve, *380*, *384*, **393–394**
Cyanosis, **1074**
Cyst(s)
branchial, *1114*
of canal of Nuck, 460
epididymal, *463*, **463**
ovarian, 656
pancreatic pseudo-cyst, 473
popliteal, 867, *867*
renal, **549**–550
sebaceous, **918**
of sebaceous glands, 969
thyroglossal duct, 1107
of wrist, **249–250**
Cystocele, **631–632**, *632*
Cystoscopy, *632*, **632**
Cystotomy, suprapubic, **632**

D

Deafness, **1154**
Deep, **8**, **9**
Deferentectomy, 639
Defibrillation, **401**
Degenerative joint disease, 29
Deglutition, **1099**, *1100*
Deltoid fascia, **164**, *165*
Deltopectoral groove, 165, **176**
Demifacets, *312*, 313
Demyelinating diseases, **1152**
Dendrites, 46
Dens
of axis (C2), *75*, **80**, *81*, 89, 92, *103*, 1087, 1096
fracture of, *110*, 114, *114*
Dental caries, *1007*, **1007**
Dental implants, **1008**, *1009*
Dentine, **991**, *993*
Dentoalveolar syndesmosis, **26**
Depression, **11**, **12**, **955**
semilunar, 383
Dermatoglyphics, **275**
Dermatome(s), **51**, **52**, *52*, *54*, *44*, 108, 110, 176
of anterolateral abdominal wall (T6-L1 dermatomes), **441**, *442*
peritoneal pain and, 465
small intestine pain and, 494
back injury and, 110
disc degeneration and, 111
of hand (C6-C8 dermatomes), 265, *267*
herpes zoster infection and, 332, *333*
L1 dermatome, 449, 464
of lower limb (L1-S2 dermatomes), 705, 734, *735*
maps, *52*
Foerster, 170, *173*, 173t, *735*
Keegan and Garret, 170, *173*, 173t, 735
of neck (C3-C5 dermatomes), 365,
of perineum (S2-S4 dermatomes), 677
pudendal nerve block and, 677, *677*
of shoulder (C3-C5 dermatomes)
diaphragmatic pain and, 465
pericardial pain and, 371
T2 dermatome, 176
T4 dermatome, *328*
T10 dermatome, *328*, 449, 459
of thorax (C2-3 to T11 dermatomes), 327, *328*
pleural pain and, 365
of trunk (C4-L1 dermatomes), 327, *328*
pericardial pain and, 371
of upper limb (C5-T21 dermatomes), 172, *173*, 173t
ureteric pain and, 553
visceral referred pain and, 506
Dermatomyotomes, 51, 52
Dermis, **14**, *14*
collagen fibers in, 14, *14*
Descending genicular artery, **789**
Development
of bones, 22–23
of cranium, 896–898
of heart, *370*
of inguinal canal, 453, *453–454*
of lower limb, **705**, *706*
of lungs, 371
of mandible, **898**
of meninges, **139**–140
of pericardium, *370*
of subarachnoid space, **139**–140
of teeth, **898**
Dextrocardia, 374
Diagnostic radiology, 4
Dialysis, peritoneal, **472**
Diaphragm, 324, *347–348*, **559**–563, 560–562, 575–576, 578
actions of, **562**–563
aperture of, **561**–562
arteries of, 560, *561*
costal attachment of, *346*
costal part of, **559**, *560*
crus/crura of, 478
dome of, *560*
left, **559**
radiographs of, *420*
right, *474*, **559**
functions of, 324, 441, 559
inspiration role of, 324
lumbar part of, **559**, *560*
lymphatic system of, *562*
nerves of, *562*
paralysis of, 321
parts of, **559**, *560*
pelvic, 432, **597**, *597–598*, *600*
posterolateral defect of, 571
referred pain from, **570**
rupture of, **570**–571
sternal part of, **559**, *560*
thoracic, 432
veins of, 560, *561*
vertebral attachment of, *346*
Diaphragm (sellar), **924**
bulging of, **932–933**
Diaphragm (urogenital), 666
Diaphysis, **23**
Diastole, **376**, 383, 394
Diencephalon, **935**, *936*, *1130*
Digestion, 475
Digestive system, **4**
Digestive tract
parasympathetic stimulation, 65t
sympathetic stimulation, 65t
Digital examination
of rectum, 639
of vagina, **654**
Digits
creases, **271**, *271*
section of, *256*
surface anatomy of, **271**, *271*
Dilator pupillae, **953**
DIP joint(s). *See* Distal interphalangeal joint(s)
Diploë, *1022*
Diplopia, 1153
Disc(s)
articular
of distal radio-ulnar joint, **289**–290
of sternoclavicular joint, *1085*
of temporomandibular joint, 975, *978*
interpubic, **591**
intervertebral, 74, *77*, 98–99, 100–101, 139, 309, 312, 591, 1087
aging of, 96, 108
function of, 98
injury to, 108
ligaments and, *99*
structure of, 98
optic, *952*, *954*, **954**, 1128
Dislocation
of acromioclavicular joints, 296–297
of atlas, **92**
of axis, 92, *94*
of biceps tendon, **244**
of cervical vertebrae, 91, *91*
of elbow joints, 300, *300*
of glenohumeral joints, 297–298, *298*
head of radius, *300*, 300–301
of hip joint, **862–863**
of lunate, 301
of manubriosternal joint, 320
of patella, **864**
of radial head, **300**

of ribs, **321**
of shoulder, 188
of sternoclavicular joints, *296*, 296–297
of temporomandibular joint, **986**
of vertebrae, 111–114
Distal, **9**
Distension
of scrotum, **685**
of vagina, 654
Diverticulum/Diverticula
ileal, *509*, **509**
of Meckel, 509
Diverticulosis, **510**–511
Doctrine, Monro-Kellie, **938**
Doppler effect, 70
Doppler ultrasonography, 70
Dorsalis pedis artery, **821**
Dorsalis pedis artery pulse, 827
Dorsiflexion, **9**, *11*
Dorsiflexors, of ankle joint, **790**
Dorsum, **9**
of foot (*see* Region(s), dorsal, of foot)
of nose, *916*
of penis, **9**
neurovasculature of, *679*, *681*
surface anatomy, *679*
Dowager hump, 115
Drainage
deep venous, **822**
Drawer sign
anterior, *865*, 866
posterior, 866, *866*
Duct(s)
alveolar, *352*, **353**
bile, *489*, *489*, 490, *515*, 520, *521*, *522*, 524, 527, 528, 529, 529, 532, 575
biliary, *515*, **527**–530
of bulbo-urethral glands, *627*, 677
cochlear, *1034*, **1035**, *1036*, **1037**
cystic, *515*, 518, 529
ejaculatory, **635**
embryonic, **650**
endolymphatic, *1034*, 1035, 1036, *1141*
of epididymis, **458**
of epoophoron, 650
frontonasal, **1020**
hepatic, *519*, 520
accessory, **536**
common, **527**, *528*
left, **527**
right, **527**
variations in, **536**
intralobular, *515*
lactiferous, *334*, **334**, *420*
lymphatic, right, *337*, 355, *412*, *1105*, 1106
mesonephric, *454*
nasolacrimal, *949*, **950**
pancreatic, *525*, 527
accessory, *515*, *525*
main, *489*, *515*, **515**
sphincter of, **515**
paramesonephric, *454*
parotid, *902*, **974**, *977*, *984*, *1143*
prostatic, **638**
semicircular, *1034*, **1035**, *1036*, **1036**–1037
submandibular, 999, *1000*, **1004**, *1004*, 1063
thoracic, 337, 355, 355, 404, 408, 410, 411, 435, 569, 570, 1049, 1078, 1085, 1106, 1106
laceration of, 419
variations of, 419
thyroglossal, **1107**, *1107*
utriculosaccular, *1034*, **1035**
Ductus deferens, *449*, 451, *452*, 453, 455, 541, 598, 603, 608, 611, 621, 635, 681
Ductus epididymis, 650
Ductus reuniens, *1034*, **1035**
Ductus venosus, 520
Duodenal cap, 69
Duodenum, *468*, *486*, **487**, *488*, 489–491, 515
ampulla of, **489**
arteries of, 489
ascending part of, *488*, **490**
computed tomography of, *576*
descending part of, 488, 514
gallstones in, **538**
horizontal part of, **489**
inferior part of, **489**
lymphatic system of, 490, *490*
magnetic resonance imaging of, *577*
parts of, 487, **489**, 489–490
superior part of, 487, *488*, **489**
ulcers of, **506**
ultrasound of, *575*
veins of, 490
Dupuytren contracture, **271**–272, *272*
Dura, arachnoid, *107*
Dura-arachnoid interface, **134**, *135*
Dural infoldings, **922**–924, *923*, *925*
Dura mater
cranial, *901*, **922**–929, *1022*
arteries of, *929*
meningeal layer of, **922**, *923*
nerves of, **928**–929, *930*
periosteal layer of, 922, *923*
venous sinuses of, 924–927, **924**–927, *927* (*see also* Sinus)
external surface of, *923*
innervation of, **134**
meningeal layer of, **922**, *923*
nerves of, **928**–929, *930*
periosteal layer of, 922, *923*
spinal, *95*, *132*, *134*, **134**
innervation of, 134
Dysarthria, 1054
Dyspareunia, 693
Dysphagia, 477, 1054, 1155
Dysphonia, 1155
Dyspnea, **332**, 563
Dysrhythmias, 401
Dystonia, cervical, 1073
Dysuria, 639

E

Ear, **1026**–1037
external, **1026**–1027, *1027*
examination of, 1038, *1038*
inflammation of (otitis externa), 1038
injury of, **1038**
internal, **1033**–1037, *1034*, *1036–1037*
middle, 1026, 1027, 1030–1032, 1030–1033, *1037* (*see also* Cavity, tympanic)
Ecchymosis, **917**
ECF. *See* Extracellular fluid
ECG. *See* Electrocardiography
ECU. *See* Extensor carpi ulnaris
Echocardiography, *395*, **395**
ED. *See* Extensor digitorum
EDB. *See* Extensor digitorum brevis
Edema, 43
EDL. *See* Extensor digitorum longus
Efferent fibers, 50
Effusion
pericardial, **373**
pleural, 359
EHB. *See* Extensor hallucis brevis
EHL. *See* Extensor hallucis longus
Ejaculation, 682, **684**
Elbow joint, *148*, **284**, *285*
articulation of, **284**
blood supply of, **286**
bursae around, **287**
bursitis of, **298–299**, *299*
capsule of, **284–285**
carrying angle of, *286*
dislocation of, *300*, **300**
extensor muscles of, 286, *286*
flexor muscles of, 286, *286*
ligaments of, **285**, *286*
movements of, *286*, **286**
muscles that move, *286*, **286**
nerves of, **287**
radiographs of, *285*
tendinitis of, **249**
Electrocardiography, 398, **398**
Electromyography, 35–36
Elements
costal, **89**
transverse, **89**
Elephantiasis, 685
Elevation, **11**, **12**, **955**
Embolism, 361
air, 1074
brain, **944**
cerebral, **944**
pulmonary, **361**
venous air, 1074

- Eminence
  - frontal, *882–883*, **887**
  - hypothenar, *248*, **254**, *269*
  - iliopubic, *450*, *587*
  - intercondylar, **716**
  - parietal, *883*, **887**
  - pyramidal, *1031*
  - thenar, *158*, *248*, 254, *256*, *266*, *269*, *271*
- Enamel, **991**, *993*
- Endochondral ossification, **22**
- Endocrine system, **5**
- Endolymph, **1035**
- Endometriosis, 656
- Endoneurium, 49
- Endoscope, **447**
- Endothelium, 39
- Endourology, 631
- Enlargement
  - cervical, 130, *131*
  - lumbar, 130, *131*
- Enteric nervous system (ENS), 30t, *63–65*, *64*, *66*, 494, 495, 553, 554, 556–558, 557, 559
- Enterocele, 673
- Entrapment
  - lower limb joints, tibial nerve, 868
  - medial plantar nerve, 827
  - renal vein, 550
  - superficial fibular nerve, **808**
  - tibial nerve, **868**
- Enucleation, 971
- EPB. *See* Extensor pollicis brevis
- Epicondyle(s), 23, 715
  - lateral
    - of femur, *149*, 156, *287*
    - of humerus, *215*, *224*, 244, 247, *247*, 285
      - avulsion of medial, 299, *299*
      - bursa of, *287*
- Epicondylitis, 249
- Epidermis, *13*, **13**
- Epididymis, 457, **458**, *681*
  - appendix of, 463
  - head of, *623*
- Epidural anesthesia
  - caudal, **93–94**
  - transsacral, 94
- Epiglottis, *994*, *997*, *999*, *1087*, *1089*, 1096–1097
- Epilepsy, 1152
- Epinephrine, 545
- Epineurium, **49**, **134**
- Epiphysis/epiphyses, **23**
  - anular, *88*, **89**
  - displacement of, 25
  - of femoral head, 722
  - fusion, 25
  - plates, **721**, 724, *724*
  - proximal humeral, fracture-dislocation of, 192
  - separation, 25
- Episiotomy, **673–674**
- Epistaxis, **1024**
- Epithelium, coelomic, 344
- EPL. *See* Extensor pollicis longus
- Eponyms, 5
- Erection, **684**
- Esophagoscopy, 1114
- Esophagus, 405, 407, 408, 410–411, 421, 435, 477–478, 994, 1051, 1051, 1087, 1097, 1103–1104
  - blockage of, 419
  - cancer, 1114–1115
  - cervical, **1104**
  - constriction of, **477**
  - constrictions in, 410
  - injuries to, 1114
  - muscles of, 478
  - nerves of, *479*
  - pyrosis of, **502**
  - varices of, 502, *503*
- Ethmoid bone, **948**
- Eversion, **11**, **12**
- Exophthalmos, 933, 967, 968
- Expansion, extensor, **237**, *824*
- Expiration, *318*
- Extension, *9*, *10*
  - of knee joint, 845t
- Extensor carpi ulnaris (ECU), *207*, *234*, 234t, 236, 237, 239, 259, 261, 266
- Extensor digiti minimi, *207*, *234*, 234t, 236, 237, 239, 259, 266, 274
- Extensor digitorum, (ED)238, *207*, *234*, 234t, 236, 237, 239, 266
- Extensor digitorum brevis (EDB), *791*, *794*, 795, 795t, **816**, 824
- Extensor hallucis brevis (EHB), *791*, *794*, 816
- Extensor hallucis longus (EHL), *790*, 792, 793t, 795, 795t, 824
- Extensor indicis, *207*, *234*, 234t, *236*, **240**, 266
- Extensor pollicis brevis (FPB), *207*, *234*, 235t, 236, 237, 240, 259, 263, 266
- Extensor pollicis longus (FPL), *207*, *234*, 235t, 236, 237, 240, 259, 266
- Extensor retinacula, **728**
- External, **9**, *11*
- External rotation, 11, 12
- Extracellular fluid, 42
- Extravasation of urine, **674–675**
- Extravascular space, 41
- Eyeball, *949*, **951**–955
  - anterior chamber of, 971
  - aqueous humor of, *952*
  - artificial, **971**
  - cornea, **951**, *952*, 954
  - fibrous layer of, **951**
  - inner layer of, **954**
  - pupil, *952*, **953**
  - refractive media of, **954**–955
  - retina of, *952*, **954**
  - sclera of, *952*
  - surface anatomy of, **964**–965
  - vascular layer of, **951**–953
- Eyebrows, **915**
- Eyelashes, **949**, 967
- Eyelids, 916, **948**–949, *949*, 967
  - infections of, 968
  - injury to, 968

F

- Fabella, **808**
- Face, **900**–922
  - arteries of, **912**, *913*, 913t
  - incisions to, **917**
  - lacerations to, **917**
  - lymphatic system of, **915**, *916*
  - muscles of, **901**–906, *902*, 902t–903t, 953, 905
    - paralysis of, **918**
  - nerves of
    - cutaneous, 906, *907*, *908*, 908t–909t
    - motor, 910
  - surface anatomy of, **915**–917
  - veins of, **913**–915, *914*, **915**
- Facet(s), **22**
  - articular
    - fibular, **715–716**
    - of vertebra(e)
      - inferior, *76*, *81*, *86*, *312*, 313
      - superior, *21*, *76* ,*81*, *86*, *312*, 313
  - for clavicle, *145*
  - costal, **80**
    - superior, *21*
  - of patella, *841*
  - of thyroid cartilage, *1092*
- Facial expressions, 901, *905*, 982t
- Facial pain, **894**
- Falciform margin, **728**
- Falx
  - cerebelli, **924**
  - cerebri, *901*, **924**, *925*
  - inguinal, *439*, **451**, *452*
- Fascia (in general), **17**
  - fusion, **467**
- Fascia (named)
  - alar, *1051*
  - antebrachial, **164**, *164*, *224*, *230*
  - axillary, **164**, *165*, *194*
  - brachial, **164**, *218*, *230*
  - buccopharyngeal, *1051*, **1053**, *1096*, *1099*, 1101
  - Buck (*see* Fascia (named), deep, of penis)
  - Camper, 434, *435*, 456t
  - cervical, 974
    - deep, 974, *1051*, **1052**, *1058*, 1101
  - clavipectoral, **164**, *165*, *198*, 327
  - Colles, 434, *440*, 457, *665*, 666
  - cremasteric, **455**, 456t
  - crural, 728, *729*
  - dartos, *440*, **456**, 456t, *665*, **666**

deep, *17*, *18*, 42, *250*, 320
  of foot, **812**
  of forearm, *250*
  of leg, *794*, *803*
  of lower limb, 728, *729*
  of penis (Buck), **678**, *679*
  of thigh, 728
deltoid, **164**, *165*
dorsal, *257*
endo-abdominal, **434**
endothoracic, 327, 344, *345*, 1053
Gallaudet, *665*
gluteal, *118*
hypothenar, *230*
iliac, 571, *605*
iliacosubfascial, 571
iliopsoas, *628*
inferior, of pelvic diaphragm, 667
infraspinous, **164**
investing, *17*, *18*, 434, *1051*, **1052**
lata, *452*, 728, **728**, *729*
obturator, **596**, *598*, *605*, *661*, *665*
orbital, 948
palmar, 165, *230*, 254, *256*
  Dupuytren contracture of, 271–272
pectineal, *833*
pectoral, **164**, *165*, *166*, *327*, **327**, 334, 334
pelvic, **603–606**
  endopelvic, **603–606**, *604*
  membranous, **603**
  parietal, **603**, *604*
  tendinous arch of, *605*
  visceral, **603**, *604*, *645*
pelvic diaphragm, *604*
perineal, *665*, **666**
  superficial, *680*
peri-ureteric, **541**
pharyngobasilar, **1100**, *1100–1101*
phrenicopleural, **344**, *345*
plantar, **812**, *813*
of popliteal fossa, **786**–787
presacral, *605*
pretracheal, **1052–1053**, *1064–1065*
prevertebral, *1051*, **1053**, *1081*, *1085*, 1096, 1099, 1106
psoas, *541*, *542*, *564*, *605*, *608*
rectal, *665*
rectosacral, *605*
renal, 541, *542*, *564*
Scarpa, 434, *665*
spermatic
  external, *452*, *681*
  internal, *452*, *457*, *628*
subserous, **18**
superficial, 13, 14, 728, *729*
supraspinous, **164**
temporal, *902*, *977*, *984*, *1022*
thenar, *230*, *246*
thoracolumbar, 118–*119*, 120, 435, *542*, 563, 564
transversalis, *118*, *435*, **435**, *437*, *438*, 440, 441, 443, 449, 452, 563, 564, 601
uterovaginal, *665*
vesical, *605*
Fascia (of regions)
  of abdominal wall
    anterolateral, **434**–435
    posterior, *564*, **565**–566
  of foot, **812**
  of levator ani, *600*
  of lower limb, **728**, *729*
  of neck, **1050**–1053
  of palm of hand, **254**
  of thoracic wall, **324**, **327**
  of upper limb, **164**–166
Fascial compartments, **17**, 35
  of foot, **812**, *813*
  of hand, 254–256, *257*
  of lower limb, 728, *729*
  of upper limb, **164**, *166*
Fascicles, *50*
Fasciitis, plantar, **826**
Fasciotomy, 741
Fat
  axillary, 193, *194*
  epidural, **132**
  in epidural space, *75*, *109*
  extradural, *107*, *109*
  intraconal, *947*
  orbital, **948**
  paranephric, **541**
  pararenal, *564*
  perinephric, **541**
  perirenal, 541, *564*, *577*
  retropubic, *694*
Fat pad
  of acetabular fossa, 832
  buccal, 917, 988, 1011
  in coronoid fossa, *285*
  extrapericardial, *347*, *409*
  gluteal, 714
  infrapatellar, *26*, 757, **838**, *839*, 867
  ischio-anal, *665*, 666
  plantar (of sole of foot), 870
  retropubic, *623*
Fauces, *994*, **994**
FB. *See* Fibularis brevis
FCL. *See* Fibular collateral ligament
FDB. *See* Flexor digitorum brevis
FDL. *See* Flexor digitorum longus
FDP. *See* Flexor digitorum profundus
FDS. *See* Flexor digitorum superficialis
Female genital cutting, **692**
Femur, *694*, **711**, *712*, 713
  angle of inclination, **711**, *712*
  fractures of, **722**
  greater trochanter of, *21*
  head of, *26–27*, *589*, *707*, 711, *712*, 715
    avascular necrosis, 862
    blood supply of, *834*
    dislocated epiphysis of, **722**
    ligament of, **832**
    necrosis of, in children, 862
  neck of, **711**, *712*
    blood supply to, *834*
    fractures, **861**–862
  proximal, 711
  shaft of, *707*, *712*, **713**, 716
  surface anatomy of, **713**–715
FHB. *See* Flexor hallucis brevis
FHL. *See* Flexor hallucis longus
Fiber(s)
  afferent (sensory), **50**
  of autonomic nervous system, **58**
  collagen, in dermis, 14, *14*
  general sensory, **54**, **56**
  glossopharyngeal nerve, **1142–1143**
  intercrural, *438*, *450*, **451**, *452*
  motor
    branchial, 1120
    of cranial nerves, 1120
    somatic, 1120
    sympathetic, *57*
  muscle, 31
  nerve
    cranial, 1128
    peripheral, 47, *49*, *50*
  parasympathetic, *554*
  postsynaptic, 391
  presynaptic, 391
    parasympathetic, 639
    sympathetic, 639
  Purkinje, 390
  sensory, of cranial nerves, 1120
  somatic efferent, general, **56**
  sympathetic, *554*
  visceral, 56
  visceral afferent
    general, 56
    pelvis, **618–619**
  zonular, *952*, **954**, *964*
Fibrillation, **401**
  atrial, 401
  ventricular, 401
Fibrin, 472
Fibrous digital sheaths, **812**
Fibula, *17*, 715, *716*, **717**
  fractures of, **724**
  functions of, 715–716
  lateral malleolus of, *21*
  shaft of, **717**
  surface anatomy of, *717*, 717–718
Fibular articular facet, **716**
Fibular collateral ligament (FCL), **838**
  Fibularis brevis (FB), *719*, *790*, *791*, 793t, *794*, *795*, 795t, **798**, *801*, *805*, 806, *851*
  Fibularis longus (FL), *719*, *790*, *791*, 793t, *794*, *795*, 795t, **797**–798, *805*, 806, *851*

Fibularis muscles, **807**
Fibularis tertius (FT), *719*, *791*, **792**, 793t, *794*
Fibular notch, **717**
Fibular trochlea, **718**
Filum terminale, *95*, *131*, **132**, *133*, *140*
Fimbriae, ovarian, **642**
Fingerprints, 271
Fingers. *See also* Digits
ischemia of, 272–273
surface anatomy of, 271, *271*
Fissure
anal, **675–676**
cerebral, longitudinal, **924**, **935**, *1121*
horizontal, of lungs, *348*, **350**, 358
oblique, of lungs, 346, *348–349*, **350**, 358
oral, **903**, **987**
orbital, *976*
inferior, 948, *1012*, *1131*
superior, 906, *940*, 948, *959*, *1120*, *1131*
palpebral, **906**, **916**, *947*, 948, 968
petro-occipital, *886*
petrosquamous, *1141*
pterygomaxillary, *1012*
sagittal
left, **520**
right, **520**
tympanomastoid, *976*
Fistula
arteriovenous, 933
branchial, 1113, *1114*
bronchopulmonary, 359
cholecystenteric, **538**
perineal, 673
rectovaginal, 655
tracheo-esophageal, 1114
urethrovaginal, 655, *655*
vaginal, **654–655**, *655*
vesicovaginal, *655*
Fixator, **35**
FL. *See* Fibularis longus
Flail chest, **319**
Flaring of nostrils, **918**
Flexion, *9*, *10*, *11*
of knee joint, 845t
lateral, **12**
of vertebral column, 104
Flexor carpi radialis (FCR), 206, *218*, 229, *230*, *231*, 231t, **232**, *241*, *246*, *248*, *259*, *261*, *263*, *266*, *274*, 292, 299
Flexor carpi ulnaris (FCU), *207*, *229*, *231*, 231t, 233, 241, 246, 248, 258, 261, 266, 299
Flexor digiti minimi, *719*, *814*, *815*, 815t, 818
Flexor digiti minimi brevis, 260t, *261*, **261**
Flexor digitorum brevis (FDB), *795*, *814*, 814t, 815, 817, 818, 850
Flexor digitorum longus (FDL), *719*, *790*, 795, 795t, 799t, 800, 800t, 801, 803, 814, 814t, 818, 852
Flexor digitorum profundus (FDP), *206*, *207*, *229*, *231*, 232t, **233**, *238*, 241, 259, 261, 263, 266, 274
Flexor digitorum superficialis (FDS), 261, 206, 229, 231, 231t, 233, 241, *246*, *258*, *259*, *263*, *266*, *274*
Flexor hallucis brevis (FHB), *795*, *815*, 815t, 817, 818
Flexor hallucis longus (FHL), 719, 795, 795t, 800, 800t, 801, 803, 852
Flexor pollicis brevis (FPB), 258, **260**, 260t
Flexor pollicis longus (FPL), *206*, *229*, *231*, 232t, *233*, *241*, *246*, *259*, 261, 263, 266
Flexor retinaculum, **798**
Flexure
anorectal, of anal canal, **628**
colic, *578*
left (splenic), *469*, *480*, *487*, *496*, 498, 500, 508, 554, 1147
right (hepatic), *469*, *487*, *496*, 498, 500, 501, 508
duodenojejunal, **487**, *487*, *488*, *489*
hepatic. (*see* Flexure, colic, left)
lateral, of rectum, **628**
sacral, of rectum, *628*, **628**
splenic. (*see* Flexure, colic, right)
Fluid
ascitic, 472
cerebrospinal (CSF), **47**, **132–137**
absorption of, **938**
circulation of, **938**
functions of, **938**
hydrocephalus, 943, *943*, 944
leakage of, **944**
otorrhea, 944
rhinorrhea, 944
secretion of, **938**
extracellular (ECF), **41**
lacrimal, 950
pericardial, 373
peritoneal, **465**
pleural, **344**
synovial, **26**
Fluoroscope, 400
Fold
alar
lateral, **838**, *839*
medial, **838**, *839*
aryepiglottic, **1088**, *1090–1091*, *1097*, 1101, 1110
axillary
anterior, 186, *187*, 193, *194*, *223*, 338, 339, 340
posterior, 186, *187*, 193, *194*
cecal, *497*
circular, *492*
conjunctival, semilunar, 968
epicanthal, *916*
glossoepiglottic, *1092*, *1110*
gluteal, **704**
ileocecal, *496*
mallear
anterior, *1029*
posterior, *1029*
mucosal, *1010*
palatine, transverse, **995**, *996*
paraduodenal, 507
peritoneal, **468**
pharyngo-epiglottic, *994*, *1097*
rectal, transverse, *623*, **628**, 633
recto-uterine, 602t, *623*, *645*
salpingopharyngeal, *994*, *1097–1098*, 1099
semilunar, *496*
spiral, **529**
sublingual, *1000*
synovial, 262, 832, *851*
infrapatellar, **838**, *839*
umbilical
lateral, *449*, 456t, 602t, *623*
medial, 602t, *623*
median, *449*, **449**, 456t, 602t
urogenital, 685
vestibular, *989*, **1088**, 1090, *1090–1091*, 1110
vocal, *1090*, **1090**, *1098*, *1110*
Fontanelles
anterior, 27, *897*, **897**
mastoid, *897*, **898**
posterior, *897*, **898**
sphenoidal, *897*, **898**
Foot, 811–827
anesthetic block of superficial fibular nerve, 827
arches of, *825*, 857–859, *858*
arteries of, *821*, 821–822
bones of
metatarsus, 718, *719*, 720
phalanges, 720
surface anatomy of, *720*, 720–721
tarsus, 718, *719*
callus of, 869
clinical importance, 811
clubfoot, **870**
contusion of extensor digitorum brevis, 826
deep fascia of, 812, *813*
dorsalis pedis artery pulse, 827
dorsal region of, **812**
dorsum of, *719*, *816*, 816t
fascia of, **812**
flatfeet, **870**
hallux valgus of, **868–869**
heel region of, **812**
hemorrhaging wounds, **827**
infections, 826
infections of, **826**
jogger's, 827
joints, **851**–853, 854t

arches, **857**–859, *858*
ligaments, **853**, 857
movements, *855*, 855t
lymphadenopathy, 827
lymphatic systems, 822, *824*
medial plantar nerve entrapment, 827
muscles, 812–813, *814*, 814t–815t, *816*, 816t, 817, 818
nerves of, 816, *820*, 820t, 821
part/region of, 812
pes planus, **870**
plantar fasciitis, 826
plantar reflex, 827
region, **705**
skeleton, 811, *811*
skin and subcutaneous tissue, 812, *813*
sole of, *804*
arteries of, **822**
central compartment of, **812**
hemorrhaging wounds of, **827**
lateral compartment of, **812**
medial compartment of, **812**
subcutaneous tissue of, **812**
sural nerve grafts, 827
surface anatomy, 824, *824*, 826
tarsus, 718
veins of, 822, *823*
Footdrop, 807–808, *808*
Foramen/Foramina (in general), 22
nutrient, 22, 23, **717**
Foramen/Foramina (named)
alveolar, posterior superior, *976*, *1012*
apical, **991**, *993*
cecum, *999*, *1097*, *1107*
cribriform, 891t
epiploic (*see* Foramen, omental)
ethmoidal
anterior, *946*
posterior, *946*
greater sciatic, **763**
infra-orbital, **885**, *946*
interventricular, *936*, *937*
intervertebral, **76**, *76–77*, *107*, *135*
jugular, *886*, *888*, 891t, *1120*, 1142, 1143–1144
lacerum, *888*, 891t, **893**, *940*
lesser sciatic, **763**
magnum, *929*, *1012*, *1141*, *1148*
mandibular, **986**, *990*
mastoid, *888*, 891t
obturator, *21*, 586, *587*, 588t
omental, **469**, *471*, *481*, *508*
optic, *940*
ovale, **379**, 910, *976*, *1012*
palatine
greater, 993, *995*
lesser, 993, *995*
parietal, *886*, **887**, *887*
rotundum, 891t, *892*, **892**, 910, 1011, *1013*
sacral, 86, *95*
anterior, *133*
posterior, *85*
sciatic
greater, 591, *591*, 597, 599t
lesser, 591, *591*, 612
sphenopalatine, *976*, *1012*
spinosum, 927, *976*, *1012*
sternal, 321
stylomastoid, *888*, **890**
supra-orbital, *881*, **885**
transversarium (transverse), **78**, 89, *1048*
vertebral, **76**, *79*, 82t, *84*, *94*
zygomaticofacial, *883*, **885**
Forearm, **228**–253
arteries of, *217*, 241–243
bones of, 152–153
compartments of, 228, *231*, 231t–232t, 232–233
cross-section of, *230*
cutaneous nerves of, 172
extensor-supinator compartment of, *236*
muscles of, 228–240, *230*
extensor, 233, 234t, 235, *247*
flexor, *247*
nerves of, 244–247
pronation of, *288*
supination of, *288*
surface anatomy of, 247–248
veins of, 243–244
Forefoot, *719*, **811**, 855t
Foreign bodies
aspiration of, **361**, **1110**–1111
in laryngopharynx, **1113**
Forensic medicine, 592
Fornix, *936*
conjunctival
inferior, **948**
superior, *947*, **948**
lateral, *641*, 646
posterior, **646**
vaginal, 643
lateral, *641*, 646
posterior, **646**
Fossa(e), 21
acetabular, **711**
axillary, **164**, *165*, *187*, 193
cerebellar, *892*, **893**
coronoid, 152
cranial
anterior, **890**, 891t
middle, **890**, 891t, *892*, 893, *940*
posterior, 891t, **893**
cubital, 218–219
boundaries of, 220
contents of, 220
cross-section of, *230*
surface anatomy of, 220, *224*, *247*, 247–248, 248
venipuncture of, 227, *227*
epigastric, 320, **338**, *458*
gallbladder, **520,** *520*
hypophysial, *889*, *892*, *924*
iliac, *565*, *587*
iliacosubfascial, **571**
incisive, 993, 995, *995*
infraclavicular, **186**, *187*
infraspinous, *151*, **151**
infratemporal, **975**, *976*
inguinal
lateral, *449*, **450**
medial, *449*, **450**
intercondylar, *708*, *712*, **713**, **716**, 838, 839
interpeduncular, 938
intrabulbar, **677**
ischio-anal, 600, 604, 612, 621, 661, *665*, **668–669**, *695*, *697*
lacrimal gland, **948**
mandibular, *978*
navicular, *623*, **677**
olecranon, *151*, **152**
oval, *379*, **379**, *382*
paraduodenal, 507
pararectal, **601**, 628, *628*
paravesical, *628*
piriform, *1091*, *1097*, **1101**, *1110*
popliteal, 785–789, *786*
abscess and tumor, 806
accessory soleus, 810, *810*
aneurysm and hemorrhage, 806–807
arteries in, **788**
calcaneal bursitis, 809
calcaneal tendinitis, 808–809
calcaneal tendon reflex, 809
common fibular nerve, 807–808
containment, 807
contents of, 785–789
cysts, 867, *867*
deep fibular nerve entrapment, 808
fabella in gastrocnemius, 808
fascia of, **786**
fibularis muscles, 807
footdrop injury, 807–808
gastrocnemius strain, 809
human foot evolution, 807
lymph nodes in, **789**
nerves in, 789
neurovascular structures, 787–789, 788, 789
plantarflexion, absence of, 809
posterior tibial pulse, 810
pulse, 806
ruptured calcaneal tendon, 809
superficial fibular nerve entrapment, 808
tibialis anterior strain, 807
tibial nerve injury, 807
veins in, **789**
venous return from leg, 809–810
pterygoid, **889**

Fossa(e) (*Continued*)
pterygopalatine, 910, *976*, **1011**–1014
contents of, **1011**, *1013*
of maxillary artery, **1011**
transantral approach to, **1014**
radial, *152*, **152**, *285*
scaphoid, *889*
subscapular, **150**
supinator, **152**
supraclavicular, *356*, **356**, 1057, *1071*
greater, 1072
lesser, *1055*, 1055t, 1070
supraspinous, 150, **151**
supravesical, *449*, **450**, **601**, *623*
temporal, *881*, *883*, **886**, **975**, *976*
tonsillar, *1098*
triangular, of antihelix, 1027
trochanteric, *712*, **713**, *750*, *768*
Fourth-degree burn, 17
Fovea
centralis, **954**
pterygoid, *978*, *1008*
Foveolae, granular, **924**
FPB. *See* Flexor pollicis brevis
FPL. *See* Flexor pollicis longus
Fractures
of atlas, **92**
avulsion, 160, 759
of axis, 92, *94*
boxer's, 162
burst, 92
calcaneal, 725, *726*
clavicle, **159**
Colles, 160
comminuted, 160, 320
compound, 722, *723*
compression, 111
of cranial base, 933
crush, 111
dancer's, 725
of dens, 114, *114*
depressed, 896
diagonal, 723, *723*
epiphysial plate, **724**
femoral, 722, *723*
of femoral neck, 861–862
fibular, 724, *724*
greenstick, 24, 160
hamate, 162
hangman's, *92*, *94*, *112*
of hip bone, **721**
humerus, **160**
hyoid bone, **1050**
impacted, 160
intercondylar, 160
Jefferson, 92
of lateral malleolus, 724
Le Fort I, **895**, *895*
Le Fort II, **895**, *895*
Le Fort III, **895**, *895*
mandibular, 895
maxillary, 895
of medial malleolus, 724
metacarpal, **162**
metatarsals, 725–726, *726*
nasal, **1023**
olecranon, 249, *249*
orbital, **968**
patellar, *759*, 759–760
pelvic, 593, *594*
of phalanges, **162**
Pott, **868**
pterion, **931**–932
radius, **160**–161
reduction of, 24
ribs, **319**
scaphoid, **162**
scapula, **160**
sesamoid bones, 726, *727*
sternal, **320**
stress, **723**
of talar neck, 725, *726*
temporal bone, **920**
tibial, **722–723**
transverse, *723*
ulna, **160**–162
of vertebrae, ***111–114***, *113*
wrist, 162, *300*, 301
Frenectomy, **1010**
Frenulectomy, *1006*
Frenulum
of clitoris, *687*
labial, *989*, **1006**
of labia minora, *687*
of prepuce, *679*, **680**
of tongue, **999**
Frontal bone, *949*
FT. *See* Fibularis tertius
Full-thickness burn, 17
Fundus
of eyeball, *952*
of stomach, **479**, *577*
of urinary bladder, *623*, **624**
of uterus, *641*, **643**, *696*
Furrow
median longitudinal, **83**
posterior median, 86, *87*, 126
Fusiform muscles, 33

G

Gag reflex, **1009**
Gait
cycle, 743, *744*, 744t–745t, 745
gluteal, 784
steppage, 808
swing-out, 807
waddling, 807
Gallbladder, *435*, 527–529, *528*
body of, **528**
fundus of, *604*
lymphatic system of, 527–529, *528*
neck of, *515*
nerves of, 529
parts of, 527–529
radiographs of, 69
sympathetic stimulation, 65t
Gallstones, **536**–538
in duodenum, **538**
Ganglion/ganglia, **50**
aorticorenal, *548*, *554*, 555t
of autonomic nervous system, **58**
celiac, *486*, 494, *526*, *541*, *548*, 555t, 556, 1147
cervical
inferior, *1081*
middle, *356*, *1081*
superior, 950, *1081*
cervicothoracic, *356*, **1082**, *1085*
block of, 1082
ciliary, *959*, **961**, *1126*, 1127t
geniculate, *1014*, *1139*, **1140**
inferior
of glossopharyngeal nerve, **1142**, *1143*
of vagus nerve, **1143**
mesenteric
inferior, *501*, 555t, **556**, *625*
superior, *486*, **494**, *501*, *526*, *548*, 1143
otic, *907*, **975**, 980, 987, *1126*, 1127t, 1143
parasympathetic
cranial, *1126*, 1127t
intrinsic, 556
paravertebral, **59**
prevertebral, **59**
pterygopalatine, *907*, *998*, *1013*, 1031, 1126, 1127t, 1135, 1134
retinal, **1128**
semilunar (*see* Ganglion/ganglia, trigeminal)
sensory, spinal, *191*
spinal, *127*, 127t, *133*, *136*, 494, *630*, *648*
spiral, *1036*, **1141**
stellate, *356*, *1085*
submandibular, *1004*, *1063*, *1126*, 1127t, 1140, 1139
superior
of glossopharyngeal nerve, **1142**, *1143*
of vagus nerve, 1143
sympathetic, *326*, *409–410*, *486*, 494, 548, 615
aberrant, *1079*
cervical, 1085, *1085*
inferior, *1085*, *1100*
middle, *1085*, *1100*
superior, 1012, **1082**, *1100*
cervicothoracic, *1079*
paravertebral, 355, 566
prevertebral, 556
thoracic, *356*
trigeminal, *907*, *978*, *990*, *1122*, **1135**, 1143
herpes zoster infection of, **919**

vagal, inferior, **1095**
vestibular, *1036*, **1036**, **1141**
Ganglion impar, 59
Gangrene, 43
Gastrectomy, 505
Gastric ulcers, 505–506
Gastrocnemius, **800**
Gastrocnemius strain, 809
Gastroenterology, 4
Gastroscopy, 505
Gemelli, **770**
General anesthesia, 656
General sensory fiber, 55, 56
General visceral efferent (GVF), 56
Genicular anastomosis, **789**, **844**
Genitalia. *See* Genital organs
Genital organs
female external, **687–690**
female internal, 640–658
male external, 677–686
male internal, **634–640**
Genu valgum, 863, *863*
Genu varum, 863, *863*
Gingiva, *988*, **989**
buccal
mandible, **989**, *1000*
maxillary, **989**
labial
mandibular, *990*
maxillary, *990*
lingual
inferior, 989
mandible, *1000*
superior, 989
nerves of, *990*
proper, **989**
Gingivitis, **1006**
Glabella, *916*
Gland(s)
areolar, 340
bulbo-urethral, *627*, *634*, **638**, *663*, 666, 677
ciliary, *947*, **949**
Cowper (*see* Gland(s), bulbo-urethral)
lacrimal, *909*, **949**, *1018*, *1139*
Littré, 677
mammary, *334*, **334**
olfactory, **1127**
palatine, **994**, *998*
parathyroid, 1085
adenoma of, 1109–1110
arteries of, 1085–1086
inadvertent removal of, 1109–1110
inferior, **1085**, *1087*, *1101*
left, *1084*
nerves of, *1087*
right, *1084*
superior, **1085**, *1087*, *1101*
para-urethral, 626, **690**
parotid, *911*, **973**–974, *996*, 1002, *1003*, 1004, 1143
abscess in, *984*
accessory, **986**
blockage of, **986**
infection of, **985**
innervation of, **974**–975, *975*
nerves of, 974–975
sialography of, **985**–986
pituitary, *1021*
tumors of, 932
prostate, 635
arterial supply of, 638
hypertrophy of, **639–640**
lobes of, **637**
salivary, **1002**, *1004*, 1004–1006
sebaceous
of breast (areolar), **335**
cysts of, 969
of skin, 14, *14*
seminal, 603, **604**, **635**, *695*
sublingual, 1002, *1002*, *1003*, *1022*, *1139*
submandibular, 974, *974*, *1003–1004*, **1004**–1006, *1063*, 1072, *1101*, *1139*
suprarenal, **545**
arteries of, **547**–548
left, *474*, *483*, *515*, *541*, *621*
lymphatic system of, *548*, **548**
nerves of, **548**–549
right, *474*, *515*, *541*, *547*
veins of, **547**–548
sweat, 13
tarsal, *947*, **948**, 967
thyroid, 1048, **1083**, *1084*, *1097*, *1100*, 1104–1105, 1105
accessory glandular tissue, 1086, 1107–1108
arteries of, **1083**
enlargement of, 1108
isthmus of, 1104
lingual, 1086
lymphatic system of, 1085, *1086*
pyramidal lobe of, 1086 veins of, 1085
vestibular, **690**
Glans
of clitoris, *687–689*, **689**
of penis, *623*, 678, *679*, **679**
Glottis, **1090**
Gluteal region, **704**, **763**, *764*
arteries of, 776–776, *777*, 778t
injections in, 784–785
lymphatic system of, 778
surface anatomy of, 779–782
veins of, **778**
Gluteal sulcus, **780**
Gluteal tuberosity, **713**
Gluteofemoral bursa, **763**
Gluteus maximus, *766*, 766–767
Gluteus medius, **767**
Gluteus minimus, **767**
Goiter, 1108, *1109*
Gomphosis, **993**
Gracilis, *751*, **751**
transplantation of, 760
Grafts
bone, 724–725
saphenous vein, 741
sural nerve, 870
Granulations, arachnoid, *923*, **924**, *937*, 938
Gray matter, 47
Gray rami communicantes, 60
Great arteries
transposition of, 374
variations in, 417–418
Great saphenous vein, **728**
Great toe, **705**
Great vessels
magnetic resonance angiography of, *424*
surface anatomy of, **402–404**
Grip
hook, **254**, *255*
power, **254**, *255*
precision, **254**, *255*
Groin pull, 760
Groove, 22
atrioventricular, **377**
bicipital, **217**, *218*
of bone, *21*
coronary, 377, *378*
costal, *326*
of ribs, *311*
deltopectoral, 165, **176**
infra-orbital, *946*
inguinal, *458*
intertubercular, *150*, 151, *194*, *215*
interventricular
anterior, **377**, *378*
posterior, **377**, *378*
for medial meniscus, *841*
nuchal, **83**, 126
occipital, **1069**
radial, *150*, **148**
for sigmoid sinus, *886*
subclavian, *145*, *147*
for tendon of fibularis longus, **718**, *719*
for tendon of flexor hallucis, **718**, *719*
for trigeminal nerve, 887
Guarding, 446
Gubernaculum
female, **453**
male, **453**
ovarian, 644
upper, *454*
Gutters, paracolic, **469**, *493*, 498
GVE. *See* General visceral efferent
Gynecology, 5
Gynecomastia, **343**

Gyrus
postcentral, *936*
precentral, *936*

H

Habit scoliosis, 117
Hair, 13, 14
arrector muscles of, **13**, **14**
follicles, 13, 14, 37
nasal, *1017*
pubic, *679*
Hair follicles, 13, *13*, 37
Hallucinations, olfactory, **1152**
Hallux valgus, 868–869
Hamate, 154, **155**, 157, 165, 274, 290
fracture of, 162
Hammer toe, 869, *870*
Hamstring injuries, 783
Hamstring muscles, **770**
Hamulus, pterygoid, *976*, *995*, 996, *997*, 1102t
Hand, 254. *See also* Phalanges; Wrist
arteries of, 244
bones of, 153–156, 254, *290*
creases of, **270**, 271
functional positions of, *255*
grip
hook, **254**, *255*
power, **254**, *255*
precision, **254**, *255*
infections of, 272
long flexor tendons in, 262
muscles of
hypothenar, **261**
short, 261–262
thenar, 256–257, 259
nerves of, 265, 268, 268t
palm of, *8*, *9*
compartments of, 256, *257*
dissection of, *258*
fascia of, 254, 256
pinching by, 254, *255*
resting position of, 254, *255*
surface anatomy of, 269–271
tendon sheaths in, 262
veins of, 265
Haustra, **494**, *496*
Haversian canal, 23
Head (in general), 22
of biceps femoris, **773**
of epididymis, **458**, 463
of femur, *26–27*, *589*, *707*, 711, *712*, 716, 717, 828
avascular necrosis, 862
blood supply to, *834*
dislocated epiphysis of, 722
ligament of, **832**
necrosis of, in children, 862
of fibula, *717*, 717–718, *758*, *805*, 806
of humerus, *21*, *149*, 151, 157, 220
of metacarpals, 270
of metatarsals, 721
of pancreas, *489*, **514**, *516*
of radius, *149*, 153, 158, *229*, *247*, 248
dislocation of, *300*, 300–301
subluxation of, *300*, 300–301
of scapula, *150*, **151**
of sternocleidomastoid, **1054**, *1056*, 1056t
of talus, **718**
of ulna, *149*, *152*, *157*, 158, *247*, 248, 270, 290
Head (region), 909
blunt trauma to, **932**
brain (*see* Brain)
cranium (*see* Cranium)
ear (*see* Ear)
face (*see* Face)
hematoma of, 933–934
injuries to, **933**–934
lymphatic system of, *1105*
magnetic resonance imaging of, *71*
nose (*see* Nose)
regions of, 916
scalp, **900**–901
surface anatomy of, 915–917
Headaches, 894
dural origin of, 933
Heart, 375, **375**
apex of, *346*, **377**, *378*, *386*, *431*, *474*
arterial supply of, 388
atrioventricular node of, *389*, **389**
auscultation of, 415
base of, **377**, *378*
borders of, *378*
cardiopulmonary resuscitation of, 401
chambers of, 375–376
conducting system of, *389*, **389–390**, 399–400
crux of, *386*
defibrillation of, **401**
development of, *370*
dextrocardia of, 374
electrocardiography of, 398, **398**
endocardium of, *368*, **376**
epicardium of, *368*, **376**
fibrillation of, **401**
fibrous skeleton of, 376, *376–377*, 380, 390
hypertrophy of, 37
innervation of, 390–391
left, 375
lymphatic drainage of, **389**
magnetic resonance angiography of, *424*
myocardium of, *368*, **376**
arrangement of, *376*
pacemaker for, **400**
percussion of, **393**
placement of, *378*
positional abnormalities of, **373–374**
referred pain, **401**
right, 375
sinu-atrial node of, *389*
sounds, **376**
surface anatomy of, 414–415
surfaces of, *378*
sympathetic stimulation, 65t
valves of
aortic, *377*, *384–385*
cusps of, **393–394**
insufficiency of, **394**
stenosis of, **394**
mitral, *375*, 384
cusps of, *384–385*
insufficiency of, **394**
pulmonary, *375*, *384*
cusps of, **393–394**
incompetence of, **394**
stenosis of, **394**
semilunar, *384–385*
tricuspid, *375*, **380**, *384*
vasculature of, **384–389**
veins of, *388*, **388–389**
walls of, 376
Heat regulation, skin's role in, 12
Heel strikes, **743**
Hegar sign, 652
Heimlich maneuver, **1110–1111**
Helicobacter pylori, **505**–506
Helix, **1026**, *1027*
Hematocele, 461, **461**, *462*
Hematoma
auricular, 1038
epidural, 933, *934*
extradural, 933, *934*
of phalanges, 162
subdural, 134, 933–934
thigh, 759
torticollis and, 1072–1073
Hemianopsia, *1153*
Hemidiaphragm, 563
Hemisacralization, 95
Hemispheres, cerebral, 924, **935**, *936*
Hemopericardium, 373
Hemopneumothorax, 359
Hemoptysis, **364**
Hemorrhage
anterior chamber of eye, **971**
intraperitoneal, 531
popliteal, 806–807
subarachnoid, 934, *934*
subconjunctival, **969**
Hemorrhagic stroke, 944
Hemorrhaging wounds, in foot, 827
Hemorrhoids, **676**
Hemothorax, *359*, **359**
Hepatomegaly, **534**–535
Hernia, 445
abdominal, 445
of canal of Nuck, 460
congenital diaphragmatic, **571**
diaphragmatic, 319, **571**
epigastric, 445
femoral, 762, *762*
hiatal, 503, 571
para-esophageal, *486*, 503

sliding, *486*, 503
incisional, **447**
inguinal, **450**–451
direct, 460, *461*
indirect, 460, *461*
paraduodenal, **507**
Spigelian, 445
supravesical, external, **450**
umbilical, 445
Herpes zoster, **332–333**, *333*, **919**
Heterotopic bones, 24
Hiatus
adductor, *750*, **751**, *756–757*, 796, 796t, 837
aortic, **409**, 548, 560, *560*, *562*, **562**, *566*
esophageal, **408**, 410, 478, 560, *560*, 562, 562, 562, 566
sacral, **86**, *86*, *95*, *136*
semilunar, *1017*, *1022*
urogenital, *598*, **599**, *600*, *663*
Hiccups, **570**
High tone deafness, 1040
Hilton's law, **28**, 834, 844
Hilum
of lungs, *349*, **350**
renal, *542*, **543**, *544*
splenic, **513**, *513*
Hindfoot, *719*, **811**
Hip
contusions, 759
region, **704**
Hip bone, **708**–709
anatomical position, *710*, 711
in children, 586
fractures of, 721
ilium, 351, 352, *353*
magnetic resonance imaging of, *577*
in infants, 352
injuries, 721, *721*
ischium, 351, 374
body of, 586
left, 373
parts of, *709*
pubertal fusion of, 586
pubis, 351, 352, 687
right, 351
Hip joints, 828–836, *829*, *830*, *831*, *833*, 834, 835
arteries of, 834
articular surfaces, 828–829, *829*, 831
blood supply of, 834
capsule of, 832
congenital dislocation of, 862
dislocation of, *862*, 862–863
flexors of, 746t
ligaments of, **832**, *833*
movements, 832, 834
nerve supply of, 834, 836
stability of, *830*
surgical replacement of, 862
Hip pointer, 761
Homeostatic, 64
Hook grip, **254**, *255*
Hook of hamate, *154*, **155**, *160*, *246*, *274*, 294
Hordeolum, 969
Hormones, **5**
parathormone, 1083
thyroid, 1083
Horn
of gray matter of spinal cord,
anterior, *49*
posterior, *49*
greater, of hyoid, **1049**, *1090–1091*
inferior, of thyroid cartilage, **1088**
lesser, of hyoid, **1049**
superior, of thyroid cartilage, **1088**
Horner syndrome, **972**
Horns, 47
Humerus, *149*, **151**–152
capitulum of, *21*
development of, 22–23
distal end of, 151
fractures of, 159–160, *161*
general images of, *20*
radial groove of, *21*
trochlea of, *21*
Humor
aqueous, *952*, **954**, *964*
vitreous, *952*, **955**
Hunter, William, 4
Hydrocele, **460**, *461*
Hydrocephalus, 943, *943*, 944
Hydrothorax, **359**
Hymen, **689**
Hyoid bone, *907*, *981*, 1001t, *1047*, **1049**, 1063, 1070, 1089, 1098, 1104
fracture of, 1050
Hyperacusis, 1039
Hyperdontia, **1007**
Hyperemia, conjunctival, **969**
Hyperextension, **9**
Hyperplasia, 37
Hypertension, 41
Hypertension, portal, 502, 536, **538**, 676
Hypertrophy, 24
of bones, 24
compensatory, 37
of muscles, 36
of myocardium, 37
of smooth muscle, 37
Hypospadias, **685**
Hypothalamus, *936*
Hypothenar fascia, *230*, *246*
Hysterectomy, 601, 619, 653–654, *654*
Hysterosalpingography, 471, **649**
Hysteroscopic sterilization, **649–650**
Hysteroscopy, 649

I

IC joint(s). *See* Intercarpal joints
Ileostomy, **510**
Ileum, 468, *474*, 487, *487*, **491**, 494
characteristics of, 492t
proximal, *492*
terminal, *492*, 497
Ileus, 508
diverticulum of, 508, **509**
gallstone, 538
Iliacus, **747**
Iliofemoral ligament, **832**
Iliopectineal arch, **752**
Iliopsoas, **747**–748
Iliotibial tract, **728**
Ilium, 351, **352**, *353*, 585–586, *587*, *694*, **709**
acetabulum, **711**
ischium, **709**
magnetic resonance imaging of, *577*
obturator foramen, **711**
pubis, **711**
Imaging
computed tomography, 68, 68–69, *70* (*see also* Computed tomography)
conventional radiography, 67, *67–68*, *68*
magnetic resonance (*see* Magnetic resonance imaging)
nuclear medicine imaging, 72
radiographs (*see* Radiographs)
ultrasonography, *69*, *70*
IMLs. *See* Intermediolateral cell columns
Impotence, **686**
Impression, cardiac, *349*, 350
Impulses, nociceptive, 356
Incisions
facial, **917**
gridiron (muscle-splitting), 447, 509
high-risk, **447**
inguinal, 447
longitudinal, **446**–447
median, 446
midline, 446
paramedian, 446–447
pararectus, 447
Pfannenstiel, *447*
suprapubic, 447
transverse, **447**
Incisure, angular, *481*
Incontinence, anorectal (fecal), **676**
Incus, 1021–1023, 1026, 1027, 1029, 1030, **1032**
Infarction, 42–43
acute cortical, 945
brain, 945
myocardial, 373, **396**
pulmonary, 364
Infections
compartments of leg, 807
eyelid, 969
of foot, 826
herpes zoster, **332–333**, *333*, **919**
in neck, 1054
of parotid gland, **985**
scalp, **917**
Inferior extensor retinaculum, **789**
Inferior gluteal artery, **776**

Inferior gluteal nerve, **775**
Inferior tibiofibular joint, **847**
Inferomedial, **9**
Infrapatellar bursae, **844**
Infrapatellar fat pad, **838**
Infrapatellar synovial fold, **838**
Infraspinous fascia, **163**
Infundibulum
  of brain, *930*, *1121–1122*
  ethmoidal, **1018**, *1018*, 1020
  of pituitary gland, *1122*
  of uterine tubes, **642**
Inguinal triangle of Hesselbach, *449*, **450**
Inion, **886**
Initial swing, **745**
Injections
  intragluteal, 784–785
  intraperitoneal, 473
Inlet
  laryngeal, **1088**, *1089–1090*, *1097*, 1101
  pelvic, 432, **586**, *586–587*, 588t, *597*
Innervation. *See also* Nerve(s)
  of bladder, *625*, **625–626**
  of bone, 23
  of dura mater, **134**
  of heart, 390–391
  of knee joint, 844
  of liver, **524**, *526*, 526–527
  of ovaries, **642**
  of pelvis, **618–619**
  of penis, **681–682**
  of periosteum, *107*
  of rectum, **629**, *630*
  of skin, 14, 53
  of teeth, *990*
  of tongue, **1000**
  of ureters, **621–622**
  of urethra, 625, **625**
  of uterus, **647–649**
  of vagina, **647–649**
  of wrist, 291
Inspiration
  diaphragm's role in, 324
  physiology of, *318*
Inspiratory stridor, 1155
Insufficiency, 394
  mitral valve, **394**
Integumentary system, **3**
  skin (*see* Skin)
Intercondylar eminence, **716**
Intercondylar tubercles, **716**
Intermediate, **9**
Intermediate cuneiform, **718**
Intermediolateral cell columns (IMLs), 58–59
Intermittent claudication, 810
Intermuscular septa, *17*, *18*
Internal, *7*, **9**
Internal pudendal artery, **819**
Internal pudendal veins, **778**
Internal rotation, 11, 12
Intersections, tendinous, **440**, 459
Intertrochanteric crest, **713**
Intertrochanteric line, **713**
Intestine(s). *See also* Colon; Rectum
  functions of, 494
  large, 475, **494**–502, *496*, *578*
    arteries of, *493*
    colonoscopy of, 510, *511*
    functions of, 494
    lymphatic system of, 498, *501*
    veins of, 498, *501*
  malrotation of, 510
  small, *487*, **487**, 489–491, *493*, *578*, *695*
    absorption in, 475
    arteries of, *493*
    duodenum (*see* Duodenum)
    ileum (*see* Ileum)
    ischemia of, **507**–508
    jejunum (*see* Jejunum)
    lymphatic system of, *486*
    nerves of, *486*, 494
    in omental bursa, 469–470, 474–475
    radiographic image of, *69*
    surgical navigation of, **507**
    veins of, *493*
Intra-abdominal pressure, 317
Intracranial pressure, 946
Intragluteal injections, *784*, 784–785
Intramembranous ossification, **22**
Intraosseous (IO) infusion, 725, *725*
Intrathoracic pressure, 317, *318*
Inversion, **12**
Investing fascia, *17*, *18*
Ipsilateral, **9**
Iris, *964*, 967, **970**–971
Ischemia, 42–43
  of fingers, 272–273
  of heart, 396
  of intestine, **507**–508
  myocardial, 396
  of peripheral nerves, 58
  of spinal cord, **140–141**
Ischemic compartment syndrome, 226
Ischemic heart disease, 396
Ischemic stroke, 944
Ischial bursa, **763**
Ischial bursitis, 783
Ischial spine, **709**
Ischial tuberosity, **709**, 714
Ischiopubic ramus, **709**
Ischium, 351, 352, 585–586, **709**
  body of, 374, 586
Islets, pancreatic, *515*
Isometric contractions, 33, *33*
Isotonic contractions, 33, *33*
Isthmus
  of fauces, **994**
  of prostate, *634*, **637**
  of thyroid gland, *1051*, 1104
  of uterine tube, **642**
  of uterus, *641*, **643**

J

Jaundice, 533, 538
Jejunum, *474*, *486*, **491**, 494
  characteristics of, 492t
  proximal, *492*
Jogger's foot, 827
Joint(s) (in general), **25**
  arthroscopy, 29
  ball and socket, **27**, **28**
  capsule, **25**
  cavity, 25–26
  classification, 25–28
  condyloid, **27**, **28**
  craniovertebral, **101–103**, *102–103*
  degenerative disease of, 29
  effusions, 867
  fibrous, **26**
  gomphosis, **26**
  hinge, **27**, **28**
  hyaline cartilaginous, 316t
  innervation of, 28
  multiaxial, 28
  neurocentral, **89**
  pivot, **27**, **28**
  plane, *27*, **27**
  plane synovial, 316t, 317
  primary cartilaginous, 26–27
  saddle, *27*, **28**
  secondary cartilaginous, 27
  syndesmosis, 26
  synovial, 25, *27*
    plane, 316t, 317
  vasculature, 28
Joint(s) (named)
  acromioclavicular (AC), *149–150*, 276, 278, 279
    articulation of, 279
    blood supply to, 279
    capsule of, *278*, 279
    dislocation of, 296–297
    ligaments of, 279, *280*
    movements of, 279
    nerves of, 279
  ankle, **849**
    articular surfaces of, **849**
    blood supply of, **851**
    capsule of, **849–850**, *851–852*
    dorsiflexion of, 850
    injuries of, 868
    ligaments of, **850**, 854t
    movements of, **850**
    nerve supply of, 851
    plantarflexion of, 850
    Pott fracture-dislocation of, 868
    radiographs of, *850*
    retinacula of, *811*
    surface anatomy of, **859**
  atlanto-axial
    central, *102*
    lateral, 101
    median, 101
    subluxation of, 114

atlanto-occipital, *101*, *103*, 1054
muscles that produce movement of, 128t
calcaneocuboid, 854t, 859
carpometacarpal (CMC), 27, 28, *148*, 294
of thumb, **293**
costochondral, *309*, *316*, 316t
costotransverse, *312*, **315**, *316*, 316t, 317, 317
costovertebral, *312*, **315**, *316*, 316t, 317, 326
crico-arytenoid, **1088**, *1089*
cricothyroid, **1088**, *1089*
cuneonavicular, 854t
elbow, *148*, **284**, *285*
articulation of, **284**
blood supply of, **286**
bursae around, **287**
bursitis of, **298**–299, *299*
capsule of, **284**–285
carrying angle of, *286*
dislocation of, **300**, *300*
extensor muscles of, 286, *286*
flexor muscles of, 286, *286*
ligaments of, **285**, *286*
movements of, **286**, *286*
muscles that move, **286**, *286*
nerves of, **287**
radiographs of, *285*
tendinitis of, 249
femoropatellar, 829
foot (*see* Foot)
glenohumeral, *148*, 186, 276, **279**
adhesive capsulitis of, 298
articulation of, 279
blood supply to, 284
bursae of, 284
capsule of, 279–280, *280*
dislocation of, 297–298, *298*
innervation of, 284
labral tears, 298
ligaments of, *281*, 281–282, *282*
movements of, 282, *283*, 283t–284t, *284*
nerves of, 282, 284
hip, 28, *705*, **828**
arteries of, **761**
articular surfaces of, **828**–829, 831
blood supply of, **834**
capsule of, **832**
congenital dislocation of, 862
dislocation of, **862–863**
flexors of, 746t
ligaments of, **832**, *833*
movements of, 832, *834*
nerves of, 834, 836
stability of, *830*
surgical replacement of, **862**
intercarpal (IC), 291, *292*, *294*
interchondral, *316*, 316t, 321
intermetacarpal, *290*, **294**
intermetatarsal, 854t
interphalangeal (IP), *148*, 294–295, 829, 854t, 855
distal (DIP), *294*
proximal (PIP), *238*, *294*, 860
intervertebral, 315, 316t, 591
cervical, *125*
muscles that move, **122–126**, *125*
knee, *705*, 836
arteries of, *804*, 844
arthroscopy of, *866*, **866–867**
articular surfaces of, **836**
articulations of, **836**
aspiration of, **867**
blood supply of, **844**
bones of, *836*
bursae of, **844**, *848*, **848**
capsule of, 836, *837*, 838, *839*
extensors of, 747t
injuries of, **864–866**
innervation of, **844**
ligaments of
extracapsular, **838**, *840*
intra-articular, **838**, **841**–844
movements of, 844
posterior part of, **705**
stability of, **836**
total knee replacement arthroplasty, 868
lumbosacral, **591–592**
of Luschka, 99
manubriosternal, **314**, *316*, *338*
metacarpophalangeal (MCP), 27, 28, 148, 257, 294, 294
metatarsophalangeal, *803*, *829*, 854t–855t, 859, *860*
midcarpal, 291
pisotriquetral, 291
radio-ulnar
distal, *148*, *266*, *288*, 289–290
proximal, *148*, *285*, 287–289
sacrococcygeal, *589*, **592**, *615*
sacro-iliac, **589–591**, *589–591*, *600*
scapulothoracic, 151
sternoclavicular (SC), *201*, **277**, *316*, 1068, 1072
ankylosis of, 296
articulation of, 277
blood supply to, 279
capsule of, 276, 277
dislocation of, *296*, 296–297
ligaments of, 277
movements of, 278, *278*
nerves of, 279
sternocostal, *316*, **317**, 321
subtalar, *726*, 851, *860*
talocalcaneal, 854t
talocalcaneonavicular, 854t
talocrural, *811*, 829
talonavicular, 859
tarsal, *852*
transverse, *852*, 853, *860*
tarsometatarsal, *719*, 851, 854t
temporomandibular, *881*, **975**–980, *977*
arthritis of, **986**
capsule of, *902*
dislocation of, **986**
movements of, 979t
muscles that move, 982t
tibiofibular, *829*, *846*, **847–849**
uncovertebral, *99*, **99**
wrist, **254**, 291
arteries of, *242*, 242t
articulation of, 291
blood supply to, 291
bones of, 153–156, *154*
capsule of, 291
cross-section of, *230*
fractures of, *161*, 301, *301*
innervation of, 291
ligaments of, 291, *292*
movements of, 291, *293*
muscles that move, 291
synovial cyst of, 249–250, *250*
zygapophysial, 75, *76*, 77, *101*, 591
degeneration of, 111
disease of, 111
injury of, 111
osteoarthritis of, 141
pain in, 111
xiphisternal, 314
Joint(s) (of regions)
of foot, *846*
of forefoot, 855t
of hand, *294*
of leg, *846*
of newborn cranium, **28**
of pelvis, *589*
of thoracic wall, **315–317**
of vertebral arches, 100
of vertebral bodies, **97–100**
of vertebral column, 97–103, *100*
Junction
anorectal, *669*, **672**
costochondral, 321
duodenojejunal, *486–488*, *489*, *491*, *493*
esophago-gastric (gastro-esophageal), *477*, **478**
ileocecal, 487, *487*, **491**
pharyngo-esophageal, *1097*, *1101*, **1103**
rectosigmoid, **626**, *669*
sclerocorneal, 951
sternal, *177*
xiphisternal, *177*

K

Kegel exercises, 693
Keloids, 15
Keratocricoid, *1089*
Kidneys, **541**–543
arteries of, 546, *546*
calculi of, **551**–552
congenital anomalies of, **550**–551
cysts of, **549**–550

Kidneys (*Continued*)
ectopic, 551, *551*
embryology of, 552
failure of, 472
function of, 543
horseshoe, 550–551
left, *474*, *576*
lymphatic system of, *548*, **548**
nerves of, **548**–549
right, *474*, *576*
supernumerary, 550
transplantation of, **549**
veins of, **547**–548
Klinefelter syndrome, 343
Klumpke paralysis, 211
Knee joints, *705*, 836. *See also* Fossa(e), popliteal
arteries of, *804*, 844
arthroscopy, 866–867
articular surfaces, 836
articulations, 836
aspiration, 867
blood supply of, 844
bones of, *836*
bursae around, 844, *848*, 848t
capsule of, 836, 838
extensors of, 747t
extracapsular ligaments, 838
injuries, 864, *864–865*, 866
innervation, 844
ligaments of
extracapsular, 838
intra-articular, 838, **841**–844
movements, 844, *845*, 845t
posterior part of, **705**
replacement, 868, *868*
stability of, **836**
total knee replacement arthroplasty, 868
Knee region, **704**–705
Kyphoscoliosis, 117
Kyphosis, 104, 105
excessive, 115

L

Labia majora, *454*, *623*, *645*, *665*, **688**
Labia minora, *641*, *645*, *665*, **688**
Labium majus, *687*
Labium minus, *687*
Labrum
acetabular, **829**
glenoid, **279**, *281*, 298
Labyrinth
bony, *1029*, *1030*, 1031, *1034*, **1035**
cochlear, *1034*, **1035**–1036
membranous, *1034*, **1035**–1036
vestibular, *1026*, *1030*, *1034*, **1035**
Lacerations, **16**
cerebral, 943
corneal, **971**
facial, **917**
of femoral artery, 761
of palmar arches, 272
of scalp, **921**
of thoracic duct, 419
Lacrimal apparatus, *949*, **949**–951
surface anatomy of, **964**–965
Lacrimal bone, *946*
Lacrimal lake, **950**, 968
Lacrimal puncta, **950**, 968
Lacteals, **491**
Lacuna, venous, lateral, *925*, 926
Lamina
capillary, of choroid, **953**, 965, *964*
of cricoid cartilage, *1090*, *1092*, *1096*, 1098
spiral, *1036*, **1037**
of vertebral arch, *99*
Laminectomy
of cervical vertebrae, 90
of lumbar vertebrae, **90**
Langer lines. *See* Tension lines of skin
Laparoscope, 656
Laparoscopic tubal sterilization, 649
Laparoscopy, **510**
pelvic viscera examined using, **656**
tubal ligation, *650*
Laparotomy, 471
Large elastic arteries, **39**–40
Large intestine, 475, *494*, **494**, *496*
arteries of, *493*
colonoscopy of, 510, *511*
functions of, 494
lymphatic system of, 498
veins of, 498
Laryngectomy, 1112
Laryngopharynx, 1088, *1090*, *1096–1098*, 1100–1101
Laryngoscopy, 1110
Larynx, 1087–1088
age changes in, **1112–1113**
arteries of, 1094
cancer of, 1112
compartments of, *1091*
contents of, 1088
folds of, *1091*
muscles of, 1092, 1093t
nerves of, *1092*, 1095
skeleton of, *1087*, 1088
veins of, 1095
Lateral, **9**
Left venous angle, 45
Leg
arteries of, 792, *793*, 793t
compartments of
anterior, *729*, 746, *772*, 789–794, *790*
artery, 792, *796*, 796t
muscles, 790, 792, *793*, 793t
nerves, 792, *795*, 795t
infections, 807
lateral, 622t, *790*, 794, 797–798
blood vessels, 798
muscles, 794, 797–798
nerves, 798
posterior, *729*, *772*, *790*, 798–805, 799, 801
arteries, *804*, 804–805
muscle, 798, *799*, 799t, 800–802, 802, 802–804, 803
nerves, 804
deep fascia of, 728
joints of, *846*
medial, *729*, *772*
muscles of, 792, *794*
nerves of, 792, *795*, 795t
surface anatomy of, *805*, 805–806
venous return from, 809–810
Leg region, **705**
Leptomeninges, *931*
Leptomeningitis, **933**
Leptomeninx, **922**, 929
Level of consciousness, 894
Ligament(s) (in general)
accessory, **100–101**
articular, **848**
extrinsic
of acromioclavicular joint, 279, *280*
of sternoclavicular joint, 302
of temporomandibular joint, 979
gluteal, **764**
intrinsic
of arch of foot, 870
of glenohumeral joint, 281
of hip joint, *830*, 832
of knee joint, 836, 838
metatarsal, superficial transverse, *165*
skin, **15**, *15*
of subcutaneous tissue, 15, *15*
Ligament(s) (named)
acetabular, transverse, 829
acromioclavicular, **282**
superior, *276*
of acromioclavicular joint, **279**, *280*
alar, *102*, 103
rupture of, 115
anococcygeal, 85, *600*, **600**, *623*, *665*, 669, 680
anterior cruciate (ACL), *839*, *841–843*, 842
anterior talofibular, **850**
anular, of radius, **285**, *285–288*, 287
subluxation of radial head from, 300–301, 300
arcuate
lateral, *560*, **560**, 563, 566, *566*
medial, *560*, **560**, 566, *566*, 567
aryepiglottic, of larynx, **1088**, *1089*
broad, of the uterus, 601, *641*, **644**, 645
calcaneocuboid, **857**
calcaneofibular, 850, *851*, 868, *869*
cardinal, *604*, **604**, *605*, 607, 609t, 644, 646, 658, 665

carpal
  palmar, *165*, *246*
  transverse, **165**
of carpometacarpal joints, **295**
cervical
  lateral, *604*
  transverse (*see* Ligament, cardinal)
check, **960**
coccygeal, 132
collateral
  fibular (FCL), **838**, *840–843*, 859
  lateral, *837*
  radial, **285**, *290–292*, **291**, *294*
  tibial (TCL), *837*, **838**, *839–841*, 843
  ulnar, **285**, *285*, *286–287*, **291**
conoid, 149, **279**, *282*
of Cooper, 451
coraco-acromial, *202*, *276*, *280*
coracoclavicular, 149, *150*, *202*, **279**
  rupture of, 297
coracohumeral, **281**, *282*
coronary, *469*, *518*, **519**
costotransverse
  anterior, 315
  lateral, *100*, *122*, **315**, *316*, *328*
  posterior, 315
  superior, *122*, **315**, *316*
craniovertebral, *102*
crico-arytenoid, *1090*
cricothyroid, 1104
  lateral, **1088**, *1090*
  median, **1088**
cricotracheal, **1088**, *1089*
cruciate
  anterior (ACL), *839*, *841–843*, **842**
  injuries to, 865
  posterior (PCL), *802*, *839*, *841–843*, 843
  of vertebrae, *102*
deltoid, 850, *851*
denticulate, *107*, *133*
falciform, *449*, **450**, 474, *481*, *508*, 518–520, 519, 575
fovea for, **711**
fundiform, of penis, *439*, *623*, **680**
gastrocolic, **467**
gastrophrenic, **467**, *469*
gastrosplenic, *513*, 514
of glenohumeral joint, **281**–282
gluteal, 594, 764
of head of femur, **661**
hepatoduodenal, **467**, *469*, 489, 520, 521
hepatogastric, **467**, *469*, 520, *521*
humeral, transverse, *184*, **212**, *215*, 276, 281
iliofemoral, **832**
iliolumbar, **563**, *565*, 565t, 590, *591*, 592
inguinal, *435*, 437, *438*, *442*, 451, *452*, 452t, 458
interclavicular, *276*, **277**
intermetatarsal, *856*
interspinous, *100*, **101**, *140*
intertransverse, 100, *100*
intra-articular, **315**, *316*, *326*
ischiofemoral, *764*, **832**
lacunar, *450*, **451**
lateral
  of the bladder, **603**, *604*
  of temporomandibular joint, *978*, **979**
longitudinal
  anterior, *76*, **99**, *99–101*, *316*, 316t, 326, 560, 1051
  posterior, *99–101*, **100**, *107*, *109*, *122*
lumbocostal, *565*
lumbosacral, *122*
Mackenrodt, *604*, **604**
meniscofemoral, posterior, *842*, 844
metacarpal, deep transverse, *294*, **295**
metatarsal, superficial transverse, *165*, **165**
nuchal, *100*, 101, 120t, *121*, *1051*, 1052
ovarian, **453**
of ovary, **644**
palpebral
  lateral, *909*, *949*, **949**
  medial, **906**, *949*
patellar, 748, 749, 757, 758, 760, 771, *781*, *794*, *805*, 806, *837*, 838, 840, 843
pectineal, *450*, **451**
pericardiacophrenic, *368*, **368**
peritoneal, 466
phrenicocolic, *469*, 498
phrenico-esophageal, *477*, **478**
pisohamate, *261*, 291
plantar, *817*, *856*, **857**
  calcaneocuboid, **857**
  calcaneonavicular, **853**
popliteal
  arcuate, *837*, 838
  oblique, **773**, **838**
posterior cruciate (PCL), *802*, *839*, 841–843, 843
posterior sacro-iliac, **763**
posterior talofibular, **850**
Poupart, 437
pubic
  inferior, **591**, *598*, *662*, *667*
  superior, *591*, **591**
pubofemoral, **832**
puboprostatic, *603*, *604*, 622, *623*, *634*, 637
pubovesical, **603**, *605*, 622, *645*
pulmonary, *349*, **350**
radiate, *316*, 316t, *326*
radiocarpal, *229*, *241*, *246*, *292*
  dorsal, **291**
  palmar, **291**
rectal, lateral, 604, 606
retinacular, **239**
round, *449*
  of liver, 450, *519*, **520**, *614*
  of uterus, **453**, *454*, *605*, *641*, **644**, 645
sacrococcygeal, *95*
  anterior, 591, *598*
  posterior, *591*, 592
sacrogenital, **603**, *604*
sacro-iliac
  anterior, *590*, **590**, *591*
  interosseous, *590*, **590**
  posterior, *590*, **590**, *591*
sacrospinous, *590–591*, 591, *600*
sacrotuberous, 590–591, *590–591*, *662*
sphenomandibular, *978*, **979**, *984*
spiral, *1036*, **1036**
splenorenal, *493*, *513*, **514**
spring, 857 sternoclavicular
  anterior, **277**, *1085*, *1106*
  posterior, **277**
sternocostal, *313*
  radiate, *313*, *316*, **317**, 320
sternopericardial, **368**
stylohyoid, 1049, *1049*, *1067*, 1067t, *1099*, 1102t
stylomandibular, *978*, **979**, 1052
subtalar, 851
supraspinous, *100*, *140*
suspensory
  axilla, **163**, *164*, *420*
  of breast (Cooper), *334*, **334**
  of eyeball, **960**, *961*
  of lens, *952*, **954**
  of ovary, 602t, *605*, *623*, *641*, **641**, 643, 645
  of penis, *623*, **680**, *681*
talocalcaneal, 816t, *851*, *852*, 854t
talocalcaneonavicular, 852
talofibular
  anterior, **850**, *851*, 868
  posterior, **850**, *851*
talonavicular, *851*
thyro-epiglottic, **1088**, *1089*
thyrohyoid
  lateral, **1088**, *1089*
  median, **1088**, *1089*
tibiofibular, *843*, 847, **848**
transverse
  of atlas, 80, *81*, *102*, *1048*
    rupture of, 115, *115*
  of knee joint, *843*, 844
  superior, *202*
trapezoid, **279**
triangular
  left, *519*, 520
  right, **519**, *519*
umbilical
  medial, *605*, 610, *611*
  median, *449*, *461*, *605*, *623*, *632*

Ligament(s) (named) (*Continued*)
uterosacral, *605*, 644
of uterus, **644**
vestibular, **1088**, *1090*
vocal, 1088, *1089*, 1090, *1091*
Ligament(s) (of regions)
of elbow joint, *285*, **285**, *286*
of foot, 850, *851*, **853**, **854t**, 857
of hip joint, **832**, *833*
of intercarpal joints, **293**–294
of intermetacarpal joints, **295**
of knee joint
extracapsular, **838**
intra-articular, **838**, 841–844
of pelvic girdle, 589–592
of pelvis, *833*
during pregnancy, 593–594
relaxation of, 593–594
of vertebral column, *100*, *107*
of wrist, **291**
Ligamentum arteriosum, *390*, **406**, *410*, 411
Ligamentum flavum, *77*, *98*, 99, *100*, *107*, 1096
Ligamentum teres, 520
Ligamentum venosum, **520**
Ligation
of ovarian artery, **619**
of uterine tubes, 656
Limb
lower
bones of, *705*, **705**, 707
arrangement, *707*, **707**, *708*
femur, **711**, *712*, 713–715, *714*, 722
fibula, *716*, **717**, 724
foot, **718**, *719*, *720*, 720–721
grafts, 724–725
hip, **708**–709, *709*
ilium, **709**, *710*, 711
patella, *715*, **715**
surface anatomy of, **713**–715
tibia, **715**–717, *716*, 722, *723*
buds, **705**
calcaneal fractures, 725
compartment syndromes, 741
contusions, **759**
coxa vara and valga, 722
cutaneous innervation, 734, *734*, 735t–736t, 736, *738*
dermatomes of, 564, *565*, **734**, *735*
development, **705**, *706*
epiphysial plates, 724
fascia, 728, *729*
fasciotomy, 741
foot (*see* Foot)
free, 704, *705*
injuries, 721
intraosseous infusion, 725
joints (*see also specific joint*)
ankle, 849–851, *850*, *851*, 868, *869*
arthroscopy of knee joint, *866*, 866–867
aspiration of knee joint, 867
bipedalism, 861
bursitis in knee region, 867
claw toes, 870, *870*
clubfoot, **870**, *871*
congruity of articular surfaces, 861
dislocation of hip, 862–863
foot, 851–859, 852, 853, 854t, 855, 855t, 856, 857, 858
fractures of femoral neck, 861–862
genu valgum and varum, 863
hallux valgus, 868–869, *869*
hammer toe, 869, *870*
hip, 828–836, 829, 830, 831, 833, 834, 835
knee, 836, 836–845, 837, 839–843, 845, 845t, 864, 864–865, 866, 868
necrosis of femoral head, in children, 862
patellar dislocation, 864
patellofemoral syndrome, 864
pes planus, 870
popliteal cysts, 867, *868*
surgical hip replacement, 862
tibial nerve entrapment, 868
tibiofibular, 845–849, *846*, *847*, 848, 848t
leg (*see* Leg)
lymphatic systems, 733, 733, *733*
lymph nodes, **742**
metatarsals, fractures of, 725–726, 726
motor innervation, 734, *737*
nerves of, 735t–736t, 734, *734*
os trigonum, 726, *727*
overview of, 704–705
popliteal fossa (*see* Fossa, popliteal)
proximal, organization of, 745–746
regional nerve blocks of, **742**
regions of, 536, *536*, 742
saphenous cutdown injury, **741**–742
saphenous nerve injury, **741**–742
saphenous vein grafts, **741**
sensory function abnormalities, **742**
sesamoid bones, fracture of, 726, *727*
subcutaneous tissue, 728
talar neck, fractures of, 725
thrombophlebitis, **741**
thrombosis, **741**
upper limb *vs*, **148**–149
varicose veins, **741**, *741*
veins of
deep, 731
superficial, 728, *729*, *741*, 731, *733*
upper
arm (*see* Arm)
arteries of (*see* Arteries, axillary)
axilla, **193**
apex of, 193, *194*
arteries of (*see* Arteries, axillary)
base of, 193, *194*
boundaries of, *194–195*
brachial plexus (*see* Plexus, brachial)
contents of, *195*
lymph nodes of (*see* Lymph nodes, axillary)
surface anatomy of, 186, 188
veins of, *199*
walls of, 178, 193, *194*
bones of, 149–162 (*see also specific bone*)
brachial plexus (*see* Plexus, brachial)
compartments of, *165*
cutaneous nerves of, 169
dermatomes of, 170, *173*, 173t
fascia of, 164–165, *165* forearm (*see* Forearm)
hand (*see* Hand)
joints of, 276–301
lower limb *vs*., **148**–149
lymphatic system of, *167*, 167
lymph nodes of (*see* Lymph nodes, axillary)
muscles of (*see also specific muscle*)
axio-appendicular, 176, 177t, *178*, 179–182
innervation of, 203t–204t
scapulohumeral, 182–185
nerves of, *167*, 203t–204t
regions of, 147, *148*
segments of, 147, *148*
superficial veins of, 165–166, *166*
veins of, 165–166, *166*, *243*
Limbus
corneal, 964
sphenoidal, *889*, **890**
Line(s), **22**
anocutaneous, *669*
anorectal, *669*
arcuate, *440*, **441**, *449*, 586, *587*
of arrested growth, 25
axial, **734**
axillary
anterior, *339*, **339**
posterior, *339*, **339**, *356*
costal, 347
left, *346*
dentate, 675
epiphysial, 23, 25
gluteal, **709**
anterior, *708*
inferior, *708*
posterior, *708*, *710*
intercondylar, *712*
intertrochanteric, *708*, **713**, *833*
jugular, *433*
median
anterior, *339*, **339**
posterior, **339**

midaxillary, **339**
midclavicular, *339*, **339**, *433*, 435, *480*
mucocutaneous, 675
Nélaton, *780*, *781*
nuchal
inferior, *127*, 127t
superior, *129*, 129t
oblique, *1067*, 1067t, *1089*
posterior, *150*
paravertebral, *356*
pectinate, *669*, **672**, 675
pectineal, *712*, **713**
pelvic pain, 618, 642, 649, 656, *681*
of pleural reflection, 346
scapular, *329*, *339*, *356*
semilunar, **433**, **459**
soleal, *21*, *708*, *716*, **718**, *800*
spino-umbilical, **435**, 447, 509
spiral, **713**
sternal, 346, **347**
supracondylar
lateral, *708*, *712*, **713**
medial, *708*, *712*, **713**, *754*
tarsometatarsal, **718**
temporal, *881*
inferior, *780*, *880*, *883*, **886**
superior, *780*, *880*, *883*, **886**
tension, 14, *14*
trapezoid, **149**
vertebral, **347**
vertical, *708*
Z-, *477*, **478**
Linea alba, *434*, **435**, *437–438*, 439, *439*, 440, 440–441, 459, 623, 681
Linea aspera, **713**
Linea nigra, **459**
Linea semilunaris, *458*
Linea terminalis, **586**
Lingula, *345*, *346*, *348*, *349*, **350**
Lip(s), **987**–988
cleft, *1006*, **1006**
cyanosis of, **1006**
ileocolic, *496*
lateral, **713**
medial, **713**
muscles of, **903**–905
squamous cell carcinoma of, **921**
Liposuction, 445
Lithotripsy, 552, 631
Liver
arteries of, 524
bare area of, *518*, **519**
bile flow in, *525*
biopsy of, **536**
blood flow in, 530
blood vessels of, **524**
cirrhosis of, 502, **535**–536, 676
computed tomography of, *576*
functions of, 517
innervation of, **524**, *526*, 526–527
left, **521**
lobectomy, 534
lobes of, *519*, *520*, **520**, *544*, *578*
lymphatic system, **524**, *526*, 526–527
nerves of, 526, *528*
parasympathetic stimulation, 65t
right, **521**
rupture of, **534**
segmentectomy, 524, **533**–534
subdivisions of, **521**, 523t, 524
surfaces of
diaphragmatic, *469*, 519, *519*
visceral, *469*, **520**
sympathetic stimulation, 65t
ultrasound of, *575*
veins of, 524
weight of, 517
Lobe(s)
of brain, **935**, *936*, *941*, *1022*
frontal, **935**, *936*, *941*, *1022*
of liver, *519*, *520*, **520**
of lung
azygos, 360
inferior, *348*
right lower, *356*
right middle, *356*
right upper, *356*
superior, *348*
variations in, **360**
occipital, **935**, *936*, *1130*
parietal, **935**, *936*
of prostate gland, **637**
temporal, **935**, 936, *936*, *941*, 1152
Lobectomy, 361, 534
Lobule(s)
of auricle, *1026*
of ear, 1026
fat, of breast, *334*
mammary gland, **334**
Locomotion, 74
Locomotor apparatus/system, **5**
Longitudinal sections, *6*, *7*
Long plantar ligament, **857**
Lordosis, 104, 105, 115, *116*, 445
Low back pain, 108
Lumbar spinal puncture, **140**, *140*
Lumina, 37
Luminal blood, **397**
Lumpectomy, 342
Lunate, *154* **154**, *274*, *290*
avascular necrosis of, 301
dislocation of, 301
Lung(s), 18, 366
apex of, *346*, *348*, **348**, *368*
appearance of, **360–361**
arteries of, **353**
auscultation of, 360
base of, **350**
border of, anterior, **350**
carbon particles inhaled into, **360–361**
collapse of, *358*, **358–359**
costal surfaces of, *348*, **350**
decortication of, 360
development of, 371
function of, 348
hilum of, 344, *349*, **350**
internal structure of, *352*
irritants inhaled into, **360–361**
left, *390*, *420*, 422, *423*, *431*
apex of, *346*
cardiac notch of, *346*
costal surfaces of, *348*
inferior lobe of, *348*
lobes of, *348*, **350**, *352*
lower, *356*
lobes of
right lower, *356*
right middle, *356*
right upper, *356*
superior, *348*, *348*
variations in, **360**
lymphatic system of, 354–355, *355*
mediastinal surface of, *348*, **350**
nerves of, **355–356**, *356*
organization of, *352*
parasympathetic stimulation, 64t
percussion of, *361*, **361**
resection of, **361**
right, *390*, *420*, 422, *423*
costal surfaces of, *348*
lobes of, **350**, *352*
roots of, 344, *348–349*, **350**
surface anatomy of, **356, 358**
sympathetic stimulation, 65t
vasculature of, **353–355**
veins of, *354*
Lunule, **383**, *385*, 394
Lymph, 43, 45
Lymphadenitis, 46
Lymphadenopathy, 827
Lymphangitis, 46
Lymphatic capillaries, 43
Lymphatic plexuses, 43
Lymphatic system, **4**
of abdominal wall
anterolateral, 443
posterior, *569*, **569**–570
of anal canal, **672–673**
of appendix, **498**
of auricle, **1026**–1027, *1028*
of bile duct, *527*, 529
of breasts, 335, *337*
of cecum, 498
of cervical region, lateral, 1064–1065
components of, *43–45*, *44*
of diaphragm, *562*
disorders of, 46
of ductus deferens, 661
of duodenum, 490
of ejaculatory ducts, 661
of face, **915**, *916*
of foot, 822, *824*
functions of, 43, 45

Lymphatic system (*Continued*)
- of gallbladder, 527–529, *528*
- of gluteal region, 778
- of head, *1105*
- of heart, 389
- of kidneys, *548*, **548**
- of large intestine, *501*
- of liver, **524**, *526*, 526–527
- of lower limb, 733–734
- of lungs, 354–355, *355*
- of neck, *1105*, **1105–1106**
- of pancreas, *517*
- of pelvis, 613–614, *615*
- of pleurae, 354–355, *355*
- of rectum, **659**–661
- of scalp, **915**, *916*
- of scrotum, *455*, **678**
- of seminal glands, *659*
- of small intestine, *486*
- of spleen, *517*
- Starling hypothesis applied to, 43
- of stomach, 482, *486*
- of suprarenal glands, *548*, **548**
- of testis, 455
- of thigh, 778
- of thyroid gland, 1085
- of tongue, **1000**, *1003*
- of upper limb, *167*, **167,** 168, *169*
- of ureters, *548*, **548**–549, 621, *632*
- of urethra, male, *659*, 661, **677**
- of urinary bladder, *632*
- of uterus, *659*, 661
- of vagina, *659*, 661
- of vulva, 690

Lymphatic trunks, 43

Lymphatic vessels, **43**
- deep, *44*
- superficial, 44, 45, **733**

Lymphedema, 46, 340

Lymph nodes, 45, *404*
- aortic arch, *355*
- apical, **199**, *200*, *337*
- axillary, *161*, 195, *337*, 443, *443*
  - anterior, **198**, *200*
  - apical, **167**, *169*
  - central, *169*, *200*
  - dissection of, 209
  - enlargement of, 209
  - humeral, *167*, **167**, 199, *200*
  - lateral, *167*, **167**
  - pectoral, 171, **198**, *200*
  - posterior, **199**, *200*
  - subscapular, *171*, **199**, *200*
- brachiocephalic, *412*, 1085
- bronchomediastinal, **355**
- bronchopulmonary, *349*, **354**, *355*
- buccal, *916*, *1028*
- cancer metastasis via, 45–46
- celiac, 478, *490*, 491, 517, 529, *562*, *569*
- central, *337*
  - superior, **491**, *494*
- cervical
  - deep, 915, 916, 974, 1002, 1003, 1028, 1047, 1063, 1086, 1095, 1104, 1105
    - inferior, *337*, *355*, **1002**, *1003*, 1085, 1086, 1095, 1105
  - superficial, *916*, *974*, **1027**, *1028*, *1086*, 1105
- clavicular, **198**
- colic
  - intermediate, 498
  - middle, *494*, **498**
  - right, *494*, **498**
- cubital, *161*, 162, *163*, *220*
- cystic, 527, *527*, 529, *569*
- deep inguinal, **734**
- deep popliteal, **789**
- deltopectoral, *167*, **167**, *169*
- diaphragmatic
  - anterior, **560**, *562*
  - posterior, **560**, *562*
- epicolic, *501*
- gastric, **482**, *486*
  - left, 478, *479*, 526
- gastro-omental, **482**, *486*, 505
- gluteal, **778**
- hepatic, 517, **524**, 527, *527*, 529, *562*, 569
- humeral, *200*, *337*
- ileocolic, **491**, *494*, 498
- iliac
  - common, 548, *569*, 569–570, **613**, 615, 659–660
  - external, *569*, **613**, *615*, *659–660*
  - internal, *569*, **613**, *615*, *659–660*, 672, 677
- lateral, 708, 716, 717, 717–720, 724, *782*, 789, 791, 794, 795t, 797, 798, 805, 806, 811, 820t, 825, *826*, *846–853*, 859, *860*, 868, 869
- medial, 708, 716, 717, 717–720, 724, 728, 730, 733, 742, 758, *782*, 789, 791, 798, *803*, 804, 805, 806, *810*–811, 816, 819, 820t, *823*, 824, 825, *826*, *846–853*, 856, 859, 860, 868, 869
- infraclavicular, **199**, *200*, *337*
- infrahyoid, *1003*, *1105*
- inguinal, *438*
  - deep, *659–660*, 677
  - enlarged, 742
  - superficial, *443*, **443**, *659*, 673, 678, 691t, 692, 733
- interpectoral, *190*, *337*
- intrapulmonary, *355*
- jugulodigastric, *1003*, **1103**, *1105*
- jugulo-omohyoid, *1003*, 1004, *1028*, *1105*
- juxta-intestinal, **491**, *494*, 498
- lumbar, 456, 560, *569*, 570, *615*, 659–660
- mastoid, *911*, *916*, *1028*
- mediastinal, posterior, *412*, 413–414, 560, 562
- mesenteric, **491**, *494*
  - inferior, 498, *499*, *569*, *615*, *659–660*
  - superior, 490, 491, 498, 491, *569*
- occipital, *916*, *1028*, *1105*
- pancreaticoduodenal, **482**, *486*, *490*, 517, 527
- pancreaticosplenic, 482, *486*, *490*, 514, 517
- paracolic, **498**
- pararectal, **613**, *659–660*
- parasternal, *325*, *337*, *412*, **443**, 526, 560, 562
- paratracheal, *355*, **1085**, *1086*, *1094*, 1095, 1101, 1104
- parotid, **915**, 974, *978*, *1028*, *1105*
- pectoral, 335, *337*
- phrenic, **526**, *569*
- popliteal, *43*, *733*, **734**, 822, *824*
  - deep, **789**
  - fossa, 789, **789**
  - superficial, **789**
- pre-aortic, 458
- prelaryngeal, **1085**, *1086*
- pretracheal, **1085**, *1086*, *1094*, 1095
- pulmonary, **354**, *355*
- pyloric, **482**, *486*, 490, *490*, 505, *527*
- retro-auricular, *1105*
- retropharyngeal, *916*, *1003*, *1028*, *1105*
- sacral, **613**, *615*, *659–660*
- sentinel, 365
- splenic, *490*
- submandibular, **915**, *916*, 988, *988*, 993, 1002, 1003, 1028, 1063, 1064, 1072, 1086, 1105
- submental, **915**, *916*, 988, *988*, *1003*, 1028, 1064, 1065, 1072, 1086, 1105
- subscapular, *337*
- superficial inguinal, **733**
- superficial popliteal, **789**
- superior, *562*
- supraclavicular, *337*, 365, 1106
- tracheobronchial, *411*, *412*
  - inferior, **354**, *355*, **389**
  - superior, **354**, *355*

Lymphocytes, 45

Lymphoid organs, 45

Lymphoid system, *43*–46, *44*

M

Macula lutea, 954

Magnetic resonance imaging (MRI), 69–73, *71*
- of larynx, *1091*
- of pelvis, **693–697**
- of thorax, *424*

Malar flush, 895

Malleolar mortise, **848**

Malleolus, **22**

lateral, 715, 716, 717, 717–720, 724, 731, *782*, 789, 791, 794, 795t, 797, 798, 805, 806, 811, 820t, 825, *826*, *846–902*, 859, *860*, 868, 869
medial, 708, 716, 717, 717–720, 724, 728, 730, 732, 742, 758, *782*, 789, 791, 798, 846, 804, 805, 806, *810*–811, 816, 819, 820t, *823*, 824, 825, *826*, *846–902*, 856, 859, 860, 866, 869
Malleus, *1026*, 1027, *1029*, *1030*, **1031**
Mammography, *341*, 342
Mandible, *880*, *881*, *883*, **885**, 903t, *904*, 909t, 911, 1026, 1087
changes in face and, *898*
development of, *897*
fracture of, 895, *895*
movements of, *979*, 979t
muscles that move, *981*, 981t
temporomandibular joint and, 1026, 975–980
Manubrium, 147, 177, 309, 313, **314**, 314–315, 316, 321, 725, 1029, 1039, 1047, 1105, 1064

Margins
costal, *309*, **310**, *311*, *314*, 336, 338, 338, 458, 578
falciform, **728**, *730*
infra-orbital, **885**
orbital, lateral, **893**
supra-orbital, **885**, *885*
Mastectomy, 342
Mastoiditis, 1039
Matter
gray, **47**
white, **47**, *49*
Maxilla, **1011**–1012, *1013*
MCP joint(s). *See* Metacarpophalangeal joint(s)
Meatus
acoustic
external, *911*, 1026, *1028*, 1027, 1027, 1029, 1068
internal, *1026*, 1027, *1029*, *1032*, 1033, 1034, 1035, 1036
internal, 1142
nasal
common, **1019**
inferior, *1017*, **1019**, *1022*
middle, *1017*, **1018**
superior, *1017*, **1018**
Medial, **7**
Median cubital veins, *166*, **165**, *169*
Median episiotomy, 674
Median sternotomy, **320**
Mediastinal shift, 361
Mediastinal silhouettes, *420*
Mediastinoscopy, **372**
Mediastinotomy, 418
Mediastinum, *419*, 367, *477*
anterior, *368*, **414**, 417
base of, *347*
biopsy of, 372
central, **361**
inferior, **367**, *368*
levels of, *368*
middle, **367**, *368*
overview, 367, 374
posterior, *368*, **404**
autonomic nerves of, 414, *414*
blood vessels of, 413–414
contents of, 404–414
esophagus, **408**, 412
nerves of, 414
thoracic aorta, 408–410
thoracic duct, **411**
subdivisions of, *368*
superior, **367**, *368*, **402**
autonomic nerves of, *414*
boundaries of, *402*
contents of, 402–414
dissection of, *404*, *414*
esophagus, **408**
great vessels of, **403–404**
nerves in, **404–406**
thymus, **402**, *403*
trachea, **406**, 422
viscera relative to, **371–372**
widening of, **372**
Mediolateral episiotomy, 674, *674*
Medium veins, **41**
Medulla oblongata, **130**, *893*, **935**, *936*, 1087
Medulla, suprarenal, **515**
parasympathetic stimulation, 65t
sympathetic stimulation, 65t
Membrane
atlanto-occipital, *101–103*
anterior, *101*, *102–103*
posterior, *101*, *102–103*, *127*, 127t
basilar, *1036*, **1037**
costocoracoid, **164**, *164*
cricovocal, **1088**
fibro-elastic, of larynx, **1088**
intercostal
external, **324**, *326*
internal, **324**, *326*
interosseous, **153**, 154, *229*
mucous, *1089*
obturator, *591*, **627**, *598*
perineal, *604*, *623*, *627*, *665*, *667*, 668, 680, 688, 677
quadrangular, **1088**, *1088–1089*, *1110*
suprapleural, **327**, **361**, *362*, **346**
synovial
of hip joint, 832
inferior, **975**
of knee joint, 838
superior, **975**
of temporomandibular joint, **975**
tectorial, *102*, **103**, **1037**, *1037*
thyrohyoid, **1088**, *1089*, 1101
tympanic, 1026, **1027**, *1029*
perforation of, 1039
secondary, *1034*, **1035**
vestibular, *1036*, **1037**
Ménière syndrome, 1040
Meninges, *901*, **922**
arachnoid mater (*see* Arachnoid mater)
development of, **139**–140
dura mater (*see* Dura mater)
function of, 922
layers of, 922
pia mater (*see* Pia mater)
spaces, **928**
spinal, 134, 136
Meningitis, 134
Menisci, movements of, **844**
Meniscus
of knee joint, 840, 844
lateral, *843*, 844
medial, *843*, 844
movements of, 844
tears of, *865*
medial, **844**
Mesenchyme, 22
Mesentery, **466**, *467*, *488*, 491
Mesiodens, 1007, *1008*
Meso-appendix, 466, *496*, 497
Mesocolon
descending, *493*
sigmoid, *487*, *493*, **500**
transverse, 466, *468*, **469**, 489, *493*, 498, 544
Mesopneumonium, 350
Mesosalpinx, **642**, 644, *647*
Mesovarium, 644
Metacarpals, *149*, 154
2nd, *290*
3rd, *238*, *290*
4th, *290*
5th, *290*
fracture of, 163
general images of, *20*
radiographs of, *290*
Metaphysis, 23 Metastasis
of breast carcinoma, 340
of bronchogenic carcinoma, 366
hematogenous, 366
of liver, 533
lymphogenic, 341
methods of, 45–46
of scrotal cancer, 463
of testicular cancer, 463
Metatarsal
1st, **718**
2nd, **718**
4th, 726
5th, **720**
fractures of, 725–726, *726*

Metatarsal (*Continued*)
  head of, *720*
  shaft of, 720
Metatarsus, **718**, 720
Micturition, 624
Midbrain, **935**, *936*, *1071*
Midfoot, **811**
Midgut, 507, **507**, *508*
Midswing, **745**
Modiolus, 903t, **905**, **1035**, *1036*
Monro-Kellie doctrine, **937**
Mons pubis, 373, *662*, **687**, *697*
Motion sickness, 1040
Motor fibers, 50
Motor nerves, 35
Motor system, somatic, **58**
Motor unit, 34, *34*
Mouth, muscles of, **903**–905
Movement terms, **8**, *9–10*, 11
Mucosa
  alveolar, *988*, *989*, **990**
  labial, 988
  nasal, **1016**
  olfactory, *1129*
  oral, *988*
  palatine, *988*
Multibellied muscles, 33
Multipolar motor neurons, 46
Mumps, 985
Murmurs, 396
Muscle(s) (in general)
  abdominal, *322*
  agonist, **35**
  antagonist, **35**
  arteries to, 35
  axio-appendicular
    anterior, 173, *174*, 174t
    posterior
      deep, 180–182
      superficial, 179–180, *179*
  bipennate, *31*, 33
  cardiac striated, 30t, **31**, **37**
  circular, 33
  contraction of, 33–36
  convergent, 33
  detrusor, **624**
  dorsiflexor, *18*
  dysfunction of, 36
  electromyography of, 35–36
  evertor, *18*
  extensor, 32
  extra-ocular, **955**–961
  fixators, **35**
  flat, *31*, **31**
  flexor, *32*
  functions of, 35
  fusiform, *31*, **33**
  gluteal, 766–767
  guarding of, 446
  hamstring, *767*, **770**, *771*, *772*
  hyoid, 1065
  hyperplasia, of smooth, 37
  hypertrophy, of myocardium, 37
  infrahyoid, 979t, 980, *981*
  insertion, 33
  involuntary, 37
  of mastication, 980, 982t
  motor unit of, **34**
  of mouth, **903**–905
  multibellied, 33
  multiheaded, 33
  multipennate, 33
  myocardial infarction, 37
  nerves to, 35
  origin, 33
  paralysis of, **918**
  pennate, 33
  phasic contraction, 33
  plantar flexor, *18*
  prevertebral, 1138
  prime mover, 35
  "pulled," 36
  quadrate, 33
  reflexive contraction, 33
  scapulohumeral, 182, 281
  shunt, **35**
  skeletal striated, **37**
    absence of tone, 36
    architecture and shape, *31*
    belly of, *31*
    cardiac muscle *vs.*, 37
    characteristics of, 30t
    concentric contractions of, **34**
    contraction, 33, 33–34, *34*
    dysfunction, 36
    eccentric contractions of, **34**, 36
    elongation of, 36
    form and features of, 31, 33
    functions, 34
    growth and regeneration of, 36
    isometric contractions of, **33**
    isotonic contractions of, **33**
    nerves and arteries, 35
    paralysis, 36
    phasic contraction of, 33–34
    pulled, 36, *36*
    reflexive contraction of, 33
    regeneration of, 36
    satellite cells of, 36
    shape of, 29, *31*
    soreness, 36
    superficial, *32*
    testing, 35–36
    tonic contraction of, 333
  smooth, **31**, 37
    characteristics of, 30t, 37
    hyperplasia of, 37
    hypertrophy of, 37
  sphincteral, 33
  spurt, **35**
  stretching of, 36
  suboccipital, *127*, 127t
  suprahyoid, 980, *981*, 982t
  synergist, **35**
  thoraco-appendicular, 173, *322*
  tonic contraction, 33
  types, 29–30, 30t, 31
  unipennate, *31*, 33
Muscle(s) (named)
  abdominal, transverse, *325*, 439, *440*, 452t
  abductor digiti minimi, *248*, 261t, *261*, 261
  abductor hallucis, *719*, *773*, *795*, 795t, 814, 814t, 817, 837
  abductor pollicis brevis, *258*, *259*, **259**, 260t
  abductor pollicis longus, *230*, *234*, 235t, 236, 237, 240, 240
  adductor brevis, 749, 751, *773*
  adductor hallucis, *719*, *754*, *815*, 815t, 817
  adductor longus, *125*
  adductor magnus, 750t, 751, *766*, *768*, 773, 782, 834, 837, 840
  adductor pollicis, *236*, *257*, *258*, *259*, 260, 261, 270
  anconeus, *151*, *207*, *215*, **216**–217, 216t, 234, 236
  arrector of hairs (pili), *12*, **13**
  articular, of knee, 749, *749*
  arytenoid
    lateral, 1092, *1092*
    oblique, **1092**, 1093t
    posterior, *1092*, 1094
    transverse, **1092**, 1093t
  auricular, *978*, *1028*
    anterior, *1022*
    superior, **900**
  biceps brachii, 32, *173*, *179*, *195*, *198*, 197, 212, 213, 214, 214, 215, 215t, 218, 219, 223, 276
    reflex testing of, 224
    surface anatomy of, 220
    tendinitis of, 224
  biceps femoris, *766 766*, *771*, 771t, 773, 784, 788, 801, 840–841
  brachialis, *207*, **214**, *215*, 215t, *223*, 229, 241, 246
  brachioradialis, *207*, *216*, *218*, **222**, *227*, 234t, 235, 236, 241, 246, 266
  buccinator, *902*, 903t, **904**, *905*, *907*, 977, 977, 984, 988, 1022
  bulbospongiosus, 646, 647, 664, 680, **682**, 683t, *689*
  chondroglossus, *1067*, 1067t
  ciliary, **956**, *966*, *1134*
  coccygeus, **597**, *598–599*, 602, *615*
  compressor urethrae, *667*, 683t
  constrictor
    inferior, **1101**, 1102t, 1103
    middle, *902*, *1100*, **1101**, 1102t, 1103
    superior, *1098*, 1102t, 1103

coracobrachialis, 178t, *178*, *207*, *213*, 214, 214, 215, 215, 215t
corrugator supercilii, *902*, *905*
cremaster, *438*, *452*, **455**
crico-arytenoid
lateral, 1093t
posterior, 1093t
cricopharyngeus, *477*, *1087*
cricothyroid, *1085*, 1092t, **1094**
dartos, **455**, *665*
deltoid, 32, 118, *178*, 179, 182–179, 179, 180, 184, *181*, 186, 187, 187, *188*, 191, *194*, 198, 198, *204*, *207*, *216*, *223*, *280*, *281*, 297, 1059
depressor anguli oris, *902*, 903t, *905*, *911*
depressor labii superioris, *902*, *905*
detrusor, *624*, **624**
digastric, *129*, 127t, 437, *928*, *977*, 982t, 984, 1022, 1032, 1065, 1066, 1067–1068, 1067t, 1079, 1100–1101
dilator pupillae, *952*, *953*, **953**, *966*
endometrium, *641*, *644*, *734*
epicranius, **900**
erector spinae, **120**, 121t, *125*, 126
extensor carpi radialis brevis, *207*, *235*, 235t, 236, 238, 266, 293
extensor carpi radialis longus, *207*, *235*, 235t, 236, 266, 293
extensor carpi ulnaris (ECU), *207*, *235*, 235t, 237, 238, 239, 261, 261, 293
extensor digiti minimi, *207*, *234*, 234t, 235, 236, 239, 245, 266, 293
extensor digitorum, (ED)238, *207*, *235*, 235t, 236, 239, 241, 293
extensor digitorum brevis (EDB), *791*, *794*, 816, 820t, 825, 826
contusion of, 826
innervation of, *207*
extensor digitorum longus, (EDL) *207*, 792, 791, 816, 825, 904, 904t
extensor hallucis brevis (EHB), *791*, *794*, **816**
extensor hallucis longus (EHL), *790*, 792, 794t, 806, 816t, 825
extensor indicis, *207*, *234*, 234t, 236, 237, 293
extensor pollicis brevis (EPB), *207*, *234*, 235t, 236, 237, 240, 266, 274, 293
extensor pollicis longus (EPL), *207*, *234*, 235t, *236*, *237*, **240**, *266*, 274
fibularis brevis (FB), *726*, *782*, *790*, 793t, 795t 798, 846, 806, 826, 851
fibularis longus (FL), *726*, *790*, 793t, 794, 795, 795t, 805, 792, 856
fibularis tertius, *726*, *790*, **792**, 793t, *793*
flexor carpi radialis (FCR), *207*, *218*, 229, 230, 231, 231t, 232, 241, 246, 248, 259, 261, 263, 266, 274, 292, 299
flexor carpi ulnaris (FCU), *207*, *229*, 231, 231t, 233, 245, 246, 251, 252, 266, 269, 299
flexor digiti minimi, *719*, *814*, *815*, 815t, 818
flexor digiti minimi brevis, 260t, *261*, **261**
flexor digitorum brevis (FDB), *795*, *814*, 814t, *815*, *817*, *818*, *807*
flexor digitorum longus (FDL), *719*, *790*, *795*, 795t, 799t, *800*, 800t, 801, 846, 814, 814t, 818, 852
flexor digitorum profundus (FDP), *207*, *207*, *229*, *231*, 232t, **233**, *238*, 241, 259, 261, 263, 266, 274
flexor digitorum superficialis (FDS), 261, *207*, *229*, *231*, 231t, **233**, 241, 246, 258, 259, 263, 266, 274
flexor hallucis brevis (FHB), *846*, *815*, 815t, 819,
flexor hallucis longus (FHL), 718, 744, 744t, 802, 801 846, 851
flexor pollicis brevis (FPB), 257, **259**, 258t
flexor pollicis longus (FPL), *207*, *229*, 231, 232t, 233, 241, 246, 259, 261, 263, 266
gastrocnemius, 32, *731*, *781*, *782*, 786, 787, 795t, 800, 801, 802, 804, 808
fabella in, 808
strain of, 806
gemellus
inferior, *765*, 765t, *768*, 776, *831*
superior, 765t, *768*, 776, *831*
genioglossus, *994*, *1001–1002*, 1001t, *1004*, *1022*, 1148
paralysis of, **1109**
geniohyoid, 982t, *994*, *1001*, *1002*, *1004*, 1022, 1062–1063, 1067, 1067t, 1070, 1096, 1098
gluteal, **763**, 764, 765t
gluteus maximus, *118–122*, *133*, *125*, *617*, 688, 695
gluteus medius, *119*, *125*, *577*
gluteus minimus, 781, 834
gracilis, *32*, 750t, *751*, *758*, *766*, *767*, 773, 788, 794, 840
transplantation of, 760
hamstrings, 770, 781
biceps femoris, *32*, *766*, *768*, *771*, 771t, 733
injuries to, 781
semimembranosus, *32*, *766*, *768*, *771*, 771t, 782, 801, 805
semitendinosus, *32*, 766, *768*, 770, 771, 771t, 782 , 801
hyoglossus, *1001*, 1001t, *1003*, *1004*, *1063*, 1067, 1067t, 1150
hypothenar, *32*, *261*, *274*
iliacus, *450*, **565**, 565t, *577*, *661*, *731*
iliococcygeus, *598–599*, **600**, *663*
iliocostalis, *119*, 120, 121t, *125*
cervicis, *121*
lumborum, *121*
thoracis, *121*
iliopsoas, *449*, **565**, 565t
infrahyoid, *32*, 980, 982t, **1066**, 1092
infraspinatus, *32*, *179*, 180t, **181**, *181*, 194, 207, 216, 281
intercostal
external, *133*, *322*, *323*, 323t, **324**, 328, 496, 1059
innermost, *323*, **324**, *326*, *328*
internal, *323*, 323t, **324**, *325*, *496*
movement of, 324
internal, *118*, *125*
interossei
dorsal, of foot, *815*, 815t, *816*
dorsal, of hand, *207*, *259*, 260t, *262*, 262
palmar, *207*, *259*, **263**
plantar, *207*, *259*, 260t, *262*, **262**
interspinales, *121*, **122**, *123*, 123t
intertransversarii, **122**, *123*, 123t
intrinsic, of tongue, **1000**, *1001*
ischiocavernosus, *664*, *680*, **682**, 684t, 689
ischiococcygeus, *663*
latissimus dorsi, 118, 126, 173, 179, 180t, *180*, *182*, *179*, *184*, *186*, 187, 189, 194, 213, 214, 223, 322, 542, 563, 564
levator anguli oris, 903t
levator ani, 597, *597*, *598–600*, 599, 605, 629, 634, 661, 663, 680, 731–695, 697
levator costarum, *122–123*, 123t, 323t, 324, 328
levator labii superioris, *902*, *912*
levator labii superioris alaeque nasii, 902, 903t, 912
levator palpebrae superioris, *951*, *949*, 950, 956, 957, 957t, 961, 1018, 1022, 1134
levator scapulae, 55, *118–119*, **180**, 180t, 182, 183, 184, 196, 205, 207, 208, 208 1057–1059, 1078
levator veli palatini, *902*, 978, *997*, 997t, 998, 988, 1042, 1102t
long flexors, of foot and ankle, *18*
longissimus, *119*, 120t, *129*, 129t
longitudinal, of tongue
inferior, **1000**, *1001*, 1002t
superior, **1000**, *1001*, 1002t
longus capitis, 1053, 1138t, *1078–1079*
longus colli, *408*, *1051*, 1053, 1138t, 1078–1079

Muscle(s) (named) (*Continued*)
- lumbricals, *238*, 260t, **262**
- masseter, *902*, *977*, 982t, *984*, *1022*
- mentalis, *902*, 903t, *905*
- multifidus, *121*, *121–122*, *123*, 123t
- musculus uvulae, *997*, 997t, *998*
- mylohyoid, *902*, 982t, *994*, *1001*, *1047*, 1063, 1065, 1070, 1096, 1098
- myometrium, *641*, **644**, *734*
- nasalis
  - alar part of, *902*
  - procerus plus transverse part of, 903t, *905*
- oblique
  - external, *118*, *125*, 322, *327*, 339, 435, 435–439, 436t, 452, 458, 542, 564
  - inferior
    - of the eyeball, *949*, *959*, *1018*
    - of the head, *127*, 127t
  - internal, *435*, 436t, **439**, *439*, *452*, 542, 564, 566
  - superior
    - of the eyeball, *949*, *1018*, *1134*
    - of the head, *127*, 127t
- obliquus capitis
  - inferior, *127*, 127t, **128**, *129*
  - superior, *127*, 127t, *129*
- obturator externus, *750*, 750t, **751**, *768*, 769, 770
- obturator internus, 597, *598–600*, *629*, 661, 655, 731–695, 697
- occipitofrontalis, **900**, *905*
  - frontal belly of, *901*, *902*, *911*
  - occipital belly of, *902*, *911*
- omohyoid, 982t, *1047*, 1053, *1055*, 1055t, 1057, 1058, 1062, 1065, 1066, 1067–1068, 1067t, 1070, 1088, 1106, 1150
- opponens digiti minimi, *261*, **261**
- opponens pollicis, *259*, **259**, 260t
- orbicularis oculi, *902*, **903**, **905**, *905*, 906, 911, 951, 977, 984
- orbicularis oris, *902*, 903t, *905*, *977*
- palatoglossus, *996*, *997*, 997t, *999*
- palatopharyngeus, *997*, 997t, *999*, *1098*, 1101, 1102t
- palmaris brevis, *207*, *229*, *246*, *256*, 258, 261
- palmaris longus, *206*, *229*, *230*, 231t, 232–234, 241, 248, 261, 266, 274, 295
- papillary
  - anterior, **381**, 383, *382*, *389*
  - posterior, **381**, 383, *382*
  - septal, **381**
- pectinate, *381*, 383
- pectineus, *450*, *695*, *697*
- pectoralis major, 157, *159*, 164, **167**, *169*, 173, 174, 174t, 173, 179, *194*, 195, 198, 198, 199, 204, *214*, 322, *334*, *336*, 339, *339*, 440, 1058
- pectoralis minor, 164, 169, 173, 174, 174t, *191*, *194*, *195*, *198*, *198*, 200, 201, 204, 208, 214, 276, 322, 334, 336
- perineal
  - deep transverse, *634*, 681t
  - in females, **691**
  - in males, **682**, 683t
  - superficial transverse, *606*, **682**, 683t, 689
- peroneus (*see* Muscle(s) (named), fibularis)
- pharyngeal, *1051*
- piriformis, 5, 597, *598–599*, 602
- plantaris, *787*, *790*, **802**, *837*
- platysma, *902*, 903t, *905*, **905**, 982t, 1106, 1051, *1052*, 1048t, 1070
- popliteus, 787, *795*, 795t, **802**–846, *840*
- procerus, *902*, *905*
- pronator quadratus, 207, 229, 231, 232t, *233*, *241*, *246*, *263*, *266*, 283, 292
- pronator teres, *207*, *218*, 229, 230, 231, 231t, **232**, *241*, *246*, *248*, *286*, *299*
- psoas major, *118*, *125*, *133*, *493*, *565*, 565, 565t, 615
- psoas minor, *565*, 565t, *566*
- pterygoid
  - lateral, *978*, *981*, 982t
  - medial, *978*, 982t, *1063*, *1100*
- pubo-analis, *599*
- pubococcygeus, *598*, *599–600*, **600**, 606, 647
- puboperinealis, *599*
- puboprostaticus, *599*
- puborectalis, *599–600*, *669*
- pubovaginalis, *599*, *647*
- pubovesicalis, *647*
- pyramidalis, **440**
- quadratus femoris, *615*, *695*, *697*
- quadratus lumborum, *122*, *125*, *541*, *542*, 564, 565–566, 565t, 566
- quadratus plantae, *719*, *846*, *814*, 814t, 852
- quadriceps femoris, 748–749
  - paralysis of, 758
  - rectus femoris, *32*, *747*, 747t
  - testing of, 748
  - vastus intermedius, 747t, *749*, **749**, 773
  - vastus lateralis, 32, 747t, *749*, **749**, 766, 773, 781, 805, 837
  - vastus medialis, *32*, 747t, *749*, **749**, 773, 801, 837
- rectovesicalis, *647*
- rectus, **956**
  - abdominis, 125, 322, 329, 435, 435, 436, 436t, 439–440, 449, 458, 487, 605, 731, 734
  - capitis
    - anterior, 1138t, *1079*
    - lateralis, 1138t, *1079*
    - posterior major, *127*, 127t, 128t
    - posterior minor, *127*, 127t, 128t, *928*
  - femoris, *32*, 747t, *766*, *781*
  - inferior, *951*, **956**, *957*, 957t, *959*, 1018, 1134
  - lateral, *949*, **956**, 957t, *959*, 1134
  - medial, *952*, **956**, *957*, 957t, *959*, 1018, 1134
  - superior, *952*, **956**, *957*, 957t, *959*, 1022, 1134
- rhomboid major, *118*, 126, *179*, 180t, 182, 182, 179, 202, 216
- rhomboid minor, *118*, 126, *179*, 170t, 182, 182, 179, 196, 202, 208
- risorius, *902*, 903t, *905*
- rotatores, *121*, **121**, *123*, 123t
- salpingopharyngeus, 1105t
- sartorius, *32*, *767*, *801*, *840*
- scalenes
  - anterior, *325*, *407*, *408*, *1051*, 1058–1059, 1073, 1138t, 1078, 1081, 1084
  - middle, *325*, *1051*, *1058*, *1060*, 1078–1079, 1079t, 1085
  - posterior, *325*, *1058–1060*, 1078t
- semimembranosus, *32*, *766*, *771*, 771t, 782, 788, 799, 799t, 801, 805, 840
- semispinalis capitis, **119**, **121**, *127*, 127t, 1058
- semispinalis cervicis, *121*, *123*, 123t, 127, 127t
- semispinalis thoracis, *121*, *123*, 123t
- semitendinosus, *32*, *766*, *768*, 770, *782*, 788, 801, 840
- serratus anterior, 125, 181, 194, 214, 322, *325*, *327*, *334*, 339–340, 458, 1059
  - paralysis, 188–189
- serratus posterior, *322*
  - inferior, **119**, *322*, *323*, 323t, *564*
  - superior, **119**, *322*, *323*, 323t
- soleus, 32, 782, 788, 790, 799, 799t, 801, 802, 805, 806, 837
  - accessory, 810
- spinalis, 121t
  - cervicis, *121*
  - thoracis, *119*, *121*
- splenius capitis, **118**, **120**, 120t, *1058*, 1078t
- splenius cervicis, *119*, **120**, 120t
- stapedius, *1031*, **1033**
- sternocleidomastoid (SCM), *119*, *125*, 902, 977, 984, 1047, 1051, 1054, 1055, 1055t–1056t, 1058–1059, 1065, 1070, 1073, 1028, 1086, 1101, 1104, 1148

sternohyoid, 325, 982t, 1051, 1062, 1064–1065, 1066, 1067, 1067t, 1028, 1086, 1091, 1106, 1150
sternothyroid, *325*, *1047*, *1051*, *1062*, 1064, 1066, 1067, 1067t, 1028–1087, 1091, 1106, 1150
styloglossus, 1001t, *1099*, *1150*
stylohyoid, *902*, 982t, *1047*, *1067*, 1067t
stylopharyngeus, 1092, *1099*, 1100–1101, 1101, 1142
subclavius, *164*, *173*, 1743t, *174*, **174**, 194, 195, 198, 204, 214, 322
subcostal, 323t, **324**, *326*
subscapularis, *173*, *179*, *181*, **181**, *194*, 195, 198, 201, 207, 213, 214, 216, 276, 281, 281
supinator, *235*, 235t, *239*, **239**, *241*, *286*
suprahyoid, 982t, *1067*, 1067t, 1092
supraspinatus, *179*, 180, *281*
  injuries to, 192
suspensory, of duodenum, 489, **490**
tarsal
  inferior, **952**
  superior, *951*, **952**, **956**, 7345
temporalis, *977*, *981*, 982t, *984*, *1022*
temporoparietalis, **900**
tensor fasciae latae, 715, 758, 765t, 766, 767, *767*, *781*, *788*
tensor tympani, *1029*, *1031*, **1033**
tensor veli palatini, *902*, *907*, *996*, *997*, 997t, *998*, 1030
teres major, 173, 179, 182, 179, 180, *184*, *184*, *186*, *187*, *194*, *196*, 207, 208, 213, 214, *217*, *223*
teres minor, *179*, 180, *182*, 184t, *194*, 207, 281, 297
thoracic, transverse, 323t, **324**, 325–326, 333, 334
thyro-arytenoid, 1093t, **1094**
thyrohyoid, 982t, 1061, 1062, 1064, **1066**, *1067*, 1067t, *1086*, *1150*
tibialis anterior, 32, 719, 790, 791, 792, 793t, 757t, 806, *814*, 814t, *851*, *856*
tibialis posterior, 719, *755*, 755t, 799, 799t, 846–804, 814, 814t, 817, *841*, *852*, *856*
trachealis, **1056**, *1057*
transverse, of tongue, 1000
transversospinalis, *120*, *122*, *125*
transversus abdominis, 436t
trapezius, 118, 126, 127, 127t, 179, 179–180, 180t, 180, 179, 187, *194*, *204*, *261*, *274*, *290*, *292*, 1047, 1055, 1055t, 1056t, 1057, 1059–1060, 1070, 1071
  paralysis of, 1074
triceps brachii, 32, 33, *179*, *207*, *214–215*, 216, 216, 215t, 223, 289, 290
  coxae, *768*, **770**
  surae, **798**, *801*, 846
vastus intermedius, 747t, *749*
vastus lateralis, *32*, 747t, *749*, 754, *754*, *762*, *772*, *780*, *782*, *805*, *837*
vastus medialis, *32*, 747t, *749*, 757, *757*, 773, 801, 837
vertebral
  anterior, **1138**
  lateral, **1138**
vertical, of tongue, 1000, 1002t
vocalis, 1090, 1093t, **1094**
zygomaticus major, *902*, 903t, *905*, *911*
zygomaticus minor, *902*, *905*
Muscle(s) (of regions or organs)
  of abdominal wall
    anterolateral, 435–441
    posterior, 565–566, *565–566*, 565t
  of arm, 212–217
  of back, 118, **118–130**
    extrinsic, **118–119**
    intrinsic, **119–126**
      deep layer of, **120–122**, *122*
      intermediate layer of, *119*, **120**, *121*
      superficial layer of, *119*, *120*, **120**
    spasm of, **129–130**
    surface anatomy of, *126*
  of cervical region
    anterior, 1066
    lateral, **1057**, *1058*
  of cheeks, **903**–905
  of esophagus, 478
  of extraocular, 948, **955**–956, *959–961*, 957t, 961
  of eyebrows, **903**, *905*
  of face, **901**–906
    paralysis of, **918**
  of foot, **812**–813, *814*, 814t–816t, *816*, 817, 818
  of forearm, *230*
  of forehead, **903**, *905*
  of larynx, 1092, *1093*
  of leg
    anterior compartment, 789, *794*
    lateral compartment, 794, 797–798
    posterior compartment, 632–633, 633t–634t, 631–633, 798–805, 799t, 800t
  of lips, **903**–905
  of mastication, **980**, 982t
  of mouth, **903**–905
  of neck, 126–127, *127*, 127t
  of orbit, *951*
  of pelvic floor, *599*
  of pelvic walls, *599*
  of pharynx, **1101**, *1102*, 1102t, 1103
  rotator cuff, *281*
    injuries to, 192, 297
    tendonitis of, 297
  of scalp, **903**, *905*
  of suboccipital, 126, *127*, 127t, 128
  thenar (of thumb), *206*, *246*, **256**–257, 260t, 301, 308
  of thigh
    anterior, *746*, 746–749, **746**–749, 746t, *747*, 747t
      iliopsoas, **747**–748
      pectineus, **747**
      quadriceps femoris, **748**–749, *749*
      sartorius, **748**
      surface anatomy of, 757, 758, *758*
    medial, **749**–751, 750t
      actions of adductor muscle group, 751
      adductor brevis, **749**, *750*, 751
      adductor hiatus, **751**
      adductor longus, **749**, *750*
      adductor magnus, *750*, 750t, **751**
      gracilis, *751*, **751**
      obturator externus, *750*, **751**
      surface anatomy of, 757, 758, *758*
    posterior, 600–601, 770–733
  of thoracic wall, **322–324**, 333
  of tongue, *1001*, 1002t
Muscle soreness, 36
Muscle testing, 35–36
Muscle tone, **36**
  absence of, 36
Muscular system, **4**
  components of, 29–36
Myelin, *46*, *47*
Myofascial pain syndromes, 323
Myofibrils, 36
Myogenic conduction, 389
Myology, 4
Myotomes, 51, 111, 164

N

Nasal bone, *880–882*
Nasion, *880–882*, **882**, 885t
Nasopharynx, *983*, *1096*, **1097**, *1097–1098*, 1099
Navicular, *390*, **720**, *721*, *811*
Navicular tuberosity, **720**
Neck (in general)
  of femur, *697*, 711, **711**, *712*, 829
    blood supply to, *834*
    fractures, 861–911
  of fibula, *717*, 806
  of gallbladder, *514*, **529**
  of humerus, *149*, **151**
  of mandible, *978*
  of pancreas, **514**, *516*
  of radius, **153**
  of ribs, *122*, **310**, *311*
  of scapula, *152*, 151
  of talus, *719*
    fractures of, 725, *726*
  of urinary bladder, **624**
  of uterus, *641*
Neck (region), 1047
  bones of, **1047–1049**
  deep structures of, **1138–1082**
  fascia of, **1106–1053**

Neck (region) (*Continued*)
- hyperextension injury of, 112, *112*
- infections in, 1054
- larynx (*see* Larynx)
- lymphatic system of, *1105*, 1105–1106
- muscles of, 126–127, 1056t
- nerve point of, 1061
- radical dissection of, 1115
- root of, **1080–1082**
  - arteries of, *1079*, **1079–1080**
  - nerves in, **1080–1082**, *1081*
  - veins of, **1080**, *1081*
- skin of, 1070
- superficial structures of, **1072**
- surface anatomy of, **1070–1073**
- trauma to, 1115
- veins of, *1060*
- viscera of
  - alimentary layer, **1096–1104**
  - endocrine layer, **1083–1086**, 1104–1105
  - respiratory layer, **1086–1096**, 1104–1105
- whiplash injury of, 91, 112, *112*

Necrosis
- avascular, 25
  - of femoral head, 911
  - of lunate, 301
- cardiac, 396
- myocardial, 37

Nélaton lines, 779, *780*

Nephroptosis, **549**

Nephroscope, 552

Nerve(s) (in general), 49
- autonomic, **617**–618
- cervical, *48*
- cranial, 59, **54**, **1118**, 1121t
  - fibers of, 1127
  - injuries to, **1150**
  - nuclei, *1127*, **1127**
- degeneration, 58
- fiber, 49
- ischemia of, 58
- lumbar, *48*
- motor, **35**
- periosteal, 23
- peripheral, 47–50, *50*, *55*
  - degeneration of, 58
  - ischemia of, 58
- vasomotor, 23

Nerve(s) (named)
- abducent, *926*, *929*, *990*, *959*, *960*, 1121–1122, 1123, 1124t
  - divisions of, *1134*
  - functions of, **1135**
  - injury to, 1153
  - lesions of, 1152t
  - nuclei of, *1127*, **1135**
- accessory (*see* Nerve(s) (named), spinal accessory)
- alveolar
  - anterior superior, *990*, *1136*
  - inferior, *907*, 980, *990*, *1022*, *1139*
  - middle superior, *990*, **1023**, *1136*
  - posterior superior, *990*, **1023**, *1136*
- anal, inferior, 673, *680–681*, 690t
- anococcygeal, **617**
- articular, 28
- auricular
  - great, 908, 909t, 910, 911, 977, 977–978, 1028, 1058, 1061, 1062
  - posterior, *911*, **911**
- auriculotemporal, *859*, 909t, 977, *977*, 980, 984, 985, 990, 1026, 1026, 1027, 1028, 1030, 1136, 1142
- axillary, *54*, *55*
  - injury to, 189–190
- buccal, *907*, *908*, 909t, *984*, *990*, *1136*
  - block of, **919**
- calcaneal, 736t
- cardiac, *390*, *1145*
- carotid sinus, **1065**
- cavernous, *681*
- cervical, transverse, *1058*, *1062*, **1069**
- chorda tympani, 980, 1000, *1029*, *1031*, 1032
- ciliary
  - long, **964**
  - short, **963**
- clunial, **773**, 775
  - inferior, 791t, 736t, 774t, **775**
  - medial, 736t, 774t, **775**
  - superior, 564t, 603t, **605**, 736t, 774t, 775
- coccygeal, **617**
- cochlear, *1026*, *1036*
- collateral, *326*
- cutaneous, *18*
  - of arm, 169
  - dorsal
    - intermediate, **819**
    - medial, **819**
  - of face, 906
  - femoral, posterior, 616t
  - of forearm, 169
  - lateral (of arm)
    - anterior branches, *327*
    - inferior, *53*, 171t
    - posterior, 171t, *327*
    - superior, *53*, *171*, 171t
  - lateral (of back), *118*
  - lateral (of forearm), *171*, *218*, *219*, 224, 244, 246t
  - lateral (of thigh), *53–54*, *566*, 567, 734, 753, 754
  - of mandibular nerve, 908t, 909t
  - of maxillary nerve, 908t–909t
  - medial
    - of arm, 330
    - of forearm, *53*, 203t, *224*, 245t, 247
  - perforating, 616t
  - posterior
    - of arm, *171*
    - of forearm, *53*, *171*, 244, *245*, 245t
    - of thigh, *53–54*, *680*, 690t, 736t, 768, 774, 775–776
  - sural
    - lateral, **788**, *795*, 795t
    - medial, **788**, *795*, 795t
  - of upper limb, 169
- deep fibular, **792**, **819**
- deep gluteal, **775**
- dorsal
  - of clitoris, *670*, *689*
  - of penis, *663*, *667*, 670, *670*, *679*, 681, 682
  - root, 50
  - scapular, 189, 202t
- ethmoidal
  - anterior, *907*, *929*, 964, *964*, **1019**
  - anterior meningeal branches of, **927**, 929
  - posterior, *929*, 964, *964*, **1019**
- of face, 906
- facial, 910–912, 911, 941, 990, 1030, 1031, 1032, 1101, 1121–1122, 1123, 1124t
  - branches of, *911*, 912, 920
  - buccal branch of, 920
  - cervical branch of, **912**, *1058*
  - distribution of, *1139*
  - functions of, **1138**
  - geniculum of, **1138**
  - injuries to, 920, 1155
  - intermediate nerve, *1121*, **1138**
  - lesions of, 1152t, 1155
  - marginal mandibular branch of, **912**, 920, *977*, *1063*
  - motor root of, **910**, 1138
  - nuclei of, *1128*, **1138**
  - palsy of, 920
  - parasympathetic innervation of, *1139*
  - primary root of, *1121*
  - temporal branch of, **912**
  - terminal branches of, *901*
  - zygomatic branch of, **912**, 920
- femoral, *438*, *449–450*, *541*, 566, *566*, 731, 752–753
- femoral cutaneous
  - lateral, *541*
  - posterior, 455, 457
- fibular (peroneal)
  - common, *54*, 775, 781, 788, *795*, 795t, 806, 846
    - injury to, 807–808
  - deep, 53, 736t, 791, 792, 795, 795t, 819, 820, 820t
  - superficial, 736t, *795*, 795t, 819, *820*, 820t, 846
    - block of, 827
    - entrapment of, 808
  - of foot, 816, 817, *818*, 818t, 819

frontal, **906**, *907*, *909*, *959*, *960*, *1136*
gastric, *1145*
genitofemoral, *541*, *566*, *628*, *681*
  genital branch of, 455, *455*, 457, 678, 690t
glossopharyngeal, *941*, **993**, 1000, *1004*, 1032, 1070, 1070, 1099–1100, 1121–1022, 1023, 1025t
  distribution of, *1142*
  functions of, **1142**
  lesions of, 1151t, **1154–1155**
  motor fibers of, 1143
  neuralgia, **1155**
  nuclei, *1128*, **1142**
  parasympathetic fibers of, 1142
  parasympathetic innervation, *1145*
gluteal
  inferior, *615*, 616t, 617
  superior, *615*, 616t, 616
great auricular, *53*, *54*
hypogastric
  left, *501*, 556, **618**, *681*
  right, *501*, 556, **618**, *625*
hypoglossal, 941, 1000, 1004, 1062–*1063*, *1064*, 1070, *1070*, *1100–1101*, 1121–1122, 1123, 1025t
  branches of, 1148, *1149*
  distribution of, *1149*
  functions of, **1148**
  injury to, **1009**, 1155
  lesions of, 1151t
  nuclei of, *1128*
  palsy, *1155*
iliohypogastric, 439–440, 442, 442, 442t, 447, **541**, *566*, **567**
ilioinguinal, 438–440, 442, 442, 442t, *452*, **541**, 566, **567**, 682
  block of, **693**
infra-orbital, 907, 908t, 910, 949, 1012, *1013*, *1022*
  block of, **918**–919
infratrochlear, 908t, *909*, **910**
intercostal, *133*, **327**, 335, *357*, *496*, 415t, 561
  1st, *325*, 330
  2nd, *325*, 330
  3rd, *325*
  4th, 335
  5th, 335
  6th, 335
  7th, 330
  8th, 330
  9th, 330
  10th, 330
  11th, 330
  anterior ramus of, *326*
  atypical, **330**
  block of, **333**, *333*
  branches of, 330
  typical, **327–330**
intercostobrachial, *191*, *194*, *327*, **330**
interosseous
  anterior, 244, *245*, 245t
  posterior, *207*, *230*, *236*, 244, 246t
labial
  anterior, **689**, 690t
  posterior, **689**, 690t
lacrimal, 907, 908t, 909, *910*, 959, 960, *1013*
laryngeal
  block of, 1112
  external, *1087*, **1056**, *1145*
  inferior, *1055*, **1056**
  injury to, 1112
  internal, **1000**, 1002, *1087*, **1056**, *1145*
  recurrent, 351, *407*, 415t, *1078*, 1081, 1084, 1087, 1092, 1103
    injury to, 418–419, 1109
    left, 348, 429, 390, 404, 405, 406, 407, 1079, 1094, 1100–1101
    right, *390*, 406, *407*, *1079*, *1094*, 1100–1101, 1145
  superior, *1086*, 1092, *1094*, *1100*, 1145
lateral plantar, **819**
lingual, *909*, **980**, *984*, *990*, *1063*, *1136*, 1139, 1141
long thoracic, *55*
mandibular, 906, 910, **929**, 980, *1120*, 1124t, **1135**, *1136*, 1136t, 1142
  anterior meningeal branches of, **927**, 929
  branches of, 1076t
maxillary, 908t, 910, 926, 929, 984, 989, 1011–1012, 1013, 1014, 1120, 1124t, **1135**, *1136*, 1136t
  anterior meningeal branches of, **927**, 929
  branches of, 1136t
medial
  of arm, *171*, 203t
  of forearm, 203t, *224*, 244, 246t
medial plantar, **819**
median, *173*, *195*, *201*, 203t, 244, *245*, 245t
  in arm, 219
  branches of, 244, *266*, *267*, 268t
  in hand, *267*, 268, 268t
  injury to, 251
  lateral branch of, *267*, 268t
  lesions of, 273
  medial branch of, *267*, 268t
  palmar cutaneous branch of, *245*, 245t, 267, 268
  recurrent branch of, *267*, 268t
  surface anatomy of, *247*
  trauma to, 273–274
meningeal, *108*, 134
mental, *907*, *908*, 909t, 980, *990*
  block of, **919**
motor root of, **910**–911
musculocutaneous, *191*, *195*, *201*, 202t, 214, 218, 218, 246
  injury to, 226
mylohyoid, *984*, *990*, *1004*
nasal, external, *908*, 909t, **910**
nasociliary, *907*, *909*, *910*, *959*, *960*, 1020, 1136
nasopalatine, **1008**, *1007*, 1020, *1136*
  block of, **1008**–1009
obturator, *567*, *598*, **615**, *615*
  accessory, **567**
  injury to, 619
  internus, **776**
occipital
  greater, *118*, *127*, 127t, *129*, 129t, 908, 909t, 910
  least, *129*, 127t
  lesser, 118, 129, 129t, 908, 909t, 910, 1058, 1061
  third, *118*, *908*, 909t, *910*
oculomotor, *929*, *940*, *941*, *959*, *960*, 1121–1122, 1123, 1124t, 1134
  compression of, **1152**
  divisions of, *1134*
  functions of, **1134**
  injury to, **1152**
  lesions of, 1151t
  nuclei of, *1128*, **1129**
olfactory, *907*, **1020**, *1121–1122*, *1123*, 1124t, 1127
  function of, **1127**
  lesions of, 1151t
  nuclei of, *1128*
  palsy of, **972**
ophthalmic, 906, 907, 1121, 1123t, **1135**, *1136*, 1136t
  branches of, 1136t
  herpes zoster infection of, **919**
ophthalmic branch of (*see* Nerve(s) (named), ophthalmic)
optic, 941, 952, 959, 960, 1121–1122, *1123*, 1124t, 1070
  demyelinating diseases and, 1151–152
  functions of, **1128**
  lesions of, 1152t
  nuclei of, *1128*
palatine
  greater, *907*, 993, **996**, *998*, *1020*, 1136
  lesser, *907*, 993, **996**, *998*, *1020*, 1136
palpebral, inferior, *909*
pectoral
  lateral, *173*, *195*, *198*, *202*
  medial, *173*, *195*, *198*, 203t
perineal, 690t
  deep, 647, **670**
  superficial, **670**
periosteal, *23*, **23**

Nerve(s) (named) (*Continued*)
  petrosal
    deep, **1012**, *1014*, *1139*
    greater, *1139*
    lesser, *1031*, *1142*
  pharyngeal, *1020*, *1136*
  phrenic, 348, 356, 388, 389, 405, 415t, 1058, 1062, 1062, 1078–1079, *1028*, *1106*
    accessory, **1062**
    block of, 1074
    crush injury of, 1074
    injury to, 434, 1074
    left, *404*, *407*, **408**, *409*, 529, 561
    right, *404*, *405*, 406, 529, 561
    section of, **570**
    severance of, 1074
  plantar
    lateral, 736t, *817*, **819**, *820*, 820t
    medial, 736t, *801*, *817*, **819**, *820*, 820t
      entrapment of, 827
    reflex testing, 656
  popliteal fossa, **787**–788
  in popliteal fossa, **787**–788
  posterior
    of arm, *171*
    of forearm, *171*, 244, *245*, 245t
    of upper limb, 169
  pterygopalatine, *907*, 1012
  pudendal, 457, *615*, 616t, *617*, *625*, 647, 679, 670, 681, 690t, 776
    block of, 657, *657*, *693*, **693**
  pulmonary, left, *405*
  quadratus femoris, **775**
  radial, *201*, 203t, *218*, *239*, *245*, 245t
    in arm, *219*
    deep branch of, 244, 246t
    in forearm, 244
    in hand, 269
    injury to, 236, 253, 275
    superficial branch of, 244, *245*, 245t
  rami communicantes, *108*, *326*, **330**, 408–409, 615, 625
  rectal, inferior, **670**
  saphenous, **752**
  scapular, dorsal, 189, 202t
  sciatic, *615*, 616t, 617, *636*
    block of, 784
  injury to, 784
  scrotal
    anterior, 455, **457**, **678**, 690t
    posterior, 455, **457**, *670*, **678**, *680*, 690t
  sinus, *1145*
  of small intestine, *486*
  spinal
    anterior rami of, *326*
    anterior root of, *1091*
    block of, *95*, 656–657
    cervical, *131*
    coccygeal, **614**
    lumbar, *110*, *131*, **566**
    meningeal branches of, **108**
    mixed, *108*
    posterior rami of, *326*
    sacral, *95*, **614**
    thoracic, *131*
  spinal accessory, 133, 941, 1032, 1059, 1060, *1060*, *1062–1063*, 1121–1122, 1123, 1125t
    distribution of, *1148*
    functions of, **1146**
    injury to, 189, 1155
    lesions of, 1074, 1151t
    nuclei of, *1128*, **1146**
  splanchnic, *413*
    abdominopelvic, **61**, 491, 541, 548, 553, 554, 555t
    abdominopelvic, **63**, 413
    greater, *356*, *408*, *409*, 478, *479*, 481, 904
    least, *356*, *554*, 555t
    lesser, *356*, *479*, *554*, 555t
    lumbar, *486*, *501*, **553**, *555*, 555t, 630, 679, 649
    pelvic, 502, 555t, **556**, *615*, 616t, 618, 630, 679
    sacral, *615*
    thoracic, **413**, *479*, 553, 555t
  subclavian, 202t
  subcostal, **327**, 415t, 442, 442t, *577*, 566, 566
  submandibular, *907*
  suboccipital, **126**, *127*, 127t
  subscapular, *55*, *202*, 203t
  superior gluteal, **775**
  superior injury, *783*, 783–784
  supraclavicular, *171*, 171t, *194*, *329*, 1061
    intermediate, *1058*
    lateral, *1058*
    medial, *1058*
  supra-orbital, **906**, *907*, 908t, *909*, *949*, 1018
  suprascapular, 202t, *214*, *1059*, 1061
    injury to, 1074
  supratrochlear, **906**, *907*, 908t, *909*, *949*
  sural, *732*, 736t, *795*, 795t, 804, *820*, 820t, 821
    calcaneal branches of, *53*
    grafts, 827
    lateral, *53*
    medial, *53*
  sympathetic, of abdominal viscera, 553
  tentorial, **927**, *929*
  thoracic
    long, *173*, *191*, 202t
    posterior ramus of, *328*
  thoraco-abdominal, 330, **441**, 442t
    anterior cutaneous branches of, *442*
    lateral cutaneous branches of, *442*
  thoracodorsal, *173*, 189, 202t
  tibial, *53*
    calcaneal branches of, *53*
    entrapment of, 825
    injury to, 807
    posterior, *819*
  tonsillar, 1141
  trigeminal, 906, *908*, *929*, *941*, *990*, 1120, 1121, 1122t
    block of, 1153
    distribution of, *907*
    divisions of, 906, *907*, *1136*
    functions of, **1134**
    injury to, **1153**
    lesions of, **919**, 1087t
    mandibular branch of (*see* Nerve(s) (named), mandibular)
    maxillary branch of (*see* Nerve(s) (named), maxillary)
    motor root of, *1121*, *1123*, **1136**
    nuclei of, *1128*, **1135**
    ophthalmic branch of (*see* Nerve(s) (named), ophthalmic)
    sensory root of, *1121*, *1123*, **1135**
    testing of, **919**–920
  trochlear, *926*, *929*, *940*, *959*, *960*, *1121*, 1124t
    divisions of, *1135*
    functions of, **1134**
    injury to, 1153
    nucleus of, *1128*, **1134**
  tympanic, *1142*
  ulnar, 159, *173*, *191*, *195*, *201*, *218*, *229*, 268t
    in arm, 220
    branches of, *245*, 268t
    compression of, 239, 275
    deep branch of, 268t
    dorsal cutaneous branch of, 241, *245*, 245t, 268t
    in forearm, 244, *245*, 245t
    in hand, 269
    injury to, 239
    palmar cutaneous branch of, *245*, 245t, 268t
    superficial branch of, 268t
  vagus, 356, 388, 389, 390, 405, 415t, 541, 529, 554, 941, 1032, 1070, 1080–1082, 1086, 1094, 1100–1101, 1121–1122, 1121, 1123t, 1143–1144
    branches of, 1082, *1145*
    distribution of, *1145*
    functions of, **1143**
    hepatic branch of, *479*, *1145*
    left, 348, 356, 390, 404, 406, 407, 479, 1078, 1080, 1145
    lesions of, 1087t, 1155
    nuclei of, *1128*, **1144**
    right, 348, 356, 390, 404, 406, 407, 479, *469*, *1078*, 1080–1081, *1056*, *1145*

summary of, 1084t
vasomotor, **23**
vestibular, *1026*
vestibulocochlear, *941*, *1026*, *1121–1122*, 1123, 1125t, 1142
functions of, **1142**
injuries to, 1155
lesions of, 1151t
nuclei of, *1126*
zygomatic, *907*, *909*, 1011, *1013*, *1136*, 1139
zygomaticofacial, *908*, 908t, *909*, *1013*
zygomaticotemporal, *908*, 909t, *909*, 1011, 1013
Nerve(s) (of regions or organs)
of abdominal wall
anterolateral, **441**–443, 442t
injury to, 446
posterior, *566*, **566**–567
of anal canal, 673
of appendix, **495**, *501*
of arm, 169
of breast, **335**
of cecum, 498, *501*
of cervical region
anterior, 1070
lateral, **1060–1062**
to coracobrachialis, *195*
cranial, **50**, **54**, *56*, **1118**
fibers of, 1127
injuries to, **1150**
nuclei, **1127**, *1128*
of diaphragm, *562*
of dura mater, **132**, **134**, **927**, *929*
of esophagus, *479*
of foot, 816–821, *820*, 820t
of forearm, 169, 244–247
of gallbladder, 529
of gingiva, *990*
of hand, 265, 268t, 269
of kidneys, **548**–549
of lacrimal gland, **950**
of larynx, 1056
of limb
upper, **169**
of liver, 526, *528*
of lungs, **355–356**, *356*
of mediastinum
posterior, 413
superior, **406–408**
of orbit, **962**–964
of pancreas, 541
of parotid gland, 977–978
of penis, 681–682
of pericardium, 388–389
of perineum, *681*, *690*
of pleura, **355–356**, *356*
of posterior mediastinum, 413
of pterygoid canal, 950
of rectum, 629, *630*
of root of neck, **1080–1082**, *1081*
sacral, *731–732*
of scalp, **861**
of small intestine, 494
spinal, *131*
of sternoclavicular joint, 266
of stomach, *479*
of superior mediastinum, **406–408**
of suprarenal glands, *548*, **548**–549
of teeth, *990*
of thoracic wall, **327–330**, 415t
of upper limb, **169**
of ureters, *548*, **548**–549
of urethra, 658, 646
of urinary bladder, *625*, 625–626
of uterus, 647
of vagina, 647
of vertebral column, **108–109**
of vulva, 689
Nervous system, **3**, 46–*47*, *48*
autonomic, **3**, **58**–*61*, 62, *63*, 65–66, 65t
functions of, 65–66, 65t
ganglia of, 58
parasympathetic division of, 62, *63*, 65
sympathetic division of, 58–*61*, *61*, *62*
visceral sensation, 66
cells of, *47*, *48*
central (CNS), 3, **46**, **47**
divisions of, 3, 46–47
enteric (ENS), 30t, **62**–65, *63*, 66, 494, *495*, 553, *554*, **556**–557, *556*, *558*
function of, 46
parasympathetic, **62**, *63*, 65
of digestive tract, 30t, **62**–65, *63*, 66, 494, *495*, 553, *554*, **556**–557, 556, 558
of heart, 65t
of liver, 65t
of lungs, 65t
of stomach, 481
of suprarenal medulla, 65t
of urinary tract, 65t
peripheral (*see* Peripheral nervous system)
peripheral (PNS), 46, *47*, *48*, *49*–57, 49–58
somatic and visceral fibers, 54, 56–57, 56–57
types of, *50*, 51, 53–*54*, *54–55*
somatic (SNS), 58
sympathetic, 58–61, *61*, 62, *62*, *62*
Nervus spinosus, *929*
Neuralgia
glossopharyngeal, **1155**
trigeminal, **919**, 1153
Neural tube defects, 97
Neuritis, optic, 972, **1152**
Neuroglia, 47
Neurolemma, 49
Neuroma, acoustic, **1155**
Neurons, 46, *46*, *47*
multipolar motor, 46
olfactory receptor, **1127**
pseudounipolar sensory, 46, 47
Neurovasculature, of thoracic wall, 316
Nipple, *334*, **335**, *340*
Nocturia, 639
Node
atrioventricular, *389*, **389**
lymph (*see* Lymph nodes)
sinu-atrial, *389*
Norepinephrine, 545
Nose
apex of, *965*
arteries of, *1019*, **1019**–1020
dorsum of, *965*
external, *1015*, **1015**–1016
fractures of, **1023**
root of, *965*
skeleton of, **1015**
vasculature of, *1019*, **1019**–1020
Nostril flaring, **918**
Notch, **22**
acetabular, **711**
angular, *480*
cardiac, *362*, 346, *347*, *348*, *431*
cardial, *476*, *478*
clavicular, *313*, **314**, *316*
costal, *313*, **314**
fibular, **717**
greater sciatic, **708**
interarytenoid, *1097*, *1110*
intertragic, *1027*
jugular, *313*, **314**, *316*, 336, *338*–*339*, 1070, 1071, 1073
lesser sciatic, **709**
mandibular, *975*, *956*
sacral, superior, *84*
sacrococcygeal, *84*
sciatic
greater, 586, *587*, 557t
lesser, 586, *587*
supinator, **153**
supra-orbital, *946*
suprascapular, *152*, **151**
suprasternal, *296*, **297**
tentorial, *926*
thyroid
inferior, **1088**
superior, **1088**
trochlear, 152, *289*, *292*
ulnar, **153**
vertebral
inferior, **74**, *75*
superior, **74**, *75*
Nuclear medicine imaging, 71
Nucleus, 47
ambiguus, *1128*
cochlear
anterior, *1128*
posterior, *1128*

Nucleus (*Continued*)
Edinger-Westphal, *1128*
of hypoglossal nerve, *1128*
mesencephalic, *1128*
motor
of facial nerve, *1128*
of trigeminal nerve, *1128*
of oculomotor nerve, *1128*
posterior, of vagus nerve, *1128*
principal sensory, *1128*
salivatory, *1128*
of solitary tract, *1128*, *1139*
spinal, *1128*
of spinal accessory nerve, *1128*
of trochlear nerve, *1128*
vestibular, *1128*
Nucleus pulposus, *76*, 98
herniation of, *110*, 110–111
Nutrient arteries, **23**
Nutrient foramen, **717**
Nutrient foramina, **23**

O

Oblique popliteal ligament, **773**, **838**
Oblique sections, **7**, *7*
Obturator artery, **755**
Obturator externus, *738*, **751**, **770**
Obturator foramen, **711**
Obturator internus, **770**
nerve to, **776**
Occipital bone, *127*, 127t, *129*, *926*, *1051*, 1097
Occlusion
carotid, 1075
coronary, 399–400
Olecranon, 220
fracture of, 249, *249*
of ulna, *150*, 152, 158
Olfactory hallucinations, **1152**
Olfactory system, *1129*
Omentum, **467**
greater, 435, 467, 468, 469, 475, 481, *487*, 489, 508
lesser, **467**, *468*, 469, 508, *517*, 520
protrusion of, 447
Open abdominal tubal sterilization, 649
Opening
external acoustic meatus, **886**
saphenous, 752
Ophthalmoscope, 4, 970
Ophthalmoscopy, **970**
Opposition, *10*, **12**
Ora serrata, *952*, **955**
Orbicular zone, **832**
Orbit, **946**, 1011, *1012*
arteries of, **963**, *964*, 964t
extra-ocular muscles of, **956**–957
eyeball, *949*, 951
anterior chamber of, **971**
aqueous humor of, *952*
artificial, **971**
cornea, 951, *952*, 955
fibrous layer of, **951**
inner layer of, **955**
pupil, *952*, **954**
refractive media of, **955**–956
retina of, *952*, **955**
sclera of, *952*
surface anatomy of, **966**–977
vascular layer of, **951**–954
eyelids, 965, **948**–949, *949*, 967
infections of, 969
injury to, 969
fractures of, **968**
muscles of, *951*
nerves of, **962**–964
pyramidal, **948**
tumors of, **968**
vasculature of, **964**–966
veins of, **964**, *966*
walls of, 948
Orchitis, 685
Organomegaly, 445
Organs
of Corti, 1037
extraperitoneal, 465
genital
female, **640–658**, *641*
male, **634–639**
intraperitoneal, 465
olfactory, **1127**
retroperitoneal, 465
subperitoneal, 465
vestibulocochlear, *1036*
Orifice
aortic valve, *382*
atrioventricular
left, *381*, *384*
right, *379*, *384*
cardial, of the stomach, *477*, 478, 479, 480, 480, 577
ileal, **494**
myopectineal, *449*, **452**
of pharyngotympanic tube, *1098*
pulmonary valve, *382*
pyloric, **480**
tricuspid valve, **380**
ureteric, *623*, **624**
urethral
external, 625, 626, 627, 634, 641, *644*, *664*, **677**, 679, *681*, *687*
internal, *623*, **624**, 626, *634*
vaginal, 626, *664*, *687*, **689**
Oropharynx, 1087, 1096–1098
functions of, 1099
Orthopedics, 4
Os
external, *641*, **643**, *676*
internal, *641*, **643**, *676*
trigonum, 726, *727*
Ossification
of clavicle, 159
of cranium, 896
endochondral, 22, 159
intramembranous, 22, 159
primary, **87–89**
primary center, 22
secondary, **89**
secondary center, 23
of vertebrae, **87–89**
Osteoarthritis, 29
of zygapophysial joints, 141
Osteoarthrosis, 96
Osteochondroses, 25
Osteology, 4
Osteons, 23
Osteopenia, 92
Osteoporosis, 24, *24*, 117
femoral neck fractures secondary to, 861
Ostium
abdominal, **642**
of maxillary sinus, *1022*, **1023**
uterine, 642
Otalgia, 1112
Otitis media, 1113
Otorrhea, 944
Otoscopic examination, *1038*, **1038**
Outflow
cranial parasympathetic, **63**
sacral parasympathetic, **63**
Outlet
pelvic, *586*, **587**, 588t, *597*, *662*
thoracic, 315
Ovaries, 453, *454*, 640–642, *734*
arteries of, **642**
innervation of, **642**
pubertal changes in, 640
veins of, **642**
Oxycephaly, *899*

P

Pacemaker, cardiac, **400**
Pachymeninx, 922
Pain
abdominal, **571**–572
anginal, 399, 401
back, 109
localized, 109
low, 109
cervical, 1106
chest, **319**
muscular, 110
myocardial infarction, 399
pararenal, **550**
peritoneal, 465
pleural, **365**
posterior abdominal, **571**–572
referred
cardiac, 400–401
diaphragm, **572**
visceral, 402
sciatica, 111

ureteric, 631
visceral referred, **506**
zygapophysial joint, 110
Palate, 1048, **1048**
cleft, *1009*, **1009**
features of, **1105**–1106
hard, 1048, 1105, 1105–1051, 1106, 1052t, 1053, 1012, 1087
soft, 1105, 1105–1051, 1106, 1052, 1052t, 1087, 1097–1099
Palatine bone, 1048, *1106*, 1011, *1012*, *1098*
Palm of hand, *7*, 8
compartments of, 255, *256*
dissection of, *525*
fascia of, **253**, 255
Palpation, **351**
of abdominal wall, anterolateral, 446
of femoral artery, 761
of radial artery, 253
of spleen, *531*
of testes, **685**
of uterus, 652
Palsy
Bell, 1154
facial nerve, 920
hypoglossal nerve, *1155*
oculomotor, 1152
Pancreas, *514*, **514**
accessory tissue of, **532**
arteries of, *541*
body of, **513**–514
cancer of, **533**, 571–572
computed tomography of, *576*
head of, *489*, **513**, *541*
lymphatic system of, *541*
neck of, **513**, *541*
nerves of, *541*
pseudocyst of, 473
rupture of, **532**
secretions produced by, 513
tail of, 516
veins of, *541*
Pancreatectomy, **533**
Pancreatitis, 532
Papilla
duodenal
major, 489, *489*, 514, *514*, *525*, 527
minor, *489*, *514*
filiform, *999*, **999**
foliate, *999*, **999**
fungiform, *999*, **999**
ileal, **469**, *471*
incisive, 1106, *1051*
lacrimal, *949*, **950**, 968
lingual, *999*, **999**
renal, *544*
vallate, *999*, **999**, *1098*
Papilledema, **970**
Pap test, 652
Paracentesis, abdominal, **472**
Paradoxical abdominothoracic rhythm, 472
Paralysis, 36
of diaphragm, **434**
of extra-ocular muscles, **972**
of genioglossus, **1009**
of hemidiaphragm, 570
Klumpke, 211
of quadriceps, 759
of serratus anterior, 188–189
of trapezius, 1074
Paraphimosis, **685–686**
Paraplegia, 141
Parasagittal, 6
Parasympathetic nervous system, 62, *63*
of abdominal viscera, 556
of digestive tract, 65t
of heart, 65t
of liver, 65t
of lungs, 65t
of skin, 65t
of stomach, 481
of suprarenal medulla, 65t
of urinary tract, 65t
Paravertebral ganglia, 59
Paresthesia, 58, 742
Parietal bone, *926*
Parotidectomy, 920, **985**
Parotiditis, 985
Part
cervical, 361
costal, 361
diaphragmatic, 361
mediastinal, 361
of parietal pleura, 361
Partial lumbar sympathectomy, **572**
Partial-thickness burn, 17
Patella, *21*, *705*, *708*, 678, **715**, *715*, **748**, 757
abnormal ossification of, 760
bipartite, 760, *760*
chondromalacia patellae, 759
dislocation of, 865
fractures of, 911
functions of, 748
ligament, **748**
surface, **713**
tendon reflex, 760, *760*
tripartite, 760
Patellofemoral syndrome, 865
PCL. *See* Ligament, posterior cruciate
Peau d'orange sign, 341
Pecten pubis, 452, 586
Pectineal line, **713**
Pectineus, **747**
Pectoral fascia, **163**, *164*, *165*
Pectoral girdle, **147**, 276, *309*
Peduncle, cerebellar, *1121*
Pelvic girdle, 148, **585**, **705**, *707*
bones of, **585–589**
features of, **585–589**
functions of, 585
joints of, 589–591
ligaments of, 589–591
orientation of, **589**
secondary functions of, 585
surface anatomy of, **713**, *714*, 714–715
Pelvic viscera, 618, **620**
urinary organs, **620–626**
Pelvis (region), **588**
android, *591*, **591**
anthropoid, 591, *591*
arteries of, **606–619**
axis of, *586*, 627, *597*
diagonal conjugate of, 591–592
diameter of, 591–592
female, *588*, 589, *623*
fractures of, 592, *593*
greater, 584–586, *586*, **587**, 588t, *597*, 628
gynecoid, *591*, **591**
interspinous distance of, *592*, **592**
joints of, *589*
lesser, 586, *586*, 589t, **590**, *592*, *628*
ligaments of, *590*, *662*
during pregnancy, 593–594
relaxation of, 593–594
lymphatic system of, 613–614, *615*
magnetic resonance imaging of, 693–697
male, *588*, 589, *623*, **639**
medical imaging of, **693–697**
neurovascular structures of, **606–619**
peritoneal reflections in, 602t, 603
veins of, 613, *614*
visceral afferent innervation in, **618–619**
walls of, 597–597, *598*
Pelvis (renal), **543**, *544*
bifid, 550
ectopic, 551, *551*
Penis, 678–682
arteries of, 679–681
body of, 678, **679**
bulb of, *627*, *634*, 671t, *731–732*
circumcision of, **685–686**
crura of, **678**, **679**, *732*
ejaculation, 682, **684**
emission from, 682, **684**
erection of, 682, **684**
glans, *623*, 677, *678*, **678**
hypospadias of, **685**
innervation of, **681–682**
nerves of, 681–682
root of, **679**
skin of, 679–680
veins of, **681**
Pennate muscles, 33
Percussion
of heart, **395**
of thorax, **361**
Percutaneous transluminal coronary angioplasty, 399, *400*
Perforating arteries, **777**

Perforating veins, **731**, **822**
Pericardial rub, **373**
Pericardiocentesis, 373, *374*
Pericarditis, **373**
Pericardium, **367**, 367–390, 374, 409
  arteries of, 388
  development of, *368*, *388*
  fibrous, 348, 367–388, *368*, *389*, *405*
    cardiac tamponade of, **373**
    functions of, 367
  hemopericardium, 373
  nerves of, *388*, 371
  pneumopericardium, 373
  serous, **367**, *368*, 388
    parietal layer of, **348**, **367**
    visceral layer of, **367**, *368*
  veins of, 388–389
Perichondrium, 20
Pericranium, **901**, *901*, *1022*
Perilymph, **1035**
Perimetrium, *641*, **644**
Perineum, **585**
  arteries of, *671*
  boundaries of, *662*
  disposition of, *662*
  episiotomy of, **673–674**
  female, *657*, *662*, *663–664*, 687–693, 691
  male, *663–664*, **677**
    distal male urethra, **677**
    lymphatic drainage of, *660*, **682**
    penis (*see* Penis)
    scrotum (*see* Scrotum)
  nerves of, *681*
  parietal, 601
Perineurium, 49
Periodontium, 989, 991, **993**
Periorbita, 948
Periosteal nerves, 23
Periosteum, 17, 20, 23, *23*, *26*, *902*
  innervation of, *108*
Peripheral nervous system (PNS), 3, 46, *47*, **47**, 48, 49–50, *49–57*, 49–58
  nerve fibers of, 49, *49–50*, *50*
  organization of, 48, 49
  somatic and visceral fibers, 54, 56–57, *56–57*
  types of, *50*, 51, 54–*54*, *54–55*
Peristalsis, **475**, 480
Peritoneal dialysis, **472**
Peritoneum, **465**, 601
  adhesions of, 472
  in females, 601
  formations, **467**–469
  intraperitoneal injection, 472
  mesentery of, **467**
  parietal, 435, *437*, *449*, **465**, *618*
    diaphragmatic, *496*
    embryology of, 466
  surgical procedures of, 471
  visceral, **465**–466
Peritonitis, **471**–472, 510, 618
Pes anserinus, **751**
Pes planus, 870
PET. *See* Positron emission tomography
Phalanges
  of foot, *719*, *811*
    general images of, *21*
  of hand
    fractures, 162
    general images of, 21
    ischemia of, 272–273
Phalanx
  distal, *149*, *294*
  middle, *294*
  proximal, *149*, *294*
Pharynx, **1097–1103**
  arteries of, 1103
  muscles of, 1101, 1102t, 1103
  parts of, 1097, 1099–1103
  veins of, 1103
Phasic contraction, 33
Philtrum, **966**, *988*
Phimosis, **685–686**
Physical examination, **351**
  instruments used in, 351
Pia mater, *95*, *134*, **928**
  spinal, *135*, **135–136**
Pilomotion, 60, *61*
PIP joints. *See* Proximal interphalangeal joints
Piriformis, **770**
Pisiform, 153, **153**, 159, 229, 246, 258, 266, 274, 290, 292, 294
Plagiocephaly, *899*
Plane(s) (in general)
  anatomical, 6–7
  fascial, 19
  interfascial, 19
  intrafascial, 19
  neurovascular, 439
Plane(s) (named)
  coronal, **6**, *7*
  frontal, **6**, *7*
  interspinous, *431*, *433*, **434**
  median, **6**, *7*, *433*, 434
  midclavicular, 432, *433*
  midsagittal, 6
  sagittal, **6**
  subcostal, **433**, *433*
  supracristal, 140
  transpyloric, **433**, *433*, **480**
  transtubercular, **433**, *433*, *480*
  transumbilical, *433*, **434**, *443*, 458
  transverse, **6**, *7*
  transverse thoracic, **367**, *368*, 371, *431*
Plantarflexion, **9**, **798**, 809
Plantar interossei adduct (PAD), **813**
Plantaris, **802**
Plaque, atheromatous, 9 4 5
Plate(s)
  cribriform, of ethmoid, *926*, 1127, *1128*
  epiphysial, **22**
  growth, 87
  horizontal, of maxillae, **887**, *839*
  perpendicular, of ethmoid, **1015**
  pterygoid
    lateral, *975*, *1106*, *1012*
    medial, *1106*, 1052t, *1053*
  tarsal, superior, *951*
  tympanic, *925*, *1012*
Plateau, tibial, 716
Pleura, **361**
  arteries of, **353**
  cervical, **361**–348, *362*, 366, *368*, *405*, 1138
    injuries to, **358**
  costal, *362*, 357, *408–409*
  cupula of, **361**, *390*
  diaphragmatic, 357
  inflammation of (pleuritis), 360
  injury to, **358**
  lymphatic system of, 354–355, *355*
  mediastinal, 356, 366, *405*, *408–409*
  nerves of, **355–356**, *356*
  parietal, *133*, **361**, *362*, *496*
    costal part of, *358*, *1078*
    lymphatic drainage from, 355
    nerves of, 356
  surface anatomy of, **356–357**
  veins of, 354
  visceral, **361**, *362*, *352*, *355*, *358*
    nerves of, *357*
Pleural adhesion, **360**
  lymphatic drainage after, **362, 364**
Pleural pain, **365**
Pleural reflection, *346–331*, **331**
Pleural rub, 360
Pleural sleeve, **350**
Pleurectomy, *360*, **360**
Pleurisy, **360**
Pleuritis, **360**, 362, 532
Pleurodesis, **360**
Plexus
  abdominal autonomic, 556
  aortic, *625*
    thoracic, **408**, *409*
  Auerbach (*see* Plexus, myenteric)
  basilar, *925*, **926**
  brachial, 169, *195*, **198**, *325*, 330, 1047, 1058, 1078
    block of, 211
    Erb-Duchenne palsy of, 210
    injuries to, 210–211
    neuritis of, 211
    roots of, **1061**
    trunks of, 198, *190*, 1061
  capillary, alveolar, *352*
  cardiac, *356*, *390*, 406, *407*, 415t, *1145*
  carotid, *1139*
    external, **975**
  celiac, 481, *486*, 514, 541, 529, 548, 556, 1145

cervical, 169, **1061**, *1062*
block of, 1074
cutaneous branches of, **1061**
motor branches of, **1061**
nerve roots of, *1150*
choroid, 922, *923*, *936*, 937, **938**, *1121*
coccygeal, **617**
dental
inferior, 980, *990*, 993
superior, *990*, 993
esophageal, *356*, 406, **406**, *407*, *408*, *413*, 415t, 478, 1144
extrinsic autonomic, **556**
hepatic, **526**, *526*
hypogastric
inferior, 553, 555, 555t, 556, 618, *625*, *630*, *617*, *657*, 673, *681*
superior, 501, 555, 555t, 556, 618, *625*, *630*, *617*, *657*
intermesenteric, *555*, 555t, **556**
intrinsic autonomic, **556**–557
limbal, **955**
lumbar, 566, *566*
lymphatic
deep, 354, *355*
of palm, *169*
pulmonary, **354**
subareolar, *190*, **335**, *336*
subepicardial, **389**
subpleural, *355*
superficial, 354
Meissner (*see* Plexus, submucosal)
mesenteric
inferior, *555*, **556**
pulmonary, *486*
superior, 490, **491**, **541**, *526*, *548*, **556**
myenteric Auerbach, *466*, 468, **556**
ovarian, 642
parotid, **912**, 977, 1138
pelvic, *9044*, **582**, *617*
peri-arterial, 479, *479*, 486, *490*, *617*, 618, 1085
peribiliary, *525*
pharyngeal, *1099*, 1103, 1142
phrenic, *541*
pterygoid, *966*, **980**, *945*, *1017*
pulmonary, 415t, *1145*
anterior, *405*
left, *356*, **406**, *407*
right, *356*, **406**, *407*
renal, 548, *548*, *555*, *1145*
sacral, *455*, 597, *598*, **615**–*617*, *630*, 648, 670
submucosal Meissner, *492*, **556**
thyroid, 1085–1086, *1086*
tympanic, 1031, *1031*, *1142*
uterine, *643*
venous
epidural, 573
pampiniform, 455, 456t, **457**, *458*, 634, 642, 681, 695
pelvic, **582**, *625*
prostatic, *614*, 625, *625*, 626, *627*, 635, 637, 638, 638, 681, 682, 731
pterygoid, *914*, *966*, **980**, 945
rectal, 614, *629*, **629**, 672, 676
submucosal, **1019**
uterine, 642, **676**–646
uterovaginal, **646**
vaginal, *614*
vesical, 621, *627*, 635, *681*
vertebral
external, **105**
internal, **105**, *135*
Pneumomediastinum, 1054
Pneumonectomy, 320, 361
Pneumopericardium, 373
Pneumothorax, 357, 496, 1073
PNS. *See* Peripheral nervous system
Podiatry, 811
Point
McBurney, *447*, 509, 510
midinguinal, **432**, *433*
semilunar, *433*
Poland syndrome, 189
Pole(s)
frontal, **935**, *936*, *942*
occipital, **935**, *936*, *942*
temporal, **935**, *936*, *942*
of thyroid gland, 1085
Polymastia, **342**
Polythelia, *339*, **342**
Pons, **935**, *936*, *1087*, *1121*
Popliteus, **802**
Popliteus bursa, **802**
Porta hepatis, *471*, *484*, *521*, **520**
Portal venous system, 42
Position
anatomical, **6**
lithotomy, *606*
prone, **6**
supine, **6**, 352
Trendelenburg, 563, 1076
Positron emission tomography (PET), 71
Posterior, *78*, **9**
Postero-anterior projections, 365, *365*, 419
Postsynaptic (postganglionic) neuron, 58
Postsynaptic sympathetic fibers, 6 0
Potentially lethal misnomer, 761
Pouch
perineal
deep, *655*, **656–658**, *657*
superficial, *655*, **656**
recto-uterine, **601**, *623*, 629, *632*, 633, 676, 676, 734
rectovesical, *468*, **603**, *623*, *628*, 628, 632, 633, 634, 731
vesicouterine, *623*, **644**, *676*, *734*
Power grip, 253, *254*
Precision grip, 253, *254*
Preganglionic neuron, 59
Pregnancy
breast changes during, 334–335
ectopic, *650*, **650**
pelvic floor injury during, **606**
pelvic ligaments during, 603–604
uterine changes during, 652, *653*
vaginal distension, **654**
Prepuce
of clitoris, *687*
of penis, *679*, 680
Presbyopia, **970**
Pressure
intra-abdominal, 300
intracranial, 945
intrathoracic, 300, *301*
Presynaptic neuron, 58
Presynaptic parasympathetic fibers, 639
Presynaptic sympathetic fiber, 59, 639
Prevertebral ganglia, 59
Primary ossification center, 22, **22**
Prime mover, 35
Process/processes
accessory, **84**
articular, 76
of cervical vertebrae, 80t, *1049*
inferior, 76, *76*, *98*, *99*, *312*, 313
of lumbar vertebrae, *84* superior, 76, *76*, *99*, *312*, 313
of thoracic vertebrae, 82t, *97*
axillary, **334**
caudate, *520*
ciliary, **953**
clinoid
anterior, *929*, *940*, *1021*
posterior, **892**, *843*
condylar, *975*
condyloid, *978*
coracoid, *152*, **151**, *153*, *155*, *157*, *158*, 174
coronoid, 152, *289*, *292*
costal, **87**
frontal
of maxilla, *882–883*
of zygomatic bone, *882–883*
jugular, *1079*
lateral, of malleus, *977*
mammillary, **83**, 87
mastoid, 118t, 977, *1012*, *1070*
of temporal bone, *975*, *993*
palatine, of maxillae, *1106*
papillary, **520**
pterygoid, *1012*
pyramidal, of palatine bone, *975*
spinous
of axis (C2 vertebra), *103*, *928*
bifid, *1049*
of cervical vertebrae, 80t, *1087*
of C6 vertebra, 1104
of C7 vertebra, *339*, 1104
of lumbar vertebrae, *82*, *118*
of L2 vertebra, *75*

Process/processes (*Continued*)
of L4 vertebra, *140*
of S2 vertebra, 85
of thoracic vertebrae, 80t, 296
of T1 vertebra, 336
of T4 vertebra, 118t
of T12 vertebra, *356*
styloid, *1101*
of 3rd metacarpal, 154, 159
of radius, *149*, 153, 159, 244, 247, 247, 286, 292
of temporal bone, *940*, *975*, *993*
of temporomandibular joint, *978*
of ulna, 152
transverse, **76**
of axis, *127*, 127t
of C4, *121*
of cervical vertebrae, 80t, *88*, *992*
of coccyx, *86*
of L2, *75*
of lumbar vertebrae, *84*, *88*
of thoracic vertebrae, 82t, *88*
uncinate, 80, *97*, *488*, 489, *516*, *575*
vaginal, *975*
xiphoid, *292*, 312–313, 313, 320, 338, *340*, *349*, *431*, *435*, *442*, *458*, 560, 577
zygomatic
of frontal bone, *834*
of temporal bone, *975*
Proctoscope, 633
Profunda brachii arteries, *191*, *196*, 187t, *208*, *213*, *216*, *206*, **206**, *219*
Profunda femoris artery, **755**
Profunda femoris vein, **755**
Projections
lateral, **366**
postero-anterior, 365, *366*, 419
Prolapse
of pelvic viscera, 673
of rectum, **675**
of uterus, *651*
Prominence
of cheek, 988
laryngeal, *1065*, *1071*, **1088**, *1089*, 1104
mandibular, 861
maxillary, 861
Promontory, sacral, **83**, 589, 589, *560*, 562
Pronation, *9*, **11**
Pronator syndrome, 251
Proprioception, **28**
Proprioceptive sensations, 54
Prosections, **351**
Protraction, *11*, **12**
Protrusion, *11*, **12**
Protuberance, **22**
mental, *965*
occipital
external, *98*, 118t, *129*, *928*, 1070
internal, *892*, **893**, *925–926*
Proximal, **8**
Pseudounipolar sensory neurons, 46, 47
Psoas, **747**
abscess, 759
sign, 572, *572*
Pterion, *975*, *1012*
fracture of, **931**–932
Ptosis, 956
Pubic crest, **711**
Pubic tubercles, **711**
Pubis, 586, **687**, **711**
Pubofemoral ligament, **832**
Pudendum, **687**
Pulmonary circulation, 39
Pulmonary embolism, 362
Pulmonology, 3–4
Pulpitis, **1007**
Pulse(s)
arterial, 3
carotid artery, **1072**, 1075
dorsalis pedis, **827**
facial artery, 920
internal jugular, 1076
popliteal, 806
posterior tibial, 767
radial artery, 251
Punchdrunk syndrome, 943. *See also* Chronic traumatic encephalopathy
Puncture
cisternal, **943**
internal jugular vein, 1076
lumbar spinal, *140*, **140**
spinal, **140**, *140*
sternal, 24
subclavian vein, 1073
Pupil, *952*, **953**, 965
Pupillary miosis, 953
Pus, **473**
Pyosalpinx, 650
Pyramid, renal, 543, *544*
Pyrosis, **502**

Q

Quadrantectomy, 342
Quadrants
of abdomen, *433*
of breasts, *340*, **340**
Quadrate muscles, 33
Quadrate tubercle, **713**
Quadratus femoris, **770**
nerve to, **775**
Quadriceps femoris, **748**–749, *749*
Quadriceps tendon, **748**
Quadriplegia, 82, 141

R

Radical mastectomy, 342
Radical prostatectomy, 640
Radiographic anatomy, 351
Radiographs
anteroposterior projections, **68**, 365, 419
chest, 365
conventional, *67*, 67–67
of elbow joint, *289*
lateral projections, **366**
mediastinal silhouettes, *399*
postero-anterior projections, **67**, **69**, 365, 366, 419
of thorax, *67*
Radiolucent, 67
Radionuclides, 71
Radiopaque, 67
Radius, 153
distal end of, 160–162
fractures of, 160–162
radiographs of, *289*
right, *153*
Ramus/rami
anterior, *54*, *84*, *108*, *136*, *326*
of brachial plexus, *1078*
of cervical plexus, *1062*
of spinal nerve C2, *928*
of spinal nerve C3, *928*
of spinal nerves, *53*, *54*
cephalic arterial, **60**
communicans/communicantes, **330**
gray, **60**, *62*
white, **59**, *61*
ischial, 586, *587*, 709, *710*
ischiopubic, **586**, *587*, **661**, *662*, 731–695, 697, 709, 750
of ischium, **709**
of mandible, *831–832*, *834*, *975*
posterior, *108*, *136*, *326*
of spinal nerves, 53
pubic, *670*
inferior, 586, *591*, *710*
superior, 586, *698*, **711**
of spinal nerve
anterior, **53**
posterior, **53**
Raphe
fibrous, *1063*, **1064**
palatine, *945*, *947*
penile, **678**, *679*
perineal, **678**, *679*
pharyngeal, *1100*, 1105t
pterygomandibular, *902*, **904**, *1099*
scrotal, **677**
Raynaud syndrome, 273
Receptors, muscarinic, 391
Recess
anterior, of ischio-anal fossae, **669**
costodiaphragmatic, 362, 346, *331*, 331, *348*, *435*, *471*, *473*, 487, *541*
costomediastinal, **331**
epitympanic, *1026*, **1027**, *1029*, *1031*, 1032, 1033
hepatorenal, *516*, **516**, 517, 543, *544*
ileocecal, *496*
lateral, *1121*
of omentum, 469

peritoneal, **468**–469
pharyngeal, *1097–1098*, **1099**
piriform, *1090*, *1097*, *1099*, 1101
sacciform
of distal radio-ulnar joint, **290**, *292*
of proximal radio-ulnar joint, **287**
sphenoethmoidal, *1017*, **1018**, *1020*
subphrenic, *516*, **516**
superior, *517*
Recta, vasa, 491, *492*, *493*
Rectum, *487*, *496*, **502**, **626–629**, *734*
arteries of, **629**
examination of, **633**
hemorrhoids, **676**
innervation of, **629**, *630*
lymphatic system of, **659**–661
prolapse of, **675**
resection of, **633**
veins of, **629**
Rectus femoris, **748**–749
Reduction of a fracture, 24
Reflex(es)
abdominal, superficial, 446
bicipital myotatic, 224
Breuer, 356
calcaneal tendon, 809
corneal, **971**
cremasteric, **461**
gag, **1009**
hammer, 33
Hering-Breuer, 356
light, 1038
myotactic, 33
patellar tendon, 760
plantar, **827**
pupillary light, **970**
Reflexive contraction, 33
Region(s)
of abdomen, 432–434, *433*
ankle, 705
buccal, 988
cervical
anterior, *1055*, 1055t, *1063–1065*, 1064, 1070, 1072
arteries in, **1066–1069**
muscles in, 1066, *1067*, 1067t
nerves in, **1069–1070**
veins in, **1069**
lateral, *1055*, 1055t, 1056, *1057*, 1070, 1072
arteries in, 1056, **1058–1059**
dissection of, *1057*
lymphatic system of, 1064–1065
muscles in, 1056, *1058*
nerve blocks in, 1074
nerves of, **1060–1062**
veins in, 1060, *1060*
posterior, *1055*, 1055t, **1057**, 1070
surface anatomy of, **1070–1073**
dorsal (dorsum), of foot, **812**, *813*, *816*, 821, 822, 824, 825
arteries of, *795*, 795t, *822*, 822–823
fascia of, 812, *813*
lymphatic drainage of, 823, *825*
muscles of, 816, 816t
nerves of, 816, *822*, 822t
surface anatomy, *811*, 825–827, *826*
venous drainage of, 823, *824*
femoral, **704**
foot, **705**
gluteal, **704**, **763**, 764
arteries of, 776–777, *777*, 778t
injections in, 784–785
lymphatic system of, 778
surface anatomy of, 779–782
veins of, **778**
hypochondriac
left, *433*
right, *433*
inguinal, **450**–454
left, *433*
right, *433*
knee, **704–705**
lateral
left, *433*
right, *433*
leg, **705**
of lower limb, **704**, *705*
oral, **953**–954
parotid, **1028**
popliteal, *615*
sternocleidomastoid, **1054–1072**
suboccipital, **126**
talocrural, **705**
thigh, 704
of upper limb, 147, *148*
Regional anatomy, 2–4
Regional anesthesia
for childbirth, 656
of lower limbs, 742
Regurgitation, 396
Renal calculi, **551**–552
Renal failure, 472
Renal transplantation, **549**
Reposition, *10*, **12**
Reproductive system, **4**
Resections
of lung, **361**
rectum, **633**
transurethral, of prostate, 640
Respiratory system, **3**–4
Retina, *953*, **955**
detachment of, *969*
Retinaculum/Retinacula, 17, 17–18, 437, 437, 450, 450, 450–452, 789
of ankle, *811*
extensor, 164, *165*, 235, *236–237*, *240*, 728
inferior, **789**, *790*, *791*, *811*, *781*
superior, **789**, *790*, *791*, *811*
fibular, *32*
inferior, **797–798**
superior, **794**, 754
flexor, *32*, **164**, *165*, *233*, *246*, *245*, *274*
lateral patellar, **748**
medial patellar, **748**
patellar
lateral, 748, *749*, *839*
medial, 748, *749*
superior extensor, **789**
superior fibular, **794**
Retraction, *11*, **12**
Retro-inguinal space, **752**
muscular compartment of, **752**
vascular compartment of, **752**
Retrusion, *11*, **12**
Rhinitis, **1024**
Rhinorrhea, 944
Rhizotomy, 57
Ribs, **310**, *1060*, *1078*
1st, 309, 310, 311, 313, 346, 405, 410, 1078
groove of, *349*
radiographic appearance of, *67*
synchondrosis of, *309*, **314**, **300**
2nd, *309*, **310**, *311*, *334*, *356*
4th, *346*
5th, *299*, *356*
6th, *309*, *334*, *346*
7th, *309*, *481*
8th, *309*, *311*, *328*
9th, *496*
10th, *309*, 310, *346*, *481*, *541*
11th, 309, *310*, *621*
12th, *309*, **310**, *311*, 314, 560, *566*, *621*
atypical, **310**, *311*
body of, 310, *311*
cervical, 93
costal cartilage of, **310**
costovertebral articulations of, *312*
counting of, 338
dislocation of, **434**
false, *309*, **310**
floating, *309*, **310**
fracture of, **319**
general images of, *20*
head of, **310**, *311*
joints of, 315
movements of, *318*
neck of, **310**, *311*
rotation of, *312*
separation of, **321**
supernumerary, **320**
surface anatomy of, *338*
true, *309*, **310**
tubercle of, **310**, *311*, *312*, 315, *316*
typical, **310**, *311*, *312*
Rider's bones, 24
Ridge(s)
mammary crest, *342*
mammary, embryonic, 109
petrous, *839*
sagittal sinus, *926*

Ridge(s) (*Continued*)
  supra-epicondylar, *236*
    lateral, *149*, *151*
    medial, *149*, *151*
  transverse, *296*
Right lymphatic duct, 45
Right venous angle, 45
Rima glottidis, **1088**, *1089–1091*
Rima vestibuli, **1092**
Rim, epiphysial, **76**, 89, 98
Ring
  common tendinous, 957
  femoral, **755**, *762*
  fibrous, **376**, 376–377, *382*
    right, *377*
  inguinal
    deep, *449*, *450*, **451**, *452*, 454, 457, 605
    superficial, *438–439*, *450*, **451**, 454
  tonsillar, 1097, 1103
  tracheal, *1089–1090*, *1092*, 1104
  umbilical, **441**
  of Waldeyer, 1103
Root(s)
  anterior, **49**, **50**
  anterior nerve, **50**
  of brachial plexus, 198, **1061**
  of cervical plexus, *1150*
  dorsal nerve, 50
  of facial nerve, **910**
  nerve, **49**, **50**
  of nose, *965*, **1015**
  of penis, **679**
  posterior, *49*, *50*, **5412**, 134
  posterior nerve, 50
  spinal nerve, 130, 132
    arteries of, *137*, *138*, *139*
    compression of, **139**
    1st cervical, *133*
    1st lumbar, *133*
    veins of, *137*, *139*
  sympathetic, of ciliary ganglion, **963**
  of teeth, **991**
  of trigeminal nerve, 910
  ventral nerve, 50
Rootlets, 50
  anterior, *49*
  posterior, *1148*
Rostral, **7**
Rotation, *8*, **11**
  of knee joint, 802t
  lateral, *9*, **11**, **956**
  medial, *9*, **11**, **956**
  of scapula, *181*
  of vertebral column, *102*
Rub
  pericardial, **373**
  pleural, 360
"Rule of Nines," 17
Runner's knee, 759
Running, **743**
Rupture
  of abdominal aortic aneurysm, **572**, 573
  of aneurysm, 945
  of appendix, 509
  of biceps tendon, **212**
  of bladder, **632**
  of calcaneal tendon, 809
  of coracoclavicular ligament, 297
  of diaphragm, **570**–571
  of liver, **534**
  of pancreas, **532**
  of spleen, **531**
  of urethra in men, **674–675**

S

Sac(s)
  alveolar, *352*, **353**
  conjunctival, 967
  dural, *95*, *131*, 132
    spinal, *136*
  endolymphatic, *1030*, *1034*, 1035, *1036*, 1036, 1141
  lacrimal, *946*, **950**
  pericardial, *388*, 373, *408*, *435*, 560
  peritoneal, 18
  pleural, 18
Saccule
  of ear, *1034*
  laryngeal, **1088**, *1090–1091*
Sacralization, 95
Sacral parasympathetic outflow, 63
Sacrospinous ligament, **764**
Sacrotuberous ligament, **764**
Sacrum, 19, 586, 587, 734
  apex of, **86**
  auricular surface of, **86**
  base of, **86**
  curvature of, 103
  dorsal surface of, **86**, *87*
  ossification of, *88*
  pelvic surface of, **86**, *87*
  surface anatomy of, 86–87, *87*
  surfaces of, 86
Saliva, 1004
Salpingitis, 649
Saphenous nerve, **752**, **816**, 819
  injury, 741–742
Saphenous open, **728**
Saphenous varix, **762**
Saphenous vein grafts, 741
Sarcomas, 45
Sartorius, **748**
Saturday night syndrome, 58
Scala tympani, *1037*, **1037**
Scala vestibuli, 1037, *1037*
Scalp, **900**
  arteries of, **912**, *913*, 913t
  infections of, **966**
  injuries to, **966**
  lacerations of, **921**
  layers of, 900–901, *901*
  lymphatic system of, **915**, *965*
  muscles of, **903**
  nerves of, **910**
  veins of, 914t–915t, **915**
  wounds to, **966**
Scalp proper, 966
Scapha, *1027*
Scaphoid, *153*, **153**, *274*, *290*, *292*
  fracture of, 160, *160*
Scapula, *20*, *27*, 146, **148**, 150–151, *309*, 474
  acromion of, *149*, 150, *150*
  arterial anastomoses around, 207–208, 208
  border of, 151, 157, *186*, 187
  fractures of, 159
  movements of, *181*, 181t
  right, *150*
  spine of, *149*, 187, *309*
  surfaces of, 150
  winged, 188
Scars, 16
Sciatica, 110
Sciatic nerve, **775**
  anesthetic block of, 784
  injury to, 784
SC joint. *See* Sternoclavicular joint
Sclera, *951*, *952*, 7345
Sclerotomes, 52
Scoliosis, *116*, 117
Scrotum, **456**–457, 677–678, *679*
  anesthetizing of, **461**
  arteries of, **678**
  cancer of, **461**
  distension of, **685**
  hematocele of, 461
  lymphatic system of, *455*, **678**
  primordial, **453**
  veins of, **678**
Secondary ossification center, 23, *23*
Second-degree burn, 16, *17*
Sections
  longitudinal, **5**, *7*
  oblique, *7*, **7**
  transverse, *7*, **7**
Segment(s)
  anterior (aqueous), of eyeball, 953, 955
  bronchopulmonary, 351–352, 352, 361–362, 365
  hepatic (surgical), *522*, **524**, 540
  of kidney (*see* Segments, renal)
  of liver (*see* Segments, hepatic (surgical))
  of lung (*see* Segments, bronchopulmonary)
  posterior (vitreous), of eyeball, *953*, **956**
  renal, *547*
Segmental atelectasis, **361–362**
Segmental nerves, 50
Segmentectomy, 361

Sellae
dorsum, *886*, *889*, *926*, *940*
tuberculum, *889*, **890**, *892*
Sella turcica, *889*, *891*, *940*
Semimembranosus, **773**
Semitendinosus, **773**
Sensory fibers, 49
Sensory system, somatic, **58**
Septal defects
atrial, 391–392
ventricular, 392–393
Septicemia, 29, 46
Septum
anterior intermuscular, **728**
atrioventricular, membranous part of, 377
carotid, 1066
femoral, **755**
fibrous
lateral, **256**
medial, **256**
interalveolar, **991**, *993*
interatrial, *379*, **379**, *381*, *382*, *389*
intermuscular
anterior, **728**
lateral, **163**, *165*
medial, **163**, *165*, *218*
posterior, **728**, *790*
transverse, **728**, *729*, *790*, 798, *846*
interradicular, **991**, *993*
interventricular, 381, **381**, *389*
membranous part of, *377*, *380*, **382**, 384, 390
muscular part of, *380*, **381**, *382*, 390
lateral fibrous, **256**
lateral intermuscular, **163**, *165*, **728**
lingual, 1000
medial fibrous, **256**
medial intermuscular, **163**, *165*, *218*
nasal, **1015**–1016, *1018*, *1020*, **1023**–1024
orbital, *951*, **953**
penis, **678**, *679*
posterior intermuscular, **728**
rectovesical, *603*, **604**, *624*, 629, *634*, 635
scrotal, 456t, **678**, *695*
Septum pellucidum, *936*
Serous membrane, **18**
Shaft
of bone, 21
of femur, **713**
of fibula, **717**
of humerus, 151, 156
fracture of, *160*
of metatarsals, 721
of phalanges, 721
of radius, *150*, 152, *165*
of tibia, **716**
of ulna, **152**
Sheath
of arachnoid, *951*
axillary, **193**, 1053
carotid, *1051*, **1053**, 1066, *1068*, 1072, 1080
dural, *951*
of eyeball, *952*
of eyeball, *951*, 948
fascial, of eyeball, 956
femoral, *753*, *754*, **755**
fibrous digital, **256**
flexor, common, 233, *250*
hypogastric, **603**, *605*
neurovascular, *18*
parotid, **977**
psoas, *564*
rectus
anterior wall, 435, *436–438*, **440**–441
posterior wall, *440*, *449*
synovial tendon, 18, *19*
tendinous
of abductor pollicis longus, **240**
of digits, *31*
of extensor carpi radialis, **235**
of extensor carpi ulnaris, *239*
of extensor digitorum, **266**
of extensor indicis, 235
of extensor pollicis brevis, **240**
of extensor pollicis longus, **240**
of flexor carpi radialis, **232**
of flexor pollicis longus, **233**
in hand, 262
of thyroid gland, *1101*
Shelf, talar, 718
Shingles, 332–333
Shin splints, 807
Shoulder, joints of. *See* Joint(s), glenohumeral
Shunt(s)
arteriovenous, 42
muscle, 35
portocaval (*see* Shunt(s), portosystemic)
portosystemic, 536, **539**
transjugular intrahepatic (TIPS), 513
Sialography
of parotid duct, **985**–986
of submandibular duct, **958**
Sialolith, 986
Sigmoidoscopy, **510**, *511*, 633
Sigmoidostomy, 510
Sign
anterior drawer, *865*, 866
Babinski, 827
Hegar, 652
peau d'orange, 341
posterior drawer, *865*, 866
psoas, 572, *572*
Trendelenburg, 911
Simple mastectomy, 342
Sinus(es)
anal, *669*, **672**
aortic
left, 383, *385*
posterior, 383, *385*
right, 383, *385*
branchial, *1058*
carotid, 1065, *1065*, *1068*
hypersensitivity, 1075
cavernous, **925**–926, *927*, *940*, *966*, 978, 1134
thrombophlebitis of, 932, 921
thrombosis of, 933
confluence of, 924, *925*, *926*
coronary, **379**, *388*
dural venous, *925*
occlusion of, 884
of epididymis, **457**, **458**, *463*
ethmoidal, 1020, *1021*
frontal, *943*, *1017*, 1018, 1020, *1021*, *1070*
intercavernous, **926**, *927*
lactiferous, **334**, *334*
maxillary, **1025**
occipital, *925*, **925**
paranasal, **1020**–1023, *1021–1022*
pericardial
formation of, 388, *389*
oblique, **388**, *389*
transverse, **388**, *389*, *373*
surgical significance of, 372–373
petrosal
inferior, *925*, *926*, **926**, *1068*, 1069
superior, *925*, *926*, **926**, *1120*
prostatic, **626**, *627*, 638
pulmonary, 374
renal, *541*, **541**
sagittal
inferior, *901*, **924**, *925*, *927*, *1120*
superior, *901*, *925*, *926*, *927*, *928*, 1022, 1120
sigmoid, **924**–925, *925*, *926*, *927*, *1120*
sphenoidal, *943*, *947*, 1017, 1020–1021, *1070*
sphenoparietal, *926*
straight, **924**, *925*, *927*
tonsillar, **943**, *943*, *1098*, 1100
transillumination of, **1024**, *1025*
transverse, **924**, *925*, *1120*
tumor metastasis to, **993**
venarum, *379*, **379**
venous, **993**
scleral, *953*, **955**, *966*
Sinusitis, **1024**
Situs inversus, 374
Skeletal striated muscle, **30**, 30t
Skeletal system, **4**
parts of, 19–20
Skeleton
appendicular, 20, 589
inferior, *149*
superior, **143**
axial, 18, 73, 142, **589**
fibrous, of heart, **376**, *377*
functions of, 377
laryngeal, **1088**, *1089*
of external nose, **1015**, 973
thoracic, 449, *309*

Skeleton (*Continued*)
ribs, **310**, *311*
surface anatomy of, **335–340**
Skier's thumb, **301**
Skin, *12*, **12**, 12–14
burns to, 16
color signs in physical diagnosis, 15
dermatomes of (*see under* Dermatomes)
dermis of, *12*, **13**
epidermis of, **12**, *12*
functions of, 12
incisions in, 15
injuries to, 15
lacerations of, 16
ligaments, *14*, **14**
map of peripheral innervation of, *58*
of neck, 1070
parasympathetic stimulation, 65t
scarring of, 15
segmental innervation of (*see under* Dermatomes)
stretch marks in, 541, *541*
subcutaneous tissue, *12*, 13–14, *14*, *327*
skin ligaments of, 14, *14*
sympathetic stimulation, 65t
tension lines of, *13*, **13**
Sleeve, pulmonary, *349*, **350**
Small arteries, 40, 40–41
Small intestine, *485*, **485**, 487–491
absorption in, 475
arteries of, *493*
duodenum (*see* Duodenum)
ischemia of, **507**–508
lymphatic system of, *486*
nerves of, *486*, 468
in omental bursa, **469**–470, 474–475
surgical navigation of, **507**
veins of, *493*
Smell, loss of, **1150–1151, 1152**
Smoker's cough, 361
Smooth muscle, 30t, **31**
SNS. *See* Somatic nervous system
Sole
central compartment of, **812**
of foot anatomy, 8, 9
lateral compartment of, **812**
medial compartment of, **812**
Soleal line, **717**
Soleus, **801**–802
Somatic fibers, 54, 56
Somatic motor fiber, 56
Somatic nervous system (SNS), 58
Somites, **52**
Space
air, **882**
of Bogros, 445, *452*
deep postanal, 675
epidural, *76*, **132**
episcleral, *951*
extradural, *106*, *135*, *140*
fascial, 445
intercostal, *309*, **310**, *326*
fourth, *334*
thoracentesis, 496
leptomeningeal, *135*
meningeal, **928**–929
midpalmar, *256*, **256**
paravesical, *604*
Parona, 272
pelvirectal, *604*, **606**
perisinusoidal, **524**, *525*
quadrangular, *196*, **197**, *216*
rectovaginal, *605*
retro-inguinal, **752**, *753*
retromammary, **334**, *334*, 341
retropharyngeal, *1051*, 1054, 1057, *1096*
retropubic, **603**, *604*, *623*, 624, *632*, *634*
retrorectal, **603**, *604*, *605*, **606**
of spinal meninges, *134*
subarachnoid, 74, 94, 106, 131, 135, 134, 140, 922, *937*, 938, *951*, *1129*
cerebral, *937*
development of, **139–140**
spinal, *937*
subcostal, **310**
subhepatic, 516, *516*
subinguinal, *450*, **451**
suprasternal, *1051*, 1052, *1065*, 1070, *1096*
thenar, *256*, **256**
vesicocervical, *605*
vesicovaginal, *605*
Special sensory fiber, **56**
Sperm, **458**
Spermatocele, *463*, **463**
Spermatogenesis, **455**
Spermatozoa, 457
Sphenoid bone, *831–832*, **889**
Sphincter
anal
external, 600, 623, 629–*630*, 634, *661*, **670**, *680*, 652t
internal, *623*, *634*, *661*, *669*, **670**, *680*
of the bile duct, **527**
esophageal, inferior, 478
hepatopancreatic, *514*
of Oddi, 514
of pancreatic duct, 514, **514**
of pupil, *1134*
pyloric, *481*
urethral
external, 598, 624, 625, 627, 646, *663*, *636*, **668**, 684t
internal, **624**, *625*
urethrovaginal, **646**, *647*, *663*, *636*, 652t
Sphincteral muscles, 33
Sphincter pupillae, **953**
Spicules, **22**
Spina bifida cystica, 97
Spina bifida occulta, 96
Spinal nerves, *50*, *51*, *52–54*
Spinal puncture, *140*, **140**
Spine (of bone), **22**
iliac
anterior inferior, *587*
anterior superior, *431*, 406, *438*, *442*, 450, 458, 458, 474, 586, 587, 589
posterior inferior, *587*
posterior superior, 86, *121–122*, 586, 587
ischial, *587*, *590*, *598*, *662*
nasal
anterior, *831–832*
posterior, **887**, *839*, *843*, *1106*
of scapula, *149*, **152**, 187
of sphenoid, *975*, *978*, *1012*
suprameatal, *975*
trochlear, *946*
Spiral line, **713**
Splanchnic nerves, 60
Spleen, *431*, 474, *487*, **487**, *552*
accessory, *531*, **531**
borders of, *487*, **514**
computed tomography of, *576*
diaphragmatic surface of, **514**
embryology of, 514
functions of, 487
lymphatic system of, *541*
needle biopsy of, **532**
palpation of, *531*
relations of, 514
rupture of, **531**
surface anatomy of, *487*
Splenectomy, **531**
Splenomegaly, **531**
Splenoportography, **532**
Spondylolisthesis, 112, 594–595, *595*
Spondylolysis, 92, 112, 594–595, *595*
Spondylosis, 141
Spongy bone, 21, *21*
Sprain
ankle, 825
back, 129–130
ligament, 821
Spurt muscle, 34
Stalk of epiglottis, **1088**
Stance phase, **743**
Standing at ease, *743*, **743**
Stapes, *977–1031*, *1030*, **1032**
Starling hypothesis, 42
Steele's Rule of Thirds, 115, *115*
Stenosis, 396
aortic valve, **395–396**
aqueductal, 943, *943*
internal carotid artery, **920**
lumbar spinal, **91–92**, *93*
pulmonary valve, **395–396**
spinal, **91–92**
Stents, intravascular, 399
Sterilization
female, **649–650**
male, **639**

Sternal puncture, 24
Sternoclavicular (SC) joint, *201*, **264**, *316*, 1068, 1072
Sternotomy, median, **320**
Sternum, *313*, **313**, *314*, *334*, 1070
  anomalies of, **321**
  biopsy through, **321**
  body of, *309*, 314, 338, *338*, *340*, *349*
  cleft of, 321
  fracture of, **320**
  general images of, *19*, *313*, *314*
  manubrium, 148, 154, *292*, 313, 314, *299*, *329*, 335, *356*, *349*, *1051*, 1079, 1115
  surfaces of, 143, 336
  xiphoid process of, *313*, **314**
Stomach, *431*, **478**
  arteries of, 481, *484*
  bed of, **481**, *481*
  blood vessels of, 480
  body of, **479**, *481*
  carcinoma of, **479**
  computed tomography of, *576*
  curvatures of, **480**, *480–481*
  displacement of, 503
  fundus of, *477*, 478, 479, **479**, *577*
  gastrectomy, **505**
  interior of, **480**
  lymphatic system of, 481, *486*
  nerves of, *479*
  parasympathetic nerve supply of, 481
  parts of, 479–480, *481*
  pyloric antrum of, *69*
  pylorospasm of, **478**
  pylorus of, *431*, 406, *474*, *481*, 514, *510*
  radiographic image of, *69*
  relations of, **480**–481
  rugae of, *69*
  surface anatomy of, 479–480, *480*
  ulcers of, **505**–506
  veins of, 481, *485*
  visceral referred pain, **506**
Strain
  back, 129 130
  gastrocnemius, 809
Stretch marks, 16, *16*
Striae
  gravidarum, 16, *16*
  olfactory, **1127**, *1128*
Strictures, urethral, 685
Stridor, inspiratory, 1155
Stroke, **395**, 1075
  hemorrhagic, 944
  ischemic, 944
Sty, 969
Subcompartment
  of leg, deep, **798**
  superficial, **798**
Subcutaneous prepatellar, **844**
Subcutaneous tissue, 13–14, *14* , 728, *729*
  of abdominal wall, anterolateral, **434**
  of foot, 769
  of lower limb, 728
  of neck, 1106
  of perineum, **635**
  skin ligaments of, 15, *15*
Sublingual absorption of drugs, **958**
Subluxation
  atlanto-axial, 114
  of radial head, 300–301
Subscapular arteries, *191*, **197**, *208*
Subtalar joint, **852**
Sudomotion, 60
Sulcus
  carotid, *889*
  central, **935**, *936*
  gluteal, *717*, *781*
  infrapalpebral, *935*, **936**
  lateral, *936*, *1121*
  mentolabial, 988, *988*
  midline, *999*
  nasolabial, **966**, *988*
  parieto-occipital, **935**, *936*
  prechiasmatic, *889*, **890**, *843*
  suprapalpebral, *965*
  terminal, 999, *999*, *1097*
Superficial, *7*, **8**
Superficial burn, *16–17*
Superior, *7*, **8**
Superolateral, **8**
Supination, *9*, **11**
Supinator
  crest, **152**
  fossa(e), **152**
  notch, **152**
Supracondylar lines, **713**
Suprapatellar bursa, **844**
Suprapubic cystotomy, **632**
Supraspinous fascia, **165**
Sural nerve, **821**
Sural nerve grafts, 827
Surface(s)
  articular, **848**
    of ankle joint, **849**
    of cervical vertebrae, 78
    of hip joint, **828**, 829, 831
    of knee joint, **836**, 838
    of lateral condyle, *841*
    of tibiofibular syndesmosis, **847**–849
  costal, of lungs, *348*, **350**
  diaphragmatic
    of heart, 377, *378*, *367*
    of liver, 517, *517*
    of lungs, *349*, **350**
  dorsal, **8**
  of heart, 377, *496*
  of hip joint, **828**, 829, 831
  of knee joint, **836**, 838
  of liver, *516*, 516–520
  mediastinal, of lungs, *348*, **350**
  palmar, **9**
  plantar, **9**
  patella, **713**
  popliteal, **786**
  pulmonary
    left, **377**, *378*
    right, **377**
  radius, 163
  sacropelvic, *587*
  of sacrum, 83
  of scapula, 152
  sternocostal, **377**, *367*
  of sternum, 148
  of teeth, **991**
  of tongue, **997**–999
Surface anatomy, 3
  of acromion, *186*
  of ankle, 781, 783, 859, *860*
  of anterolateral abdominal wall, **458**–458
  of arm, 220
  of axilla, 181, 187
  of back muscles, *126*
  of biceps brachii muscles, 220
  of cervical region, **1070–1073**
  of clavicle, 181
  of coccyx, 85–86, *86*
  of cubital fossa, 220 of eyeball, **966**–967
  of face, **915**–916
  of femoral triangle, *752*
  of fingers, 258, *258*
  of foot, 781, 783, 859, *860*
  of forearm, 247–248
  of fossa(e) cubital, 220, *224*
  of gluteal region, 779–782
  of great vessels, **403–404**
  of hand, 269–258
  of head, 915–966
  of heart, 414–415
  of knee, 859, *860*
  of lacrimal apparatus, 949 of leg, *805*, 805–806
  of limb upper, axilla, 181, 187
  of lumbar vertebrae, 84–85, *85*
  of lungs, *356*, **356–357**
  of medial thigh muscles, 757, 758, *758*
  of median nerves, *247*
  of neck, **1070–1073**
  of pleura, *356*, **356–357**
  of sacrum, 84–85, *85*
  of spleen, *487*
  of stomach, 479–480, *480*
  of thigh,
    anterior, 757, 758, *758*
      medial, 757, 758, *758*
      posterior, **779**–782, *780*, *781*, *782*
  of thoracic wall, 335–339, 342
Surgery
  endoscopic, **447**
  extrapleural intrathoracic access, **332**
  lumpectomy, 342
  mastectomy, 342
  minimally invasive, **447**

Surgery (*Continued*)
open-chest, 496
peritoneal, 471
Sustentaculum tali, **718**
Suture(s)
intermaxillary, *995*
interpalatine, *995*
Swallowing, 1099, *1100*
Swing phase, **743**
Sympathectomy, **572**
Sympathetic nervous system, of abdominal viscera, 553, 557
Symphysial surface, **711**
Symphysis
mandibular, *27*, 1064, *1065*
pubic, *19*, 432, 434, *435*, 458, *552*, 586, 586–586, 588, 590, 590, 597, 605
Synchondroses
of 1st rib, *292*, **314**, **317**
sternal, 314
Syndesmosis
dento-alveolar, **942**
tibiofibular, *829*, **847**
Syndrome(s)
carpal tunnel, 250, 273, 301
compartment, 741
cubital tunnel, 239
Horner, **971**
ischemic compartment, 226
jugular foramen (Vernet), 1155
Klinefelter, 342
Ménière, 1040
myofascial pain, 323
painful arc, 297
patellofemoral, 821
Poland, 188
pronator, 251
punchdrunk, 943
Raynaud, 273
renal entrapment, **550**
Saturday night, 58
tarsal tunnel, 825
thoracic outlet, **321**
Synergist, 35
Synostosis, 314
System
alimentary, **4**, 475
articular, **4**
cardiovascular, **4**, 38
circulatory, **4**
endocrine, **4**
genital, **464**
integumentary, **4**, 12
locomotor, **4**
lymphatic/lymphoid, **4**, 43
muscular, **4**
nervous, **4**, 46
autonomic, **58**
central, **47**
enteric, **62**
peripheral, **47**, 49
somatic, 58
somatic motor, **58**
somatic sensory, **58**
portal venous, **42**
reproductive, **46**
respiratory, **4–5**
skeletal, **4**, 19, 20
urinary, **46**
Systemic anatomy, 4–5
Systemic arteries, 39
Systemic circulation, 39
Systemic veins, 39
Systole, **376**, 381

T

TA. *See* Tibialis anterior
Tail
of epididymis, **458**, *463*
of pancreas, 541
Talipes equinovarus, 870, *828*
Talocrural region, **705**
Talus, 670, *671*, **718**, *811*
head of, 718, *718–719*, *719*, 859
trochlea of, **718**
Tamponade, cardiac, **373**
Tarsal bones, *20*
Tarsal tunnel syndrome, 825
Tarsometatarsal line, **718**
Tarsus, **718**
Taste sensations, 1000
TCL. *See* Tibial collateral ligament
Teeth
accessory, **1007**, *1008*
arteries of, 992
canines, 989, *991*, *1008*
caries, **1007**
deciduous, **989**, *992*
development of, 897, 899
extraction of, **1007–1008**
functions of, 989
incisors, 989, *990*, *991*
innervation of, *990*
mandibular, **886**
maxillary, *977*
maxillary sinus and, **1025**
molars, *988*, **989**, *990 991*, 1007, 1008
nerves of, *990*
parts of, 989
permanent, **989**
premolars, *1008*
secondary, **989**, *990*
sections of, *992*
supernumerary, **1007**, *1008*
types of, 989
Tegmen tympani, 975, *1012*, 1027, *1029*, **1030**, 1039
Temporal bone
fractures of, **920**
petrous part of, *926*, *936*, *1141*
squamous part of, *926*, *936*, *1141*
Tendinitis
biceps, 224
calcaneal, 808–809
calcific supraspinatus, 297
elbow, 249
Tendon(s) (in general), 451, 456t, *598*
Tendon(s) (named)
abductor pollicis longus, *269–270*
adductor, *750*
biceps brachii, 212, *218*, *223*, *281*
dislocation of, 224
rupture of, 225
surface anatomy of, 220
biceps femoris, *782*, 806, 859
calcaneal, *34*, *782*, *794*, 799, 799t, *846*, 806, 837, 851, 859, 860
reflex, 809
ruptured, 809
central, 560, *560*
digastric, *907*, 1053, 1066
extensor digitorum, *238*, 270
extensor digitorum longus, 806
extensor hallucis brevis, 806
extensor hallucis longus, 806, 855t
extensor pollicis longus, *240*
fibularis longus, *782*, *800*, 781, 783, *813*
flexor carpi radialis, 269, *269*
flexor carpi ulnaris, 269, *269*
flexor digitorum brevis, *800*, *846*, *817*
flexor digitorum longus, 800t, *801*, *846*, 814, 814t, 817
flexor digitorum profundus, *238*, 256, *250*
flexor digitorum superficialis, 256, *250*
flexor hallucis brevis, *846*
flexor hallucis longus, 800t, *846*, *814*, 814t, 817
flexor pollicis longus, *274*
of forearm, *237*
gastrocnemius, *846*, *840*
of hand, *237*
long extensor, *34*
long flexor, *32*
palmaris longus, *165*, *246*, *248*, 256, 266, 269
pes anserinus, 755, *837*, *840*
plantarflexor, 846
popliteus, *839–840*
psoas, *450*
quadriceps, **748**, *749*, *841*
sartorius, *841*
semimembranosus, *782*, *805*, *837*
semitendinosus, *782*
supraspinatus, *296*
tibialis anterior, *846*, 806, *837*
tibialis posterior, 795t, *801*, *846*, *837*
triceps, 219
Tenosynovitis, 272
Tension lines of skin, *14*, *13*
Tensor fasciae latae, **767**, *768*, 770

Tentorial herniation, 932
Tentorium, cerebellar, *1120*
Tentorium cerebelli, *924*
Terminal arteries, 41
Terminal filum. *See* Filum terminale
Terminalis
  crista, **379**, *379*, *389*
  sulcus, *378*, 379 *389*
Terminologia Anatomica, 46
Terminology, anatomicomedical, 5-12
  abbreviation of, **5**
  anatomical planes, 6–7, *7*
  anatomical position, **6**
  laterality terms, 9
  movement terms, 9, *10-11*, 12
  relationship and comparison terms, 7, *8*, 9
  structure of, 5
Terms
  laterality, 9
  of laterality, **9**
  of movement, 9, *10-11*, 12
  of relationship and comparison, 7, 8, 9
  structure of, **5**
Testis, 457, **457**–458, *695*
  appendix of, 463, *463*
  cancer of, 463
  descent of, *453*
  hematocele of, **461**, *462*
  hydrocele of, 460, *462*
  lymphatic system of, *455*
  maldescent of, 458
  mediastinum of, **457**
  palpation of, **685**
  primordial, 453
  rete, **457**
Tetany, 1109
Thenar eminence, *159*, *248*, *253*, 255, 266, 269, 271
Thenar fascia, *230*, *266*
Thigh
  abductors of, *765*, 765t, *766*
  abnormal ossification of patella, 760
  accessory obturator artery, 764, *764*
  adductor longus, injury to, 760–761
  anterior muscles, *746*, **746**–749, 746t, 747, 747t
    iliopsoas, **747**–748
    pectineus, **747**
    quadriceps femoris, **748**–749, *749*
    sartorius, **748**
    surface anatomy of, 757, 758, *758*
  in anteromedial
    adductor canal, *757*, **757**
    femoral artery, **755**, *756*, 756t, *757*
    femoral nerve, **752**, 753
    femoral sheath, **753**, 755
    femoral triangle, *752*, **752**, *753*, *754*
    femoral vein, **755**, 757
  arteries of, 776–777, *777*, 778t
  chondromalacia patellae, 759
  contusions, 759
  fascia lata of, *452*
  fascial compartments of, *772*
  femoral artery
    cannulation, 761
    laceration, 761
  femoral hernias, 762
  femoral vein
    cannulation of, 762
    location of, 762
  gluteal region
    anesthetic block of sciatic nerve, 784
    buttocks, **763**–764, *764*
    hamstring injuries, 783
    intragluteal injections, 784–785
    ischial bursitis, 783
    muscles of, **764**–770, *765*, 765t, *766*, 767, 767, 768
    neurovascular structures, **773**–778, 774, 774t–775t, 776, 777, 778
    superior nerve injury, *783*, 783–784
    surface anatomy of, **778**–782, *779*, 780, 782
    trochanteric bursitis, 783
  gracilis, transplantation of, 760
  groin pull, 760
  hematoma of, 759
  hip and thigh contusions, 759
  lymphatic system of, 778, *778*
  medial muscles, **749**–751, *750*, 750t
    actions of adductor muscle group, **751**
    adductor brevis, **749**, *750*, 751
    adductor hiatus, **751**
    adductor longus, **749**, *750*
    adductor magnus, *750*, 750t, **751**
    gracilis, *751*, **751**
    obturator externus, *750*, **751**
    surface anatomy of, 757, 758, *758*
  muscles of
    anterior, **749**–751
    posterior, **770**–773
    testing of, 753
  paralysis of quadriceps, 759
  patellar fractures, 759–760
  patellar tendon reflex, 760
  posterior region, **770**–773, *772*
    anesthetic block of sciatic nerve, 784
    biceps femoris, **773**
    hamstring injuries, 783
    intragluteal injections, 784–785
    ischial bursitis, 783
    neurovascular structures, **773**–778, 774, 774t–775t, 776, 777, 778
    semimembranosus, **773**
    semitendinosus, **773**
    surface anatomy of, **778**–782, *780*, 781, 782
    trochanteric bursitis, 783
  potentially lethal misnomer, 761
  proximal lower limb, organization of, 745–746
  psoas abscess, 759
  region of, 745–746
  rotators of, *765*, 765t, *769*
  saphenous varix, 762
  surface anatomy of, 757–758
  veins of, 7778
Thoracentesis, *496*, **496**
Thoracic outlet syndrome, **321**
Thoracoscopy, *360*, **360**
Thoracotomy, *319*, **319–320**, 372
Thorax, 414, **415**
  computed tomography scans of, 420–424
  dimensions of
    anteroposterior, 317
    transverse, 317, *318*
  elements of, 449
  flail chest, **319**
  great vessels (*see* Great vessels)
  heart (*see* Heart)
  magnetic resonance imaging of, *424*
  mediastinum (*see* Mediastinum)
  nerves of, 327, 330, 415t
  percussion of, **361**
  radiography of, *366*
  viscera of, *431*
  wall of
    anterior aspect of, *325*, *334*
    apertures, **315**
    arteries of, **330–331**
    breasts (*see* Breast(s))
    dermatomes of, 327, *328*
    fascia of, *327*
    joints of, **315–317**
    movements of, **317**, *318*
    muscles of, **302–304**
    nerves of, **327–330**, 415t
    overview of, 308, *312*
    posterior aspect of, *328*
    ribs, **310**, *311*
    skeleton (*see* Skeleton, thoracic)
    sternum, *313*, **313–314**
    surface anatomy of, 335–339, 342
    thoracic vertebrae (*see* Vertebrae, thoracic)
    thoracotomy, *319*, **319–320**
    vasculature of, 330–332
    veins of, 331–332, *332*
Thrills, 396
Thromboembolism, pulmonary, 741
Thrombokinase, 399
Thrombophlebitis, 932, 972
Thrombosis, 509
  deep venous, 741
Thumb(digit 1 of hand)
  bull rider's, 301
  gamekeeper's, 301
  movements of, 9, *257*
  skier's, 301

Thymus, **402**, *404*, 419, *1113*
Thyroidectomy, 1109
TIAs. *See* Transient ischemic attacks
Tibia (shin bone), *20*, 714, *715*, 716–717
  anterior border of, **717**
  anterolateral tubercle of, **728**
  fractures of, 722–724
  functions of, 715–716
  general images of, *17*
  nutrient artery of, **805**
  right, *716*
  of shaft, **716**
  surface anatomy of, *717*, 717–718
Tibial collateral ligament (TCL), **838**
Tibial fractures (TF), 722, *724*
Tibialis anterior (TA), **792**
Tibialis anterior strain, 807
Tibialis posterior, **847**
Tibial nerve, injury to, 807
Tibial tuberosity, **717**
Tibiofibular joints, **845**, **847**
  tibiofibular, 847
  tibiofibular syndesmosis, 847
Tic douloureux, 919
TIPS procedure. *See* Shunt(s), portosystemic
Tissue(s)
  connective, extraperitoneal, *754*
  lymphoid, **43**
Toes, **705**
  claw, 870
  great, **705**, *732*, 733, *811*, 859–860
  hammer, 869
  little, *732*, *811*
Tomography
  computed (*see* Computed tomography)
  positron emission, **71**
Tongue, *988*, **997**, **999**, *999*, *1087*, *1098*, 1107
  arteries of, 1000
  innervation of, **1000**
  lymphatic system of, **1000**, *1003*
  mucosal surface of, *1087*
  muscles of, **997**–1000, *1000*, 1001t, 1002t
  nerves of, 1000
  parts of, **997**–999
  surfaces of, **997**–999, *1087*
  veins of, 1000
Tonic contraction, 33
Tonsil
  lingual, *999*, **999**, *1098*, **1103**
  palatine, *965*, **993**, *993*, *995*, *996*, *999*, 1100, 1105
  pharyngeal, *965*, *1087*, *1096*, *1098*, 1099, 1105
  tubal, *1098*, **1099**
Tonsillectomy, 1113
Tonsillitis, 1103
Tonus, 33
Tooth sockets, 989
Torsion angle, **713**
Torticollis, *1058*, 1072–1073
Torus of pharyngotympanic tube, **1099**
TP. *See* Tibialis posterior
Trabecula
  arachnoid, *135*, 928
  septomarginal, *380*, **382**, *389*
Trabeculae carneae, **380**, 383, *382*
Trachea, 362, 348, 351, 361, 390, 390, 404, 408, 421–422, 993, 1047, 1085, 1087, 1056–1059, 1110
  septomarginal, *380*, **382**, *390*
Tracheostomy, 1112
Tract
  alimentary, arterial supply to, 475, *476*
  gastrointestinal, **475**
  iliopubic, *449*, **450**–451, *452*, 452t
  iliotibial, **728**, *729*, *758*, *765–766*, 765t, 773, 781, 781, 805, 837, 840
  nerve of, **47**
  olfactory, *941*, **1020**, *1121–1122*, **1127**, 1128
  optic, *1121*, **1134**
  urinary
    parasympathetic stimulation, 65t
    sympathetic stimulation, 65t
  uveal, 902
Tragus, *1026*, *1027*
Transient ischemic attacks (TIAs), **945**, 1075
Transillumination, 461
Transplantation
  corneal, **971**
  renal, **549**
Transvaginal sonography, 69
Transverse acetabular ligament, **829**
Transverse intermuscular septum, **728**
Transverse sections, **7**, *53*
Transverse tarsal joint, **853**
Trapezium, *153*, **153**, *160*, *165*, *246*, *261*, 274, 290, 292
Trapezoid, *153*, **154**, *160*, *165*, *274*, *276*, 290
Trauma
  blunt, **932**
  to bone, 23
  to head, **932**
  to median nerve, 273
  to neck, 1115
  to peripheral nerves, 58
  to vulva, **687**
Tree
  bronchial, *362*
  tracheobronchial, *350*, **350**, 351, *351*, 366–367
T1 relaxation, 71
T2 relaxation, 71
Trendelenburg sign, 862
Trendelenburg test, 784
Triad, portal, **520**, *521*, *522*, 524, *525*, 527
Triangle
  anal, **661**, **668–673**
  of auscultation, *118*
  carotid, *1055*, 1055t, **1065**, 1070, 1074–1075
  clavipectoral, *157*, 167, *167*
  cystohepatic, *514*, **529**
  deltopectoral, *157*, *327*
  digastric, *1055*, 1055t
  femoral, *752*, **752**
    structures of, 754
  lumbocostal, *560*, 571
  muscular, *1055*, 1055t, **1066**
  occipital, 126, *1055*, 1055t, **1057**, 1072
  omoclavicular, *1055*, 1055t, **1057**, 1071
  omotracheal, *1055*, 1055t
  posterior, *204*
  sacral, *86*, **86**
  sternocostal, *560*, **562**
  submandibular, *1055*, 1055t, 1072
  submental, *1055*, 1055t, 1064, 1072
  suboccipital, *127*, 127t
  urogenital, **663**, **664–668**
Triceps coxae, **770**
Triceps surae, **798**
Trigone
  of bladder, **624**
  fibrous, **377**
    left, *377*
    right, *377*
  lumbocostal, *566*
Triquetrum, *153*, **153**, *160*, *274*, *290*, *292*
Triradiate cartilage, **709**
Trochanter, **22**
  greater, *21*, *712*, **713**, 715, 780, *781*, 784, 829
    fracture of, 722
  lesser, *565*, **713**
Trochanteric bursa, **763**
Trochanteric bursitis, 783
Trochlea, **22**
  fibular, **718**, 720, *829*
  of humerus, *21*, *289*
  of talus, *720*, 720
Trochlear, notch, 152, *286*, *288*
Trunk(s)
  of brachial plexus, 1059
    anterior, *201*, 204
    inferior, **763**, *763*, *201*, **201**
    infraclavicular part of, *198*, 202t, **204**
    middle, 201, **201**
    parts of, *763*, 766, 201, *201*
    supraclavicular part of, *201*, 202t, **204**
    variations of, 209–210
  brachiocephalic, *329*, *496*, *390*, *404*, 405, 406, 407, 1060, 1068, 1079, 1080, 1086
  bronchomediastinal, 411
    left, *355*
    right, *355*

celiac, *476*, *484*, 484t, *488*, *493*, *521*, 541, 555, 569, 575
collecting, *411*
costocervical, *329*, *410*, *1060*, *1079*, **1080**
jugular, *411*
left, *336*
lumbosacral, *566*, *567*, *598*, **615**, *625*, 681, 695
lymphatic
bronchomediastinal, 335, *336*, *1059*
intestinal, *494*, *569*
jugular, 335, *336*, *1059*, *1105*, **1106**
subclavian, *169*, *200*, *1059*
left, *336*
right, *336*, *355*
thoracic, *543*
pulmonary, 353, 389, 377, 378, 382, *367*, 421–422
subclavian, *200*, *411*
sympathetic, *133*, *326*, 330, *356*, *404*, 408–409, 486, 526, 548, 566, 566, 681
abdominal, 566, *566*
cervical, 1069, 1082
lesion of, 1082
sacral, 617
thoracic, *414*, **414**, 478
thoraco-acromial, *336*
thyrocervical, *196*, 197t, *329*, *1060*, 1078–1079, 1080, 1084, 1094
vagal, 478
anterior, 481, *486*, *526*, 556, **1144**, 1145
posterior, *356*, 481, *484*, *486*, *526*, 548, 556, 1144, 1145
Tubal sterilization, **649**
Tube
chest, insertion of, **496–360**
heart, 368, *388*
pharyngotympanic, *978*, *994*, *997*, *1017*, 1025, 1026, 1027, 1027–1028, 1029, 1029, 1030, 1038, 1097–1099
blockage of, 1039
uterine, *641*, 642
arteries of, **642**
blockage of, **471**
ectopic pregnancy, *650*, **650**
innervation of, **642**
ligation of, 656
parts of, 642
patency of, **471**, **649**
Tubercle, 22
adductor, *708*, *712*, **713**, 715, *750*
anterior, of cervical vertebrae, 77, *80*, 89
articular, *975*, *1012*
of bone, 21, 22
carotid, *1078–1079*
conoid, **148**
corniculate, *1090–1091*
cuneiform, *1090–1091*
deltoid, 151
dorsal, of radius, **153**
epiglottic, *1090–1091*
Gerdy, *752*, *766*, 859, 864
greater, of humerus, *149*, 151, 156, 187
iliac, 432, *433*
infraglenoid, *215*
intercondylar, **716**, *841*
lateral, of tarsus, 718, *719*, 720
lesser, of humerus, 151, 156
of lip, 965
medial
of calcaneus, 720
of tarsus, *719*, 720
mental, *832*, *834*
pharyngeal, 1105t
posterior, of cervical vertebrae, 77, *80*, 88
postglenoid, *975*, *977*
pterygoid, *839*
pubic, 437, *438*, *450*, *458*, 458, 586, *587*
quadrate, *712*, **713**
radial, dorsal, *149*, 159, *237*
of rib, *122*
scalene, **310**, *311*
of scaphoid, **153**, *156*, *274*, *292*
supraglenoid, *215*
tibial, anterolateral, **716**, *717*, *692*, *766*
of trapezium, 159
Tuberculosis, 571
Tuberosity, **22**
of 5th metatarsal, *720*, **720**–721
calcaneal, **718**, *719*, 799, *860*
of cuboid, **718**, *719*
deltoid, *149*, **151**
gluteal, *708*, *712*, **713**, *750*, *766*
ischial, 586, *598*, *600*, *662*, *695*
of maxilla, *1012*
navicular, **718**, *819*, 720, *846*, *837*
radial, **153**, *286*
tibial, *716*, 717, *758*, 805, *836*, *846*
of ulna, **153**
Tubule
seminiferous, **457**, *458*
straight, **457**, *458*
Tumors
orbital, **994**
pituitary, 932
Tunica adventitia, **39**
Tunica albuginea, **457**, *458*, **678**, *679*
Tunica intima, 39
Tunica media, 39 Tunnel
carpal, 272
osseofibrous, **262**

U

Ulcer(s)
corneal, **971**
duodenal, **506**
Ulcerative colitis, 510
Ulna, *20*, 152
fractures of, 160–162
radiographs of, *289*
right, *153*
Ulnar, notch, **153**
Ultrasonography (US), **69**
of abdomen, *575*
of aorta, *575*
Doppler, 69
of duodenum, *575*
of liver, *575*
Umbilicus, *440*, **458**
Umbo, **1027**, *1029*
Uncus, of body, 80t Unilateral, **9**
Ureters, *474*, **543**, *544*, *605*, 621, **621**
arteries of, **621**
bifid, 550
calculi of, **551**–552, **631**
congenital anomalies of, **550**–525
iatrogenic injury to, **619**
innervation of, **621–621**
lymphatic drainage of, 621
lymphatic system of, *548*, **548**–549
nerves of, *548*, **548**–549
retrocaval, 550, *551*
veins of, **621**
Urethra, *695*, *697*
female
arterial supply of, **626**
male urethra *vs.*, **633**
veins of, **626**
innervation of, *625*
male, *678*
arterial supply of, **626**
catheterization of, **684–685**
distal, **677**
female urethra *vs.*, **633**
innervation of, *625*, **626**
intermediate part of, 84, 627t, 674
intramural part of, 627t
parts of, 627t prostatic, 627t
proximal, **626**
rupture of, **674–675**
spongy, *627*, 627t, *634*, *664*, 675, 676
veins of, **626**
spongy, *627*, 627t, *634*, *664*, 675, **676**
Urinary bladder, **924**
apex of, **624**
arteries of, **624–625**
body of, **624**
in children, 621
cystocele, **631–632**, *632*
cystoscopy of, *632*, **632**
fundus of, *621*, **624**
in infants, 621
innervation of, *624*, **625–626**
interior of, *626*
lymphatic system of, *659*
micturition, 624
neck of, **624**
rupture of, **632**
trigone of, **624**
uvula of, **624**
veins of, 625

Urinary system, **4**
Urine extravasation, **674–675**
Urology, 4
US. *See* Ultrasonography
Uterus, **642**
  age-related changes in, 652, *653*
  anteflexed, *651*
  anteverted, *651*
  arteries of, *643*, **646**
  bicornate, **650**, *651*
  bimanual palpation of, 652
  body of, *641*, **642**, *734*
  cancer of, 460–461
  cervix of, **642**, *734*
  disposition of, **650**–652, *651*
  endometrium of, *641*, **644**, *734*
  examination of, 652, *652*
  fundus of, *641*, **642**, *734*
  hysterectomy of, **653–654**, *654*
  innervation of, **647–649**
  ligaments of, **644**
  lymphatic system of, *659*, 661
  menopause-related changes in, 652
  multiparous, 652, *653*
  myometrium of, *641*, **644**
  neck of, *641*
  perimetrium of, *641*, **644**
  position of, 643, 644
  postpartum changes in, 652, *653*
  pregnancy-related changes in, *653*
  prolapse of, *651*
  pubertal changes in, 652
  relations of, **644**
Utricle
  of ear, **1035**, *1036*
  macula of, **1035**
  prostatic, *623*, **626**, *634*
Uveitis, **970**
Uvula, **624**, *998*, *1009*, 1010, 1097–1099

V

Vagina, 646, *734*
  arteries of, **610**, 647
  culdocentesis of, 655
  digital examination through, 654
  distension of, **654**
  fistulae of, 654–655, *655*
  functions of, 646
  innervation of, **647–649**
  lymphatic system of, *659*, 661
  ostium of, *623*
  veins of, *642*, **647**
  walls of, *641*
Vaginalis
  processus, **453**, **456**, **460**
  tunica, *453*, *457*, **457**
Vaginismus, **693**
Vagotomy, **505**–506
Valleculae, *1091*, *1110*
Valsalva maneuver, 41, 1110
Valve
  anal, **672**
  aortic, *377*, *382–383*
    cusps of, *383*
    insufficiency of, **396**
    stenosis of, **396**
  mitral, *375*, *382*
    cusps of, *382–383*
    insufficiency of, **396**
  pulmonary, *375*, 383
    cusps of, **395**
    incompetence of, **396**
    stenosis of, 396
  semilunar, **383**
  tricuspid, *375*, 380, *382*
  venous, 731
Valve prostheses, 395
Valvular heart disease, **396**
Valvular sinuses, **41**
Valvuloplasty, 395
Variations
  anatomical, 12–13
  of bony pelvis, 561
  in lobes of lungs, **360**
  of sacrum, 95
  of stomach disposition and shape, *480*
  of transverse colon disposition, *502*
Varicella-zoster virus, 332
Varices, esophageal, 502, *503*
Varicocele, **463**
Varicose veins, 43, *43*
Varix, saphenous, 762
Vasa nervorum, 58
Vascular sheath, **41**
Vasectomy, 639
Vasoconstrictors, 355
Vasomotion, 65
Vasomotor nerves, 23
Vastus intermedius, **749**
Vastus lateralis, **749**
Vastus medialis, **749**
Vastus muscles, **749**
Vein(s) (in general)
  accompanying, *41*, **41**
  arteries and, comparisons between, 41
  articular, 28
  azygos/hemi-azygos system of, 341, *411*, 412–414, 478, 574
  collecting, 524
  communicating, *819*
  compression of, 41
  countercurrent heat exchanger, 41
  flap valves of, 41
  large, **41**
  medium, **41**
  nutrient, *23*
  superficial, *18*, *40*, *218*
  varicose, 43, *43*, 538, *741*, 762
Vein(s) (named)
  accessory saphenous, **731**
  accompanying, **731**
  angular, *914*, 914t
  antebrachial
    intermediate, *42*
    median, **167**, *218*, *224*
  anterior cutaneous, **731**
  anterior tibial, **731**
  appendicular, *476*
  auricular, posterior, *914*, **915**, 1060, 1060
  axillary, *167*, *195*, 198, *198*, 204, *325*, 336–336, 421–422, 1059
    injury to, 209
    right, *1073*
    in subclavian vein puncture, 209
  azygos, *332*, 354, *408*, **413**, *435*, *530*
    arch of, *420*, 421–422
  basilic, 165, *167*, **167**, *198*, 218, 220, 224
  basivertebral, **108**
  brachiocephalic, *40*, *325*, *405*, *914*, 1059, 1060, 1060, 1069
    groove for, *349*
    left, *332*, *336*, *388*, *496*, *404*, *405*, 408, 411, 421–422
    right, 331, 336, 496, 404, 405, 407, 408, 411, 421–422
  bronchial, *354*, **354**
  bronchomediastinal, left, *337*
  cardiac, **388**, *405*
    anterior, *388*, 389
    great, 388, *388*
    middle, 388, *388*
    small, *388*, 389
  central, 524, 525, *525*, **527**
    of retina, 955, *966*
  cephalic, 165, *167*, **167**, 168, *168*, *169*, 173, 191, 195, 198, 213, 218, 224, 248, 327, 336
  cerebral
    great, 924, *926*, **940**
    inferior, **940**
    middle, **940**
    occlusion of, **836**
    superior, **940**
  cervical
    deep, *129*
    transverse, *1060*, *1064*
  ciliary, anterior, 955
  colic
    left, *476*, *501*
    middle, *476*, *501*
    right, *476*, *488*, **498**, *501*
  cubital, median, *167*, **167**, *169*
  cutaneous
    anterior, *732*, **733**
    lateral, *722*, **733**
  cystic, *476*, *528*, **529**
  deep
    of arm (*see* Vein(s) (named), profunda brachii)
    of thigh (*see* Vein(s) (named), profunda femoris)

digital, plantar, **822**
dorsal
  of clitoris, 625
  of great toe, 728, *732*
  of little toe, 731, *732*
  of penis, *614*, *634*, *636*, *679*, **681**, *681*
dorsal metatarsal, **822**
emissary, 926, **927**–928
  frontal, **928**
  mastoid, **928**, *930*
  parietal, **928**
  posterior condylar, **928**, *930*
epigastric, *530*
  inferior, 443, *449*
  superficial, *438*, 443
esophageal, *530*
facial, *911*, *914*, 914t–915t, **915**, *924*, 926, 1060, 1068, 1069
  common, *914*, *1063*
  deep, *914*, 914t, **915**, *924*
  thrombophlebitis of, **932**
  transverse, *978*
femoral, *40*, *438*, 419, *697*, *732*, 733, 753, 755, 758, 773, 789
  cannulation of, 762
  lateral circumflex, *732*
  location of, 762
  superficial, 761
of foot, 822, *823*
gastric
  left, *476*, 478, **484**, *459*, *530*
  right, **484**, *487*
  short, *476*, **484**, *487*, *516*
gastro-omental
  left, *476*, **481**, *487*
  right, **481**, *487*
gluteal
  inferior, *614*, 778, *778*
  superior, *614*, 778, *778*
of gluteal, **778**
great saphenous, **728**
hemi-azygos, *332*, **412**–414, 421–422, 546
  accessory, *332*, *409*, **414**
hepatic, 522, **524**, *541*, *577*
ileal, *476*
ileocolic, *476*, **497**, 501 iliac
  common, *541*, **613**, *614*
  deep circumflex, *732*
  external, *449–450*, *541*, *605*, *614*, *597*
  internal, *605*, **613**, *614*, *615*
iliolumbar, **613**
intercostal, **341**
  anterior, **341**, *342*
  left superior, **341**, *405*, *409*, *411*
  posterior, *108*, *326*, 340t, **341**, *342*, 412
  right superior, **341**, *342*, *405*
internal pudendal, **778**
interventricular
  anterior, 388, *405*
  posterior, *405*
intervertebral, 105–106, *106*, *135*, *139*
jejunal, *476*
jugular
  anterior, *1060*, *1064*, *1068*, **1080**
  external, 911, 914, 915, 965, 977, 1028, 1047, 1059, 1060, 1060, 1068, 1070, 1071
    prominence of, 1073
    severance of, 1074
  internal, 332, 336–336, 346, 355, 407, 558, 914, *926*, 977, *984*, *1003*, *1051*, *1058–1059*, *1064*, 1068, 1069, 1078, 1101, 1106
    left, *1105*
    pulse taking, 1076
    puncture of, 1076
    right, *1105*
labial
  inferior, *914*
  superior, *914*
laryngeal, *1055*, 1056
left, *1047*, *1068*, *1078*, *1105*, *1113*
of leg, 822, *823*
lingual
  deep, **1000**, 1009
  dorsal, **1000**
lobar, *353*
lower limb
  deep, 731
  superficial, 728, *730*, 731
mammary
  lateral, *336*
  medial, *336*
marginal
  lateral, **822**, *823*
  left, *388*
  medial, **822**
maxillary, *914*, *924*, *1060*
medial marginal, **822**
median, of forearm, *167*
meningeal, middle, 926
mesenteric
  inferior, *476*, *488*, *501*, *516*, *530*, *541*, 578
  superior, *476*, *488*, 489, *501*, *516*, 530, 541, 544, 575, 578
metatarsal, dorsal, *40*, **822**, *833*
middle lobe, **354**
nasal, external, *914*
oblique, of left atrium, 388, *388*, *393*
obturator, *614*
occipital, *928*, *1060*, *1068*, *1069*
ophthalmic
  inferior, *914*, *925*, *961*, *962*, **964**, *966*
  superior, *914*, *915*, *925*, **964**, *966*
ovarian, *614*, **642**
palatine, *1099*, 1103, 1113 palpebral
  inferior, *914*
  superior, *914*
pancreatic, *516*, 541
pancreaticoduodenal, *476*, *516*
parathyroid, **1086**
paratonsillar, 1103
para-umbilical, *449*, *530*
perforating, **167**, *218*, *224*, **731**
pericardiacophrenic, *388*, 389
pharyngeal, 1069
phrenic
  inferior, **560**
  superior, **560**
plantar, *732*, **733**
plantar digital, **822**
popliteal, *732*, 733, *734*, *788*, **789**
portal, 478, *488*, *489*, *490*, *493*, *501*, *516*, 517, 520, 529–530, 575–577, 614
prepyloric, **482**, *485*
profunda brachii, 219
profunda femoris, *732*, 733, 777
pudendal
  external, *438*, 678, 681
  internal, 689
pulmonary, *349*, *353*
  left, *353*, *388*, *496*, *382*, *382*
  left inferior, *496*, *382*, 421–422
  left superior, *496*, *382*
  right, *388*, *382*, *382*
  right superior, *496*
radial, *40*
rectal
  inferior, *530*, *629*
  middle, *614*, *629*
  superior, *476*, *501*, *530*, *614*, *669*
rectosigmoid, *501*
renal, *544*, *614*
  entrapment syndrome, **550**
  left, *516*, *538*, *541*, *575*, 642
  right, *332*, *546*, *577*
retromandibular, *914*, **915**, 866t, 977, 977, 1060, 1060, 1063
retroperitoneal, *530*
right, *1068*, *1094*
sacral
  lateral, *614*
  median, **613**
saphenous
  accessory, **731**
  cutdown, 742
  grafts, 741
  great (long), 399, 731, 732, 753, 754, *757*, 758, 762, *780*
  injury to, 741–742
  small (short), *40*, *728–729*, **731**, *732*, 789, 822
saphenous, great (long), 399, *438*, *440*
segmental, *353*
sigmoid, *476*, *501*
small saphenous, **731**
spinal
  anterior, **135**, *139*
  posterior, *137*, *139*
splenic, 502, 503, 501, 514, 514, 541, 530, 530, 575, 614

Vein(s) (named) (*Continued*)
subclavian, *325*, *336–336*, *346*, *388*, 496, 408, 914, 965, 1047, 1059–1060, 1076, 1080, 1106
left, *355*, *569*, *1078*
puncture of, 1073
right, *1073*
subcostal, **331**, *332*
sublingual, **1000**, *1003*
submental, *914*
supra-orbital, *914*, 914t, *915*, *924*, *926*, *966*
suprarenal
left, 548
right, 548
suprascapular, *198*, *204*, *1059–1060*
supratrochlear, *914*, 914t, **915**
temporal
deep, **915**
middle, *914*
superficial, *914*, **915**, 866t, *1060*
testicular, *452*, **458**, *541*
left, **457–458**, *614*
right, **457–458**
thoracic
internal, *325*, 330t, *332*, **332**, *336*, 405, 407, 408
lateral, *417*
thoraco-acromial, *198*
thoraco-epigastric, *198*, *417*, **417**
thyroid
inferior, *405*, *1047*, *1068*, **1085**, 1085–1086, 1094, 1096, 1104
middle, *1047*, *1068*, **1085**, *1086*, *1094*
superior, *1047*, *1068*, **1085**, *1086*
tibial
anterior, *990*, *732*, *780*
posterior, *732*, **733**, 789, *780*
ulnar, *40*
umbilical, *482*, 520
postnatal patency of, 458
of upper limb, 165–168
uterine, *614*, 642, *643*, **646**
vaginal, *643*
valves, **733**
ventricular, left posterior, *388*
vorticose, *952*, *966*
Vein(s) (of regions or organs)
of abdominal wall
anterolateral, 417
posterior, 567–570
of anal canal, **672–673**
of brain, **940**
of cervical region, lateral, 1060, 1060
of diaphragm, 560
of ductus deferens, 635
of duodenum, *490*
of ejaculatory ducts, 635
of face, *914*
of foot, 822, *823*
of forearm, 243–244
of hand, 289
of heart, *388*, *405*
of kidneys, **547**–548
of larynx, 1056
of liver, 521, *528*
of lower limb
deep, 733
superficial, *732*, 733
of lungs, 354
of neck, *1060*
of orbit, **964**, 966, *966*
of pancreas, *516*
of pelvis, 613, *614*
of pericardium, 349
of pharynx, 1103
of pleurae, 354
of popliteal fascia, **786**
of prostate gland, 638
of rectum, **629**
of root of neck, 1080, *1081*
of scalp, 914t–915t, **915**
of scrotum, **678**
of seminal glands, 635
of small intestine, *493*
of spinal cord, *137*, *139*
of spinal nerve roots, *139*
of stomach, *481*, **481**
of suprarenal glands, *546*, 547
of teeth, *942*
of thigh, 778
of thoracic wall, 331–332, *332*
of thyroid gland, 1085
of tongue, **1000**
of upper limb, 165–168
of ureters, **621**
of urethra
female, **626**
male, **626**, **646**
of urinary bladder, 625
of vagina, *642*, **647**
of vertebral column, *104*, 104–108
of vulva, 689
Vena cavae, 582, *614*, 642
inferior, *315*, *388*, *378*, *379*, *407*, *408*, 418, 426, 487, 492, 514, 533, 533
caval opening, **561**
groove for, *349*, **520**
magnetic resonance imaging of, *577*
obstruction of, 419
surgical exposure of, 373
superior, *331*, *388*, *375*, *378*, *379*, *382*, 386, 405, 407, 1070, 1073, 1076
computed tomography of, 421–422
groove for, *349*
obstruction of, 419
radiographic appearance of, *67*
surface anatomy of, *336*
surgical exposure of, 373
Venous drainage, superficial, **822**
Venous network
dorsal, *167*, *248*, 265, 270, **822**
plantar, **822**
Venous plexuses, **41**
Venous stasis, 741
Venous valves, **41**
Ventricles
of brain
1st, 935
2nd, 935
3rd, *923*, *936*, **936**, *937*, *943*
4th, *923*, **936**, *938*, *1087*, *1121*
lateral, *937*, *938*
of heart
left, *375*, **375**, *378*, *382*, *382*, *389*
right, *376*, **376**, *378*, 379–382, *384*, 404, 421–422
laryngeal, **1088**, *1089–1090*
Ventricular fibrillation, 401
Ventricular septal defects, 392–393
Venules, **41**
Vertebrae, 73, **73**
abnormal fusion of, **95**
aging effects on, **95–96**
anomalies of, **96–98**
cervical, *20*, 1047–1049, *1048*
atypical, 1049
C1 (*see* Atlas)
C2 (*see* Axis)
C3-C7, 79, *99*, *1087*
C7, 356
characteristics of, 77–78
dislocation of, 90, *90*
features of, 77–78, 80t
typical, 1049
characteristics of, 77–78
dislocations of, **111–114**
fractures of, 111–114
function of, 75–77
laminae of, **76**
lumbar, 83, 85, *88–89*
abnormal fusion of, 95
body of, *542*
L2, *75*
L5, 84
ossification of, *87*
stenosis of, 91, *93*
surface anatomy of, 86–87, *87*
ossification of, 87–89
pedicles of, **76**
structure of, 75–78
T4, 422
T5, 422
T6, 422
T8, 422
thoracic, 79, **80–82**, **310**, 313
facets of, *312*, **313**
features of, 313
ossification of, *88*
spinous processes of, *312*, 313
T1, 82, *308*, *312*
superior costal facets of, 313
T3, 80

T4, 82
T5, 80
T6, 80, *312*
T8, 80
T10, 80, 82, 313
T11, 80, 82, 313
T12, 80, 82, *308*, *314*
costal facets of, *312*, 313
variations in, **89–90**, 97
vasculature of, *106*, 106–107
Vertebral column, *73*, *74*, **76**, **96–117**
arteries of, 107–108
cervical, 1106
curvatures of
abnormal, 115–117, *116*
normal, 104–105, *113*
flexibility of, 73
flexion of, 104
hyperflexion injury of, 112
injuries of, 1106
joints of, **97–103**
ligaments of, *108*
movements of, **104–105**
nerves of, **108–109**
regions of, *75*
rotation of, *104*
vasculature of, **106–108**
veins of, *106*, 106–108
Vertebra prominens, 1105
Vertex, **7**, **887**
Vertigo, 1155
Vesicles
optic, **969**
seminal, *632*
Vessels
deep lymphatic, 45
Vestibule
aortic, *382*, 383, *382*
of bony labyrinth, *1030*, **1035**
laryngeal, **1088**, *1090*, *1110*
of nose, **1015**, 1016, *1017*, *1096*
oral, 988, *988*, *997*, 1000, *1000*, *1022*
of vagina, *676*, **646**, *687*, **689**, *697*
Vestibulocochlear, *941*, *1026*, 1035, *1036*
View, anteroposterior, 68
Villi, intestinal, **491**
Viscera
abdominal, 426, **426**, **474**–477
innervation of, **553**–557
parasympathetic innervation of, **553**, 556
physiology of, 475
sympathetic innervation of, **553**, 557
of neck
alimentary layer, **1096**–1104
endocrine layer, **1083–1086**, 1104–1105
respiratory layer, **1086–1096**, 1104–1105
pelvic, **620**
urinary organs, **620–626**
pleura, **361**, *362*, *349*, *352*, *355*
nerves of, *356*
surface anatomy of, 356–357, 414–415, 424
of thoracic cavity, 342–*350*
Visceral afferent fiber, 66
Visceral fibers, 56
Visceral motor fiber, 56
Visceral sensory fiber, 56
Viscerocranium, 879, *880*
Visual fields, **1134**
defects in, **1152**
Volkmann contracture, 226
Volvulus, 472, *511*, **511**
Vomer, **1015**, *1016*
Vulva, **687**, 688, 690
Vulvar trauma, **692**

W

Wall(s)
abdominal (*see* Abdominal wall)
of axilla, *164*, **193**, *194*, *198*, *214*
of bladder, 624
capillary, 42
of heart, 376
of orbit, *946*, 948
of pelvic cavity, *597*, 647
of rectus sheath, 435, *437–440*, 440–441, 449
of thorax, 449, 310–314
of vagina, *641*
Wallerian degeneration, 58
Whiplash, 92, 112, *112*
White matter, 47, *49*
White rami communicantes, 59
Window
oval, *1029*, **1031**, *1034*
round, *1027*, *1034*, **1035**
Wing
greater, of sphenoid, *926*, *1028*, 1011, 1012, 1022
of ilium, 586
lesser, of sphenoid, **889**, 890, 926, 946
Wounds
palmar arch, 275
scalp, **917**
sole of foot, 827
Wrist, **253**, 291. *See also* Joints (named), Wrist
arteries of, *242*, 242t
articulation of, 291
blood supply to, 291
bones of, 153–155, *154*
capsule of, 291
cross-section of, *230*
fractures of, *161*, 301, *301*
innervation of, 291
ligaments of, 291, *292*
movements of, 291, *293*
muscles that move, 291
synovial cyst of, 249–250, *250*

X

X-rays, 67, 67–68, **366**

Y

Yoke muscles, **961**

Z

Zone
orbicular, 832
transitional, of lips, 988
Zygomatic bone, *880–882*, 884, *948*, *976*